Atlas of Anatomic Pathology

Series Editor
Liang Cheng

For further volumes:
http://www.springer.com/series/10144

Anthony W.H. Chan • Alberto Quaglia
Beate Haugk • Alastair Burt

Atlas of Liver Pathology

Springer

Anthony W.H. Chan, BMedSc, MBChB, FRCPA, FHKCPath, FHKAM (Pathology)
Prince of Wales Hospital
The Chinese University of Hong Kong
Hong Kong

Alberto Quaglia, MD, PhD, FRCPath
Institute of Liver Studies
King's College Hospital
Denmark Hill, London
UK

Beate Haugk, MD, FRCPath
Department of Cellular Pathology
Royal Victoria Infirmary
Newcastle upon Tyne
UK

Alastair Burt, BSc(Hons), MBChB, MD(Hons), FRCP, FSB
School of Medicine
The University of Adelaide
Adelaide
Australia

ISBN 978-1-4939-4353-1 ISBN 978-1-4614-9114-9 (eBook)
DOI 10.1007/978-1-4614-9114-9
Springer New York Heidelberg Dordrecht London

Printed on acid-free paper

Springer is part of Springer Science+Business Media (www.springer.com)

Series Preface

One Picture Is Worth Ten Thousand Words

– Frederick Barnard, 1927

Remarkable progress has been made in anatomic and surgical pathology during the last 10 years. The ability of surgical pathologists to reach a definite diagnosis is now enhanced by immunohistochemical and molecular techniques. Many new clinically important histopathologic entities and variants have been described using these techniques. Established diagnostic entities are more fully defined for virtually every organ system. The emergence of personalized medicine has also created a paradigm shift in surgical pathology. Both promptness and precision are required of modern pathologists. Newer diagnostic tests in anatomic pathology, however, cannot benefit the patient unless the pathologist recognizes the lesion and requests the necessary special studies. An up-to-date Atlas encompassing the full spectrum of benign and malignant lesions, their variants, and evidence-based diagnostic criteria for each organ system is needed. This Atlas is not intended as a comprehensive source of detailed clinical information concerning the entities shown. Clinical and therapeutic guidelines are served admirably by a large number of excellent textbooks. This Atlas, however, is intended as a "first knowledge base" in the quest for definitive and efficient diagnosis of both usual and unusual diseases.

The *Atlas of Anatomic Pathology* is presented to the reader as a quick reference guide for diagnosis and classification of benign, congenital, inflammatory, nonneoplastic, and neoplastic lesions organized by organ systems. Normal and variations of "normal" histology are illustrated for each organ. The Atlas focuses on visual diagnostic criteria and differential diagnosis. The organization is intended to provide quick access to images and confirmatory tests for each specific organ or site. The Atlas adopts the well-known and widely accepted terminology, nomenclature, classification schemes, and staging algorithms.

This book Series is intended chiefly for use by pathologists in training and practicing surgical pathologists in their daily practice. It is also a useful resource for medical students, cytotechnologists, pathologist assistants, and other medical professionals with special interest in anatomic pathology. We hope that our trainees, students, and readers at all levels of expertise will learn, understand, and gain insight into the pathophysiology of disease processes through this comprehensive resource. Macroscopic and histological images are aesthetically pleasing in many ways. We hope that the new Series will serve as a virtual pathology museum for the edification of our readers.

Liang Cheng, MD, Series Editor

Preface

This atlas is designed to be a primer for students and residents and for general pathologists in the interpretation of liver biopsy histology. The liver is subjected to a wide range of insults but has a relatively limited repertoire of histopathological changes. Optimal interpretation of liver biopsy specimens requires accurate recognition of the morphological abnormalities and an ability to put these into the appropriate clinical context.

We have deliberately not tried to be comprehensive in this atlas but rather sought to cover an approach to the most common forms of liver disease in which biopsy interpretation remains an important part of the diagnostic workup or indeed in prognostication. We set the scene with the first two chapters by covering normal liver and variants and basic patterns of injury. This forms a basis for a greater understanding of the impact of different disease processes on liver microarchitecture described in the remaining chapters.

All four of the authors remain fascinated by the changes that can be seen by microscopy in liver tissues; we hope that our enthusiasm for the subject will rub off on those who read and use this book. We are each indebted to our respective mentors and to histopathological and hepatological colleagues who continue to share their interesting and challenging cases with us. Finally all four authors would like to acknowledge the incredible support of their respective families during the preparation of this atlas.

Hong Kong
London
Newcastle
Adelaide

Anthony W.H. Chan
Alberto Quaglia
Beate Haugk
Alastair Burt

Contents

1 Normal, Variants, and Methods . . . 1
- 1.1 Normal Liver Landmarks . . . 1
- 1.2 Normal Variants and Artefacts . . . 5
- 1.3 Routine Handling and Histochemical Staining . . . 8
- 1.4 Ancillary Tests . . . 15

2 General Processes . . . 19
- 2.1 Inflammation . . . 19
- 2.2 Cellular Damage . . . 23
- 2.3 Intracellular/Extracellular Accumulations . . . 28
- 2.4 Regeneration . . . 34
- 2.5 Fibrosis . . . 36

3 Developmental Abnormalities . . . 39
- 3.1 Normal Development . . . 39
- 3.2 Fibrocystic Liver Disease and Choledochal Cyst . . . 41
- 3.3 Paucity of Intrahepatic Bile Ducts and Biliary Atresia . . . 46
- 3.4 Miscellaneous Anatomic and Vascular Anomalies . . . 47

4 Metabolic Liver Disease . . . 49
- 4.1 Disorders of Iron Metabolism . . . 50
- 4.2 Disorders of Copper Metabolism . . . 53
- 4.3 Disorders of Carbohydrate Metabolism . . . 55
- 4.4 Endoplasmic Reticulum Storage Disorders . . . 58
- 4.5 Disorders of Amino Acid Metabolism . . . 60
- 4.6 Lysosomal Storage Disorders . . . 62
- 4.7 Primary Mitochondrial Hepatopathy . . . 64
- 4.8 Disorders of Bile Acid and Bilirubin Metabolism . . . 66
- 4.9 Miscellaneous Metabolic Disorders . . . 68

5 Fatty Liver Disease . . . 71
- 5.1 Alcoholic Liver Disease . . . 71
- 5.2 Nonalcoholic Fatty Liver Disease . . . 76
- 5.3 Focal Fatty Change . . . 84

6 Viral Liver Disease . . . 85
- 6.1 Hepatotropic Viral Hepatitis . . . 85
- 6.2 Grading and Staging of Chronic Viral Hepatitis . . . 91
- 6.3 Nonhepatotropic Viral Hepatitis . . . 101

7 Nonviral Infectious Liver Disease . . . 105
- 7.1 Bacterial Infection . . . 105
- 7.2 Mycobacterial Infection . . . 107
- 7.3 Rickettsial Infection . . . 109
- 7.4 Fungal Infection . . . 110

7.5 Protozoal Infection ... 112
7.6 Helminth Infection ... 115

8 Drug-Induced Liver Injury ... 119
8.1 Necroinflammatory Injury ... 119
8.2 Cholestatic Injury ... 125
8.3 Steatosis and Steatohepatitis ... 129
8.4 Vascular Lesions ... 132
8.5 Neoplasm and Tumour-like Lesions ... 135
8.6 Adaptive Change ... 136

9 Autoimmune Hepatitis ... 139
9.1 Autoimmune Hepatitis ... 140
9.2 Overlap and Variant Syndromes ... 147

10 Biliary Disease ... 149
10.1 Primary Biliary Cirrhosis ... 150
10.2 Primary Sclerosing Cholangitis ... 154
10.3 Other Biliary Diseases ... 157

11 Vascular Disorders ... 163

12 Premalignant Lesions ... 171

13 Neoplasm-like Liver Lesions ... 179

14 Epithelial Liver Neoplasms ... 185
14.1 Hepatocellular Epithelial Neoplasms ... 186
14.2 Biliary Epithelial Neoplasms ... 198
14.3 Combined Hepatocellular–Cholangiocarcinoma ... 204
14.4 Other Epithelial Neoplasms ... 207

15 Nonepithelial Liver Neoplasms ... 209
15.1 Benign Mesenchymal Neoplasms ... 209
15.2 Malignant Mesenchymal Neoplasms ... 214
15.3 Haematolymphoid Neoplasms ... 217

16 Obstetric Liver Disease ... 221

17 Transplantation Pathology ... 225

Index ... 241

Normal, Variants, and Methods

1

A sound knowledge of normal liver microscopic anatomy is essential for the correct interpretation of pathological changes. The severity and the progression of acute and chronic liver injury often are defined on the basis of how the injury affects the lobular architecture and the normal anatomic vascular relationships. The classical models of the Kiernan lobule and Rappaport acinus commonly are used to describe the distribution, extent, and possible causes of some types of liver injury. The appearance of some normal components varies according to the location (e.g., the connective tissue of small and large portal tracts) and age (e.g., periportal accumulation of iron and copper in neonates). A sound knowledge of liver biopsy techniques, specimen processing, and staining helps in evaluating the adequacy of a biopsy sample, recognising artefacts, and choosing the most appropriate set of histochemical and immunohistochemical stains to answer specific clinical questions. This chapter covers all these aspects, illustrating the normal liver architecture and its variants, common technical artefacts, sampling size variation in relation to biopsy technique, and the application of the common histochemical and immunohistochemical stainings.

1.1 Normal Liver Landmarks

Recognition of normal liver landmarks helps in the assessment of the integrity of the overall hepatic architecture and the distribution of pathologic changes, and hence in the formulation of histopathologic diagnoses (Figs. 1.1 to 1.10).

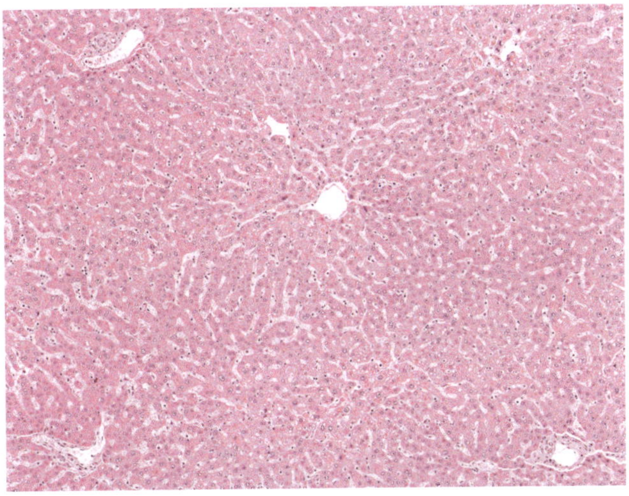

Fig. 1.1 Normal histology; low-power view of normal liver parenchyma. Two terminal hepatic venules (central veins) are located in the centre and at the right-hand side of the image. Three portal tracts also are seen; each one is separated from the others by a similar distance. The overall hepatic architecture is best assessed under low magnification. An even distribution of portal tracts and terminal hepatic venules indicates preserved hepatic architecture. The normal distance between portal tract and terminal hepatic venule is approximately 0.5 mm (0.4–0.75 mm). Distortion of hepatic architecture can be manifest by approximation of the portal tract and terminal hepatic venules (indicating parenchymal collapse), the absence of portal tracts or terminal hepatic venules, or the presence of fibrosis.

A.W.H. Chan et al., *Atlas of Liver Pathology*, Atlas of Anatomic Pathology,
DOI 10.1007/978-1-4614-9114-9_1, © Springer Science+Business Media New York 2014

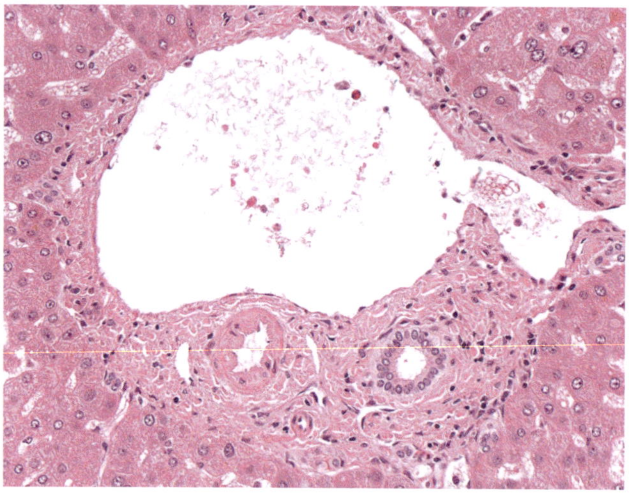

Fig. 1.2 Normal portal tract. A normal portal tract contains a portal venule, a hepatic arteriole, and an interlobular bile duct, which collectively are called a portal triad. A few lymphocytes and macrophages frequently are present in normal portal tracts. Not all portal tracts contain all three components of the portal triad. One recent study demonstrated that 6.2%, 10.2%, and 9.2% of portal tracts do not contain a bile duct, hepatic artery, or portal vein, respectively. The hepatic artery is accompanied by a nearby (within a distance two to three times that of its diameter) interlobular bile duct of similar diameter in >90% of portal tracts. This so-called parallelism of hepatic arteries and bile ducts is the basis of recently proposed criteria for ductopaenia.

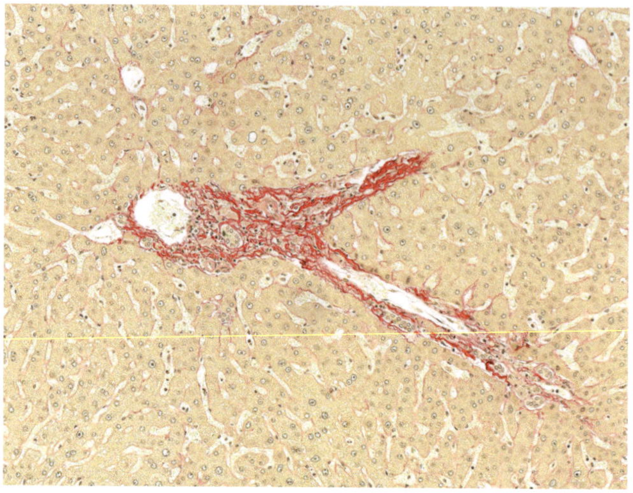

Fig. 1.4 Normal portal tract (picrosirius red stain); normal branching small-sized portal tract. A portal venule and interlobular bile duct are present in the branching connective tissue stroma. One of the pitfalls in assessing fibrosis is misinterpretation of branching or tangentially cut portal tracts as periportal or even bridging fibrosis. Branching or tangentially cut portal tracts can be recognized correctly by the presence of vessels and/or bile ducts travelling along thin fibrous "septa."

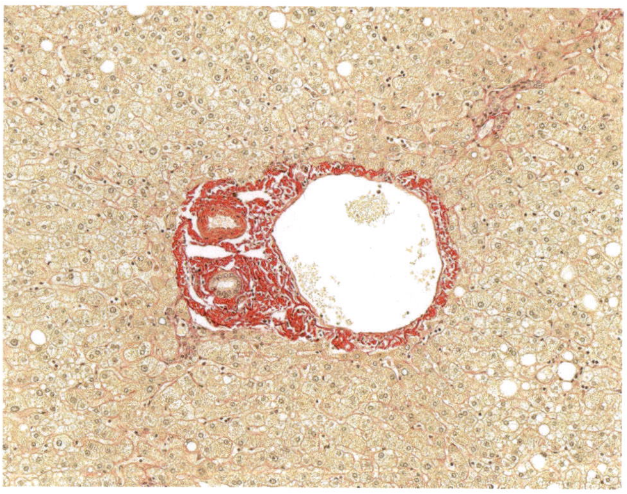

Fig. 1.3 Normal portal tract (picrosirius red stain). A normal medium-sized portal tract contains a portal vein branch, a hepatic arteriole, and an interlobular bile duct. Normal portal tracts contain a certain amount of connective tissue to support their constituent structures. The amount of connective tissue is proportional to the size of the vascular and biliary components and, hence, the size of the portal tract. An appreciation of normal amounts of portal connective tissue is crucial in being able to assess abnormal excessive deposition of connective tissue (i.e., fibrosis). Portal tracts in older people may contain more connective tissue, slightly more lymphocytes and macrophages, and/or hyalinised arterioles.

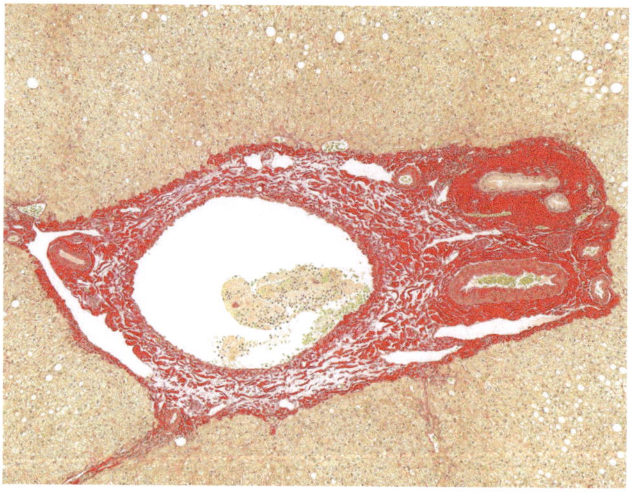

Fig. 1.5 Normal portal tract (picrosirius red stain); normal large-sized portal tract containing a portal vein branch, hepatic artery, and septal bile duct, which are embedded in a normal amount of connective tissue. Another pitfall in the assessment of fibrosis is misinterpretation of normal large-sized portal tracts as portal fibrosis. Identification of larger vessels or septal bile ducts may clarify this potentially misleading appearance. A further problem is that septal bile ducts normally are surrounded by denser connective tissue than are smaller ducts, and this may be mistaken for periductal fibrosis.

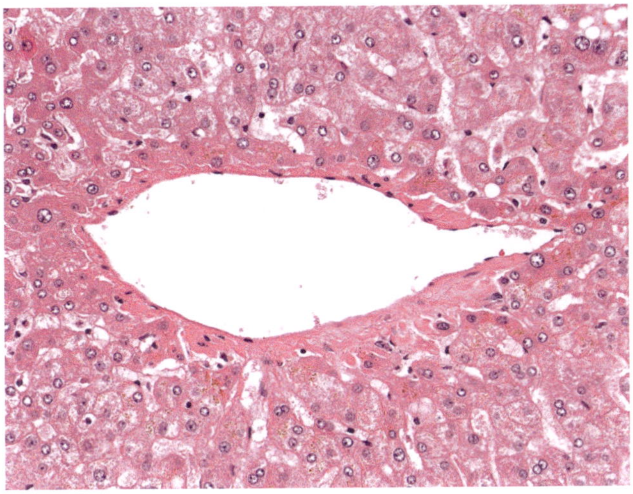

Fig. 1.6 Normal perivenular region. A normal terminal hepatic venule (central vein) is shown. The hepatocytes surrounding the venule contain some golden-yellow fine granular pigment (lipofuscin) in their cytoplasm. Identification of lipofuscin might be useful in the identification of perivenular regions. The distinction between perivenular and periportal areas sometimes may be problematic in small biopsies in which there are ductopaenic conditions (especially chronic allograft rejection in which hepatic arteries may also be lost) and confluent necrosis associated with ductular reaction. Immunostaining for glutamine synthetase, however, serves as a better tool for highlighting perivenular hepatocytes in such conditions.

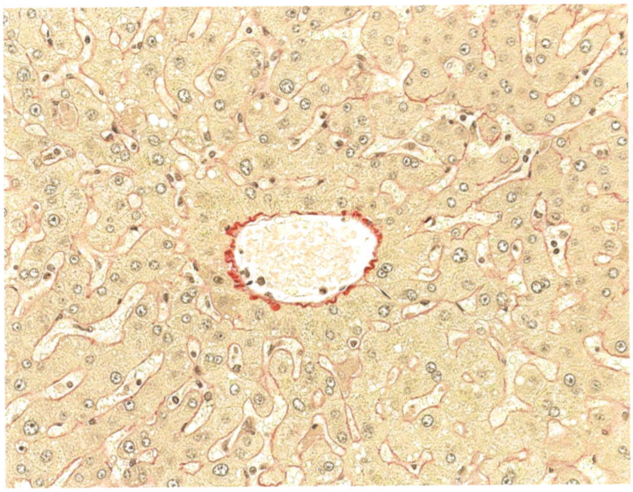

Fig. 1.7 Normal terminal hepatic venule (picrosirius red stain). A normal small-sized terminal hepatic venule is surrounded by a thin rim of connective tissue. Some irregularity of perivenular fibrous tissue is a normal finding and should not be mistaken for perivenular fibrosis. The absence of thick perivenular fibrous tissue and/or pericellular scarring may avoid overestimation of perivenular fibrosis.

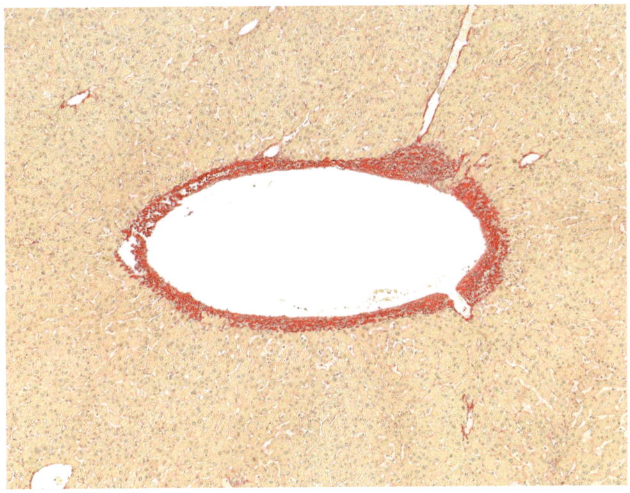

Fig. 1.8 Normal hepatic vein (picrosirius red stain). A normal large-sized hepatic vein is surrounded by a thicker rim of connective tissue. Similar to portal tracts, the amount of connective tissue surrounding the hepatic vein correlates with the size of the vein. A large hepatic vein sometimes may be mistaken for perivenular fibrosis.

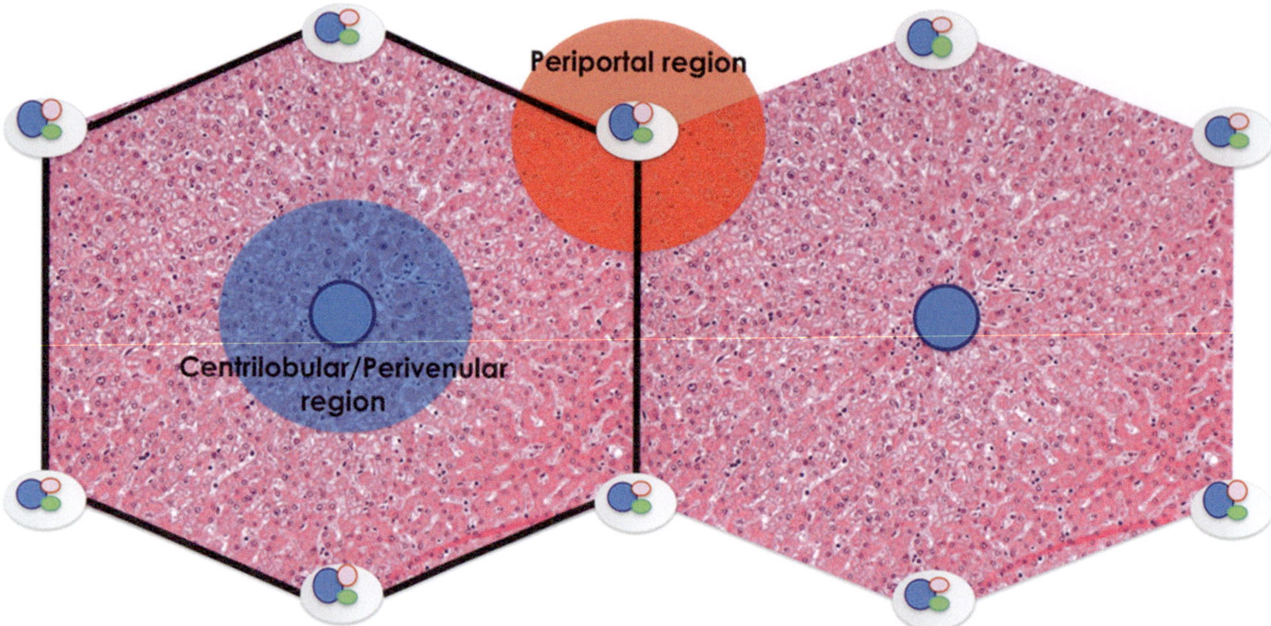

Fig. 1.9 Classic lobular architecture. The classic lobule was described by Kiernan in 1833. A hepatic lobule is a roughly hexagonal structure containing a central vein (terminal hepatic venule) at its core with plates of hepatocytes radiating centrifugally towards portal tracts (three to six) at the corners. The lobule is divided into three regions: a centrilobular/perivenular region around the central vein, a periportal region around the portal tract, and a midlobular region situated in between. This concept is easy to understand, and the microanatomy of the liver is easy to appreciate under the microscope. It still is very common for pathologists to use the terminology of this lobular concept to describe the distribution of pathologic changes.

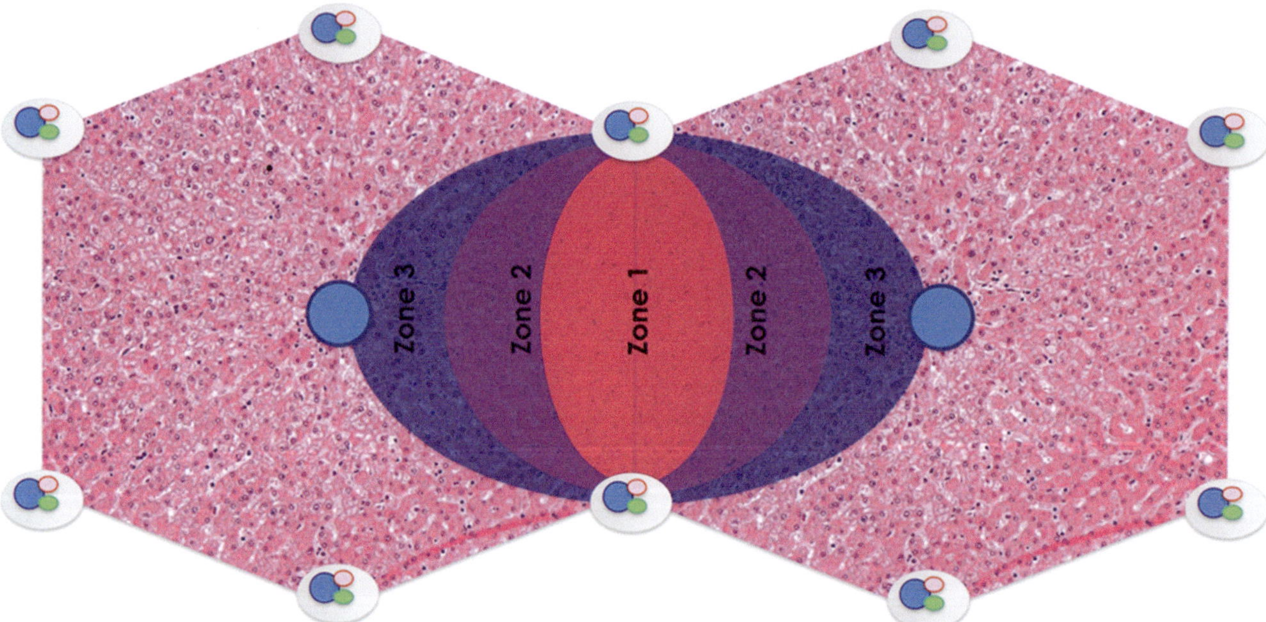

Fig. 1.10 Rappaport acinar architecture. The acinar structure was proposed by Rappaport in 1954. A simple acinus is a berry-shaped structure with a central axis formed by the terminal branches of a portal venule, a hepatic arteriole, and an interlobular bile duct. Blood from the terminal branches of portal venules and hepatic arterioles drains through the hepatic sinusoids into several terminal hepatic venules at the periphery of the acinus. The acinus is divided into three zones (zones 1, 2, and 3) according to the proximity to the terminal branches of vessels. The three zones differ in their tissue oxygenation, metabolic activity, and enzyme distribution. The acinar concept explains the zonal predilection of certain liver injuries. Portal–central and portal–portal bridging necrosis/fibrosis can be better appreciated as extensive zone 3 and zone 1 necrosis/fibrosis, respectively.

1.2 Normal Variants and Artefacts

Some normal variants and morphologic alterations by various artefacts may be alarming and give the erroneous impression of a pathologic abnormality. Awareness of such changes minimizes potential misinterpretation during histologic assessment (Figs. 1.11 to 1.18).

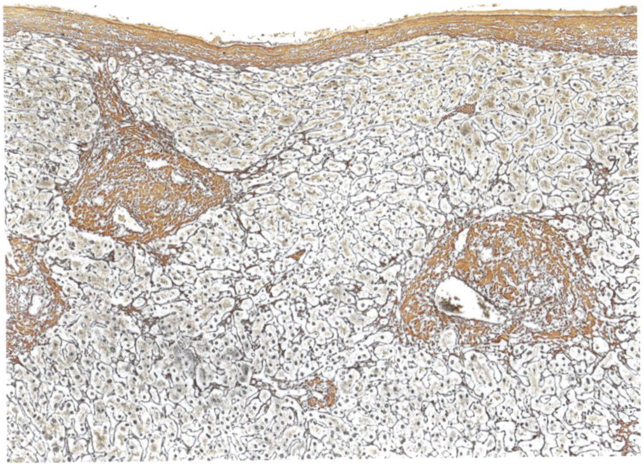

Fig. 1.11 Subcapsular liver (Gordon and Sweets stain for reticulin). A fibrous band extends from Glisson's capsule into a portal tract located in the subcapsular region. The amount of fibrous tissue varies in the subcapsular region of normal liver (within 2 mm of Glisson's capsule). It is not uncommon to find thin and occasionally thick fibrous bands extending from Glisson's capsule and sometimes joining portal tracts in this area. This phenomenon may lead to misinterpretation of bridging fibrosis, particularly in assessment of superficial tangentially obtained needle liver biopsies.

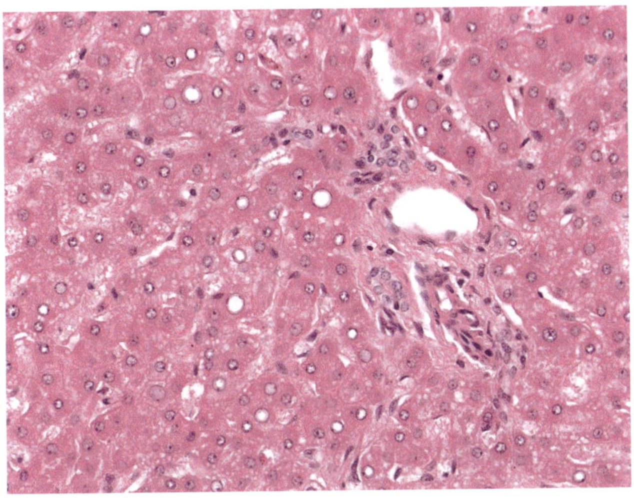

Fig. 1.12 Normal liver of an adolescent. Some periportal hepatocytes possess glycogenated nuclei. Physiologic hepatic nuclear glycogenation is common in children, adolescents, and young adults (11% and 4% in the 20s and early 30s, respectively).

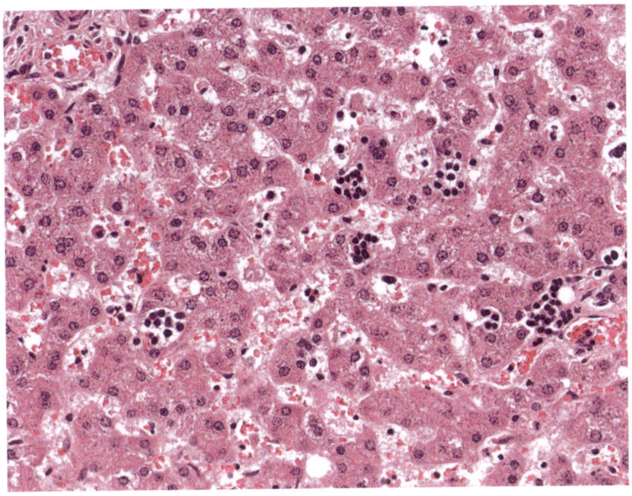

Fig. 1.13 Normal liver of an infant. Foci of extramedullary haematopoiesis are present. Extramedullary haematopoiesis is a normal physiologic finding during fetal development. It normally ceases within a month after birth. Erythropoiesis tends to occur along hepatic sinusoids, whereas leucopoiesis and thrombopoiesis are found more commonly in portal tracts. The presence of these immature haematopoietic cells should not be misinterpreted as lobular or portal inflammation, or as an atypical haematolymphoid infiltrate. Hepatocyte plates in children before the age of five are two cells thick and become one cell thick around that time. Therefore, a twin-cell hepatocyte plate in infants does not indicate regenerative activity, as it would in adults.

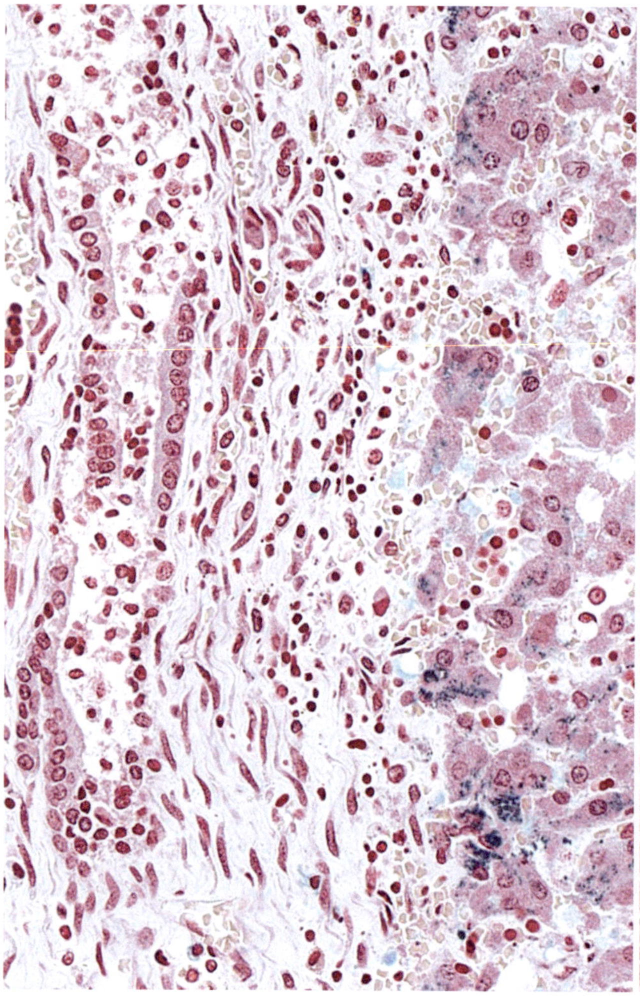

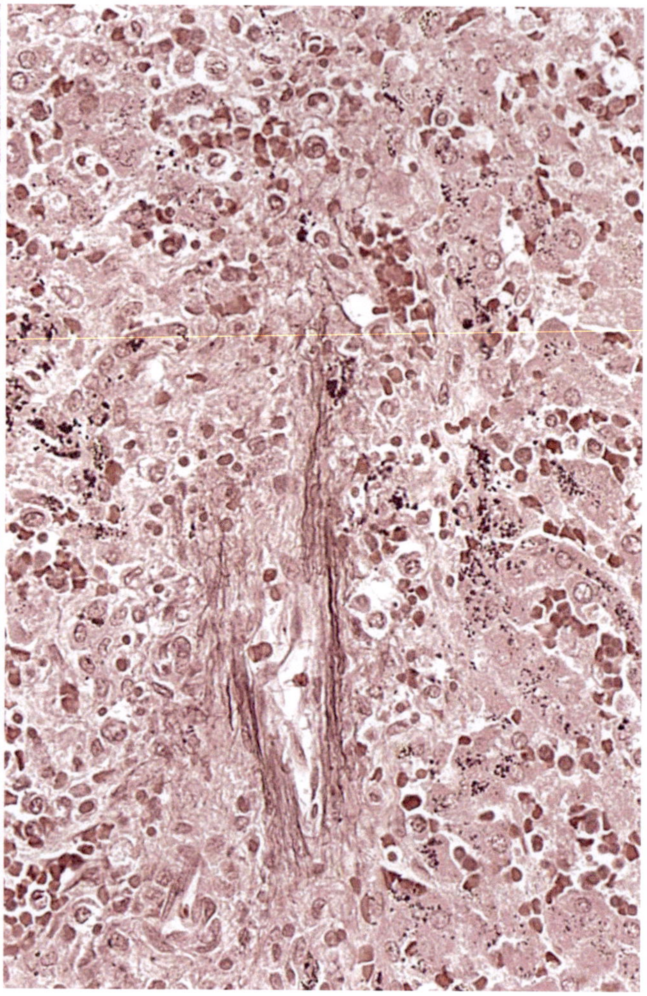

Fig. 1.14 Normal liver of an infant (*left*: Perls stain; *right*: orcein stain). Deposition of haemosiderin and copper-associated protein is seen in the periportal hepatocytes of a neonatal liver. The presence of stainable iron and copper in these cells is a physiologic phenomenon during the fetal and infantile periods (up to 3 months old) and should not be misinterpreted as a pathologic feature of iron or copper overload.

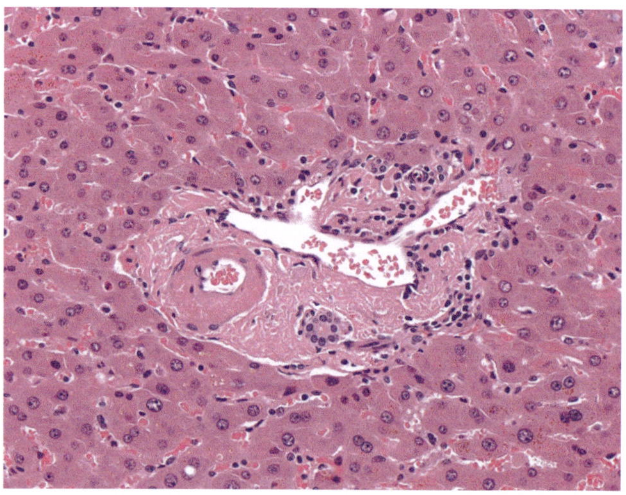

Fig. 1.15 Normal liver of an elderly individual. In this liver tissue from an octogenarian without any chronic liver disease, a portal tract contains a hyalinised hepatic arteriole and there is a mild increase in lymphocytes. The hepatocytes show mild anisonucleosis and occasional binucleation. In the elderly liver, anisonucleosis, ploidy, and increased lipofuscin deposition commonly are observed in the hepatocytes, whereas hyaline arteriosclerosis (not necessarily associated with systemic hypertension), an increase in portal tract collagen, and a lymphocytic infiltrate are not infrequently present in portal tracts.

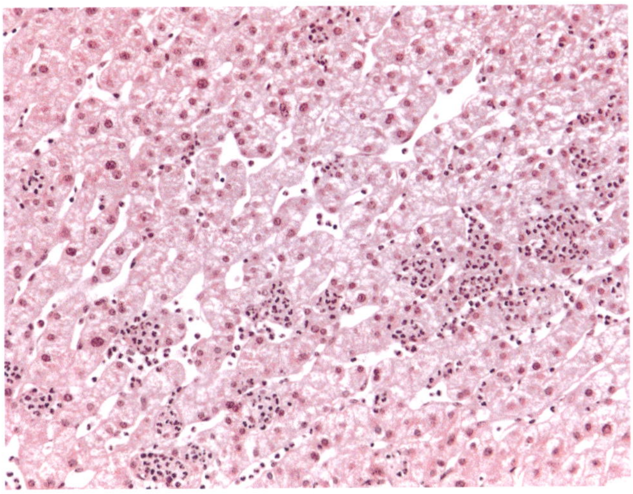

Fig. 1.16 "Surgical hepatitis." Clusters of neutrophils are scattered in the sinusoids without any associated hepatocytic injury or necrosis. Surgical hepatitis is a nonspecific finding commonly seen in specimens taken during a surgical procedure. The neutrophils are irregularly scattered but often concentrated in the perivenular or subcapsular region. Surgical hepatitis is not a genuine hepatitis and does not carry any clinical significance. It should not be confused with other conditions with sinusoidal neutrophilic infiltrates, such as alcoholic hepatitis, cytomegalovirus infection, and sepsis.

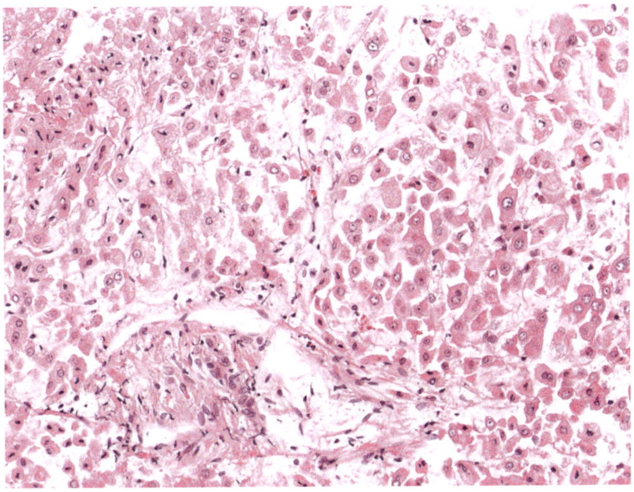

Fig. 1.17 Artefact by immersion into saline. In liver biopsy tissue submitted in normal saline, hepatocytes demonstrate a prominent artefactual discohesive appearance.

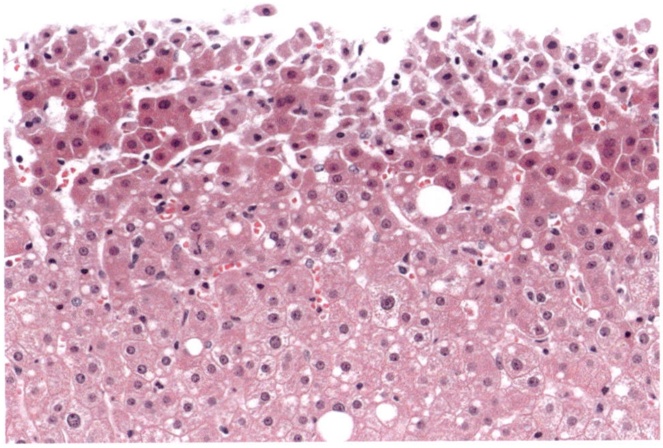

Fig. 1.18 Drying artefact. In liver biopsy tissue submitted by being placed on dry blotting paper, hepatocytes on the edge show a drying artefact with nuclear hyperchromasia and pyknosis, cellular shrinkage, and discohesion.

1.3 Routine Handling and Histochemical Staining

Proper handling and processing of liver tissue are fundamental steps for histological assessment of hepatic diseases. Understanding the use and pitfalls of various common histochemical stains used in liver pathology allows accurate interpretation of their morphologic findings (Figs. 1.19 to 1.39).

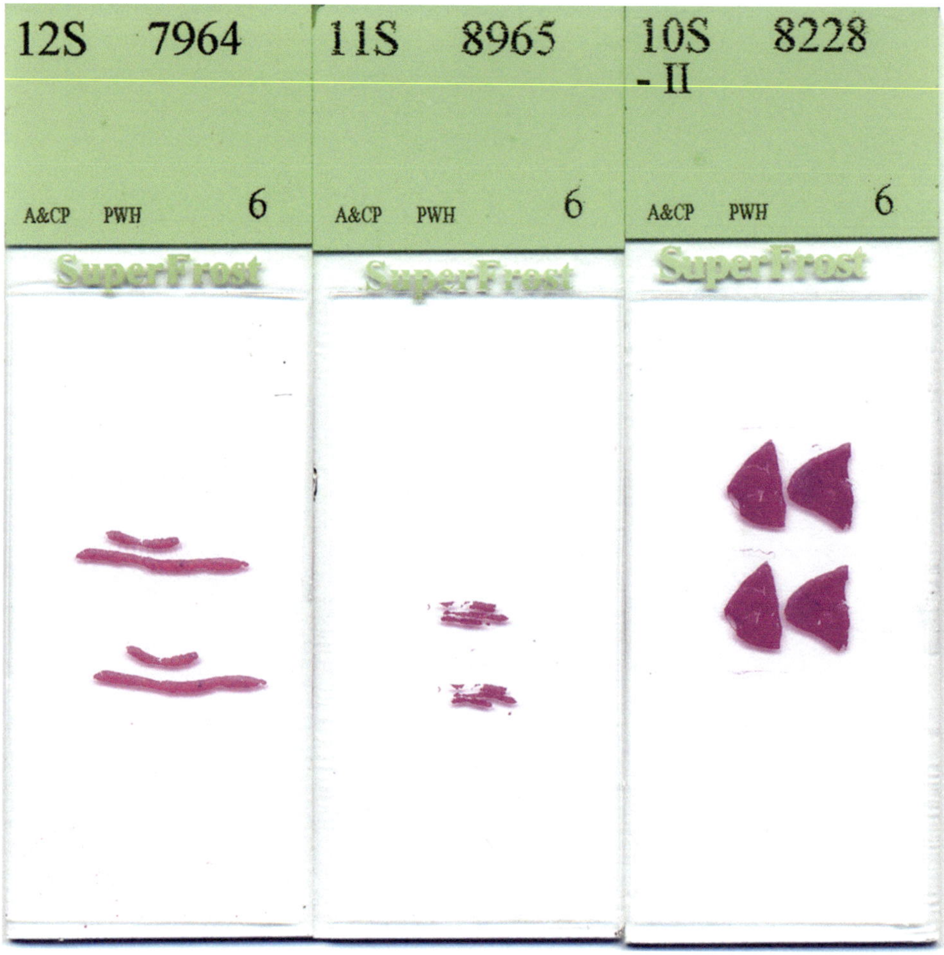

Fig. 1.19 Different types of liver biopsy. Liver biopsy samples are obtained from three common routes: percutaneous (*left*), transjugular (*middle*) and open/laparoscopic wedge (*right*). Percutaneous liver biopsy with or without imaging guidance is the commonest form of liver biopsy. Transjugular liver biopsy is suitable for patients with significant coagulopathies due to cirrhosis or other diseases. Tissue cores taken through the transjugular route are thinner and may be fragmented. Wedge biopsies obtained intraoperatively provide a good way to assess focal hepatic lesions over and just beneath the hepatic capsule. However, the liver tissue acquired by wedge biopsy is suboptimal for the assessment of medical liver diseases because of the thick fibrous tissue in the subcapsular region, artefactual surgical hepatitis, and cauterization effects.

Order # : OR
Lab # : **12S**

Request Date : 03/04/2012
Request By :
Report Loc : (PWH/MED/HEP)
Admit Dx : Suspected cirrhosis

Name :
Sex/Age : F/50Y
DOB :
Ward/Bed/Spec :
Admission Date : 02/04/2012
Copy to :

HKID :

Case # :

Test	Specimen	Spec #	Spec status	Collect time
Biopsy, Liver	Liver, right lobe, punch	PWHSP	A	03/04/2012 10:25

1. Clinical History, Symptoms and Signs: DM, HT, dyslipidaemia, psychosis. Mildly raised ALP and GGT. USG showed coarse liver echotexture.
2. Drug history: Metformin, Gliclazide, Trifluoperazine, Lorazepam
3. Smoking history: None
4. Alcoholic consumption: None
5. Alb : 42
6. TB : 6
7. ALP : 110
8. ALT : 25
9. GGT : 100
10. Ferritin : 211
11. HBsAg : –
12. Anti-HCV : –
13. Hb : 11.5
14. PLT : 290
15. WCC : 7.2
16. INR : 0.98
17. ANA : + (1:320)
18. AMA : –
19. SMA : –

Preparation/Remark:
PWHSP : Formalin fixed

Fig. 1.20 Form to request liver biopsy for medical liver disease. Clinicopathologic correlation is crucial in the assessment of nonneoplastic liver disease. To ensure that essential clinical information and laboratory results are adequately provided, a properly designed request form is strongly recommended.

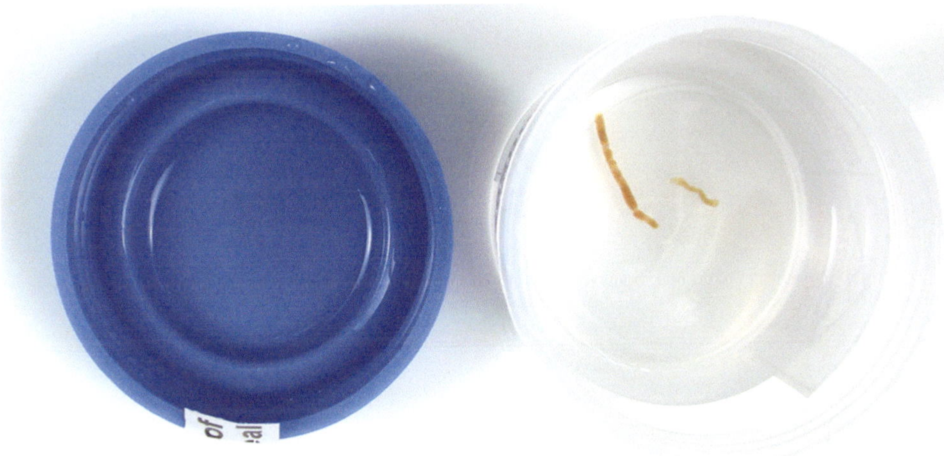

Fig. 1.21 Fixation of liver biopsies. Two cores of liver tissue are seen here in a specimen bottle containing 10% buffered formalin. The routine fixative for liver biopsies is 10% neutral buffered formalin. It allows the subsequent application of most histochemical, immunohistochemical, and some molecular investigations. Prompt fixation is crucial to achieve good preservation and allow optimal histologic preparation. A core needle liver biopsy requires at least 2 to 4 hours for adequate fixation. Placing fresh liver biopsy tissue on a dry blotting paper or gauze is not recommended because it causes marked drying and autolytic artefacts. Submitting liver biopsy tissue in normal saline also should be avoided, as it results in artefactual discohesion of cells.

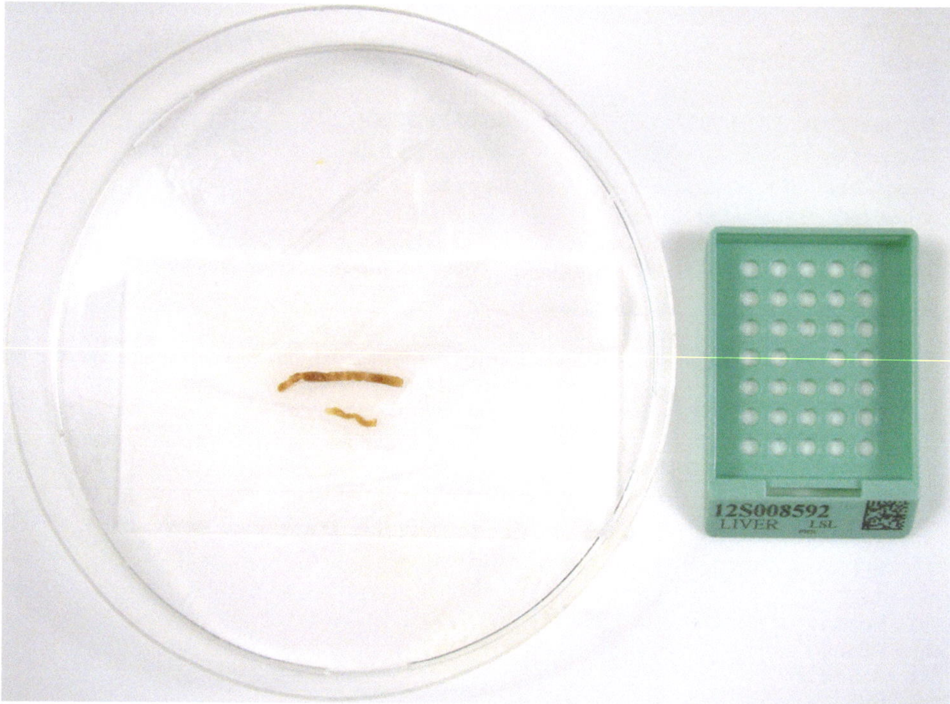

Fig. 1.22 Wrapping of liver biopsy. Two cores of liver tissue are transferred from the specimen bottle onto a piece of wet lens paper on a Petri dish. They are wrapped and placed into a cassette for embedding. Packing liver biopsy tissue between foam sponges into a cassette is not recommended because it leads to artefactual tissue distortion with triangular spaces.

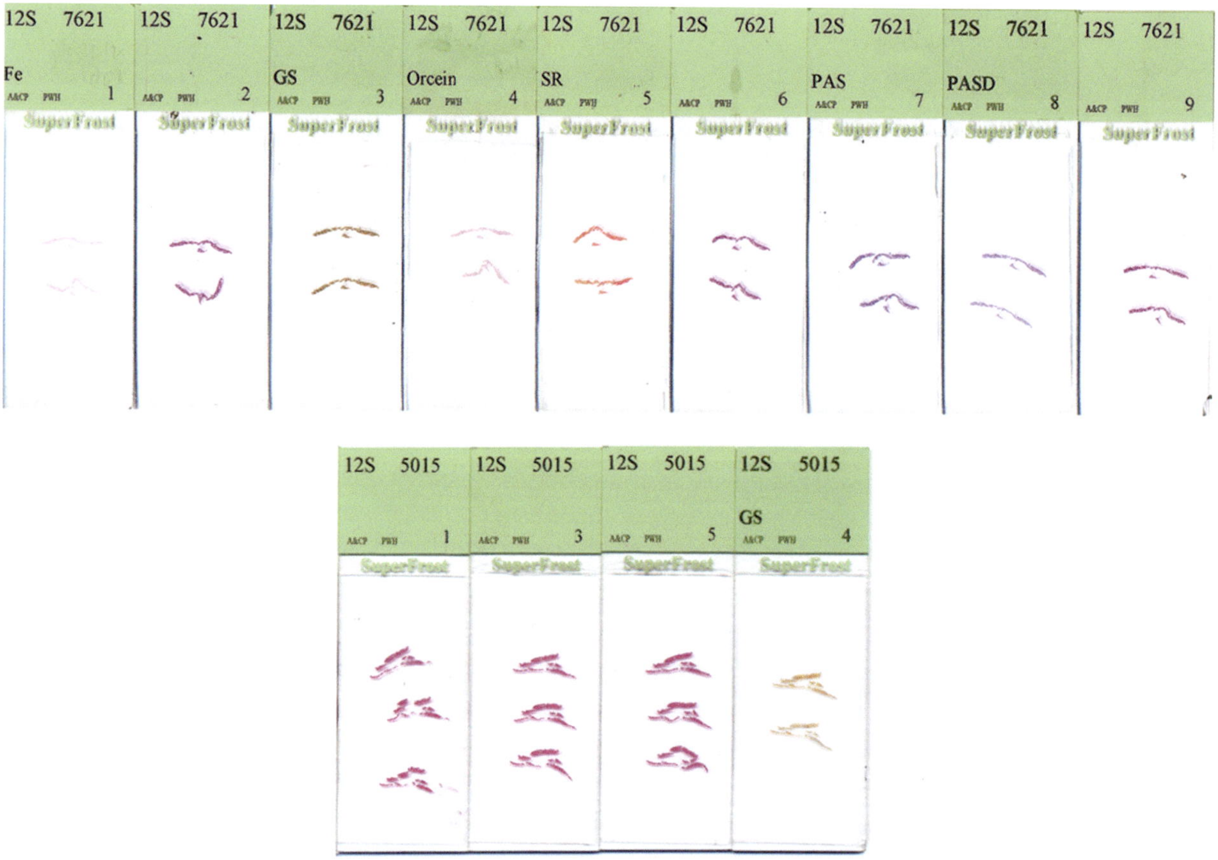

Fig. 1.23 "Liver panel." Panels of stains are performed for evaluating nonneoplastic (*upper*) and neoplastic (*lower*) liver diseases. There is no standard recommendation regarding stains for liver biopsies. Two to three levels of haematoxylin and eosin (H&E) are minimal to evaluate both nonneoplastic liver disease and focal hepatic mass lesion. For the assessment of a focal hepatocytic lesion, reticulin stain helps highlight the thickness of hepatocyte cords, the integrity of the reticulin framework, and the nodular architecture. For the assessment of medical liver diseases, stains for connective tissue, reticulin framework, iron, and copper, as well as periodic acid-Schiff with diastase (PASD) stain, constitute the minimally essential panel.

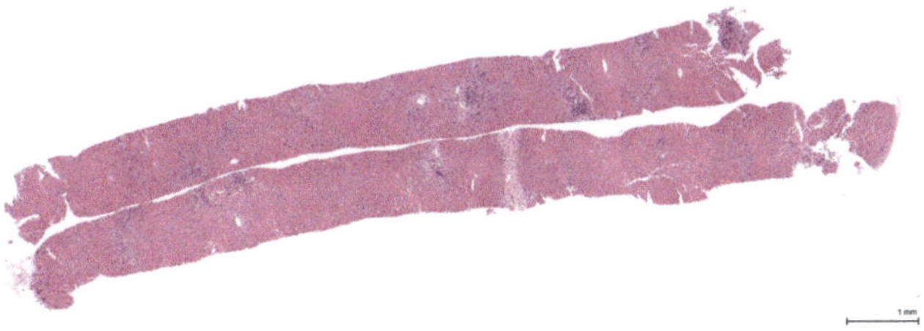

Fig. 1.24 Adequacy of a needle liver biopsy. Traditionally, a liver biopsy core 1.0 to 1.5 cm long with four to six portal tracts was thought to be adequate for assessing medical liver diseases. Currently, it is accepted that a core about 2 cm long with 11 to 15 portal tracts is more appropriate for proper evaluation. Inadequate sampling may underestimate necroinflammatory activity (grade) and degree of fibrosis (stage) of the liver disease.

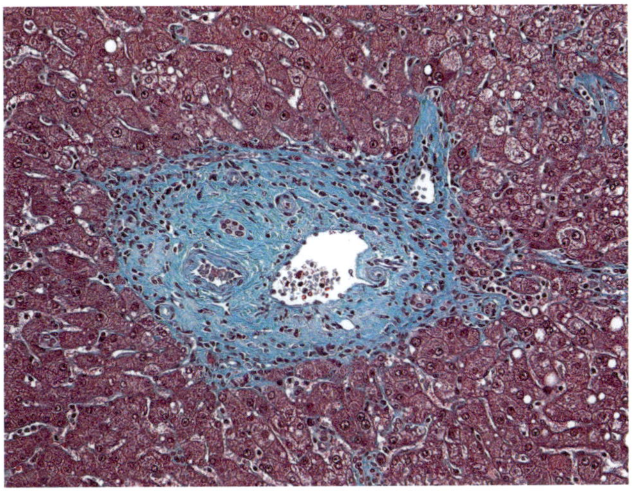

Fig. 1.25 Masson trichrome stain. A normal portal tract is highlighted by this histochemical stain. Masson trichrome is one of the connective tissue stains widely used in hepatopathology. Its main purpose is to highlight type I collagen (greenish/bluish) in turn to identify normal structures (portal tracts and terminal hepatic venules), evaluate the overall hepatic architecture, assess the degree of fibrosis, and distinguish between necrosis and fibrosis. In the last situation, a good trichrome stain may demonstrate a characteristic two-tone appearance with darker staining in the residual normal structure and lighter staining in the necrotic region. Its miscellaneous applications include highlighting Mallory-Denk bodies (red), giant mitochondria (red), and amyloidosis (pale homogenous green/blue).

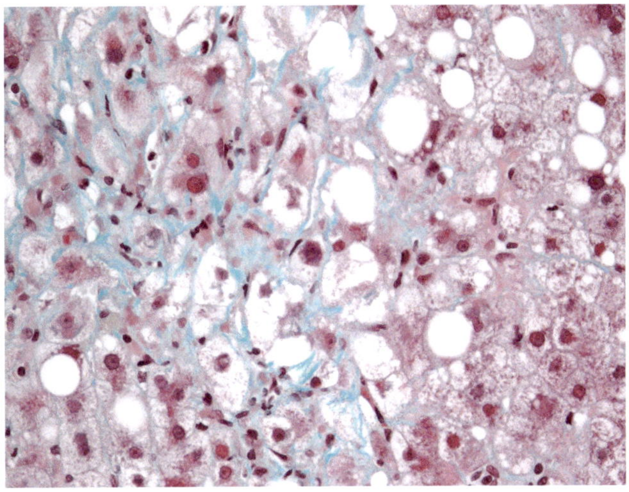

Fig. 1.26 Masson trichrome stain. The hepatocytes are surrounded by delicate pericellular or perisinusoidal fibrosis. A good trichrome stain requires an adequate step of differentiation (usually by phosphomolybdic acid). Inadequate or excessive differentiation leads to over- or understaining, which may lead to over- or underestimation of the degree of fibrosis. Without a good trichrome stain, necrosis and bridging fibrosis cannot be differentiated readily.

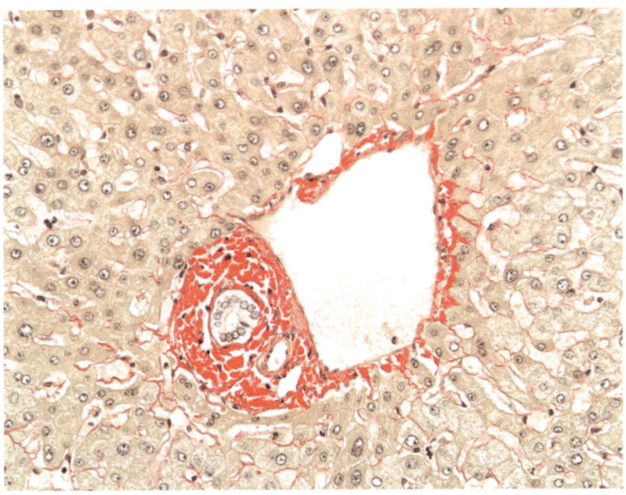

Fig. 1.27 Picrosirius red stain. Picrosirius red is another connective tissue stain providing an alternative to trichrome stains for highlighting type I collagen. It is recommended for morphometric quantitation of fibrosis because it provides highly detailed and contrasted staining and is more sensitive in identifying mild pericellular fibrosis

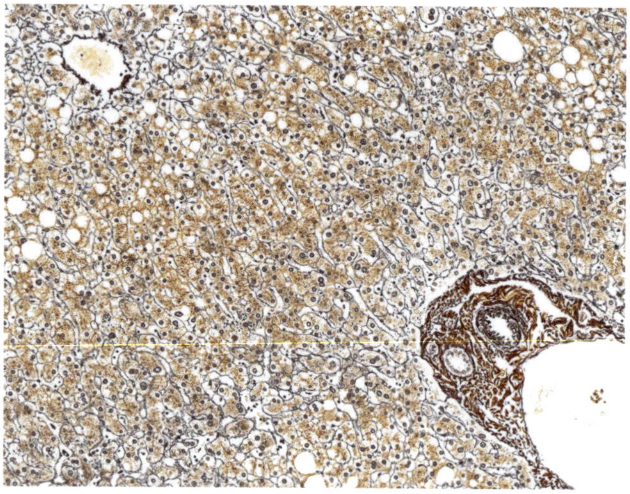

Fig. 1.28 Gordon-Sweets reticulin stain. Normal liver architecture is demonstrated by highlighting the portal tract and the terminal hepatic venule (connective tissue rich in type I collagen appears golden yellow, when the Gordon and Sweets technique is left untoned) and radiating cords of hepatocytes one cell thick (reticulin fibres along the sinusoids appear black). The reticulin stain is helpful in identifying type III collagen (reticulin fibres), which is essential in the assessment of hepatocyte cord thickness, the integrity of the reticulin framework, and the presence of any nodular architecture. In some centres, reticulin stain is the only connective tissue stain used routinely in liver biopsy because it also can highlight type I collagen, as trichrome or picrosirius red stain does for the assessment of fibrosis.

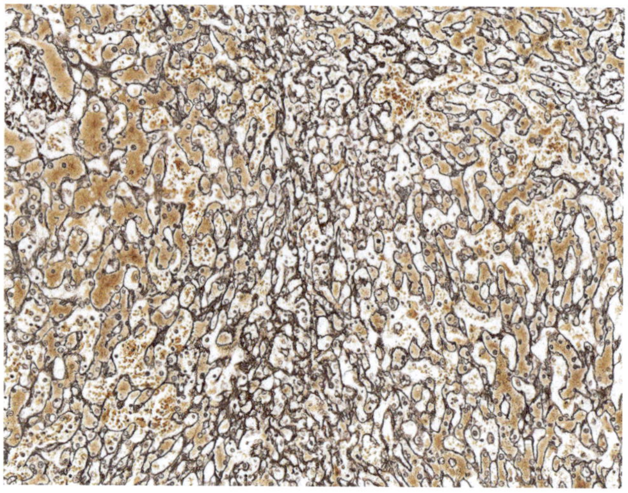

Fig. 1.29 Gordon-Sweets reticulin stain. Condensation of the reticulin framework is demonstrated easily in the area of parenchymal collapse (*middle*). The reticulin stain is helpful in demonstrating subtle parenchymal collapse, which may be overlooked in H&E-stained sections. It also is valuable in differentiating bridging necrosis from bridging fibrosis by showing condensation of residual loosely aggregated reticulin fibres in the former.

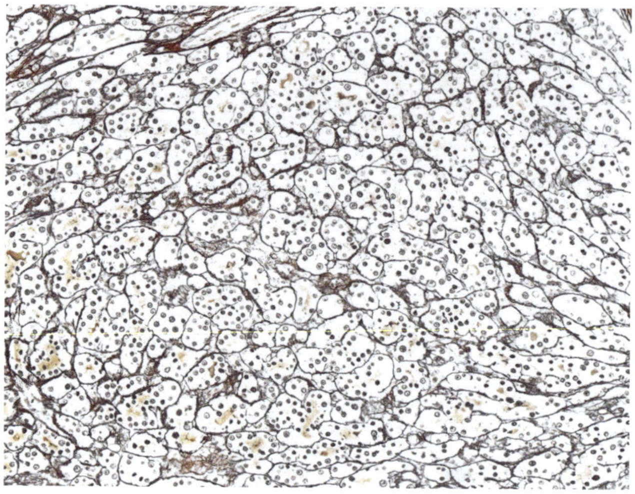

Fig. 1.30 Gordon-Sweets reticulin stain. Increased trabecular thickness with a distorted pattern in a hepatocellular carcinoma is highlighted. The reticulin stain is crucial in discriminating benign from well-differentiated malignant hepatocellular neoplasms. It may help demonstrate the characteristic peripheral condensation of reticulin fibres in nodular regenerative hyperplasia, which might be subtle in H&E sections. Hence, it is recommended that this method be performed routinely in assessing liver mass lesions.

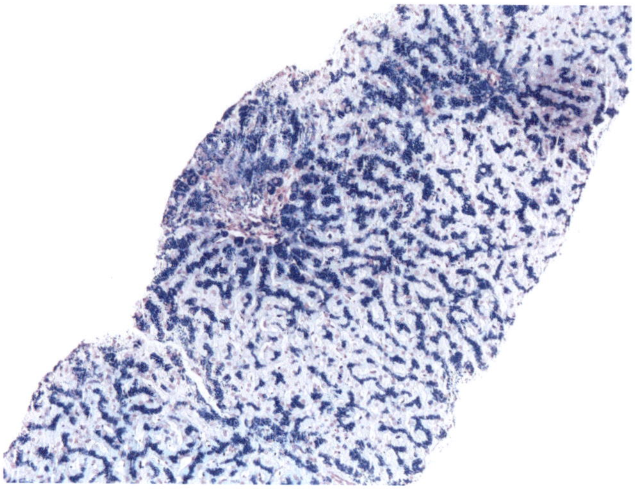

Fig. 1.31 Perls stain. Diffuse iron deposition (haemosiderin) is shown in the cytoplasm of hepatocytes with a pericanalicular pattern. Perls stain, or Perls Prussian Blue stain, is helpful in highlighting iron deposition in the liver to assess both the distribution and degree of iron overload. There are two storage forms of iron in liver: haemosiderin and ferritin. Haemosiderin and ferritin are stained intensely and faintly by Perls stain, respectively. One should not overinterpret the nonspecific faint staining by ferritin, as ferritin is an acute-phase protein and may be seen in many active inflammatory conditions unrelated to iron overload.

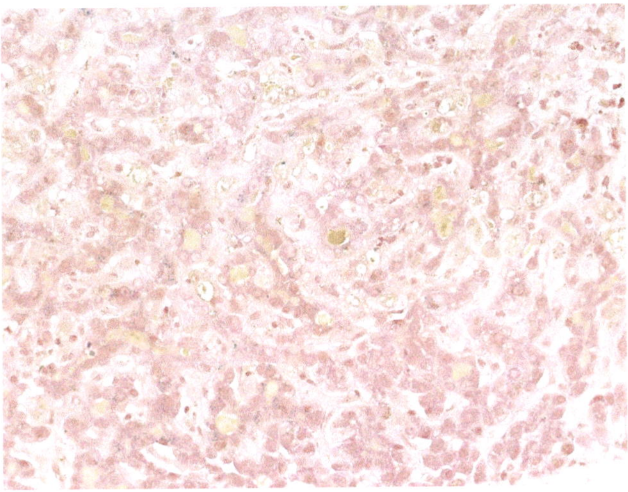

Fig. 1.32 Perls stain. Pale greenish yellow canalicular bile plugs are noted in this Perls stain. An auxiliary practical use of Perls stain is to better visualize subtle bilirubinostasis in the background of pale nuclear and cytoplasmic counterstaining.

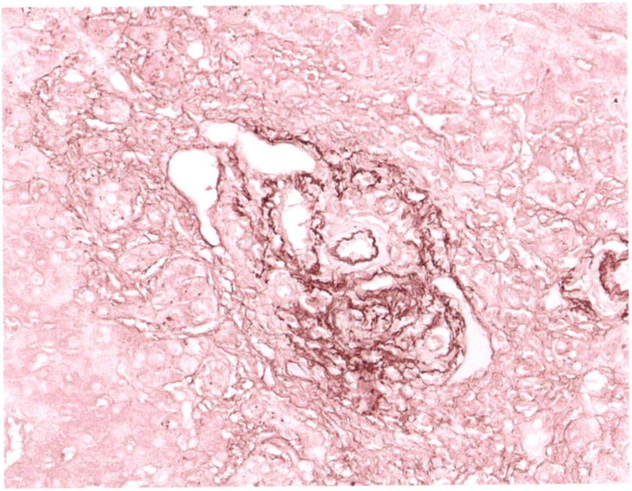

Fig. 1.33 Orcein stain. Scattered tiny copper-associated protein deposits in the periportal hepatocytes are highlighted. Normal elastic fibres in the portal tract also are shown. Orcein stain and its alternative, Victoria blue stain, are the indirect methods for identifying copper by highlighting copper-associated protein (metallothionein). They are superior to the direct stains of copper (rhodanine and rubeanic acid) because copper is highly soluble, especially in poorly buffered formalin. Orcein also is good for highlighting elastic fibres. Normal fibrous tissue, such as that in large portal tracts, and well-established fibrotic tissue contain elastic fibres. This phenomenon makes the Orcein stain helpful in delineating bridging necrosis from bridging fibrosis by demonstrating the absence of elastic fibres in the former.

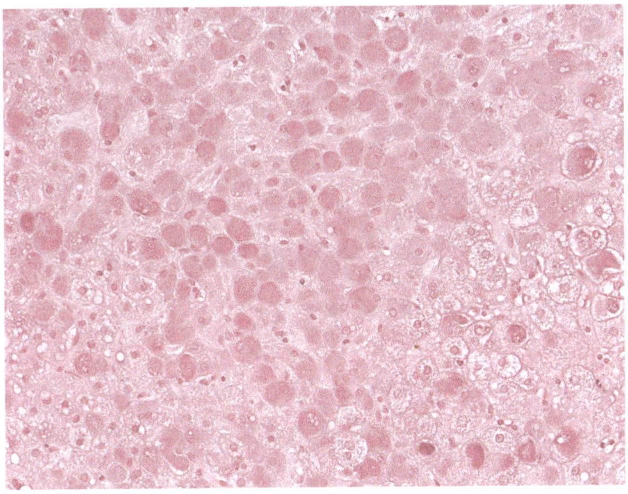

Fig. 1.34 Orcein stain. Numerous hepatitis B surface antigen (HBsAg)-containing cells are highlighted. The orcein stain confirms the nature of ground-glass inclusions of HBsAg type and differentiates them from other forms of ground-glass inclusion (such as polyglucosan inclusions), pale bodies, oncocytic hepatocytes, and hepatocytes with enzyme induction.

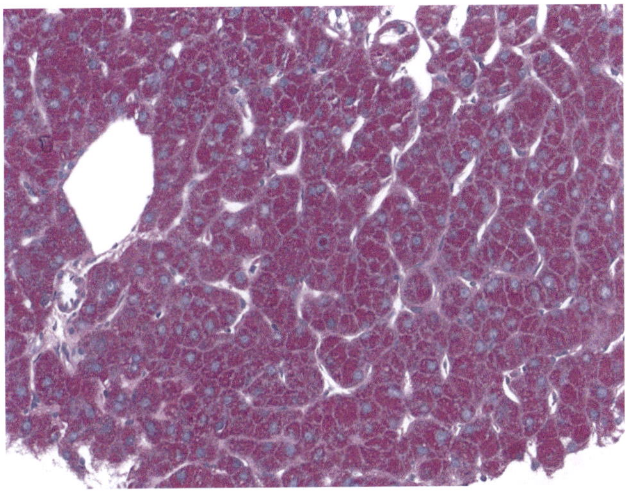

Fig. 1.35 Periodic acid-Schiff (PAS) stain. Cytoplasmic glycogen of hepatocytes and one glycogenated nuclei (*centre*) are shown. PAS stain has a relatively limited role in liver biopsy assessment and is not always performed routinely. PAS stain highlights the glycogen content in the hepatocytes, but glycogen is highly soluble, giving rise to inconsistent staining results. It may be helpful in identifying parenchymal granulomas (which stand out as PAS negative) and in assessing confluent necrosis. Furthermore, it may be helpful in identifying microorganisms such as *Entamoeba histolytica*.

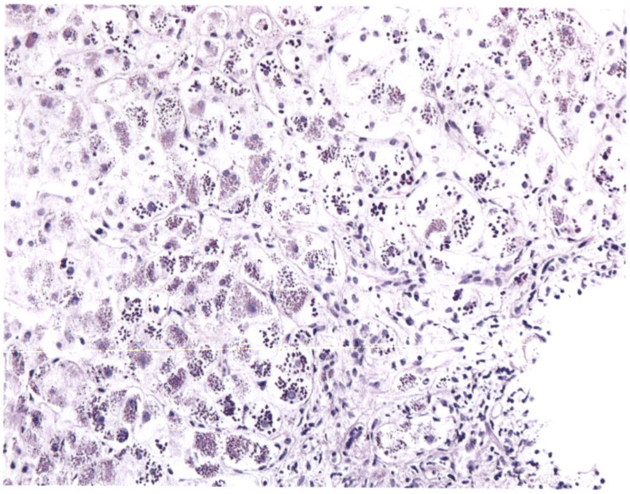

Fig. 1.36 Periodic acid-Schiff with diastase stain. Numerous α_1-antitrypsin cytoplasmic globules are shown. Residual glycogen in the hepatocytes due to incomplete diastase digestion may mimic α_1-antitrypsin cytoplasmic globules. However, the residual glycogen appears granular instead of globular. The equivocal case may be differentiated by immunostaining for α_1-antitrypsin.

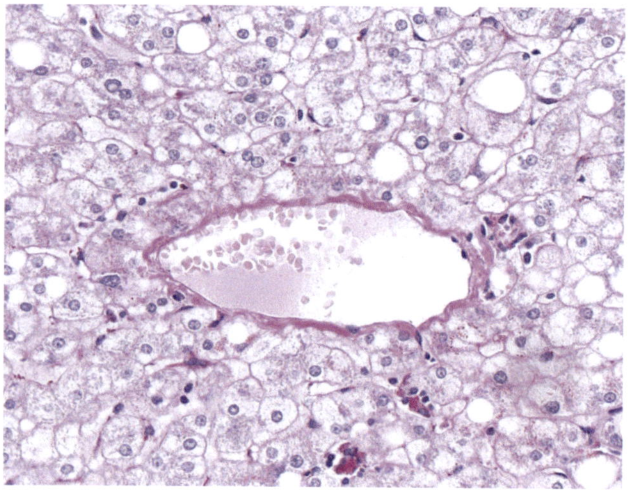

Fig. 1.37 Periodic acid-Schiff with diastase stain. Several ceroid-laden Kupffer cells are illustrated. Ceroid represents early-stage lipofuscin; it results from digestion of engulfed necroinflammatory debris and signifies recent active liver injury.

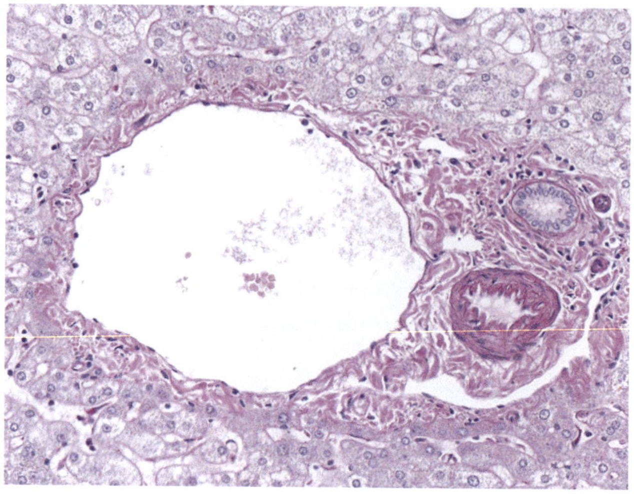

Fig. 1.38 Periodic acid-Schiff with diastase stain. A delicate basement membrane of an interlobular bile duct is highlighted. The PASD stain may be used to assess the integrity and thickness of the basement membrane of bile ducts. Disruption of the basement membrane by an inflammatory infiltrate indicates bile duct injury, whereas a thickened basement membrane in atrophic bile ducts is seen in some chronic biliary diseases, most notably primary sclerosing cholangitis.

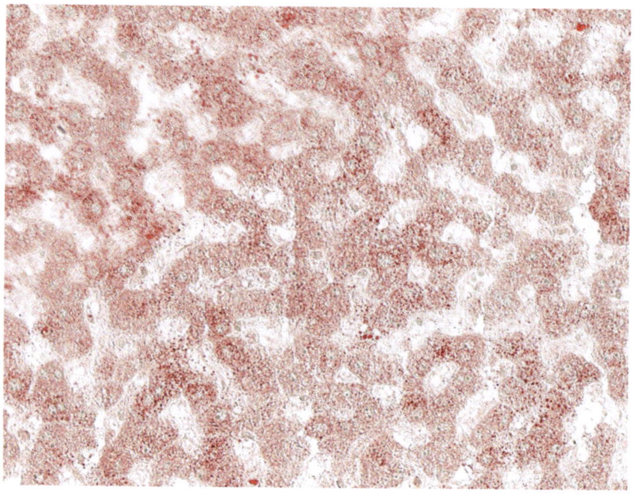

Fig. 1.39 Oil red O stain. Multiple minute fat droplets are highlighted in the hepatocytes. The oil red O stain is important for establishing the presence of microvesicular steatosis if fat droplets are too tiny to be appreciated in paraffin-embedded material. However, it requires a frozen section of the specimen (preferentially fresh) before paraffin embedding.

1.4 Ancillary Tests

Immunohistochemistry is almost a routine laboratory procedure in assisting the diagnosis of a wide range of non-neoplastic and neoplastic liver diseases. For the evaluation of nonneoplastic liver diseases, immunohistochemistry is useful in (1) identifying causative infective agents, (2) determining the nature of inclusion bodies, (3) highlighting biliary epithelium of bile ducts and ductules and the presence of cholate stasis, and (4) detecting aberrant expression of bile acid transport proteins. For the assessment of neoplastic liver diseases, immunohistochemistry is helpful in the (1) distinction of hepatocellular carcinoma from cholangiocarcinoma and metastatic carcinoma; (2) differentiation between hepatocellular carcinoma and benign hepatocellular lesions (hepatocellular adenoma, focal nodular hyperplasia, regenerative nodule and dysplastic nodule); (3) identification of subtypes of hepatocellular carcinoma with poorer prognosis; (4) subclassification of hepatocellular adenoma; (5) identification of the lineage of differentiation of nonepithelial neoplasms; and (6) determination of the primary origin of metastatic tumours.

In situ hybridization, other molecular tests, and ultrastructural studies may provide additional valuable information in some cases (Figs. 1.40 to 1.50).

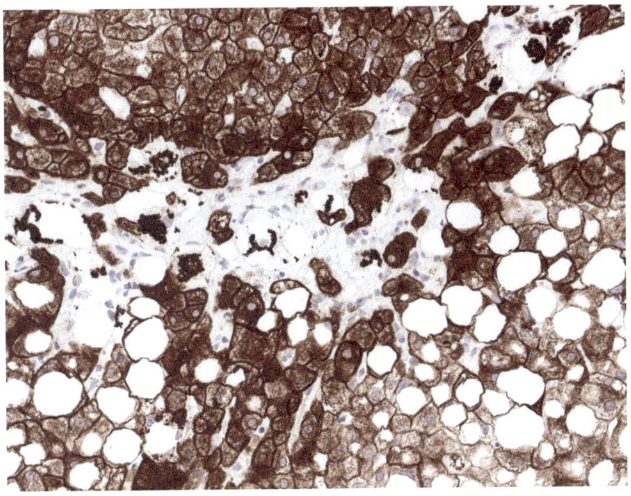

Fig. 1.41 Immunostain for cytokeratin 8/18 (CK8/18). Ballooned hepatocytes lose cytoplasmic expression of CK8/18, whereas the residual immunoreactivity is confined to their Mallory-Denk bodies. Immunostaining for CK8/18 highlights normal hepatocytes. Ballooned hepatocytes and cells with feathery degeneration show a characteristic diminished expression of CK8/18. This stain may be helpful in differentiating ballooning degeneration from steatosis and glycogen-rich hepatocytes. Moreover, immunostaining for CK8/18 highlights Mallory-Denk bodies, which also are immunoreactive to p62 and ubiquitin. Additionally, immunohistochemistry is valuable in highlighting other inclusion bodies, including α_1-antitrypsin globule, intracellular hyaline bodies (p62), and pale bodies (fibrinogen).

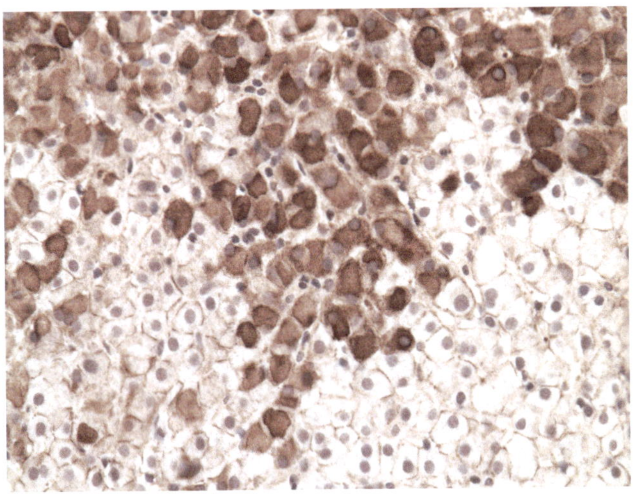

Fig. 1.40 Immunostain for hepatitis B surface antigen. Half the hepatocytes show membranous positivity, whereas the other half show intracytoplasmic positivity highlighting ground-glass hepatocytes. Immunostaining for HBsAg confirms the diagnosis of chronic hepatitis B. Extensive membranous staining indicates a high viral replicative rate, whereas diffuse intracytoplasmic staining suggests a low replicative state. Immunostaining for hepatitis B core antigen (HBcAg) shows mainly nuclear staining and, less commonly, cytoplasmic or membranous staining. The presence of immunoreactivity to core antigen signifies high viral replication, which correlates with serum hepatitis B DNA level.

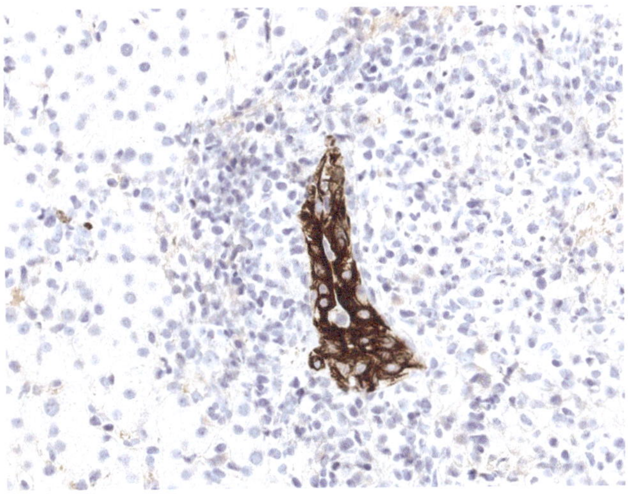

Fig. 1.42 Immunostain for cytokeratin 19 (CK19). A damaged interlobular bile duct with lymphocytic infiltrate is highlighted. Immunostaining for CK7 or CK19 highlights biliary epithelial cells (cholangiocytes) and is useful for assessing the integrity and number of bile ducts. It demonstrates subtle bile duct injury more obviously, and confirms ductopaenia by aiding the assessment of the total number of bile ducts.

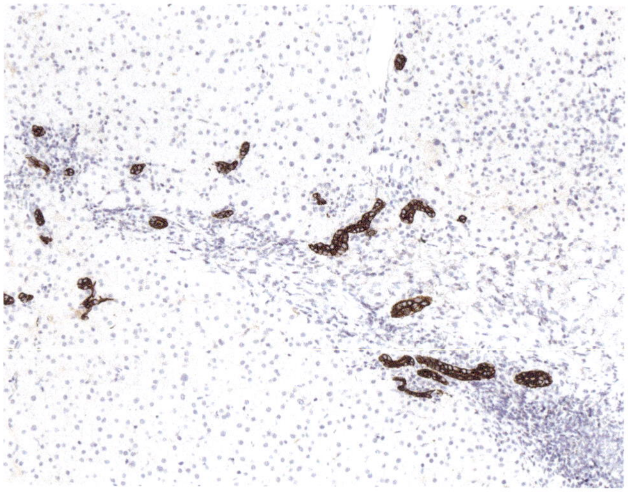

Fig. 1.43 Immunostain for cytokeratin 19. Irregular angulated bile ductules (cholangioles) are shown, and these are mainly located at the portal–parenchymal interface. Immunostaining for CK7 or CK19 highlights biliary epithelial cells of bile ductules and helps illustrate the degree of ductular reaction. Immunostaining for CK19 also may demonstrate biliary differentiation in classical-type combined hepatocellular-cholangiocarcinoma and poorly differentiated cholangiocarcinoma, and a prognostic marker indicating more aggressive hepatocellular carcinoma. The presence of a ductular reaction highlighted by immunostaining for CK7 or CK19, associated with "entrapped" hepatocytes in the intratumoural septum or portal tract, helps differentiate high-grade dysplastic nodule from early hepatocellular carcinoma.

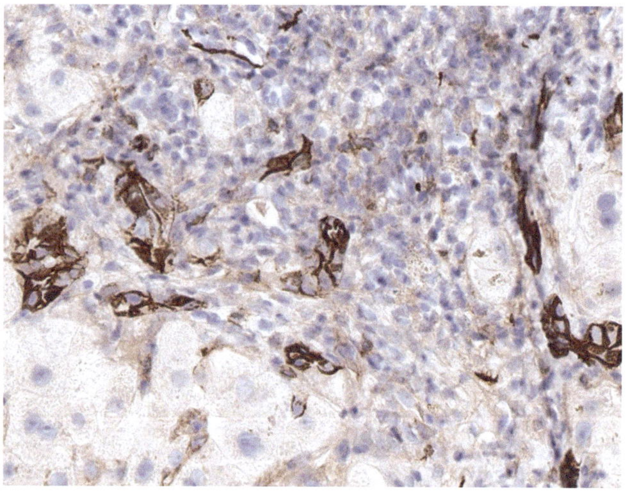

Fig. 1.44 Immunostain for CD56/neural cell adhesion molecule (NCAM). Irregular angulated bile ductules are shown; these are located mainly at the portal–parenchymal interface. Immunostaining for CD56/NCAM highlights biliary epithelial cells of bile ductules but not those of interlobular or other larger bile ducts. Therefore, it is helpful in assessing the degree of ductular reaction and differentiating between bile ductules and atrophic or compressed interlobular bile ducts. Immunostaining for CD56/NCAM is one of the "stem cell" markers, which also include epithelial cell adhesion molecule (EpCAM), CD133, and c-kit/CD117. It is used to diagnose combined hepatocellular-cholangiocarcinoma with stem cell features. Small nerve fibres, which are invisible in H&E sections, in portal tracts, and along sinusoids, also are immunoreactive for CD56/NCAM.

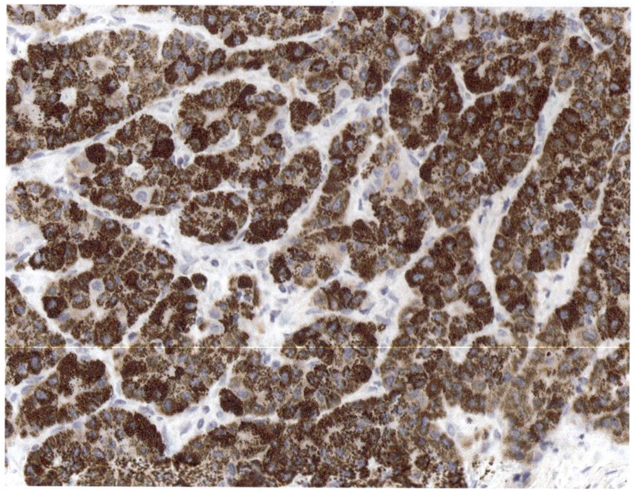

Fig. 1.45 Immunostain for hepatocyte paraffin-1 (HepPar-1). The malignant tumour cells in a moderately differentiated hepatocellular carcinoma are highlighted with a granular cytoplasmic pattern. Immunostaining with HepPar-1 is useful for demonstrating hepatocellular differentiation by reacting with carbamoyl phosphate synthetase in liver mitochondria. About 85% of well- and moderately differentiated hepatocellular carcinomas are immunoreactive to HepPar-1, whereas less than 40% of poorly differentiated carcinomas are positive. The staining pattern also tends to be heterogeneous and patchy, particularly in less-differentiated hepatocellular carcinomas. Moreover, this immunostaining is not entirely specific because it also stains hepatoid adenocarcinoma from other primary sites, as well as a small portion (<5%) of cholangiocarcinomas.

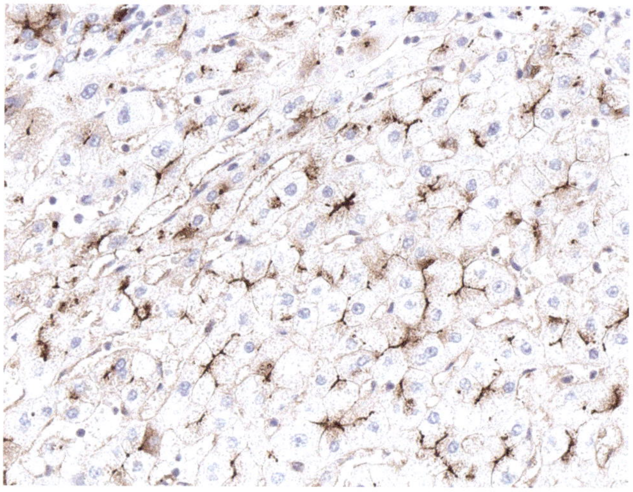

Fig. 1.46 Immunostain for carcinoembryonic antigen (polyclonal antibody). The malignant tumour cells in a well-differentiated hepatocellular carcinoma are highlighted by a prominent canalicular pattern. Canalicular immunoreactivity for pCEA is helpful in demonstrating hepatocellular differentiation by reacting with biliary glycoprotein I in bile canaliculi. The overall sensitivity and specificity are 70% (60%–95%) and nearly 100% in detecting hepatocellular carcinoma. Similar to HepPar-1, its immunopositivity rate is reciprocal to the differentiation of hepatocellular carcinoma. Immunostaining for CD10 also demonstrates a similar canalicular immunoreactivity in tumours with hepatocellular differentiation, with sensitivity and specificity comparable to those of pCEA.

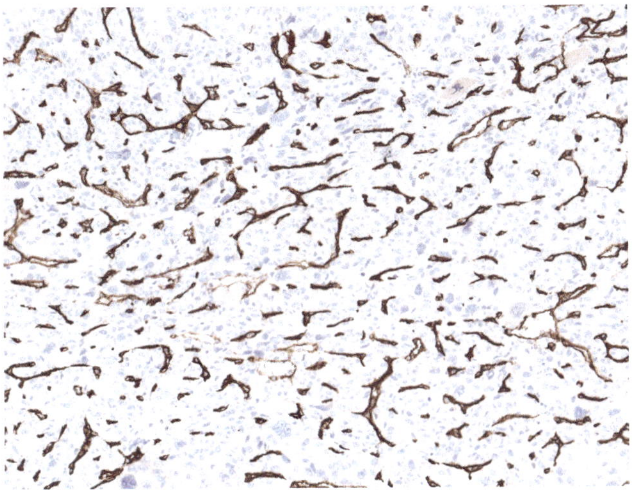

Fig. 1.47 Immunostain for CD34. Diffuse sinusoidal expression of CD34 is demonstrated in a moderately differentiated hepatocellular carcinoma. Sinusoidal endothelium in normal liver is devoid of CD34 immunoreactivity. However, many nonneoplastic and neoplastic liver diseases lead to distortion of the normal hepatic microcirculation and the formation of aberrant new vessels, resulting in sinusoidal capillarization. Two distinct patterns of capillarization may be demonstrated by immunostaining for CD34: complete and incomplete patterns. The former is characterized by a diffuse sinusoidal expression of CD34 within the entire lesion, whereas an incomplete pattern is featured by focal and preferentially peripheral sinusoidal expression in the lesion. The complete pattern of CD34 staining is helpful in differentiating hepatocellular carcinoma from benign hepatocellular lesions, with an overall sensitivity of 93.2% and specificity of 96.2%.

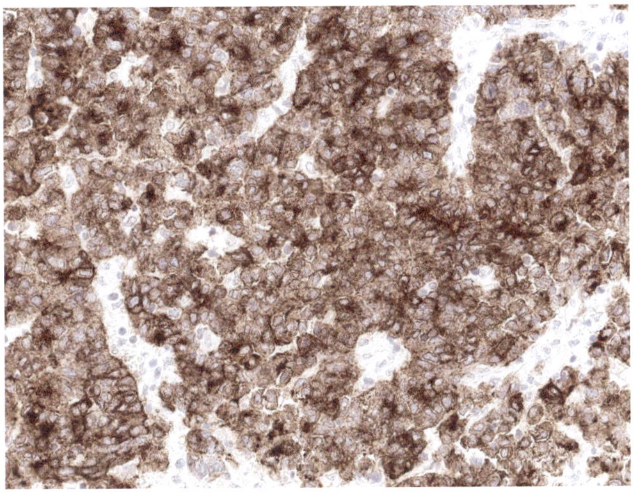

Fig. 1.48 Immunostain for glypican-3 (GPC3). The malignant tumour cells in a moderately differentiated hepatocellular carcinoma are highlighted with both membranous and cytoplasmic staining patterns. GPC3 is a member of the glycosylphosphatidylinositol-anchored heparin sulphate proteoglycans, and is expressed normally in fetal but not adult liver. It promotes the growth of hepatocellular carcinoma by activating Wnt/β-catenin and insulin-like growth factor signalling pathways. It differentiates hepatocellular carcinoma from benign hepatocellular lesions with an overall sensitivity of 78.6% and specificity of 92.9%. Other markers (glutamine synthetase, heat shock protein 70, and clathrin heavy chain) may be used independently or in combination with the others to help in the distinction between benign and malignant hepatocellular lesions.

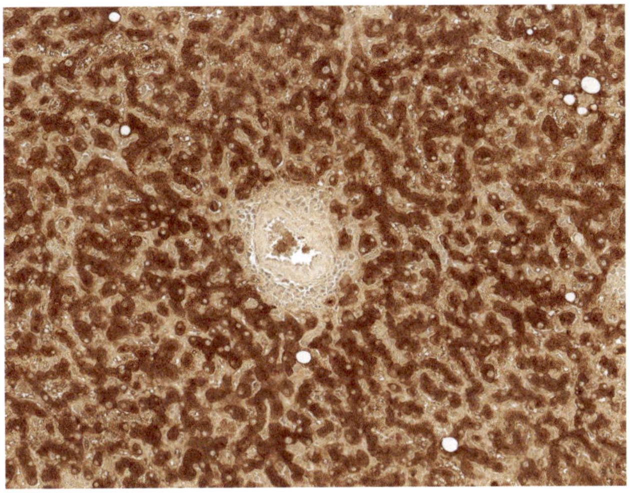

Fig. 1.49 Immunostain for serum amyloid A (SAA). The tumour cells in an inflammatory-type hepatocellular adenoma are highlighted. Hepatocellular adenomas are now known to be a heterogeneous entity and are subdivided into four main groups by genotype and phenotype. Each subtype has different clinical and pathologic features. A combination of immunostains for SAA/C-reactive protein), liver fatty acid-binding protein, glutamine synthetase, and β-catenin has been used to differentiate inflammatory, hepatocyte nuclear factor 1–inactivated, β-catenin–activated, and unclassified subtypes of hepatocellular adenoma.

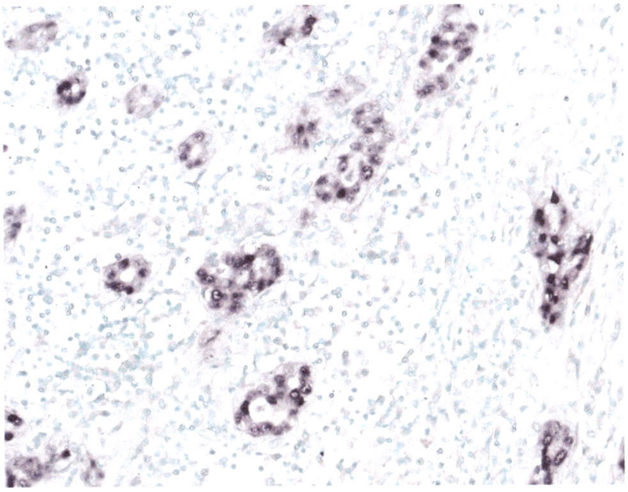

Fig. 1.50 In situ hybridization for Epstein-Barr virus–encoded RNA (EBER). The malignant tumour cells in a lymphoepithelioma-like cholangiocarcinoma are highlighted. Epstein-Barr virus (EBV) is involved in benign and malignant liver diseases, including EBV hepatitis, post-transplant lymphoproliferative disorder, and various primary and metastatic EBV-associated epithelial, mesenchymal, and haematolymphoid neoplasms.

2 General Processes

The liver exhibits only a limited repertoire of morphologic changes in response to a wide variety of infectious, metabolic, immune-mediated, circulatory, or neoplastic injuries. Many such changes are neither pathognomonic nor specific and may be caused by a variety of disorders; however, recognition of the principal pattern(s) of injury is central to making a clinical diagnosis. By systematic examination and interpretation of the morphologic changes, together with correlation of clinical, biochemical, serologic, and radiologic, information, an accurate pathologic diagnosis, or at least differential diagnoses, normally can be achieved.

Common morphologic changes of liver injury may be categorized as (1) inflammation, (2) cellular damage, (3) intracellular/extracellular accumulation, (4) regeneration, (5) fibrosis, (6) preneoplastic, or (7) neoplastic change. Preneoplastic and neoplastic changes are illustrated in chapters 12 and 14, respectively.

2.1 Inflammation

To evaluate the inflammatory process in the liver, one should determine the predominant pattern of inflammation according to its distribution (portal inflammation, interface hepatitis, or lobular inflammation) and cellular component (lymphocyte predominant, plasma cell rich, eosinophil rich, neutrophil rich, or granulomatous). Recognition of the major inflammatory pattern helps narrow down the differential diagnoses.

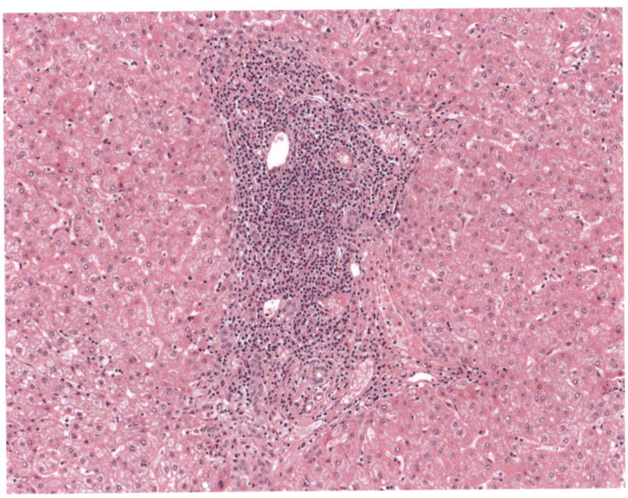

Fig. 2.1 Portal inflammation, lymphocyte predominant. This portal tract is expanded by a moderate amount of lymphocyte-predominant inflammation. Portal inflammation of this sort commonly is associated with chronic viral hepatitis, autoimmune hepatitis, and chronic biliary disease but may be observed in many other conditions, including drug-induced liver injury. It is essential to look for other associated findings, such as ground-glass hepatocytes in chronic hepatitis B, prominent interface hepatitis and hepatocyte rosettes in autoimmune hepatitis, and bile duct damage and loss in chronic biliary disease, to achieve the definite diagnosis.

A.W.H. Chan et al., *Atlas of Liver Pathology*, Atlas of Anatomic Pathology,
DOI 10.1007/978-1-4614-9114-9_2, © Springer Science+Business Media New York 2014

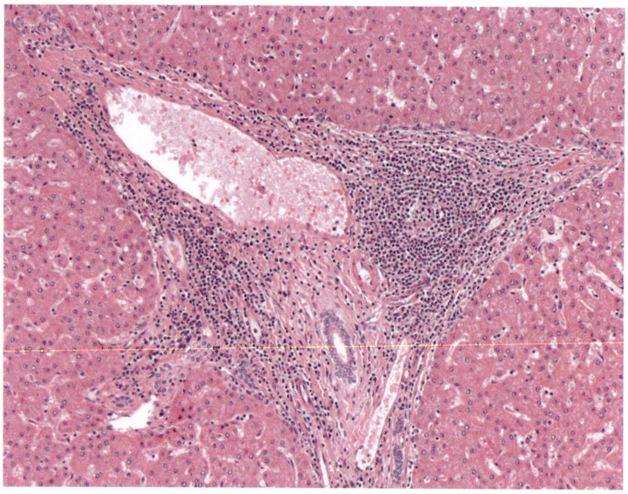

Fig. 2.2 Portal inflammation, lymphocyte predominant. This portal tract is expanded by a moderate lymphocyte-predominant inflammatory infiltrate with a reactive lymphoid follicle. Portal lymphoid follicles are a characteristic feature of chronic hepatitis C, but may be found in many other liver diseases, such as chronic hepatitis B, autoimmune hepatitis, and primary biliary cirrhosis.

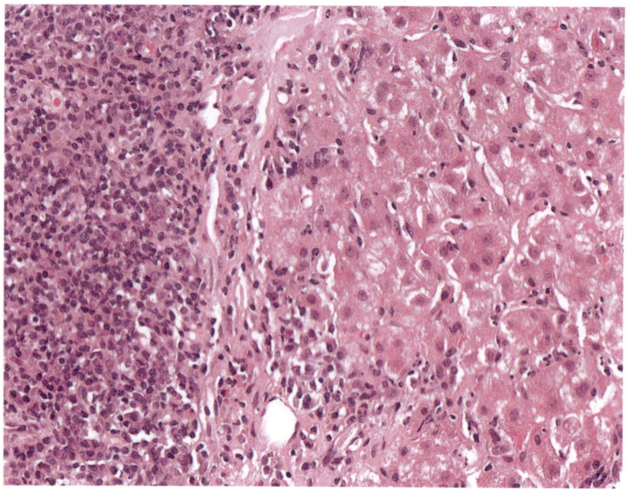

Fig. 2.3 Portal inflammation, plasma cell rich. This portal tract is expanded by a prominent lymphoplasmacytic infiltrate. A few scattered eosinophils also are noted, but this is a relatively nonspecific finding. Plasma cell–rich portal inflammation typically is associated with immune-mediated liver diseases, including autoimmune hepatitis, primary biliary cirrhosis, and immunoglobulin G4-related disease in the liver. Acute hepatitis A, chronic hepatitis B, drug-induced liver injury, and plasma cell dyscrasia are other less common causes of this pattern of inflammation.

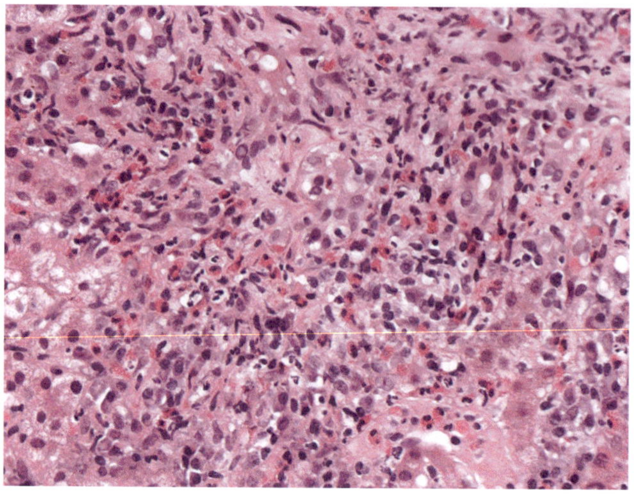

Fig. 2.4 Portal inflammation, eosinophil rich. This portal tract is expanded by an inflammatory infiltrate in which there are a significant number of eosinophils. Parasitic infestation, inflammatory myofibroblastic tumour, inflammatory pseudotumour-like follicular dendritic cell tumour, Hodgkin disease and Langerhans cell histiocytosis are the major differential diagnoses that must be considered. However, one should note that the presence of a few scattered eosinophils in the portal tract is rather nonspecific and not uncommonly seen in a wide range of liver diseases.

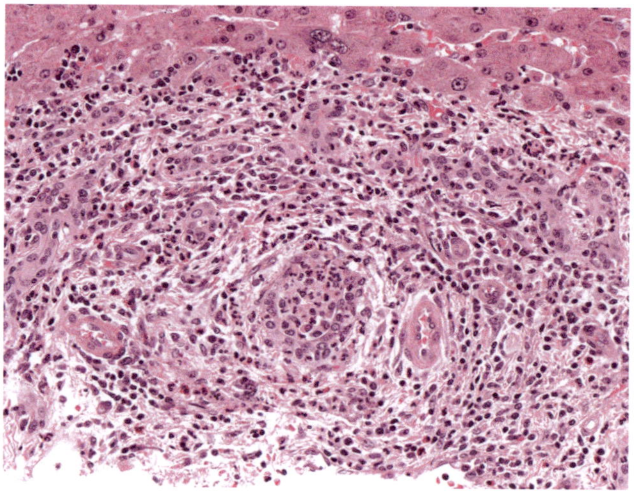

Fig. 2.5 Portal inflammation, neutrophil rich. This portal tract is expanded by a mixed inflammatory infiltrate with a significant number of neutrophils. An interlobular bile duct is infiltrated and distended by neutrophils (acute cholangitis). A prominent ductular reaction is noted at the edge of the portal tract. The presence of portal neutrophils is not diagnostic of acute large duct obstruction or acute ascending cholangitis per se. Neutrophils commonly are associated with proliferating bile ductules and are one of the components of ductular reaction (sometimes referred to as "cholangiolitis"). Conditions with a prominent ductular reaction in portal regions, including chronic intrahepatic biliary disease and adjacent space-occupying lesion, thus may have a significant portal neutrophilic infiltrate.

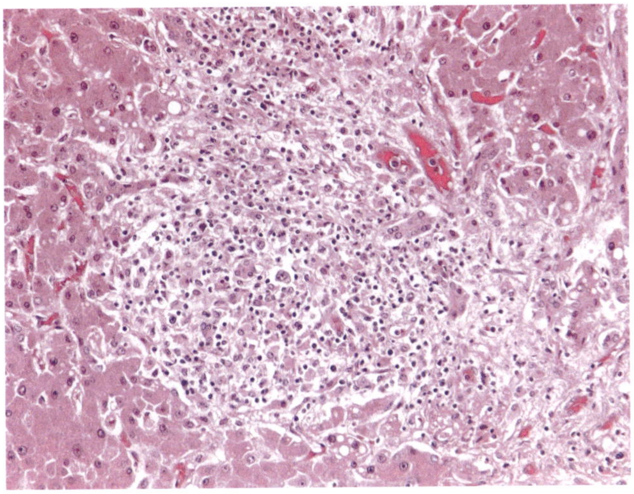

Fig. 2.6 Portal inflammation, atypical lymphoid infiltrate. This portal tract is expanded by atypical lymphoid cells. The presence of atypical lymphoid cells within portal tracts is associated with lymphoma, leukaemia, and posttransplant lymphoproliferative disorder. Benign conditions, including Epstein-Barr virus (EBV) infection, also must be considered.

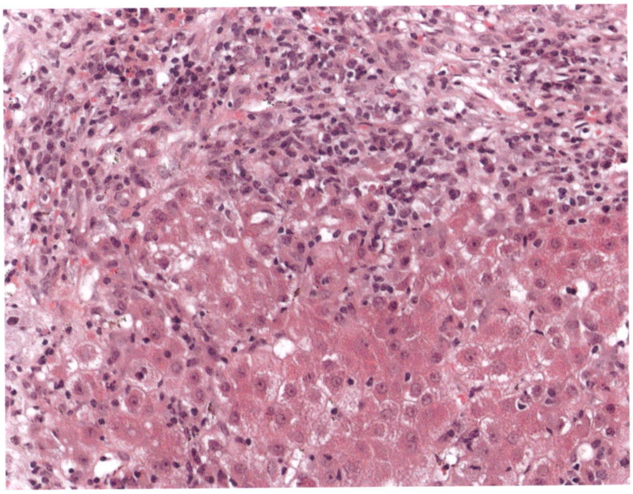

Fig. 2.7 Interface hepatitis. Lymphoplasmacytic cells erode through the interface between portal tract and liver parenchyma and surround individual and small groups of periportal hepatocytes with evidence of liver cell apoptosis. Interface hepatitis, formerly known as piecemeal necrosis, differs from the simple spillover of portal inflammatory infiltrate in acute hepatitis by the presence of periportal hepatocellular damage.

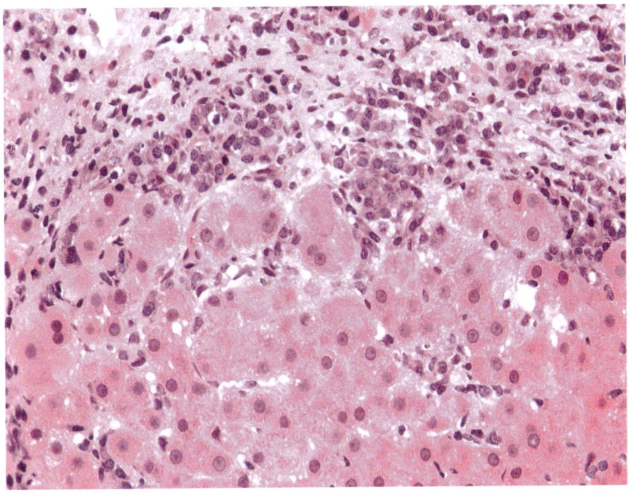

Fig. 2.8 Interface hepatitis. A moderate interface hepatitis and prominent portal plasma cell–rich inflammation are present. Significant interface hepatitis, as seen here, is the hallmark feature of autoimmune hepatitis. However, interface hepatitis also may be observed in chronic viral hepatitis, primary biliary cirrhosis, Wilson disease, α_1-antitrypsin deficiency, and drug-induced liver injury.

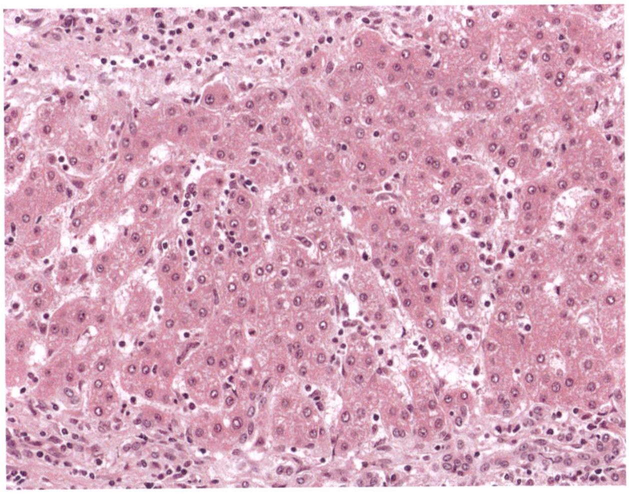

Fig. 2.9 Lobular inflammation with minimal hepatocellular damage. The sinusoids contain a moderate mononuclear cell infiltrate, but there is no significant hepatocellular injury or necrosis. The major differential diagnoses of a predominantly mononuclear infiltrate in the lobule include viral hepatitis C, EBV infection, drug-induced liver injury, nonspecific reactive hepatitis, extramedullary haematopoiesis, leukaemia, and non-Hodgkin lymphoma, whereas a predominantly neutrophilic infiltrate is seen in alcoholic hepatitis, sepsis, cytomegalovirus infection in immunocompromised patients, drug-induced liver injury, and "surgical hepatitis".

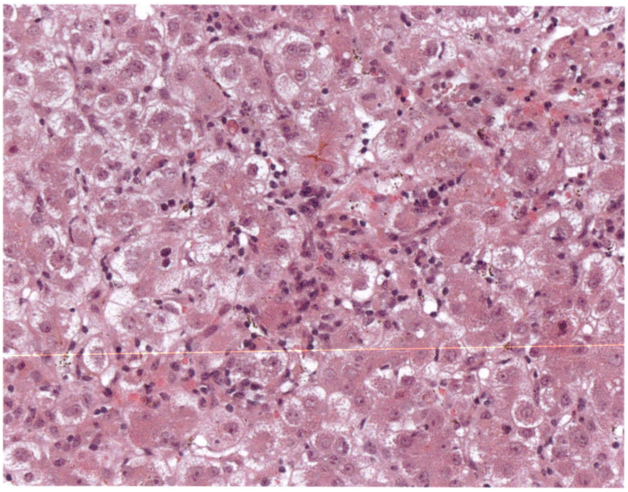

Fig. 2.10 Lobular inflammation associated with significant hepatocellular damage (lobular disarray). Here, there is a lobular mononuclear infiltrate accompanied by many swollen and enlarged hepatocytes and several apoptotic bodies.

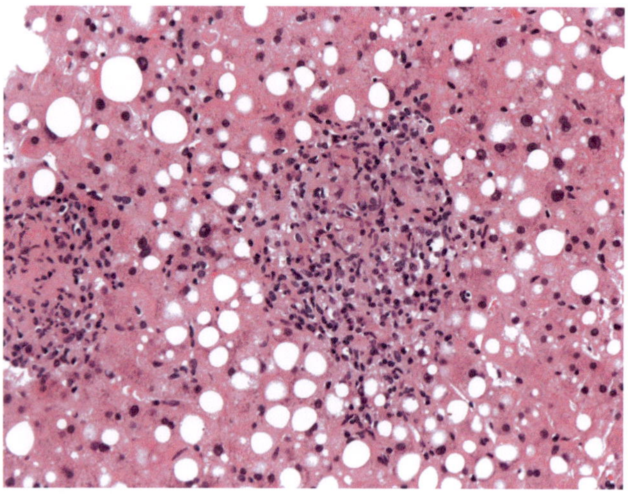

Fig. 2.11 Lobular epithelioid granulomas. Two noncaseating epithelioid granulomas are present; these are composed of discrete aggregates of histiocytes, lymphocytes, and plasma cells in the absence of any necrosis. Hepatic granulomas are a relatively common finding and said to be present in up to 10% of all liver biopsy specimens. They are seen in a very wide range of conditions. The morphologic type of hepatic granulomas may provide certain diagnostic hints. Other than epithelioid granulomas, there are also lipogranulomas, fibrin ring granulomas, foamy macrophage aggregates, and suppurative granulomas. Suppurative granulomas are characterised by granulomatous inflammation with stellate abscess formation or suppurative inflammation and are associated with bartonellosis, yersiniosis, tularaemia, listeriosis, melioidosis, actinomycosis, and fungal infection.

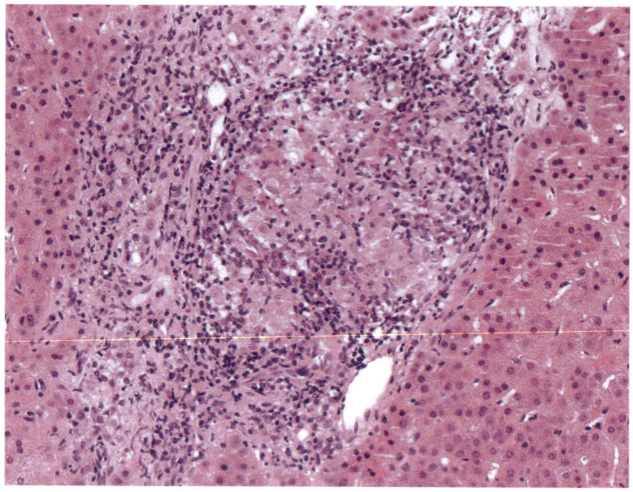

Fig. 2.12 Epithelioid granuloma. A large portal noncaseating epithelioid granuloma is seen. Epithelioid granulomas may be classified as caseating or noncaseating according to the presence of necrosis. Caseating granulomas normally are associated with infections, most notably tuberculosis. The underlying causes of epithelioid granuloma are divided into infectious (e.g., mycobacterial infection, tertiary syphilis, parasitic infestation, fungal infection, and, rarely, viral infection) and noninfectious (e.g., primary biliary cirrhosis, drug-induced liver injury, foreign body reaction, sarcoidosis, Hodgkin lymphoma, and chronic granulomatous disease).

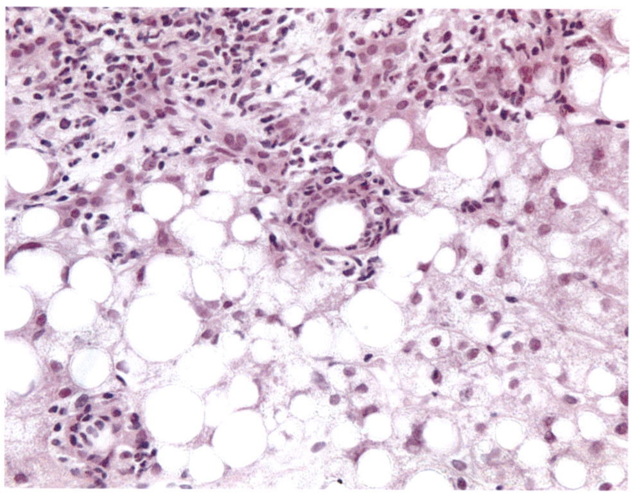

Fig. 2.13 Fibrin ring granuloma. A granuloma is seen with a central fat globule and surrounded by a circumferential rim of fibrin. Fibrin ring granulomas, sometimes referred to as doughnut granulomas, may resemble lipogranulomas superficially. Their key discernible feature, the fibrin ring, may be highlighted by phosphotungstic acid–haematoxylin stain, Martius scarlet blue stain, or immunostaining for fibrin. Fibrin ring granulomas classically are associated with Q fever (*Coxiella burnetii*), but now are considered rather nonspecific. Other associations include mycobacterial infection, staphylococcal bacteraemia, leishmaniasis, toxoplasmosis, cytomegalovirus infection, EBV infection, acute hepatitis A, lupus, giant cell arteritis, allopurinol toxicity, and lymphoma.

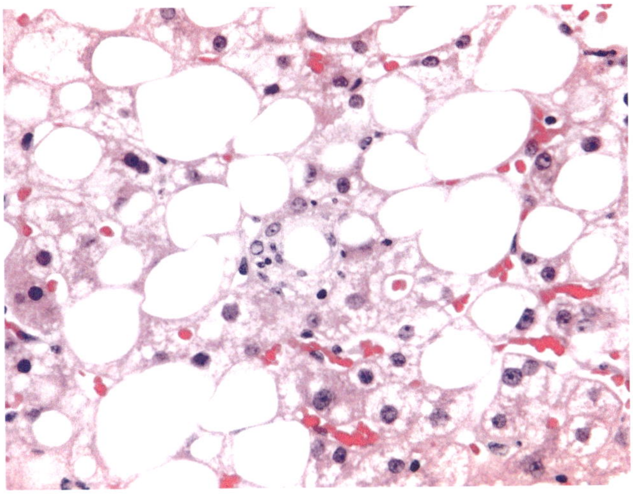

Fig. 2.14 Lipogranuloma. A loose aggregate of lymphocytes and macrophages surround a central fat globule in the absence of any fibrin ring. Lipogranulomas are associated with alcoholic and nonalcoholic fatty liver disease, as well as ingestion of mineral oil in food and medication.

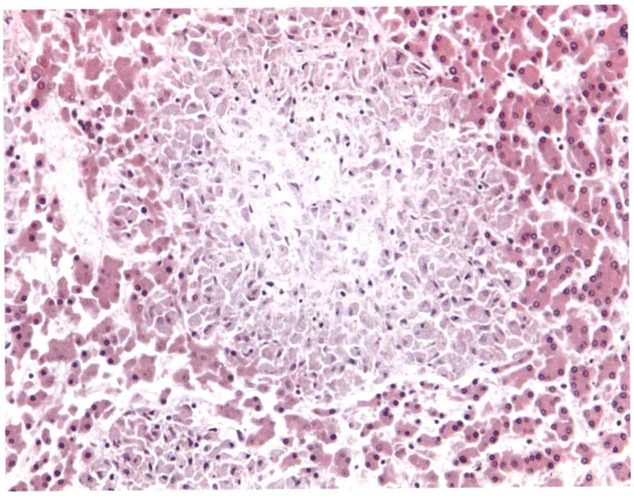

Fig. 2.15 Foamy macrophage aggregates. Large aggregates of pale-staining macrophages are noted within the lobule without any significant necrosis or other accompanying inflammatory infiltrate. Foamy macrophage aggregates usually are found in immunocompromised patients and are caused by *Mycobacterium avium-intracellulare*, Whipple disease, and lepromatous leprosy.

2.2 Cellular Damage

Hepatocytes and cholangiocytes are subjected to different sublethal and lethal injuries in a wide range of liver diseases. The recognition of different morphologies of cellular damage provides diagnostic hints to the underlying aetiology.

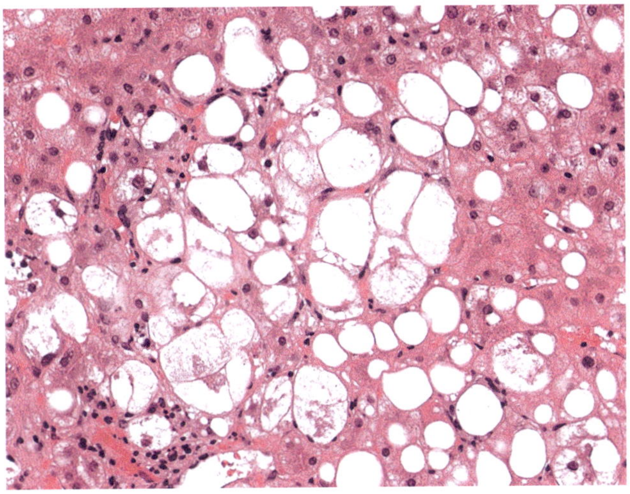

Fig. 2.16 Ballooning degeneration. There are many ballooned hepatocytes, which are characterized by cellular swelling, rarefaction of the cytoplasm, and clumped strands of intermediate filaments. The mimickers of ballooning degeneration are feathery degeneration, steatosis (particularly the microvesicular form), and glycogen-rich hepatocytes. Feathery degeneration is almost indistinguishable from ballooning degeneration, but one can differentiate between them by the presence of cholestasis and/or cholate stasis, frequently associated with feathery degeneration. Macrovesicular and microvesicular steatosis are characterised by hepatocytes distended by well-formed discrete fat droplets. Glycogen-rich hepatocytes in glycogen storage disease or glycogenic hepatopathy show diffuse cytoplasmic enlargement and clearing and sometimes contain glycogenated nuclei and giant mitochondria.

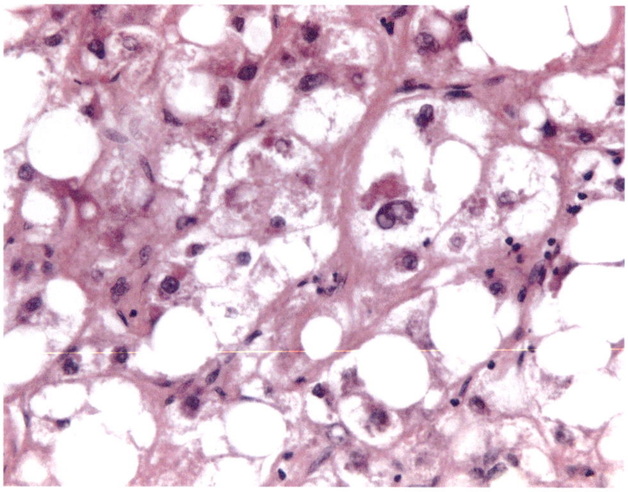

Fig. 2.17 Ballooning degeneration. Several ballooned hepatocytes are present, and one of these contains a Mallory-Denk body. One should note that Mallory-Denk bodies often, but not always, are found in ballooned hepatocytes; however, not all ballooned hepatocytes contain such inclusions. Ballooning degeneration is considered a hallmark feature of alcoholic and nonalcoholic steatohepatitis, but it also occurs in acute viral hepatitis, chronic hepatitis C with concurrent steatohepatitic features, autoimmune hepatitis, neonatal giant cell hepatitis, drug-induced liver injury, and ischaemia/reperfusion injury in liver allograft.

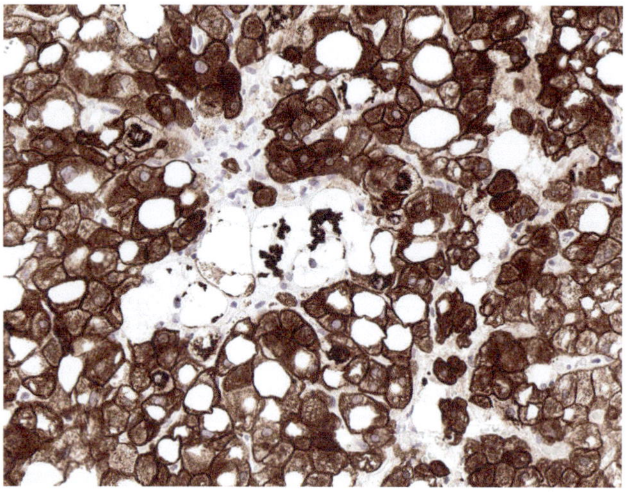

Fig. 2.18 Ballooning degeneration (cytokeratin 8/18 [CK8/18] stain). Ballooned hepatocytes lose cytoplasmic expression of CK8/18, whereas the residual immunoreactivity is confined to their Mallory-Denk bodies. Such characteristic diminished expression of CK8/18 is observed in ballooned hepatocytes in alcoholic and nonalcoholic steatohepatitis, chronic hepatitis C with concurrent steatohepatitic features, and ischaemia/reperfusion injury in liver allograft. However, ballooned cells in acute viral hepatitis, autoimmune hepatitis, neonatal giant cell hepatitis, and drug-induced liver injury retain normal cytoplasmic expression of CK8/18. Immunostaining for CK8/18 may be helpful to differentiate ballooning degeneration from steatosis and glycogen-rich hepatocytes.

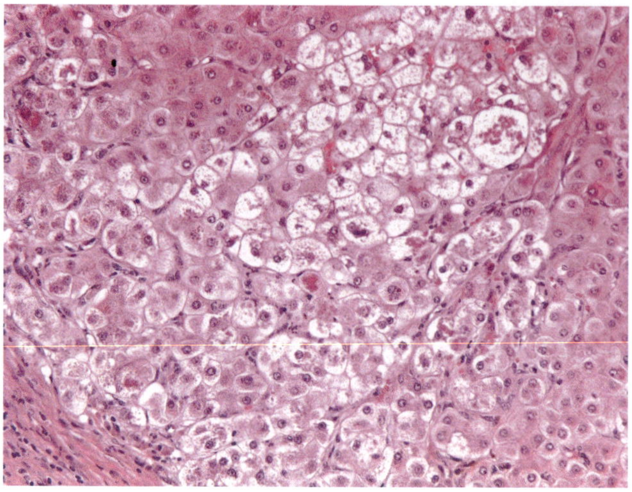

Fig. 2.19 Feathery degeneration. Shown here are numerous injured hepatocytes with marked cellular swelling and rarefaction of the cytoplasm. Several Mallory-Denk bodies also are noted. Feathery degeneration results from the detergent effect of retained bile salts (cholate stasis) in cholestatic conditions. It is almost identical to ballooning degeneration in light microscopy, particularly feathery degenerated hepatocytes containing Mallory-Denk bodies. Moreover, both of them fail to express cytoplasmic CK8/18. The distinction may be made by identifying other histologic features associated with feathery degeneration, such as bilirubinostasis, bile infarcts and/or hepatocyte rosette in acute cholestatic diseases (cholestatic rosettes), and copper-associated protein deposition, ductopaenia, and/or biliary-type fibrosis in chronic cholestatic diseases.

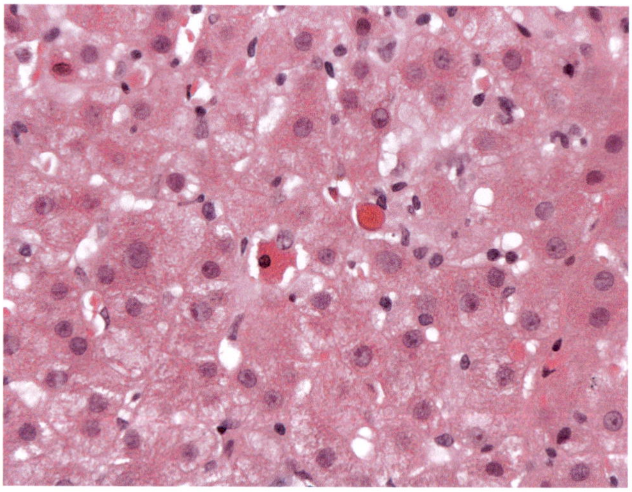

Fig. 2.20 Apoptosis. An apoptotic hepatocyte (*left*) contains a pyknotic nucleus and shrunken angulated hypereosinophilic cytoplasm. To the *right* is a structure sometimes referred to as an acidophilic body or Councilman body; this is a small, mummified, and rounded remnant of an apoptotic hepatocyte. Apoptosis is one of the two principal forms of cell death and is characterized by cytoplasmic shrinkage, chromatin condensation and fragmentation, and formation of cytoplasmic blebs and apoptotic bodies. This active form of cell death results from the activation of caspases and endonucleases through two overlapping signalling pathways: the extrinsic death receptor-initiated pathway and the intrinsic mitochondrial pathway.

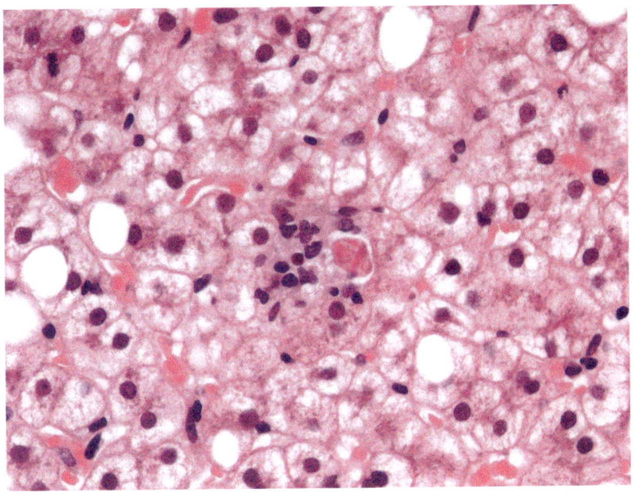

Fig. 2.21 Apoptotic body. Here, an apoptotic body is associated with a small group of mononuclear inflammatory cells. Apoptotic bodies are a nonspecific finding occurring in a very wide range of acute and chronic liver diseases, and sometimes may be observed in normal liver.

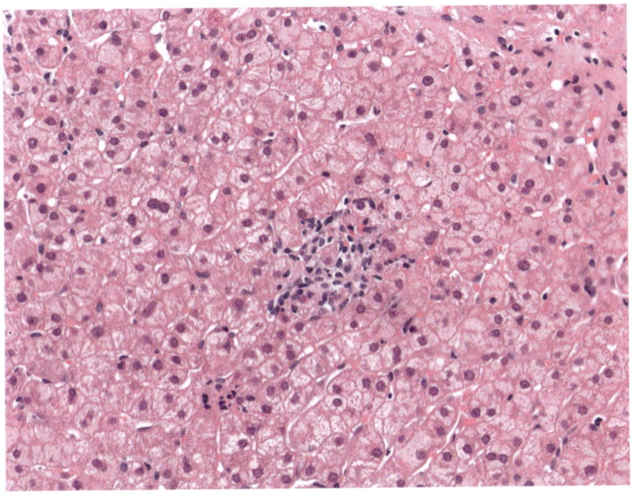

Fig. 2.22 Spotty necrosis. A small focus of lymphocytes and activated Kupffer cells/macrophages is noted in the lobule and fills the gap in which there has been liver cell drop-out. Necrosis, the other main form of cell death, is characterised by cell swelling, karyolysis, cell lysis, and release of cellular contents. Spotty necrosis, also known as focal necrosis, lytic necrosis, and oncotic necrosis, represents necrosis of an individual or small number of hepatocytes. However, the necrotic hepatocyte very often is not identifiable, although its resultant parenchymal collapse, condensation of reticulin framework, and associated mononuclear inflammatory cells may be recognised.

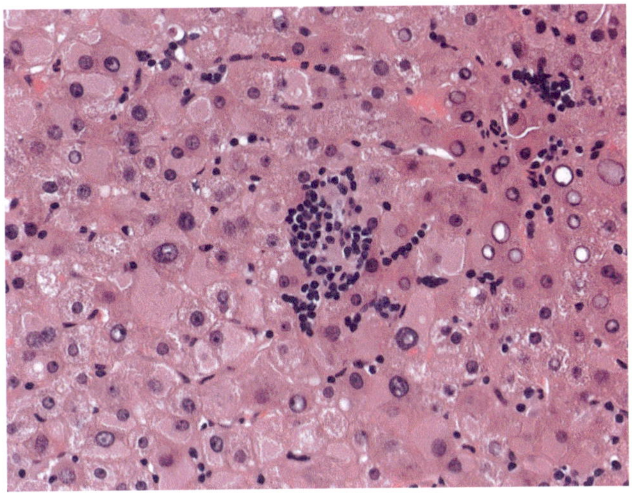

Fig. 2.23 Spotty necrosis. Two small foci of lymphocytes and activated Kupffer cells/macrophages are noted in the lobule. Hepatocytes with prominent ground-glass changes also are seen in this case of chronic hepatitis B. Like apoptotic bodies, spotty necrosis is a nonspecific finding associated with a very broad range of liver diseases.

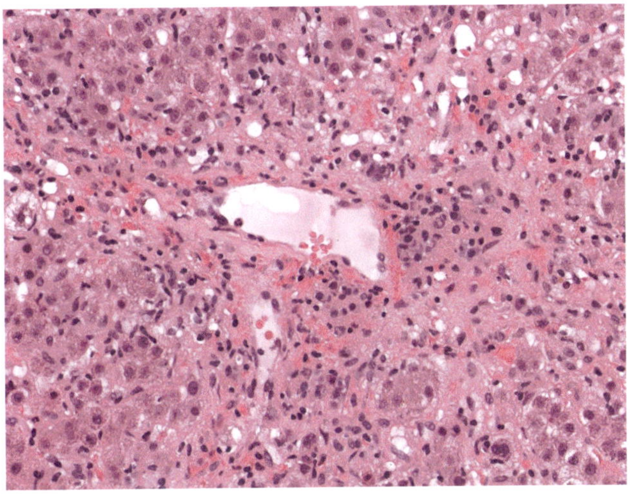

Fig. 2.24 Confluent necrosis. A large group of hepatocytes has been lost in this perivenular region. Confluent necrosis represents necrosis of a large group of contiguous hepatocytes, and commonly occurs in the perivenular (zone 3)/centrilobular region. It signifies a more active and severe injury to the liver parenchyma than spotty necrosis and typically is associated with acute viral hepatitis, drug-induced liver injury, autoimmune hepatitis, and Wilson disease. Less commonly, it may be seen in chronic viral hepatitis, including cases in which there is seroconversion in chronic hepatitis B and superinfection with hepatitis D.

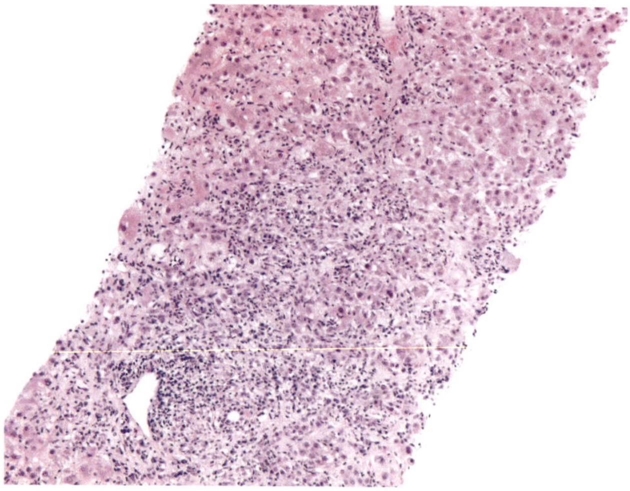

Fig. 2.25 Bridging necrosis. An extensive area of hepatocyte loss with inflammatory infiltrate bridges a terminal hepatic venule (*top*) with a portal tract (*bottom*). In the classical lobular concept, such bridging necrosis may be labelled "portal–central" bridging necrosis. In the Rappaport acinar concept, it represents an extensive zone 3 confluent necrosis. Bridging necrosis signifies very active and severe damage to the liver parenchyma, and may occur in acute viral hepatitis, drug-induced liver injury, autoimmune hepatitis, and Wilson disease. It also may be seen in chronic viral hepatitis, particularly in the context of seroconversion in chronic hepatitis B; it is usually not a feature of hepatitis C infection.

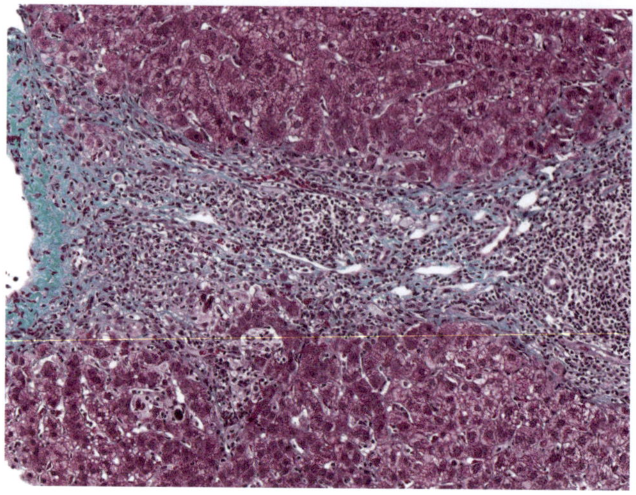

Fig. 2.27 Bridging necrosis (Masson trichrome stain). Bridging necrosis is demonstrated by a characteristic two-tone appearance, with darker staining in the wall of the terminal hepatic vein (*left*) and lighter staining in the bridging region of recent collapse. A ductular reaction also is noted within the bridging region.

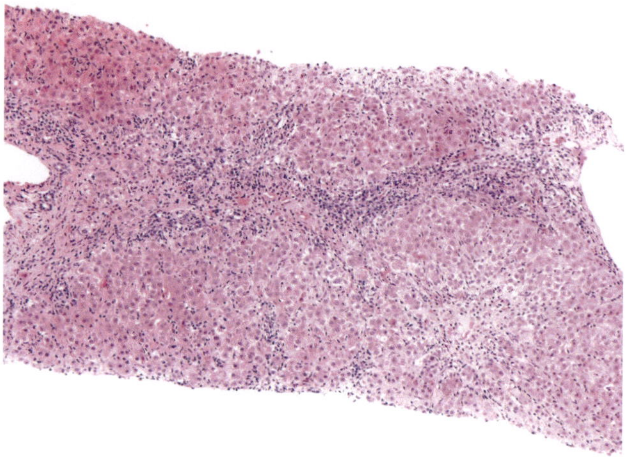

Fig. 2.26 Bridging necrosis. Shown is an extensive area of lobular collapse with an associated inflammatory cell infiltrate; this bridges a terminal hepatic venule (*right*) and portal tract (*left*). Differentiation between bridging necrosis and bridging fibrosis may be challenging. Several histologic features favour the former: (1) the bridging region is more congested and haemorrhagic, and contains more ceroid-laden macrophages, (2) any ductular reaction is present within the bridging region rather than at the parenchymal–stromal interface, (3) trichrome stains show a characteristic two-tone appearance with darker staining in the residual portal tract and terminal hepatic venule wall and lighter staining in areas of recent collapse, (4) reticulin stains show condensation of residual loosely aggregated reticulin fibres, and (5) the orcein stain fails to highlight the presence of elastic fibres.

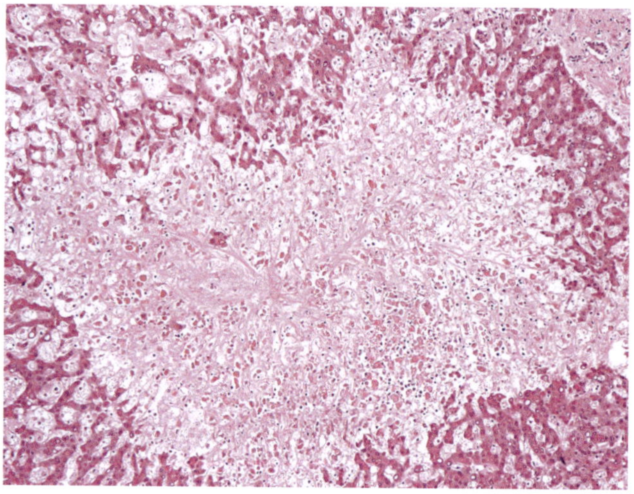

Fig. 2.28 Panacinar/panlobular necrosis. The entire acinus/lobule of hepatic parenchyma is almost necrotic. There are other, closely related terms, namely *multiacinar/multilobular necrosis*, *submassive necrosis*, and *massive necrosis*. *Multiacinar necrosis* is designated for necrosis of multiple adjacent acini. The terms *massive* and *submassive hepatic necrosis* are used to describe necrosis of >70% and 30% to 70% of the entire liver, respectively. Panacinar or multiacinar necrosis differs from parenchymal extinction in cirrhosis by the absence of fibrotic scar tissue.

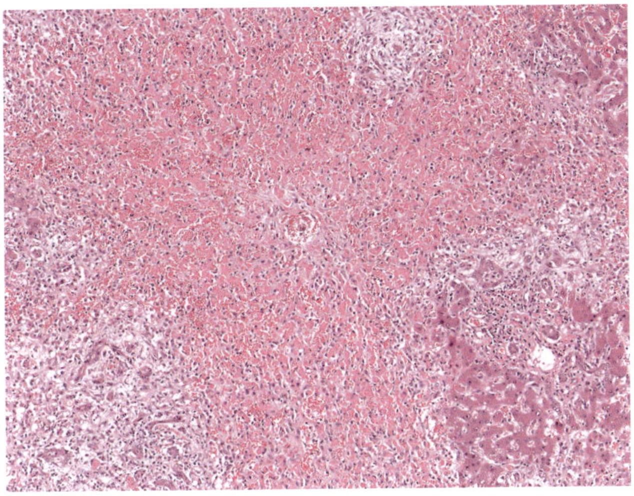

Fig. 2.29 Panacinar necrosis. Here, the entire acinus/lobule of hepatic parenchyma shows haemorrhagic necrosis. The differential diagnosis of panacinar necrosis depends on the amount of any associated inflammatory infiltrate. Panacinar necrosis with minimal inflammation typically is associated with acute nonhepatotropic viral hepatitis, dose-dependent drug-induced liver injury, and vascular disorders, whereas panacinar necrosis with marked inflammation usually is found in acute hepatotropic viral hepatitis, idiosyncratic drug-induced liver injury, autoimmune hepatitis, and Wilson disease.

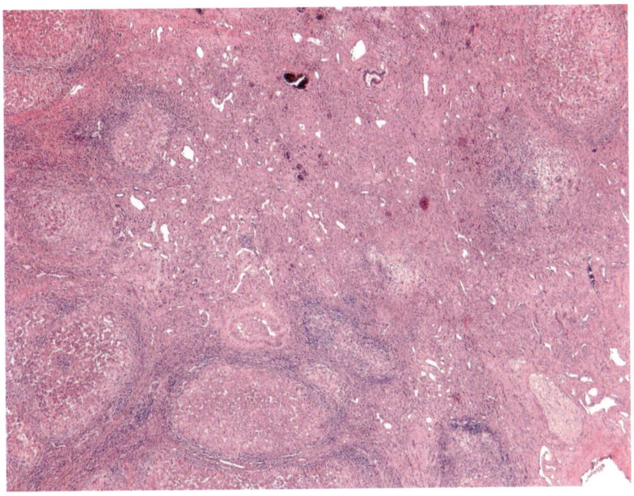

Fig. 2.30 Parenchymal extinction. Parenchymal extinction is defined as focal loss of contiguous hepatocytes, resulting from focal ischaemia by vascular obstruction in cirrhotic livers. It may involve a small portion of an acinus, larger units of one or more adjacent acini, or even an entire lobe, depending on the size of the blocked vessels. Parenchymal extinction is distinguished from panacinar or multiacinar necrosis by the cirrhotic background.

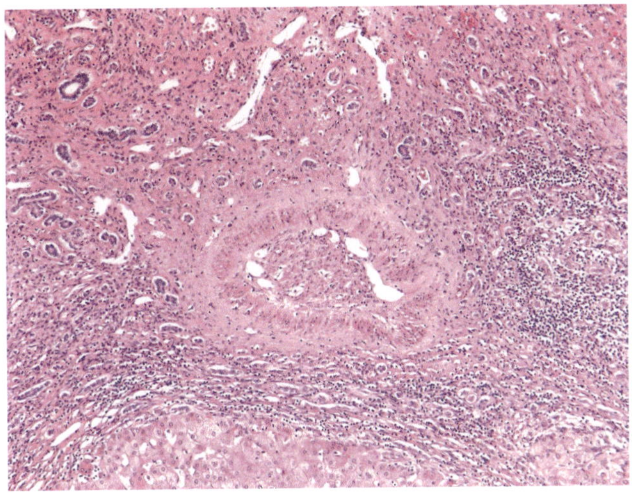

Fig. 2.31 Parenchymal extinction. Focal loss of contiguous hepatocytes here is associated with an old and recanalising thrombotic vein in a cirrhotic liver. Most parenchymal extinction lesions are formed by the obstruction of veins larger than 100 μm. Formation and accumulation of parenchymal extinction may continue after cirrhosis has already developed and may explain the slowly progressive deterioration of liver functional reserve even when the primary causative injury has ceased.

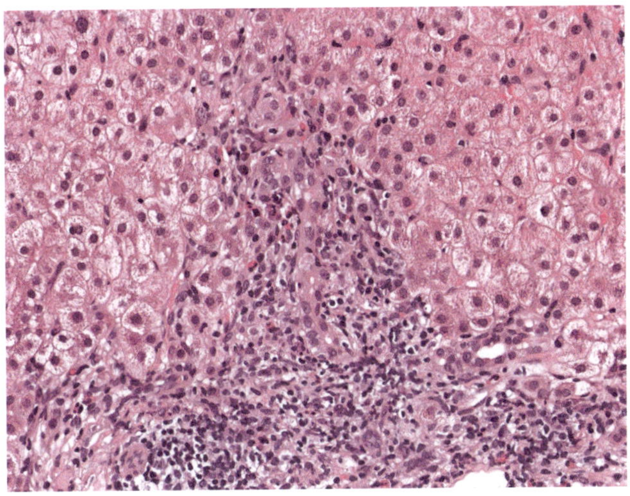

Fig. 2.32 Bile duct damage. An interlobular bile duct is infiltrated by lymphocytes and shows varying degrees of epithelial disarray. The major differential diagnoses are primary biliary cirrhosis, chronic viral hepatitis C, drug-induced cholangiopathy, and acute cellular rejection in liver allograft. Other possible causes include autoimmune hepatitis (focal bile duct injury may be found up to 24% of classical autoimmune hepatitis), primary sclerosing cholangitis, HIV-associated cholangiopathy, Langerhans cell histiocytes and Hodgkin lymphoma, and graft-versus-host disease.

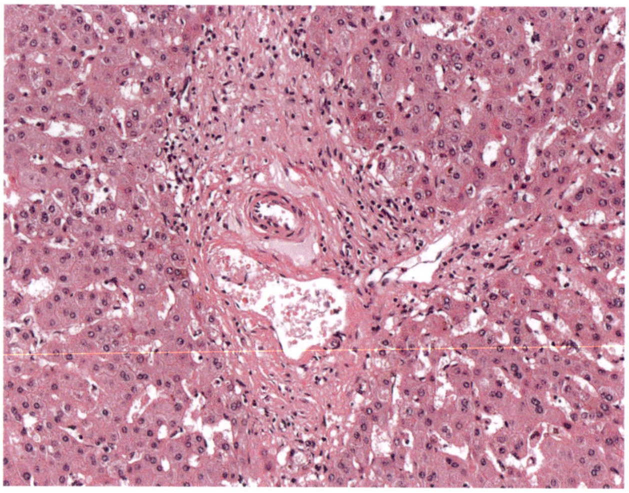

Fig. 2.33 Ductopaenia. An unpaired hepatic artery without a bile duct is noted in a portal tract. Ductopaenia traditionally is defined as the loss of interlobular duct in more than 50% of portal tracts in an adequate sample containing at least 10 portal tracts or 5 complete portal tracts, although alternative definitions recently were proposed. The principle aetiologies in adults are primary biliary cirrhosis, primary sclerosing cholangitis, sarcoidosis, drug-induced cholangiopathy, chronic rejection in liver allograft, chronic graft-versus-host disease, and idiopathic adult ductopaenia. Less commonly ductopaenia also can occur in the context of ischaemia, certain infections (e.g. CMV and cryptosporidium), and neoplastic conditions (e.g. Hodgkin lymphoma). The major aetiologies in children are extrahepatic biliary atresia, α_1-antitrypsin deficiency, paucity of the intrahepatic ducts, and primary sclerosing cholangitis.

2.3 Intracellular/Extracellular Accumulations

In various physiologic and pathologic conditions, there are different intrahepatic depositions, including fat (steatosis), glycogen, intracytoplasmic and intranuclear inclusions, pigments, and other extracellular materials. Some intrahepatic depositions on their own may be relatively specific to the underlying diseases (e.g., abundant accumulation of α_1-antitrypsin globules in α_1-antitrypsin deficiency), whereas some depositions in combination with other features may help point to the underlying causes (e.g., presence of macrovesicular steatosis, Mallory-Denk bodies, glycogenated nuclei, and giant mitochondria in steatohepatitis).

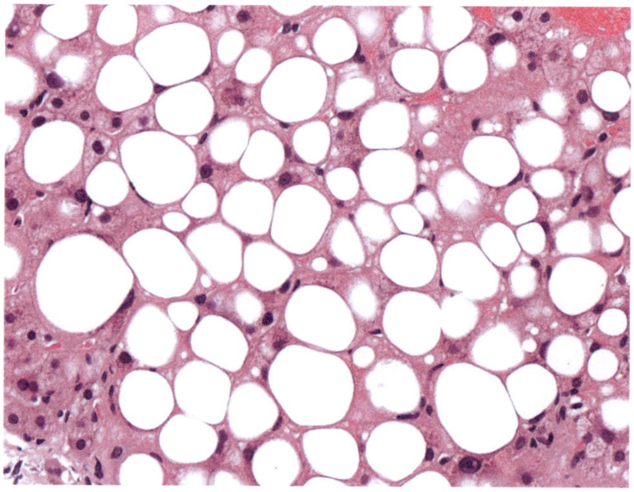

Fig. 2.34 Macrovesicular steatosis. Hepatocytes contain a single large fat droplet, which displaces the nucleus to the periphery. Macrovesicular steatosis is associated with a wide range of liver diseases, such as alcoholic and nonalcoholic fatty liver disease, chronic hepatitis C, Wilson disease, drug-induced liver injury, and various nutritional, metabolic, and endocrine disorders.

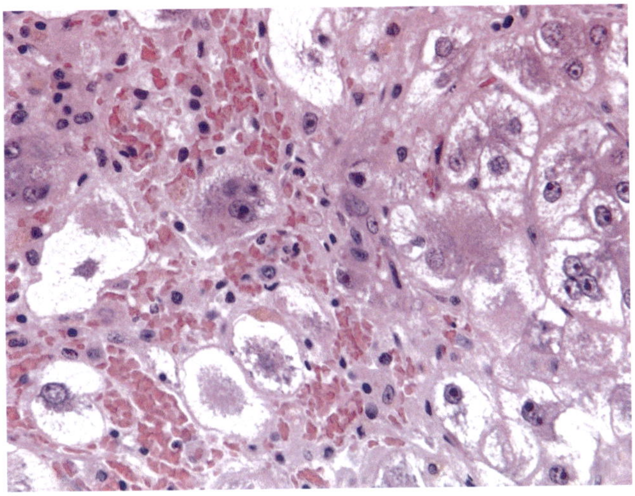

Fig. 2.35 Microvesicular steatosis. Hepatocytes contain multiple small fat droplets, which do not displace the nucleus. Diffuse microvesicular steatosis is uncommon and associated with serious mitochondriopathies with fatty acid oxidation defects, acute alcoholic foamy degeneration, acute fatty liver of pregnancy, toxaemia of pregnancy, drug/toxin-induced liver injury, and various primary mitochondrial hepatopathies.

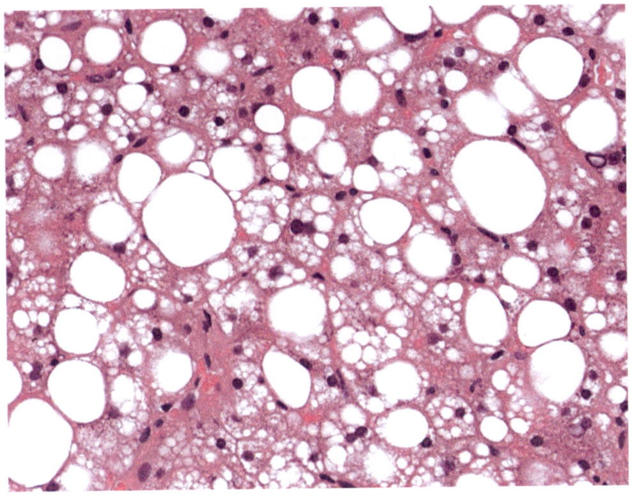

Fig. 2.37 Macrovesicular and "mediovesicular" steatosis. Many hepatocytes contain multiple medium-sized fat droplets, in addition to some with macrovesicular steatosis. The formation of a single large fat droplet in macrovesicular steatosis from fusion of multiple small fat droplets in microvesicular steatosis was first demonstrated in animal models. Mediovesicular steatosis may represent the intermediate step in such conversion. It is not uncommon to find microvesicular or mediovesicular steatosis admixed with macrovesicular steatosis. The term *mixed macrovesicular/microvesicular* or *macrovesicular/mediovesicular* steatosis may be applied. The latter term may be preferable to reserve the use of *microvesicular steatosis* specifically for clinically critical conditions with fatty acid oxidation defects.

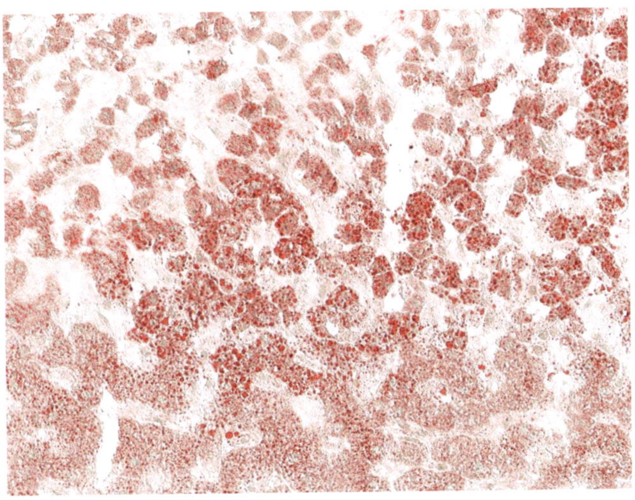

Fig. 2.36 Microvesicular steatosis (oil red O stain). Multiple minute fat droplets are seen in the hepatocytes. Such fat droplets occasionally are so small that hepatocytes appear swollen with a fine foamy cytoplasm, which may mimic ballooning degeneration, feathery degeneration, and glycogen-rich hepatocytes. Although the oil red O stain can highlight these droplets, it requires a frozen section of the specimen, which usually is not available routinely. Immunostaining for CK8/18 is useful for differentiating ballooning degeneration from microvesicular steatosis by the loss of cytoplasmic expression in the former.

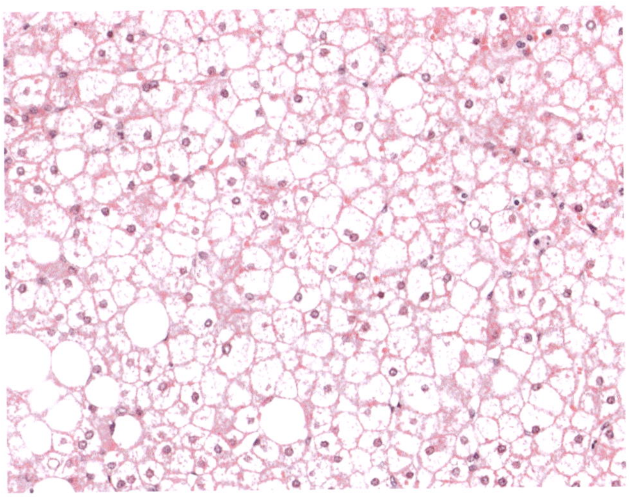

Fig. 2.38 Glycogen-rich hepatocytes. Almost all hepatocytes in this section are enlarged with cytoplasmic clearing as the result of excessive accumulation of cytoplasmic glycogen. Glycogen-rich hepatocytes may be confused with ballooned hepatocytes in steatohepatitis. The distinction may be complicated further by the fact that glycogenated nuclei and giant mitochondria frequently are found in glycogen-rich hepatocytes. However, diffuse involvement of hepatocytes and minimal steatosis distinguishes glycogen-rich hepatocytes from cells with ballooning degeneration. Glycogen-rich hepatocytes are found in glycogen storage diseases, urea cycle defects, and the so-called glycogenic hepatopathy of poorly controlled type 1 diabetes mellitus (Mauriac syndrome).

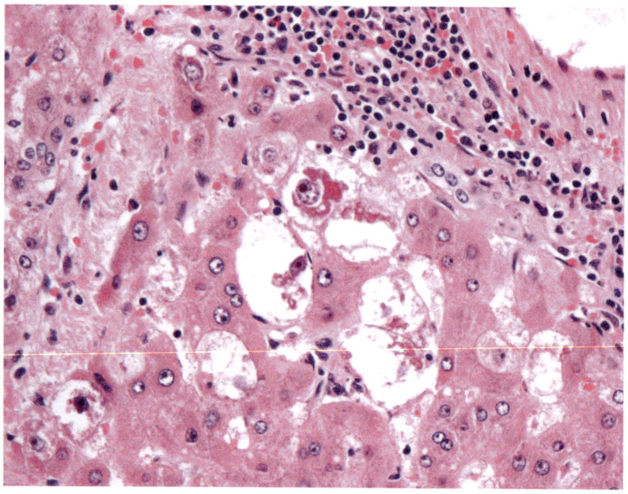

Fig. 2.39 Mallory-Denk bodies. Some deeply eosinophilic ropey intracytoplasmic inclusions are present within ballooned hepatocytes. Mallory-Denk bodies, previously known as Mallory bodies and Mallory hyaline, represent misfolded and aggregated intermediate filaments (mainly CK8/18) combined with other, different classes of proteins, including p62 and ubiquitin. They often (although not always) are found in ballooned hepatocytes. Ballooned hepatocytes possessing Mallory-Denk bodies sometimes are surrounded by neutrophils (satellitosis).

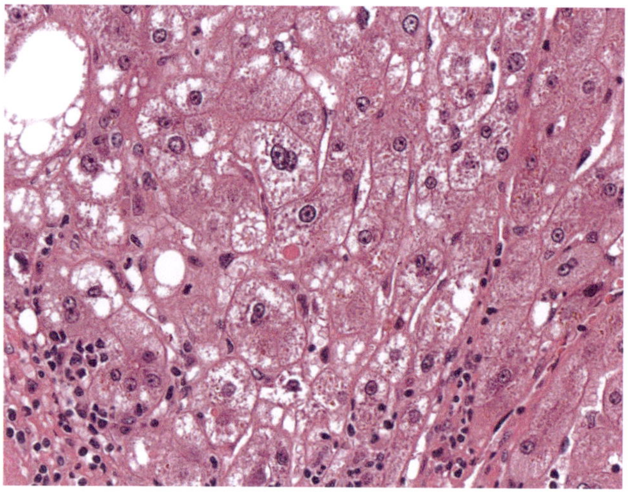

Fig. 2.40 Giant mitochondria. An oval-shaped eosinophilic intracytoplasmic inclusion is noted. Giant mitochondria, also called megamitochondria, are eosinophilic oval or needle-shaped intracytoplasmic inclusions. They represent enlarged and distended mitochondria with paracrystalline inclusions ultrastructurally. They should be distinguished from other eosinophilic globular intracytoplasmic inclusions, particularly α_1-antitrypsin globules. The latter are periodic acid-Schiff (PAS) positive, diastase resistant, and immunoreactive to α_1-antitrypsin, whereas the former are not. Misplaced red cells can occasionally be mistaken for giant mitochondria. The targetoid shape of the former differentiates them from the more homogenous giant mitochondria. Giant mitochondria are observed in a wide variety of physiologic and pathologic conditions, such as aging, alcoholic and nonalcoholic steatohepatitis, acute fatty liver of pregnancy, glycogen storage diseases, urea cycle defects, and glycogenic hepatopathy.

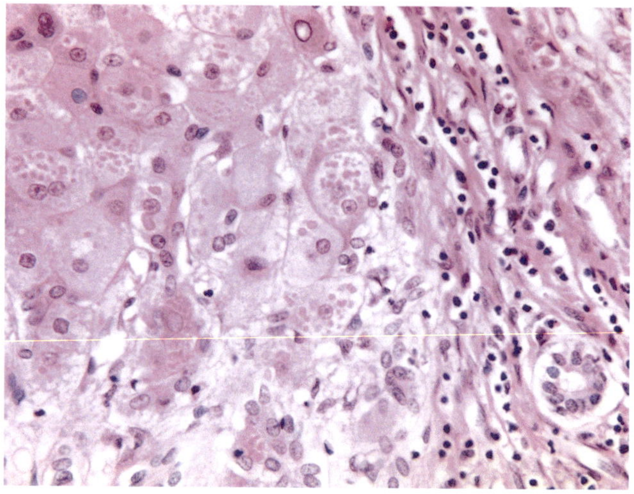

Fig. 2.41 α_1-Antitrypsin globules. In this section, there are numerous lightly eosinophilic globular intracytoplasmic inclusions in the periportal hepatocytes. α_1-Antitrypsin globules may be distinguished from other eosinophilic globular intracytoplasmic inclusions by demonstration of intense positivity with the PAS plus diastase (PASD) stain and immunostain for α_1-antitrypsin. In contrast, a closely related intracytoplasmic inclusion, α_1-antichromotrypsin, appears finely granular rather than discretely globular in haematoxylin and eosin (H&E) sections, and shows weak positivity with PASD stain and immunoreactivity to α_1-antichymotrypsin. α_1-Antitrypsin globules are not pathognomonic of α_1-antitrypsin deficiency, as they also appear in cirrhoses of other aetiologies and in critically ill elderly patients with high serum α_1-antitrypsin levels.

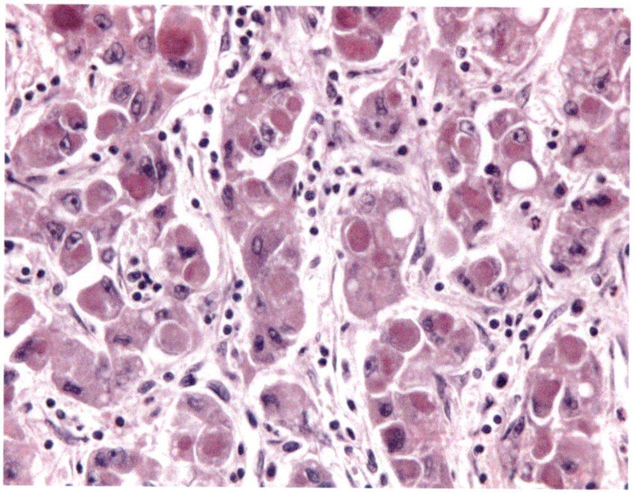

Fig. 2.42 Intracellular hyaline bodies. Intracellular hyaline bodies are deeply eosinophilic globular intracytoplasmic inclusions usually surrounded by a clear halo. Intracellular hyaline bodies are distinguished from other eosinophilic globular intracytoplasmic inclusions by demonstrating negativity on PASD staining and immunoreactivity to p62. Intracellular hyaline bodies are observed in hepatocellular carcinoma, cholangiocarcinoma, and, rarely, idiopathic copper toxicosis.

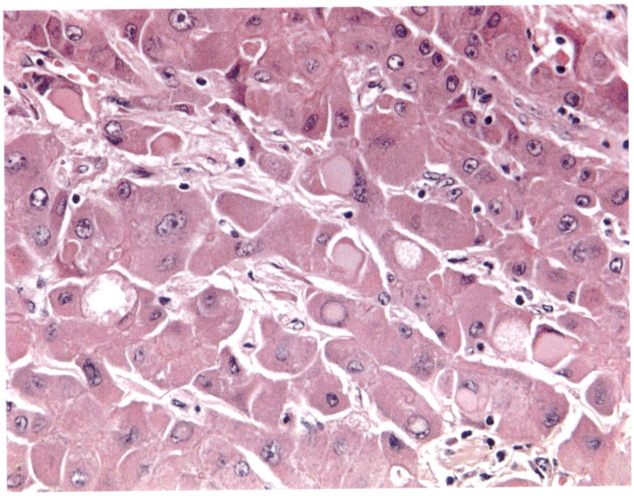

Fig. 2.43 Pale bodies. In this section, there are many lightly eosinophilic globular homogenous intracytoplasmic inclusions in malignant hepatocytes. Pale bodies may vary from lightly to deeply eosinophilic and may resemble large α_1-antitrypsin globules, intracellular hyaline bodies, and ground-glass hepatocytes. Immunoreactivity to fibrinogen is the key discriminating feature. Pale bodies are found in fibrolamellar hepatocellular carcinomas and in fibrinogen storage disease.

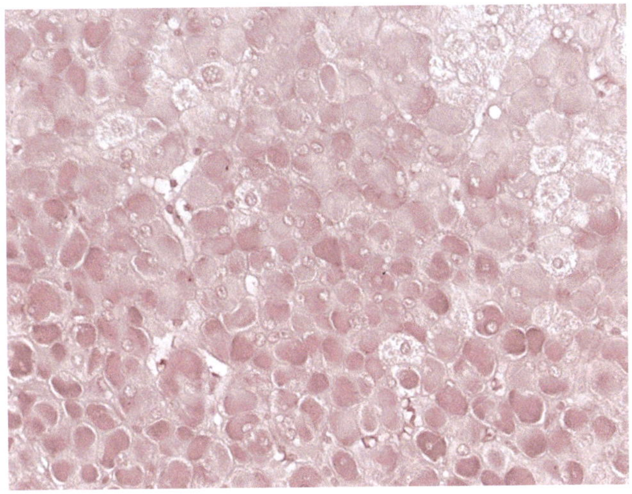

Fig. 2.45 Ground-glass hepatocytes (orcein stain). Ground-glass hepatocytes containing abundant HBsAg are highlighted by orcein stain. Victoria blue stain and immunostain for HBsAg are alternative confirmatory tools.

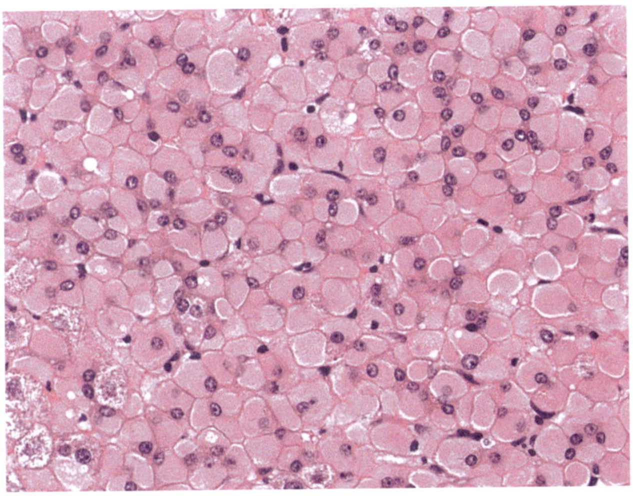

Fig. 2.44 Ground-glass hepatocytes. Shown are numerous ground-glass hepatocytes, characterised by their palely eosinophilic, finely granular intracytoplasmic inclusions with an occasional surrounding clear halo. Ground-glass inclusions represent endoplasmic reticulum containing abundant hepatitis B surface antigen (HBsAg); they are highlighted by orcein or Victoria blue histochemical stains and by immunostaining for HBsAg. These special stains help differentiate ground-glass hepatocytes from pseudo–ground-glass inclusions, pale bodies, oncocytic hepatocytes, and hepatocytes in which there is enzyme induction. Pseudo–ground-glass inclusions may be found in glycogen storage disease type IV, Lafora disease, cyanamide-induced injury, and immunocompromised patients on multiple medications.

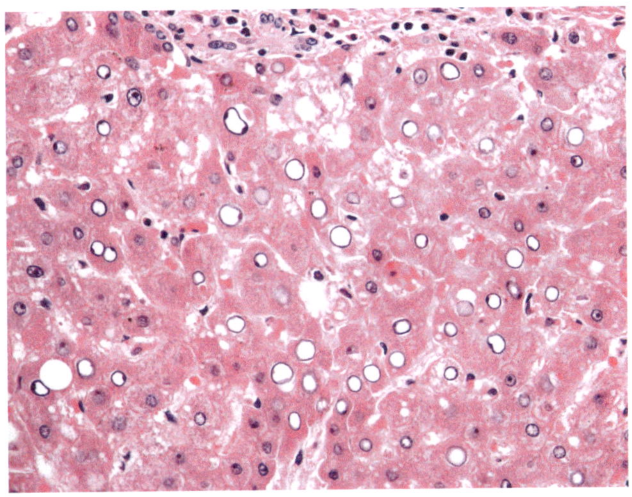

Fig. 2.46 Glycogenated nuclei. Many hepatocytes exhibit nuclear clear vacuolation due to glycogen accumulation. Physiologic hepatic nuclear glycogenation is common in children, adolescents and young adults. Originally described in patients with diabetes, pathologically, nuclear glycogenation is associated with nonalcoholic fatty liver disease, chronic hepatitis C with steatohepatitic features, glycogen storage disease, Wilson disease, and other copper overload disorders.

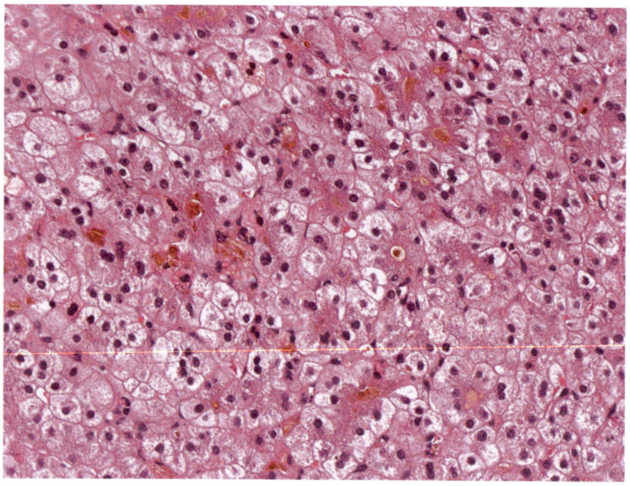

Fig. 2.47 Bilirubinostasis. Many bile plugs are present within dilated bile canaliculi. Some Kupffer cells and a few hepatocytes also contain yellowish brown granular bile pigments. Bile accumulates predominantly in the perivenular region and appears as yellowish to greenish brown granular pigment. The presence of bile plugs in canaliculi delineates bile from other cytoplasmic pigments. The Fouchet stain may be applied to highlight bile pigments in difficult cases. Bilirubinostasis commonly is associated with acute cholestasis. Four distinct patterns of acute cholestasis have been described: (1) bland cholestasis (minimal portal or parenchymal change), (2) cholestasis in acute large duct obstruction (portal oedema, portal neutrophilic infiltrate, and ductular reaction), (3) cholestasis in intrahepatic bile duct disease (bile duct damage and/or ductopaenia), and (4) acute cholestatic hepatitis (lobular necroinflammation).

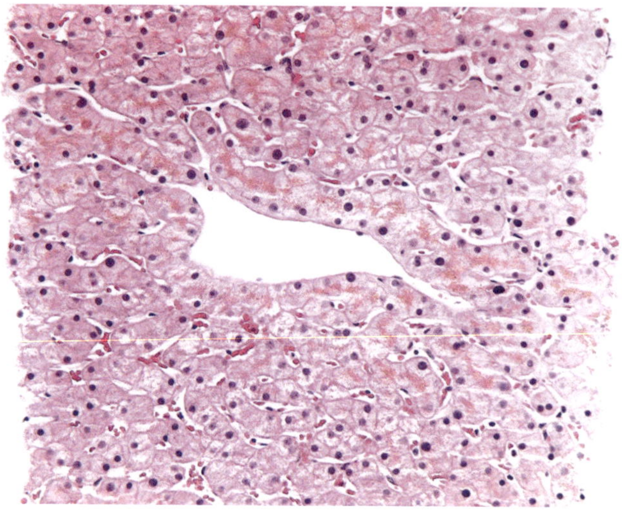

Fig. 2.49 Lipofuscin. There are many golden yellow finely granular pigments in the pericanalicular cytoplasm of perivenular hepatocytes. Lipofuscin is a "wear-and-tear" pigment produced by lysosomal oxidation of lipids and lipoproteins. Although it may be highlighted in PASD (variable), Sudan black, and long Ziehl-Neelsen stains, it is easily appreciated in H&E-stained sections. Dubin-Johnson pigment resembles lipofuscin and shares similar staining properties, but it appears dark brown and more coarsely granular. It also is more widely distributed in the lobules. Lipofuscin has no functional or clinical importance. A minor practical issue regarding identification of lipofuscin is that it may help in orienting the perivenular regions in a biopsy.

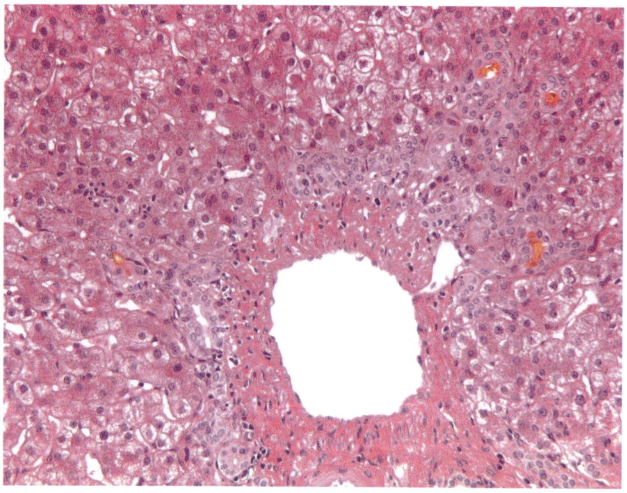

Fig. 2.48 Ductular cholestasis. Some bile ductules are distended by inspissated bile concretions. Ductular cholestasis, also referred to as cholangitis lenta, is a pathognomonic feature of sepsis. It is encountered uncommonly in routine liver biopsies, but when present, it should stimulate prompt communication with the relevant clinicians to guide appropriate management of the septic or (impeding septic) patient. However, there are potential pitfalls, especially if only a small biopsy specimen exists. The edge of a von Meyenburg complex, congenital hepatic fibrosis, or other ductal plate malformation containing irregular dilated bile ducts inspissated with bile concretions may be confused with ductular cholestasis.

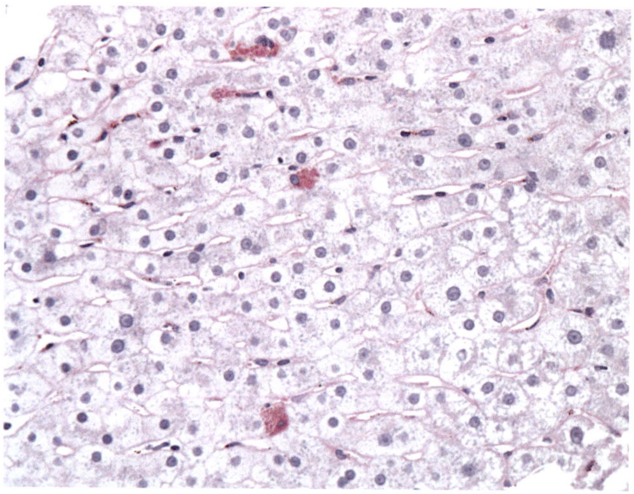

Fig. 2.50 Ceroid/ lipofuscin (periodic acid-Schiff with diastase stain). Some ceroid-laden Kupffer cells are present. Ceroid represents early-stage lipofuscin and results from digestion of engulfed necroinflammatory debris by Kupffer cells or portal macrophages. In contrast to lipofuscin deposition in hepatocytes, the presence of ceroid-laden Kupffer cells or portal macrophages signifies recent active liver injury.

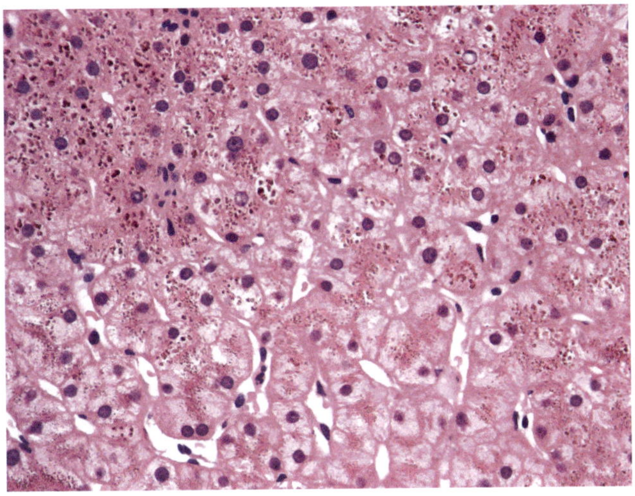

Fig. 2.51 Iron. Many brownish, refractile, finely to coarsely granular pigments are present in the hepatocytes. In the liver, iron is stored in two forms: ferritin and haemosiderin. Ferritin normally is invisible in H&E and Perls stains, but it sometimes may be appear as diffuse and pale positivity in Perls stain in conditions with hyperferritinaemia (including any inflammatory condition). Haemosiderin appears as brown, refractile, coarsely granular pigment in H&E sections and stains intensely in Perls stain.

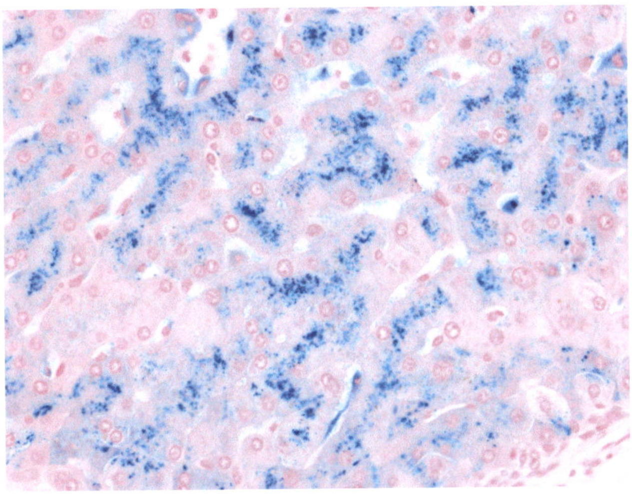

Fig. 2.52 Iron (Perls stain). Iron accumulation with pericanalicular accentuation is noted in the hepatocytes. The differential diagnosis of iron overload may be helped by evaluating the distribution among hepatocytes (parenchymal) and Kupffer cells/portal macrophages (mesenchymal). Parenchymal iron overload is associated with early hereditary haemochromatosis, acaeruloplasminaemia, ferroportin disease type B, nontransfused ineffective erythropoiesis, and cirrhosis of other causes. Mesenchymal iron overload is associated with ferroportin disease type A, blood transfusions, and inflammatory syndromes. A mixed pattern of iron overload is seen in late hereditary haemochromatosis, transfused ineffective erythropoiesis, chronic viral hepatitis, steatohepatitis, Wilson disease, and porphyria cutanea tarda.

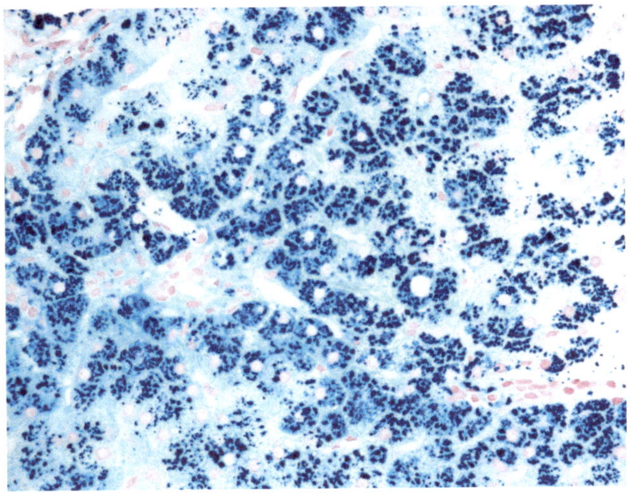

Fig. 2.53 Iron (Perls stain). Marked iron accumulation is widely noted in the hepatocytes. Many grading systems have been proposed to evaluate the severity of iron overload. Two commonly adopted grading systems are the modified Scheuer system:

- 0: iron granules absent/barely seen at 400×
- 1+: iron granules resolved at 250×
- 2+: iron granules resolved at 100×
- 3+: iron granules resolved at 25×
- 4+: iron deposits visible at 4× or by the naked eye

and the modified LeSage system:

- 0: iron granules absent
- 1+: iron granules in <25% of hepatocytes
- 2+: iron granules in 26% to 50% of hepatocytes
- 3+: iron granules in 51% to 75% of hepatocytes
- 4+: iron granules in >75% of hepatocytes

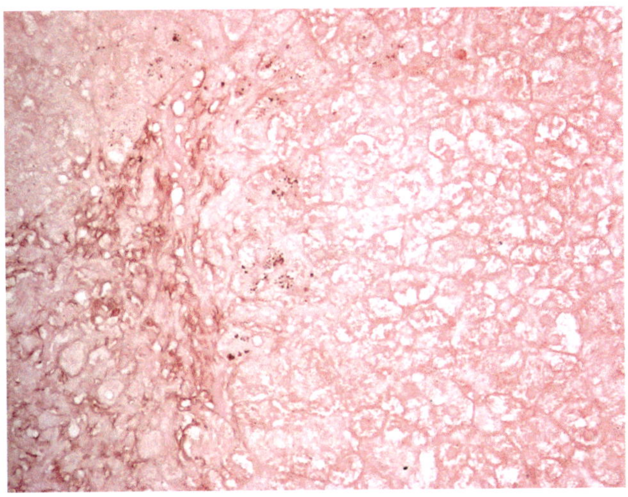

Fig. 2.54 Copper-associated protein (orcein stain). Some periportal hepatocytes contain copper- associated protein. Orcein and Victoria blue stains are indirect methods used for illustrating the presence of copper by highlighting metallothionein (copper-associated protein). They are superior to direct copper stains (rhodanine and rubeanic acid) because copper is highly soluble, especially in poorly buffered formalin. Accumulation of copper is caused mainly by Wilson disease, Indian childhood cirrhosis, idiopathic copper toxicosis, and chronic cholestatic disease. However, one should note that focal mild copper deposition may be present physiologically in infants younger than 3 months and pathologically in the periseptal hepatocytes in advanced fibrosis or cirrhosis of any cause, which probably is related to altered bile flow. Moreover, the absence of copper does not exclude Wilson disease or chronic biliary disease.

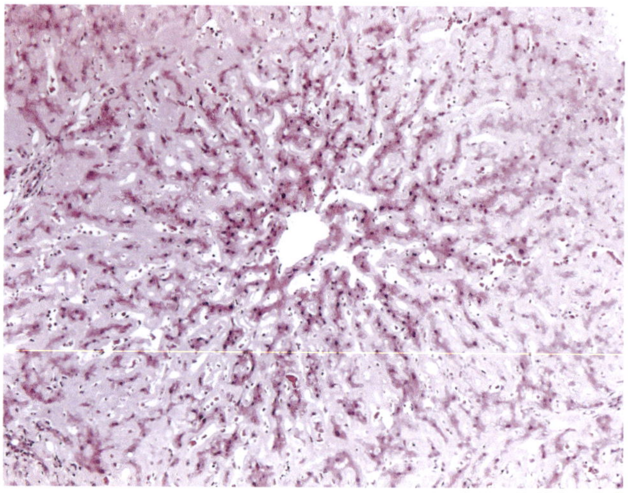

Fig. 2.55 Amyloidosis. Extensive amorphous eosinophilic extracellular deposits are present within the hepatic sinusoids in a linear manner and with compression of the cords of hepatocytes. The presence of amyloid may be confirmed by a Congo red stain (pinkish in light microscopy with apple-green birefringence under polarized light). The liver commonly is involved in systemic amyloidosis. There are three main histologic patterns of amyloid deposition in the liver: vascular (in the wall of blood vessels), sinusoidal (in the sinusoids beneath the space of Disse in either a linear or globular manner), and stromal (in portal tract connective tissue). Vascular, linear sinusoidal, and stromal patterns of amyloidosis should be differentiated from fibrosis, whereas globular sinusoidal pattern must be distinguished from ground-glass hepatocytes, pseudo–ground-glass inclusions, and pale bodies.

2.4 Regeneration

The liver is renowned for its incredible regenerating capacity, having the ability to restore approximately three-quarters of its own mass within half a year. In mild to moderate parenchymal necrosis, mitotic division of hepatocytes is adequate to replace the cellular loss and results in architectural changes of the hepatocyte plates with some cytologic alterations of the liver cells. In severe parenchymal damage, there is activation and replication of stem or progenitor cells, which are derived from bipotential cells thought to be reside in the canal of Hering. Proliferation of bipotential cells of the canal of Hering with the associated stromal response is manifest as the ductular reaction histologically.

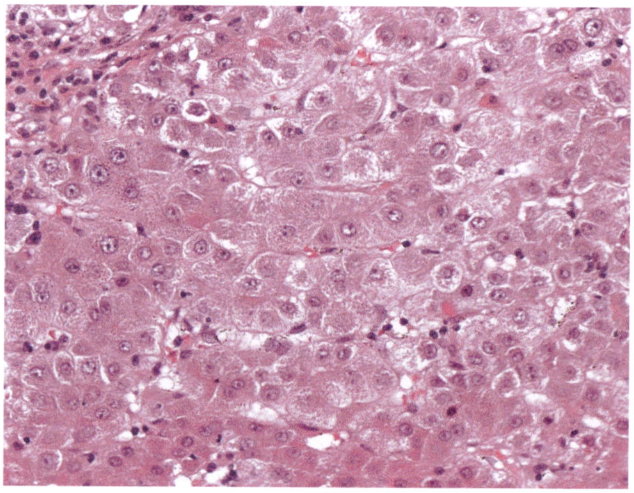

Fig. 2.56 Twin-cell plate. Regenerating hepatocytes are arranged in thickened cords two cells thick. Hepatocytes in normal adult liver normally are arranged in single-cell plates. In the regenerating process, the hepatocyte plates are thickened to twin-cell plates as the result of replication of regenerating hepatocytes. Hepatocellular neoplastic processes also may lead to thickening of the hepatocyte plate. However, regeneration rarely produces hepatocyte plates more than two cells thick.

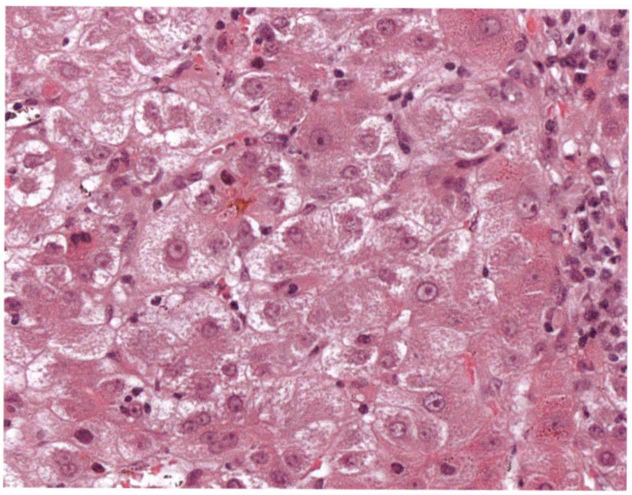

Fig. 2.57 Hepatocyte rosette. Regenerating hepatocytes are arranged in rosettes or pseudo-acini. In an active regenerating process, the hepatocyte plate is distorted to form a rosette, pseudo-acinus, or pseudo-gland.

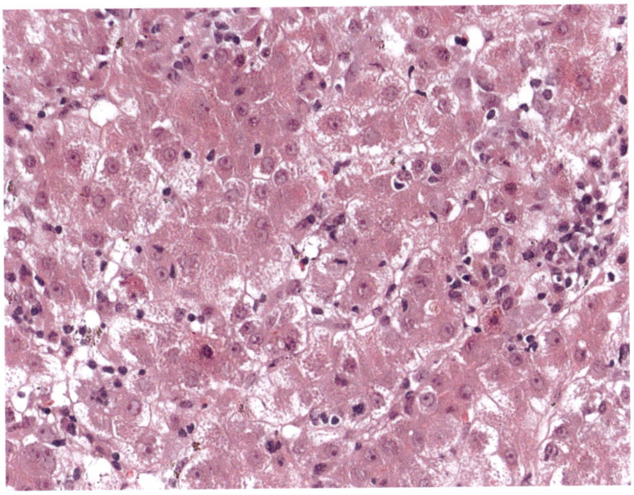

Fig. 2.58 Mitotic activity. A mitotic figure (*centre*) is present in a dividing hepatocyte in response to acute hepatitis. Replication of hepatocytes through mitotic division is a key part of regenerative responses in liver and is evident in mild to moderate cellular loss. Of course, mitotic activity also may be prominent in hepatocellular neoplasms. However, atypical mitotic figures are never encountered in regeneration.

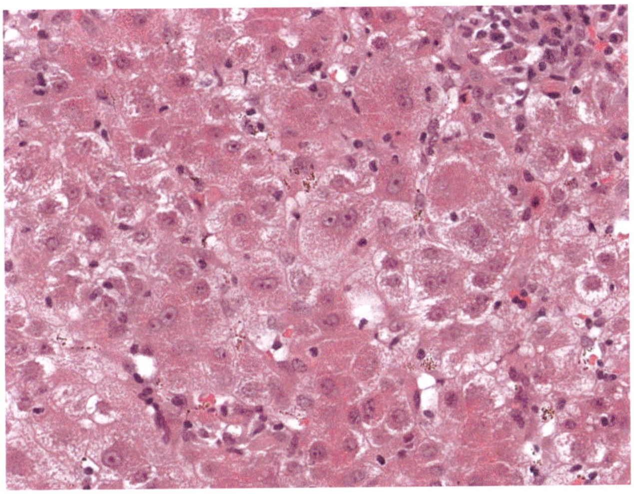

Fig. 2.59 Ploidy. Regenerating hepatocytes may show binucleation, vesicular chromatin, and prominent nucleoli. Ploidy may represent one stage (telophase) of mitotic division and is evidence of replication of regenerating hepatocytes. However, binucleated hepatocytes are not uncommonly found in liver biopsies, especially in the elderly. Such aging hepatocytes usually contain lipofuscin, in contrast to those in active replication.

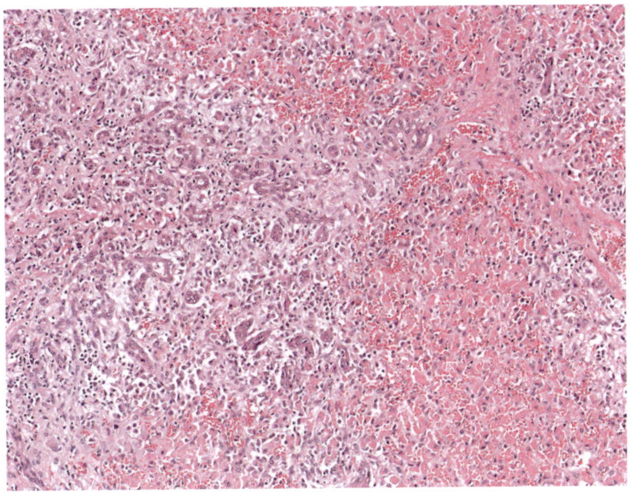

Fig. 2.60 Ductular reaction. There is prominent proliferation of bile ductules (cholangioles) in an oedematous stroma associated with an inflammatory infiltrate, in response to multiacinar necrosis. Ductular reaction is associated with acute hepatitis with bridging/panacinar necrosis, chronic hepatitis with bridging fibrosis/cirrhosis, large duct obstruction, sepsis, acute ascending cholangitis, chronic intrahepatic biliary disease, focal nodular hyperplasia and inflammatory hepatocellular adenoma.

2.5 Fibrosis

When chronic persistent liver injury exceeds the regenerative capacity of the liver, deposition of fibrous connective tissue occurs, which is essentially scarring the damaged tissue loss. Fibrosis is a dynamic and bidirectional process resulting from the balance between fibrogenesis and fibrolysis. The degree of fibrosis indicates the chronicity (or "stage") of the liver disease, and its pattern sometimes may be helpful in giving diagnostic clues to the underlying disease.

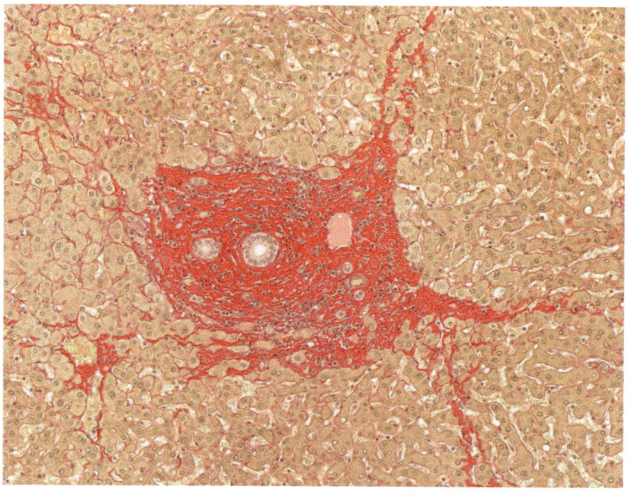

Fig. 2.61 Portal and periportal fibrosis (picrosirius red stain). Fibrous tissue expands a portal tract and extends into the periportal region as short fibrous septa. Portal fibrosis is related to activation of portal macrophages and possibly epithelial–mesenchymal transition of cholangiocytes. This pattern of fibrosis typically is seen in portal-based diseases such as chronic viral hepatitis, autoimmune hepatitis, and chronic biliary disease.

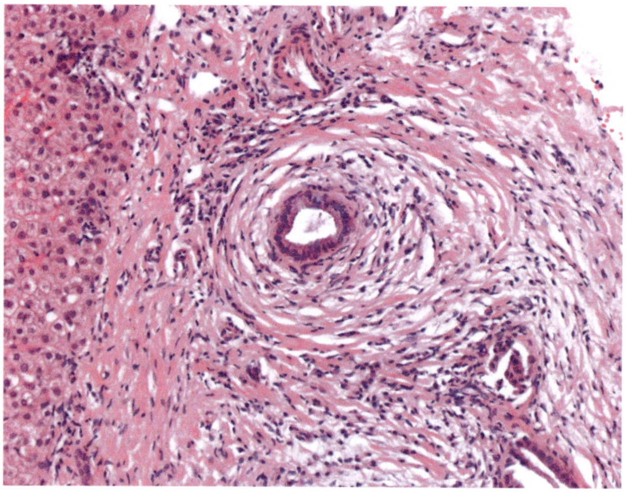

Fig. 2.62 Periductal fibrosis. A bile duct is surrounded by "onion-skin" concentric fibrous tissue. Periductal fibrosis is related to activation of peribiliary macrophages and epithelial–mesenchymal transition of cholangiocytes. Periductal fibrosis is a characteristic finding in primary sclerosing cholangitis, secondary sclerosing cholangitis, and ischaemic cholangitis.

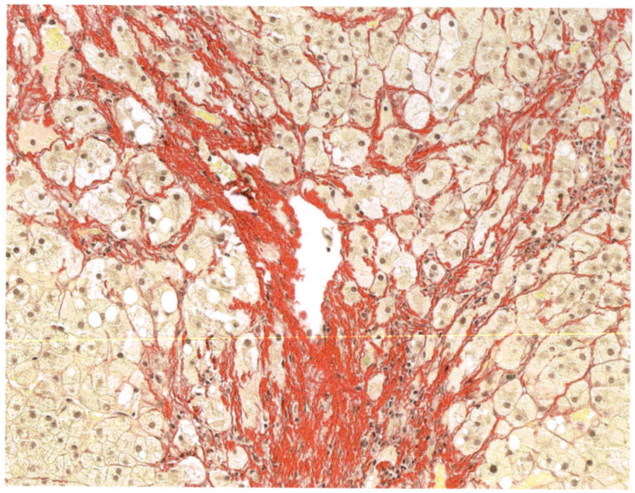

Fig. 2.63 Perivenular and pericellular (perisinusoidal) fibrosis (picrosirius red stain). Delicate fibrous strands are deposited around the terminal hepatic venule with extension into sinusoids and appear to be wrapping around hepatocytes. Perivenular and pericellular fibrosis commonly is found in alcoholic and nonalcoholic steatohepatitis, but also may be seen in congestive heart failure, Budd-Chiari syndrome, sinusoidal obstruction syndrome, and sickle cell disease.

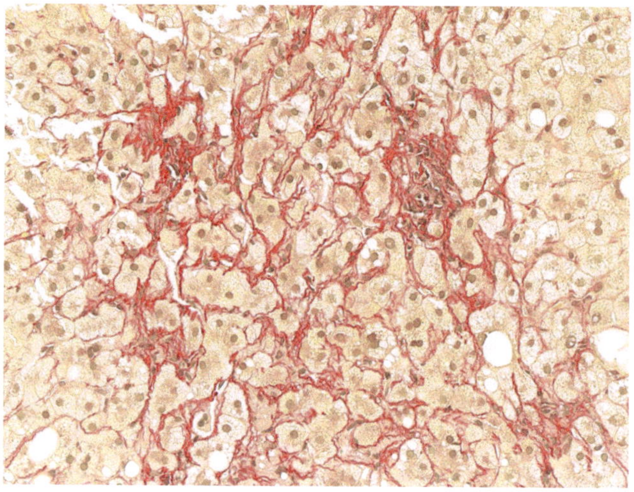

Fig. 2.64 Pericellular fibrosis (picrosirius red stain). Delicate fibrous strands are deposited along the sinusoids and around hepatocytes. Pericellular fibrosis represents the deposition of fibrous tissue in the space of Disse and is related to activation of stellate cells. Pericellular fibrosis typically is observed in alcoholic and nonalcoholic steatohepatitis but also is associated with fibrosing cholestatic hepatitis B/C, total parenteral nutrition, Wilson disease and other copper overload disorders, tyrosinaemia, hereditary fructose intolerance, mucopolysaccharidoses, Down syndrome, visceral leishmaniasis, and congenital syphilis.

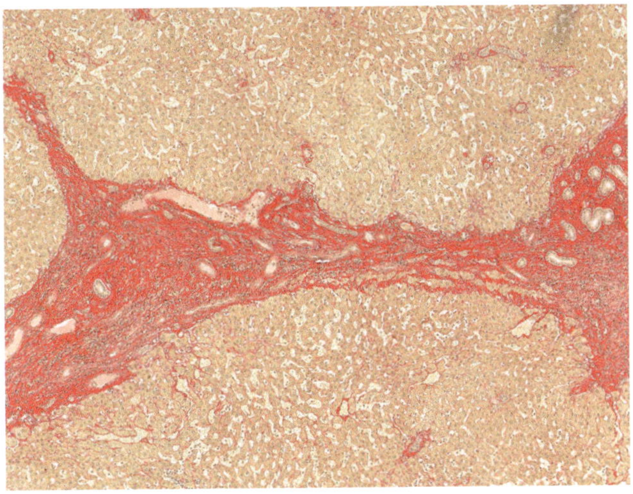

Fig. 2.65 Bridging fibrosis (picrosirius red stain). A thick fibrous septum bridges two portal tracts with minimal inflammatory infiltrate and mild ductular reaction. Bridging fibrosis represents a more severe and chronic form of fibrosis with expansion of connective tissue linking between portal tracts and/or terminal hepatic venules.

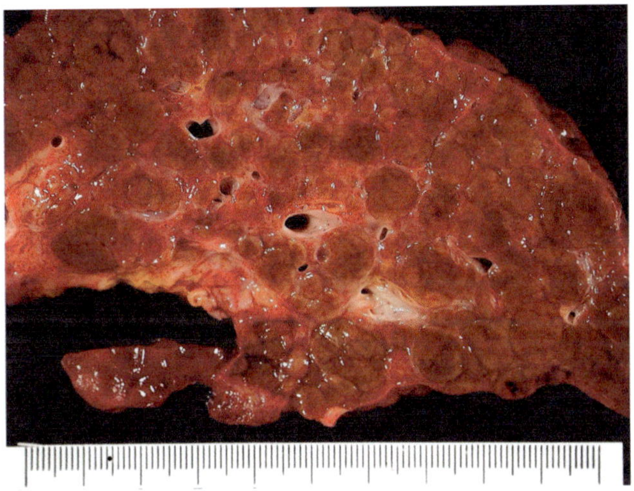

Fig. 2.66 Cirrhosis. The entire liver is diffusely replaced by regenerative nodules of varied sizes. Traditionally, cirrhosis was classified into macronodular (regenerative nodules >3 mm), micronodular (regenerative nodules up to 3 mm), and mixed types. Macronodular cirrhosis typically is associated with chronic viral hepatitis, whereas micronodular cirrhosis usually is the result of alcoholic liver disease. However, this classification is of limited value in evaluating the underlying aetiology because it has been well recognised that transformation between two types is not uncommon. Micronodular cirrhosis in alcoholic liver disease, for example, transforms to a macronodular pattern following abstinence.

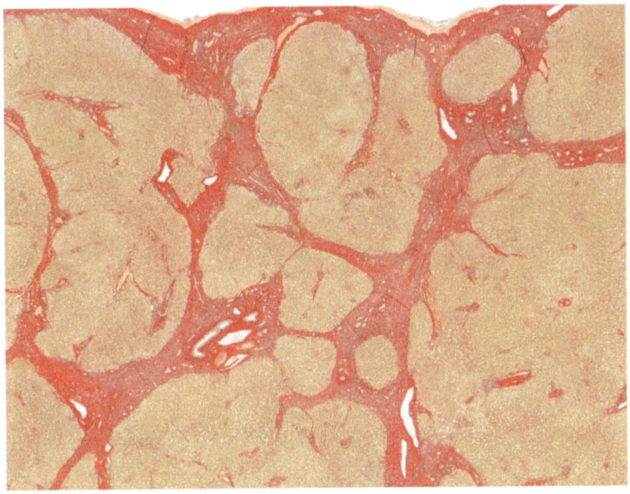

Fig. 2.67 Cirrhosis (picrosirius red stain). The entire liver parenchyma is subdivided into regenerative nodules of varying sizes by fibrous septa. Cirrhosis is a diffuse process characterised by fibrosis and the conversion of normal liver architecture into structurally abnormal nodules. The morphologic changes are contributed to by the accumulation of confluent parenchymal extinction lesions secondary to widespread imbalanced intrahepatic circulation. The traditional concept of cirrhosis as an end-stage and irreversible process was widely accepted. However, it has been clearly demonstrated that cirrhosis is neither static nor persistently progressive, but rather a dynamic and bidirectional process, and most would now accept that under some circumstances, cirrhosis may be reversible.

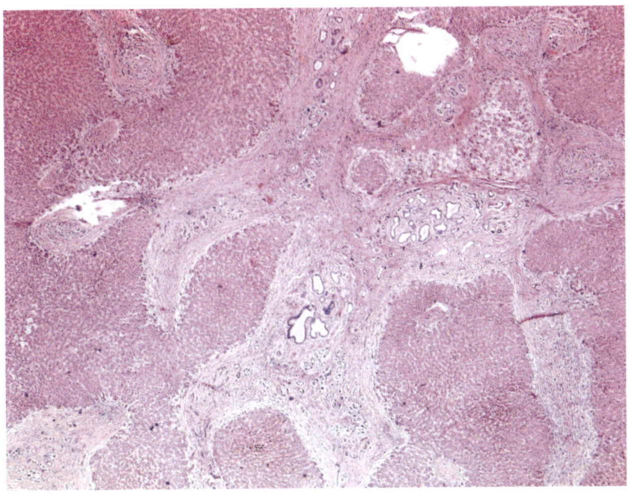

Fig. 2.68 Biliary cirrhosis. Irregular regenerative nodules with a jigsaw puzzle appearance and a peripheral pale biliary halo are surrounded by thick fibrous septa. Irregular regenerative nodules with a peripheral biliary halo are typical of biliary cirrhosis. The halo is the result of periseptal oedema, loosely packed fibrous tissue at the interface, and periseptal hepatocytes with feathery degeneration. Common causes of biliary cirrhosis include primary biliary cirrhosis, primary sclerosing cholangitis, ischaemic cholangitis, chronic large duct obstruction, α_1-antitrypsin deficiency, biliary atresia, cystic fibrosis, and type III progressive familial intrahepatic cholestasis.

3 Developmental Abnormalities

Human liver development begins at around 3 weeks, when part of the hepatic diverticulum composed of endodermal cells buds from the primordial duodenum and merges with the mesenchymal cells of the septum transversum to form the primordial liver. The rest of the hepatic diverticulum gives rise to the extrahepatic biliary tree, from which the ventral pancreas also originates. The intrahepatic biliary tree later derives from the hepatoblasts through the formation of the ductal plate and its remodelling after the development of the hepatic arteries, in a centripetal fashion, beginning at the hilum and spreading to the periphery. The developing liver serves as the haematopoietic organ of the fetus. Until birth, the umbilical vein blood is shunted to the inferior vena cava through the ductus venosus. Bile starts flowing through the biliary tree at birth.

This brief summary sets the scene for this chapter, which illustrates aspects of normal development, and the main, yet rare, developmental abnormalities, including ductal plate malformation, Alagille syndrome, and biliary atresia. The various aspects of normal development also remind us of the close relationships among the liver, pancreas, gastrointestinal tract, and haematopoietic system, and between hepatocytes and the biliary epithelium. This, in turn, helps our understanding of the mechanisms of liver regeneration, tumour origin, shared disorders, and their similarities.

3.1 Normal Development

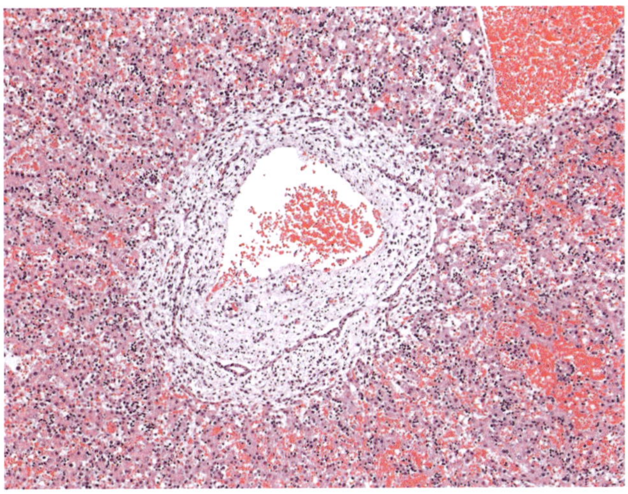

Fig. 3.1 Bile duct development in a fetus at the 14th week of gestation. There is a double-layered ductal plate surrounding a portal vein. Intrahepatic bile duct development begins in the 8th week of gestation. It commences around large portal venous branches at the hilum and proceeds centrifugally along smaller portal veins. A layer of hepatoblasts at the outer boundary of the portal tracts is induced by portal mesenchyme to acquire a biliary phenotype with expression of cytokeratin 19 (CK19) and to form a single-layered ductal plate. A second layer of hepatoblasts immediately adjacent to the single-layered ductal plate subsequently gains a biliary phenotype to produce a double-layered ductal plate. Remodelling of the double-layered ductal plate starts from the 12th week of gestation to acquire lumina to produce a wreath of discrete tubular spaces.

A.W.H. Chan et al., *Atlas of Liver Pathology*, Atlas of Anatomic Pathology,
DOI 10.1007/978-1-4614-9114-9_3,

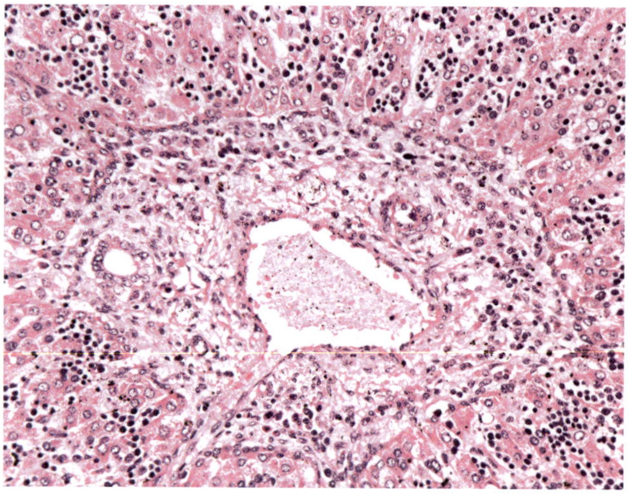

Fig. 3.2 Bile duct development in a fetus at the 20th week of gestation. An interlobular bile duct is present. The double-layered ductal plate at the periphery becomes fragmented and less conspicuous by the remodelling process. Interlobular bile ducts are formed by further remodelling of the ductal plate through production of portal mesenchymal tissue, separation of tubular structures from the interface between the portal tract and liver parenchyma, and absorption of excessive ductal structures. Bile duct epithelial cells begin to express another biliary cytokeratin (CK7) from the 20th week of gestation, whereas uninvolved hepatocytes in the ductal plate lose CK19.

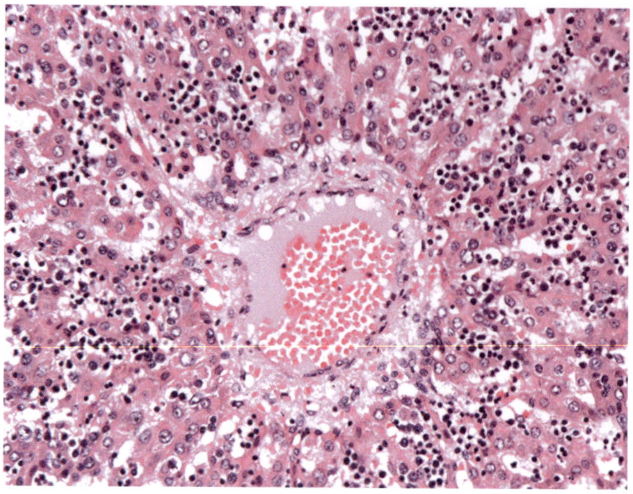

Fig. 3.4 Extramedullary haematopoiesis in a fetal liver. Extensive sinusoidal extramedullary haematopoiesis is present among a twin-cell plate of hepatocytes. Extramedullary haematopoiesis is a normal physiologic finding during fetal development and normally ceases within a month after birth. Erythropoiesis tends to occur along the hepatic sinusoids, whereas leucopoiesis and thrombopoiesis are found more commonly in portal tracts. The presence of these immature haematopoietic cells should not be misinterpreted as lobular or portal inflammation, or as an atypical haematolymphoid infiltrate. Hepatocyte plates in children younger than 5 years are two cells thick and become one cell thick thereafter. Twin-cell hepatocyte plates in infants do not indicate regenerative activity.

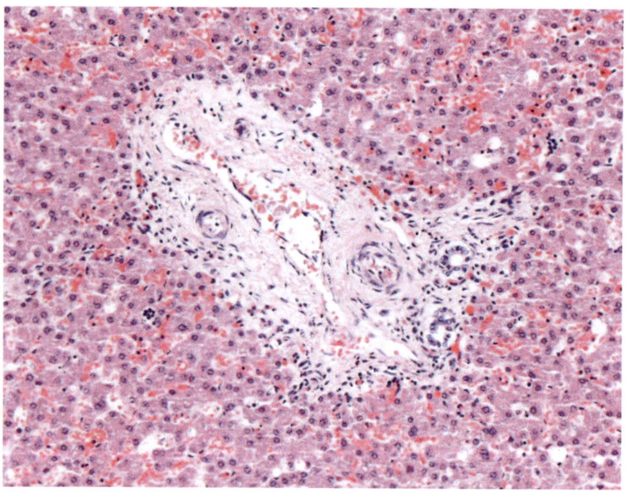

Fig. 3.3 Bile duct development in a fetus at the 24th week of gestation. An interlobular bile duct is present. By this stage in the growth of the portal tract, the ductal plate is completely absorbed by the remodelling process. Remodelling starts around large portal venous branches at the hilum and proceeds centrifugally along smaller portal veins. The entire process is incomplete until the first month of life ex utero. It is normal to find residual ductal plate remnants in the liver of neonates, particularly preterm ones.

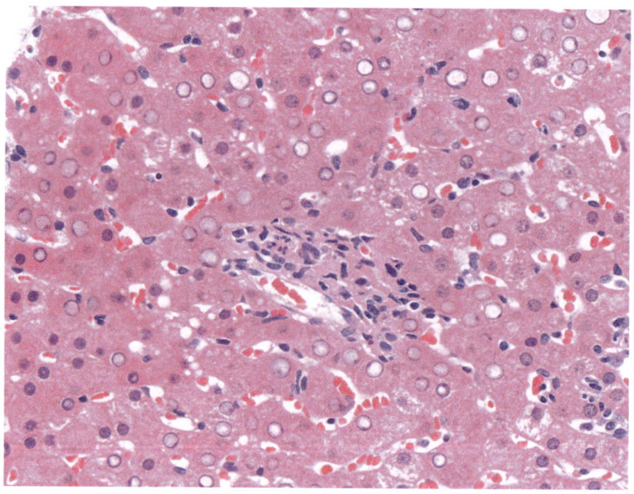

Fig. 3.5 Normal liver of an infant. Periportal hepatocytes possess glycogenated nuclei. Physiologic hepatic nuclear glycogenation is common in children, adolescents, and young adults (11% and 4% in the 20s and early 30s, respectively). Pathologically, nuclear glycogenation is associated with nonalcoholic fatty liver disease, chronic hepatitis C with steatohepatitic features, glycogen storage disease, Wilson disease, and other copper overload disorders.

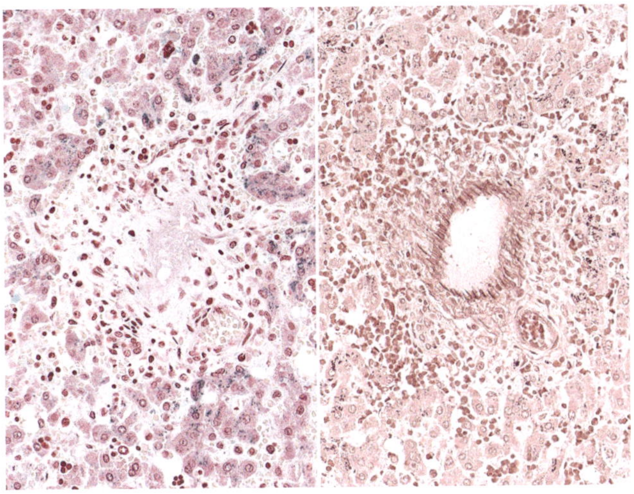

Fig. 3.6 Normal liver of an infant (*left*: Perls stain; *right*: orcein stain). Deposition of haemosiderin and copper-associated protein is noted in the periportal hepatocytes. The presence of stainable iron and copper in periportal hepatocytes is a physiologic phenomenon during fetal and infantile periods (up to 3 months old) and should not be misinterpreted as a pathologic feature of iron or copper overload.

3.2 Fibrocystic Liver Disease and Choledochal Cyst

Fibrocystic liver disease comprises a heterogeneous group of diseases with varying degrees of cystic dilatation of intrahepatic bile ducts and hepatic fibrosis. It is believed to be associated with defective remodelling of ductal plates and, hence, also is known as ductal plate malformation. There is a full spectrum of morphologic changes, ranging from von Meyenburg complex, solitary bile duct cyst, Caroli disease, and congenital hepatic fibrosis to polycystic liver disease. Caroli disease sometimes is considered one form (type V) of choledochal cyst; thus, choledochal cyst also is included in this section. The pathogenesis of Caroli disease, congenital hepatic fibrosis, and polycystic liver disease is associated with mutations in genes encoding proteins on primary cilia; hence, fibrocystic liver disease also may be regarded as a ciliopathy.

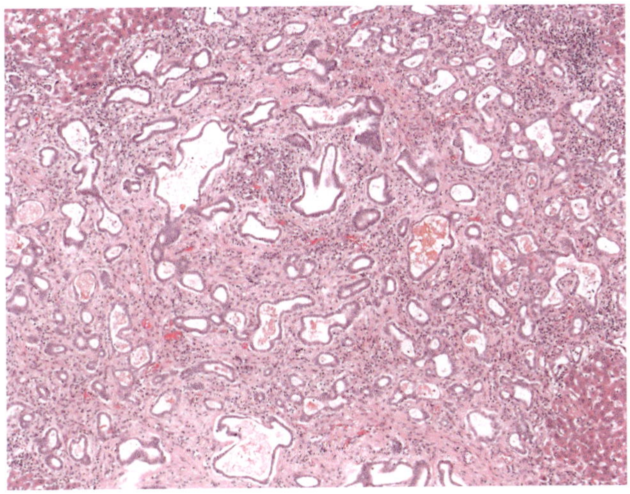

Fig. 3.7 von Meyenburg complex. Numerous irregularly dilated ductal structures are present in a fibrous stroma and are lined by a single layer of bland cuboidal epithelial cells. Some ductal structures are filled with inspissated bile or eosinophilic material. von Meyenburg complex, also known as bile duct (micro)hamartoma, is a localized form of ductal plate malformation. It may be an incidental finding in normal individuals or patients with nondevelopmental liver diseases. It also is present abundantly in other forms of fibrocystic liver disease.

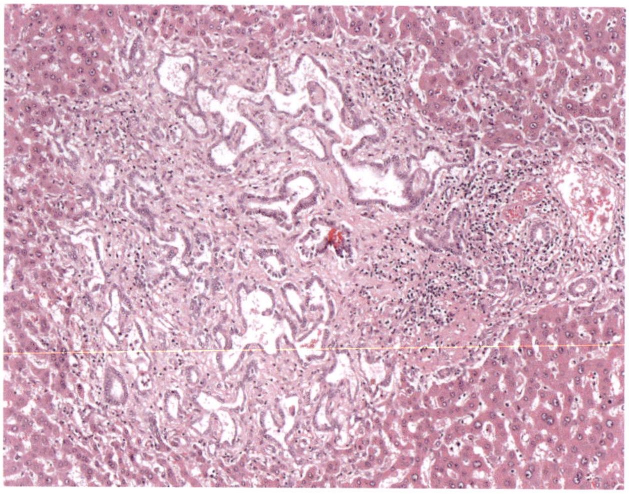

Fig. 3.8 von Meyenburg complex. Numerous irregularly dilated ductal structures are present in a fibrous stroma and are lined by a single layer of bland cuboidal epithelial cells. von Meyenburg complexes are composed of a cluster of irregularly dilated ductal structures in a fibrous stroma. The ductal structures are lined by attenuated, cuboidal, or, rarely, columnar cells. Their lumina may contain inspissated bile or eosinophilic material. von Meyenburg complex may be single or multiple but tends to be more frequent when associated with other forms of fibrocystic liver disease. It usually is situated in the subcapsular region and, not uncommonly, the target of frozen section during abdominal operations to exclude metastatic malignancy.

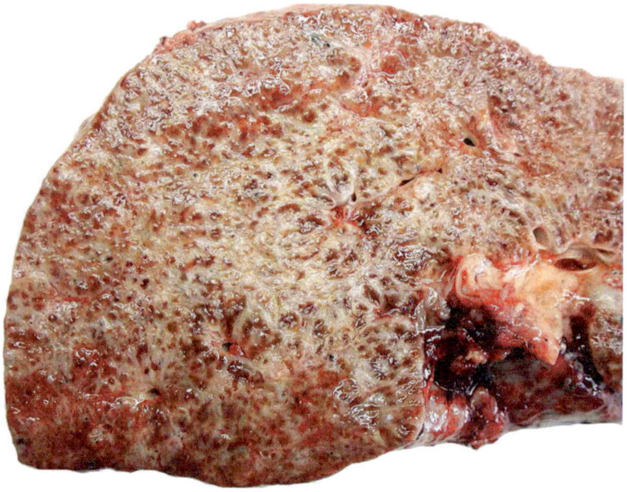

Fig. 3.9 Congenital hepatic fibrosis. The liver is enlarged with multiple nodules separated by thick fibrous bands. No cystic dilatation of bile ducts is noted grossly. Congenital hepatic fibrosis is mostly the hepatic presentation of a multisystem disorder, and rarely presents in isolation. Juvenile or adult presentation of autosomal recessive polycystic kidney disease accounts for majority of congenital hepatic fibrosis. Other hepatorenal ciliopathies (e.g. Meckel-Gruber syndrome, Joubert syndrome, COACH syndrome, nephronophthisis, renal-hepatic-pancreatic dysplasia and rarely autosomal dominant polycystic kidney disease) and ciliary skeletal dysplasia (e.g. Jeune syndrome and Ellis-van Creveld syndrome) are also associated with congenital hepatic fibrosis. Many cases have concurrent Caroli disease-type changes and are designated as Caroli syndrome.

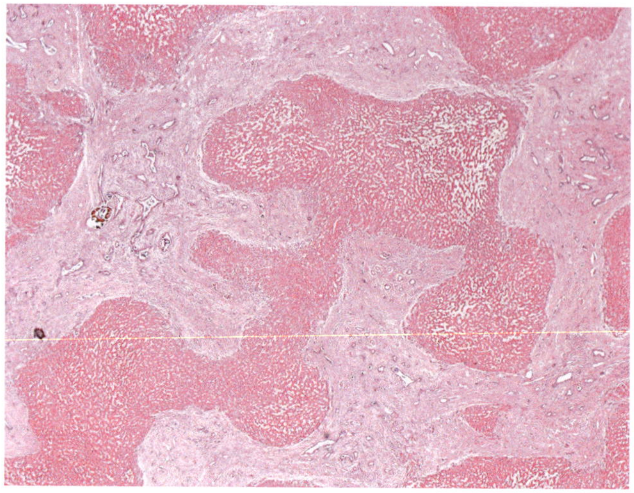

Fig. 3.10 Congenital hepatic fibrosis. Irregular hepatic nodules with a jigsaw puzzle configuration are surrounded by thick fibrous septa. This low-power appearance resembles a biliary-type cirrhosis. Clinical manifestations of congenital hepatic fibrosis are hepatomegaly and those of portal hypertension, including splenomegaly, hypersplenism, and bleeding oesophageal varices. Liver function derangement, ascites, and encephalopathy are not typical. Cholangitis and hepatolithiasis may occur, particularly in patients with Caroli syndrome.

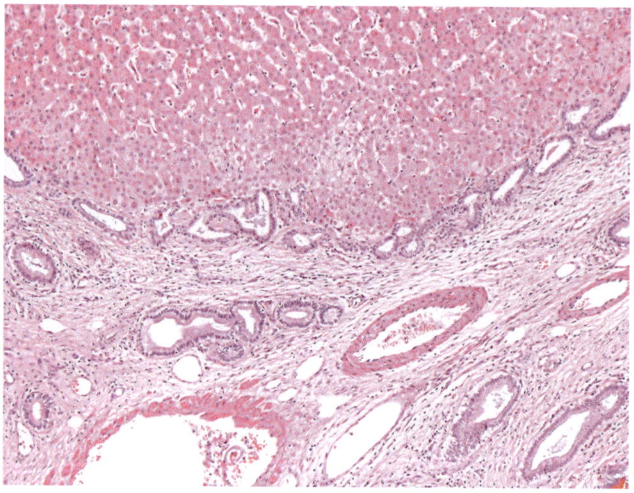

Fig. 3.11 Congenital hepatic fibrosis. There are many irregularly dilated ductal structures at the portal–parenchymal interface. Congenital hepatic fibrosis is characterised macroscopically by hepatomegaly with multiple nodules separated by thick fibrous bands. Histologically, the entire liver is divided into irregular hepatic nodules with a jigsaw puzzle appearance by diffuse periportal and portal-portal bridging fibrosis, and resembles biliary-type cirrhosis. Fibrous septa contain numerous irregularly dilated ductal structures at the portal–parenchymal interface. The ductal structures are lined by cuboidal or columnar cells and may contain inspissated bile or eosinophilic material. Obliterative portal venopathy and von Meyenburg complexes commonly are found. Septal inflammation typically is minimal, unless it is complicated by acute cholangitis. Multiple cystically dilated bile ducts are present in Caroli syndrome.

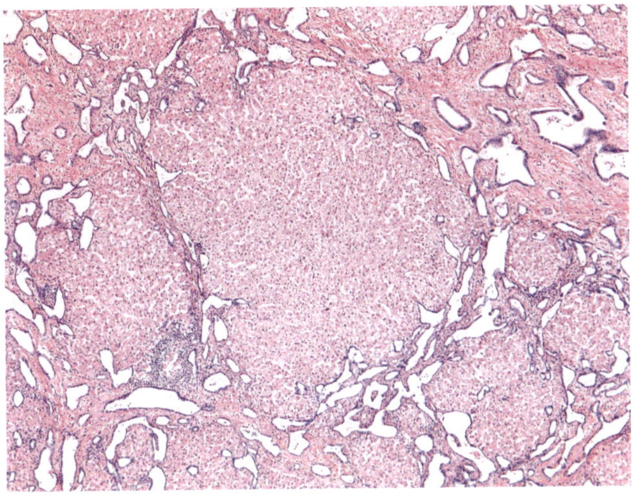

Fig. 3.12 Congenital hepatic fibrosis. Irregular hepatic nodules are surrounded by many irregularly dilated ductal structures at the portal–parenchymal interface. Pathologically, congenital hepatic fibrosis may mimic cirrhosis, especially the biliary type. The differentiation may be challenging even on liver biopsies. Identification of irregularly dilated ductal structures at the portal–parenchymal interface (ductal plate malformation) is essential to establish the correct diagnosis.

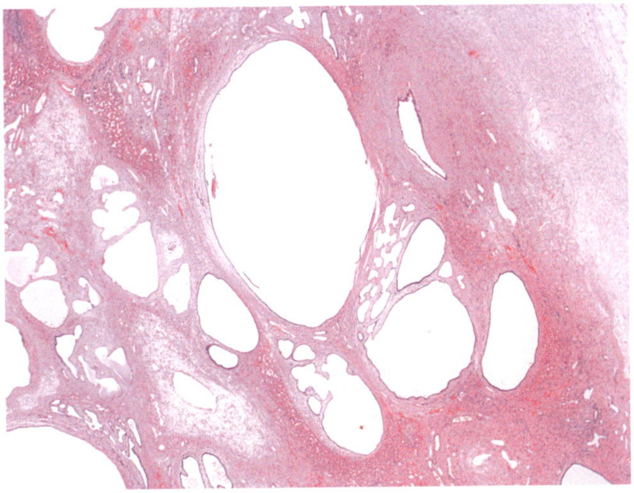

Fig. 3.13 Polycystic liver disease. There are multiple hepatic cysts of varied sizes. Polycystic liver disease most commonly is associated with autosomal dominant polycystic kidney disease (ADPKD) but may be an isolated form without kidney abnormalities. The latter is a rare autosomal dominant disease with mutations in the gene encoding for hepatocystin (PRKCSH) and Sec63 (SEC63) proteins, which are not ciliary proteins, in contrast to hepatorenal ciliopathies. Both forms of polycystic liver disease are manifested as right upper quadrant pain, nausea, and early satiety with normal liver function. Cystic haemorrhage, infection, and rupture are possible complications. ADPKD rarely is associated with congenital hepatic fibrosis and Caroli disease.

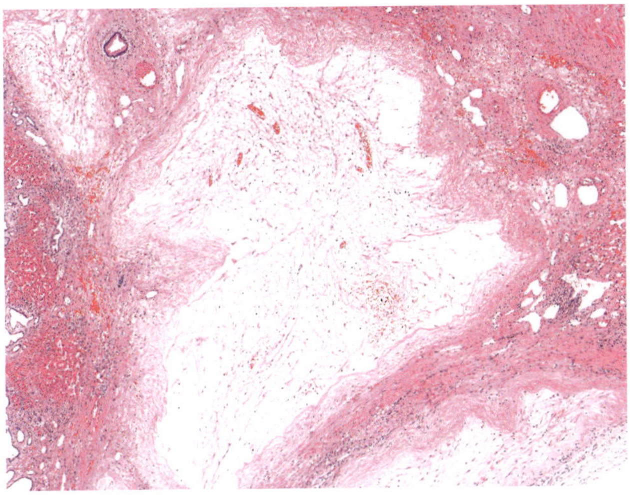

Fig. 3.14 Polycystic liver disease. Collapsed cysts contain corrugated walls and are filled by loose fibrous tissue. Polycystic liver disease is characterised pathologically by the presence of multiple hepatic cysts of varied sizes. The cysts are lined by attenuated, cuboidal, or, rarely, columnar cells. Most cysts are completely isolated from the intrahepatic biliary tree, but a few may arise from von Meyenburg complexes, which commonly are present in polycystic liver disease. Some collapsed cysts are filled by loose fibrous tissue and may resemble ovarian corpora albicantes. A neutrophilic infiltrate may be seen in the presence of cyst rupture and inflammation.

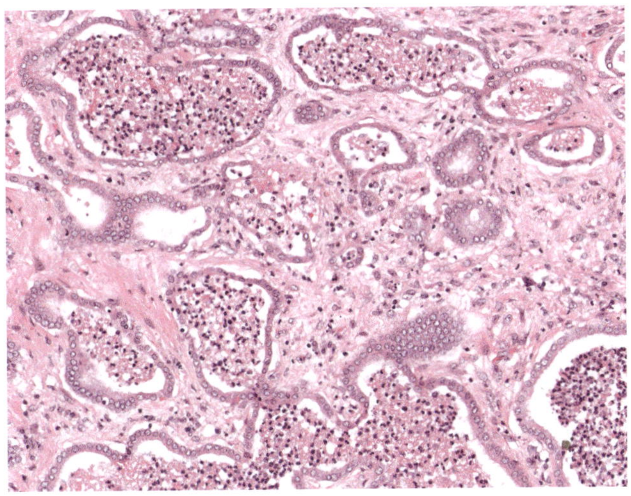

Fig. 3.15 Polycystic liver disease. Dilated ductal structures are filled by neutrophils. Clinical and radiologic correlations for identifying renal involvement are essential for differentiating the two forms of polycystic liver disease, because both share the same pathologic features. Genetic tests are confirmatory but are not widely available.

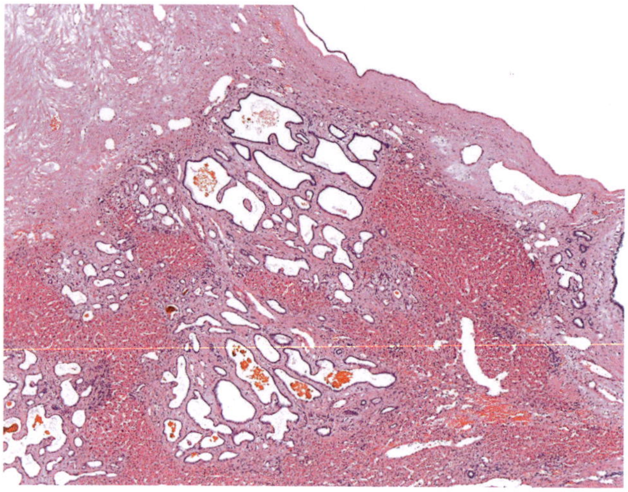

Fig. 3.16 Polycystic liver disease. There are von Meyenburg complexes adjacent to a dilated hepatic cyst. Cystic structures in polycystic liver disease typically are isolated from the intrahepatic biliary tree, whereas those in Caroli disease and infantile presentation of autosomal recessive polycystic liver disease represent cystically distended bile ducts.

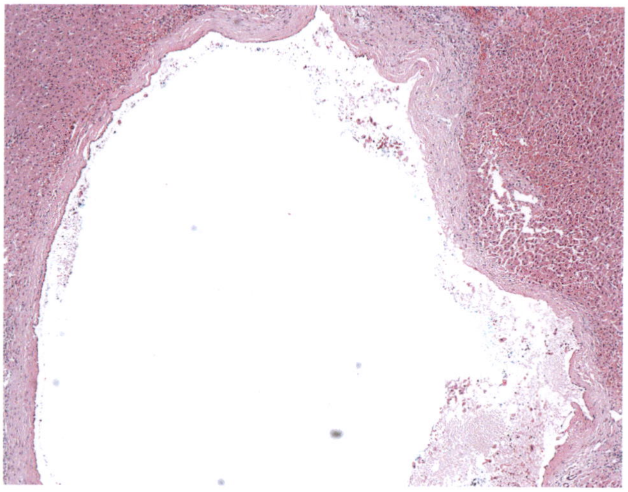

Fig. 3.17 Solitary bile duct cyst. A unilocular cystic lesion is lined by a single layer of bland nonciliated cuboidal cells. Solitary bile duct cyst, also known as solitary hepatic cyst and solitary nonparasitic cyst, usually is an incidental finding. It may represent a limited form at one end of the spectrum of fibropolycystic liver disease (ductal plate malformation). The usual age of presentation is 30 to 50 years. Most (95%) of solitary bile duct cysts are unilocular. They are lined by a single layer of nonciliated cuboidal, columnar, or attenuated cells, which are immunoreactive to CK7 and CK19. Malignant transformation is extremely rare.

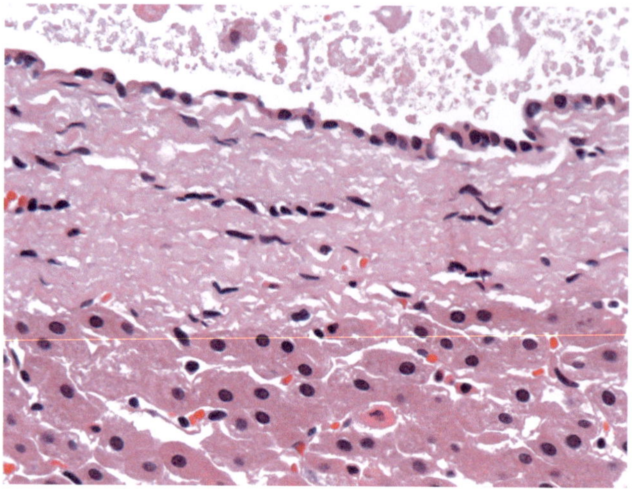

Fig. 3.18 Solitary bile duct cyst. A unilocular cystic lesion is lined by a single layer of bland nonciliated cuboidal cells. Differential diagnoses include other epithelial lined benign cystic lesions: ciliated foregut cyst, mucinous cystic neoplasm, and cystic forms of intraductal papillary neoplasm of bile duct (IPNB). Ciliated foregut cyst is lined by pseudostratified ciliated columnar cells. Mucinous cystic neoplasm is lined by mucinous epithelial cells with variable cytologic and architectural atypia, and the characteristic ovarian-type stroma. The cystic type of IPNB is characterised by cystic ductal dilatation by mucinous epithelial cells with variable cytologic and architectural atypia, with prominent intraductal mucin accumulation, direct luminal connection to the bile ducts, and absence of the ovarian-type stroma.

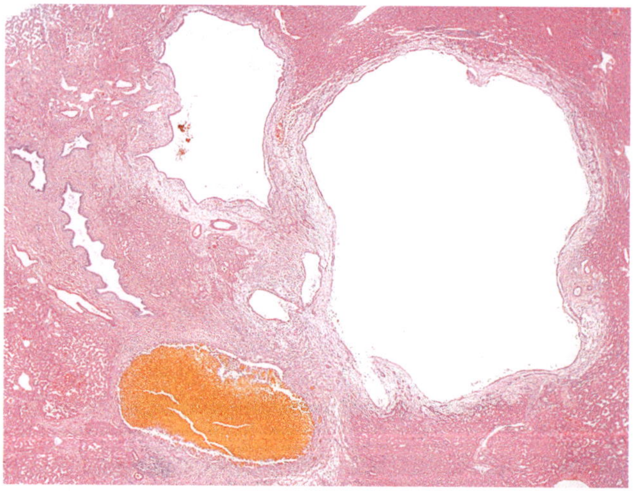

Fig. 3.19 Caroli disease. Cystically dilated bile ducts with irregular contours are present. One of these (*right*) contains an intraluminal protrusion of ductal wall with a fibrovascular core. Caroli disease mostly commonly is associated with autosomal recessive polycystic kidney and, rarely, ADPKD. More than half of Caroli disease cases have concurrent congenital hepatic fibrosis and are designated as Caroli syndrome. Caroli disease may be associated with extrahepatic biliary dilatation and is considered one form (type V) of choledochal cyst. Clinical presentations are associated with the principal complications, namely acute cholangitis and hepatolithiasis. Portal hypertension occurs in Caroli syndrome and usually precedes episodes of acute cholangitis. Caroli disease is associated with an overall risk of 7% to 15% for developing cholangiocarcinoma.

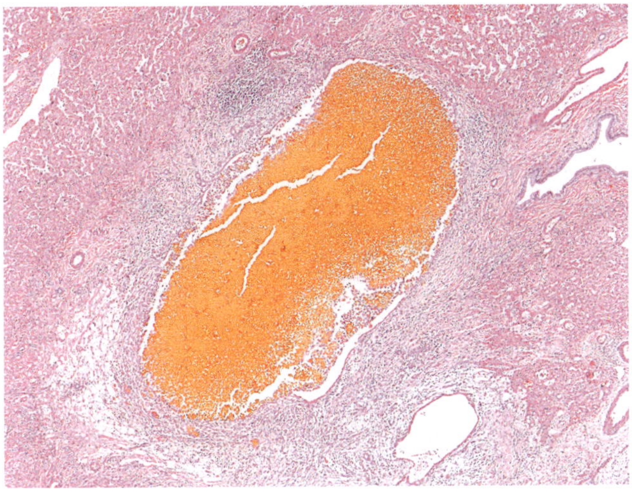

Fig. 3.20 Caroli disease. A cystically dilated bile duct is eroded and filled with inspissated bile sludge. Caroli disease is characterised by multiple segmental dilatations of the intrahepatic biliary tree. Intraluminal protrusion of the duct wall with a fibrovascular core is a typical finding. Cystically dilated bile ducts are lined by cuboidal or columnar cells and may be complicated by ulceration, acute cholangitis, and pyogenic abscess. Periductal fibrosis and inflammation of varying degrees may be found. Premalignant lesions, namely biliary intraepithelial neoplasm or intraductal papillary neoplasm of bile duct, and cholangiocarcinoma may occur in longstanding disease.

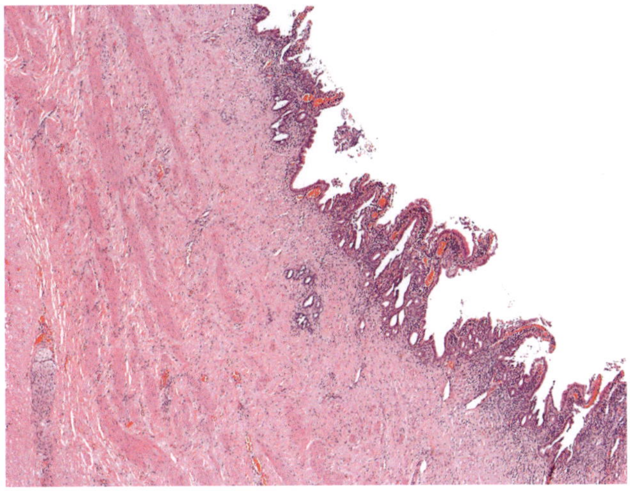

Fig. 3.22 Choledochal cyst. The cystically dilated bile duct is lined by reactive columnar cells, and here it is seen to be associated with a mild chronic inflammatory infiltrate and periductal fibrosis. Choledochal cyst was classified into five types by Todani in 1977 according to location, morphology, and number of dilatation: type I (saccular or fusiform dilatation of extrahepatic bile duct), type II (diverticulum of extrahepatic bile duct), type III (dilatation of duodenal portion of common bile duct; choledochocele), type IV (multiple dilatations of extrahepatic bile duct with or without involvement of intrahepatic bile ducts), and type V (Caroli disease). The overall frequencies of different types of choledochal cysts are 50% to 80% for type I, 2% for type II, 1% to 5% for type III, 15% to 35% for type IV, and 20% for type V.

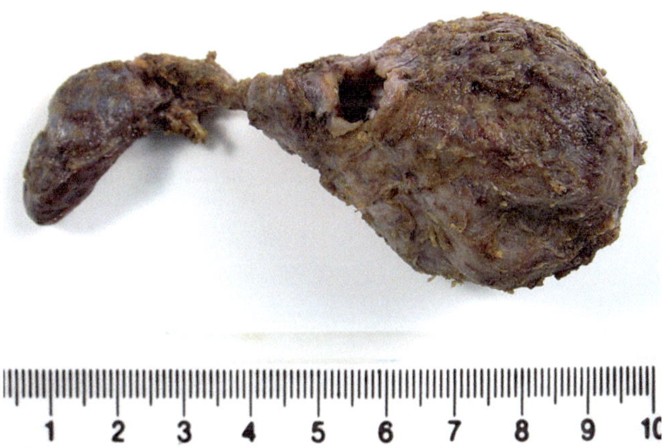

Fig. 3.21 Choledochal cyst. A large saccular dilatation of the common bile duct (*right*) is seen connected to the gallbladder (*left*) in this case. The opening represents the resected margin of the common bile duct. Choledochal cyst is a developmental abnormalities of the biliary tree. It is common in Asian populations but much less frequent in Western populations. The female-to-male ratio is 3:1. The presence of an abdominal mass, right upper quadrant pain, and jaundice are classical clinical features. Choledochal cyst is associated with an overall cancer risk of 10% to 15%.

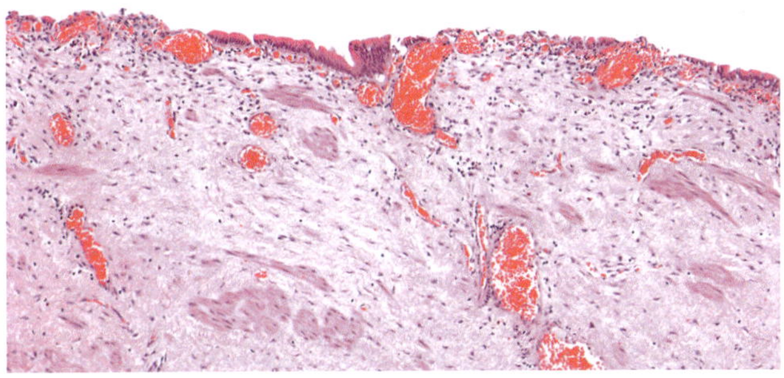

Fig. 3.23 Choledochal cyst. This cystically dilated bile duct is lined by columnar cells. Focal denudation and underlying congestion are noted. Choledochal cyst is a cystically dilated bile duct lined by biliary-type epithelial cells with varying degrees of erosion, ulceration, and regenerative and metaplastic change. Periductal fibrosis and inflammation of varying degrees also may be found. Choledochal cysts can contain a smooth muscle layer allowing distinction from the inflamed, dilated common bile duct observed in obstruction. Premalignant lesions may occur and progress to invasive malignancy, most commonly cholangiocarcinoma, less frequently anaplastic carcinoma and squamous cell carcinoma.

3.3 Paucity of Intrahepatic Bile Ducts and Biliary Atresia

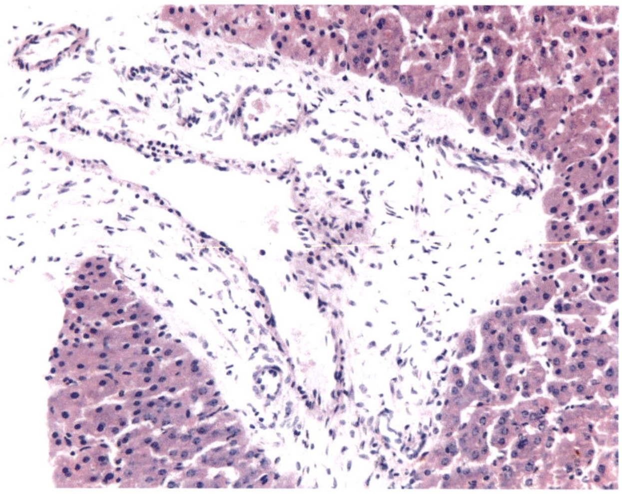

Fig. 3.24 Nonsyndromic paucity of intrahepatic bile ducts. This portal tract is devoid of an interlobular bile duct (ductopaenia). Portal inflammation and ductular reaction also are absent. Paucity of intrahepatic bile ducts may be congenital or acquired and affects a wide range of age groups. It is classified into syndromic (Alagille syndrome) or nonsyndromic forms. Nonsyndromic forms may be caused by a variety of conditions, including biliary diseases (e.g., biliary atresia and secondary sclerosing cholangitis), infection (e.g., congenital rubella and cytomegalovirus infection), and metabolic disease (e.g., α_1-antitrypsin deficiency). The term *nonsyndromic paucity of intrahepatic bile ducts* often is designated for idiopathic ductopaenia in children.

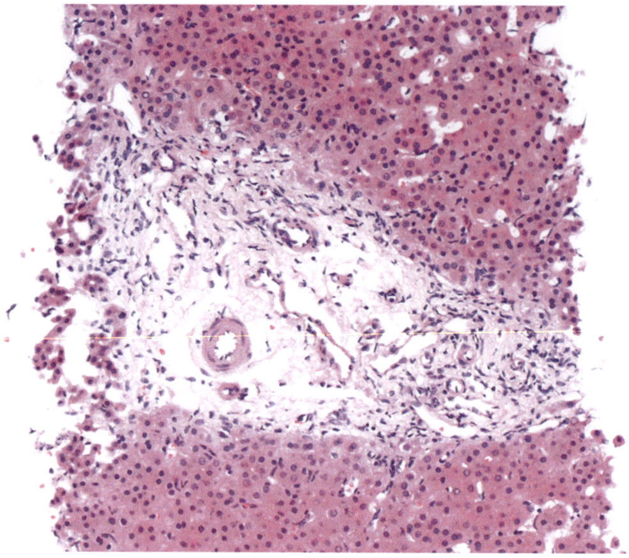

Fig. 3.26 Alagille syndrome. This portal tract is devoid of an interlobular bile duct (ductopaenia). Portal inflammation and ductular reaction also are absent. Alagille syndrome is an autosomal dominant disease with a highly variable clinical picture and nearly complete penetrance. It is associated with mutation of the *JAG1* or *NOTCH2* gene. About 30% to 40% of cases are inherited, but the remaining ones are sporadic as the result of spontaneous germline mutation. The complete syndrome is characterised by paucity of interlobular bile ducts, pulmonary artery stenosis, butterfly-like vertebrae, posterior embryotoxon, and a peculiar face. Pathologically, absence of CD10 among canaliculi of hepatocytes is typical in Alagille syndrome, although lack of CD10 expression is physiological until about seven years of age.

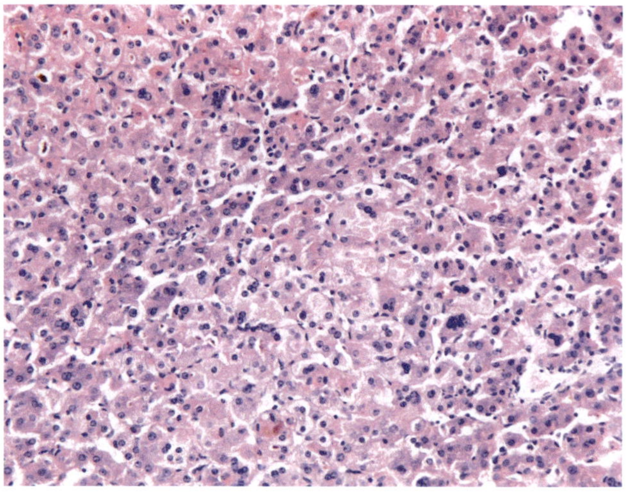

Fig. 3.25 Nonsyndromic paucity of intrahepatic bile ducts. Canalicular and cytoplasmic bilirubinostasis is seen here accompanied by focal giant cell transformation. Full-blown paucity of intrahepatic bile ducts, both syndromic and nonsyndromic, is characterized by ductopaenia and varying degrees of bilirubinostasis. Chronic cholate stasis may occur, but ductular reaction, portal inflammation, and lobular necroinflammatory activity typically are absent. Giant cell transformation, a nonspecific reaction in paediatric livers, may be present. Portal fibrosis typically is mild, but bridging fibrosis and cirrhosis may be seen in some cases.

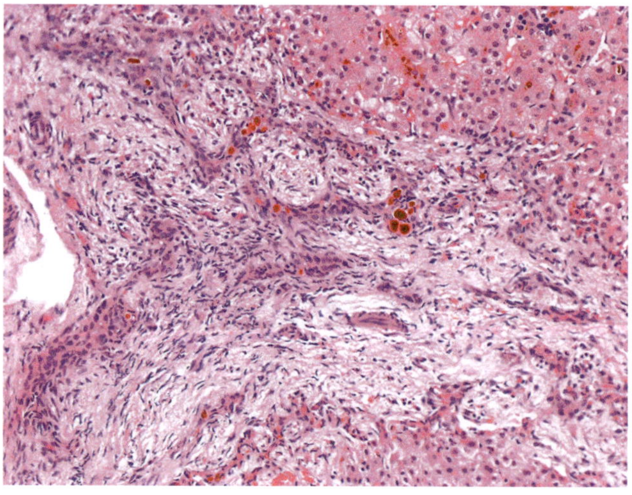

Fig. 3.27 Biliary atresia. A florid ductular reaction is accompanied by canalicular and ductular cholestasis. Biliary atresia is an idiopathic, destructive biliary disease leading to progressive obliteration of bile ducts and secondary biliary cirrhosis. Its pathogenesis is uncertain but believed to be multifactorial. It is classified into two forms: perinatal (70%–80%) and embryonal (20%–30%). The embryonal form is often is associated with extrahepatic malformations (e.g., polysplenia, preduodenal portal vein, gut malrotation, congenital heart disease, and laterality and situs anomalies of internal organs). Abdominal ultrasound, hepatobiliary iminodiacetic acid (HIDA) scan, and cholangiogram are important radiologic diagnostic tools.

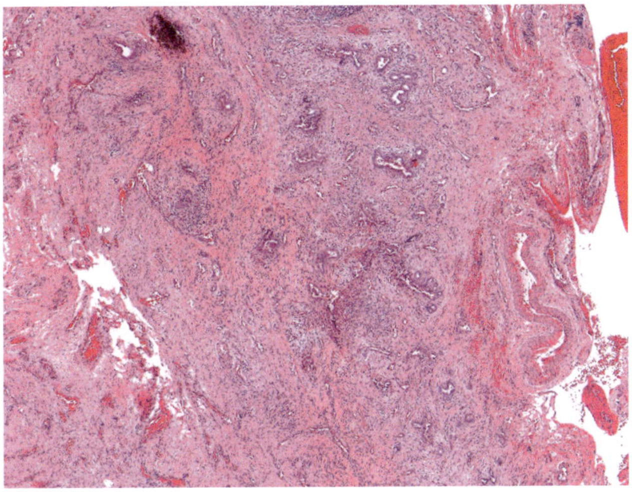

Fig. 3.28 Biliary atresia. This excised atretic porta hepatis contains multiple small duct remnants. The pathologic features of biliary atresia are influenced by the timing and location of specimens obtained. More than 90% of cases are the result of obliteration of the common hepatic duct at the porta hepatis. The peripheral liver exhibits changes of large duct obstruction. The early stages are characterised by perivenular bilirubinostasis, portal oedema and inflammation, and a prominent ductular reaction. Later stages show ductopaenia, chronic cholate stasis, and progression of portal fibrosis to bridging fibrosis and biliary cirrhosis. In the porta hepatis excised during Kasai operations, varying degrees of destruction and fibro-obliteration of the common hepatic duct are observed. Duct remnants previously were classified into different types to predict the prognosis; however, such classifications have very limited clinical value.

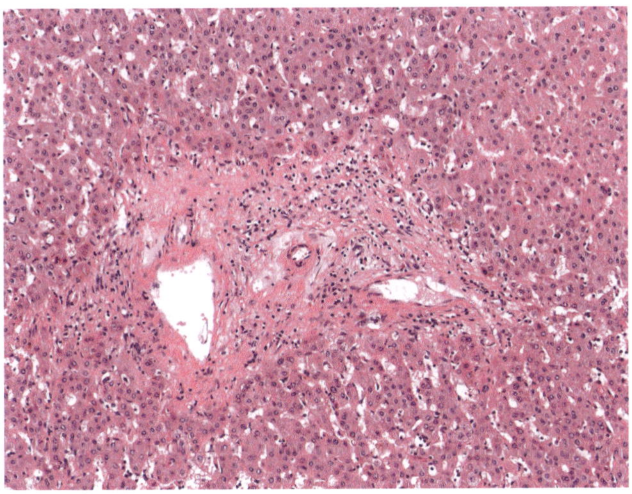

Fig. 3.29 Biliary atresia. In this liver explant from a patient who underwent a Kasai operation several years previously, ductopaenia and portal fibrosis are observed. Destruction and fibro-obliteration of intrahepatic bile ducts continue even after Kasai operations in which there has been satisfactory bile drainage. Development of biliary fibrosis and cirrhosis is almost unavoidable, but the time course is unpredictable.

3.4 Miscellaneous Anatomic and Vascular Anomalies

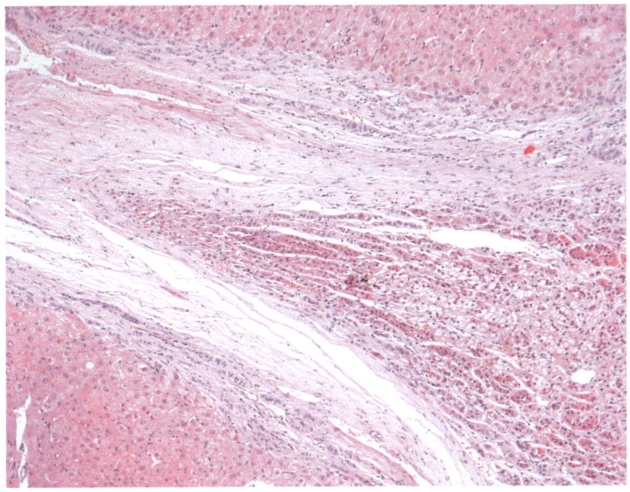

Fig. 3.30 Adrenal–hepatic fusion. Adrenal cortical tissue is present within a liver. Adrenal–hepatic fusion, which is referred to as adrenal heterotopia by some authors, is a common finding of uncertain clinical significance. It was reported in 9.9% of unselected autopsy cases, with a higher incidence in older age groups, suggesting it may be a phenomenon of aging.

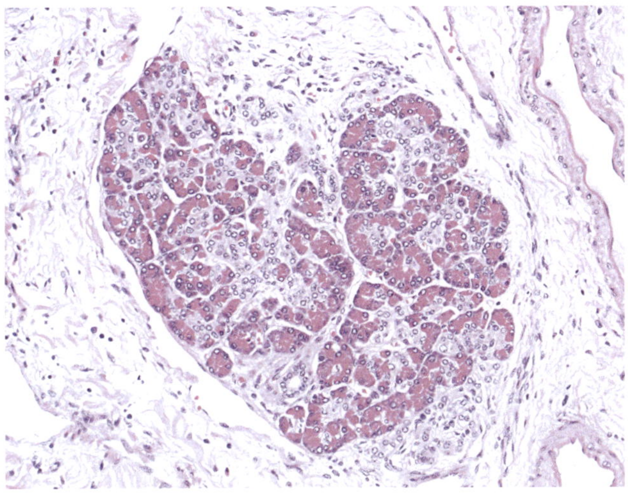

Fig. 3.31 Pancreatic heterotopia. Pancreatic acini and small ducts are present without islets of Langerhans. Pancreatic heterotopia may be found virtually anywhere along the gastrointestinal tract. The most frequent sites are the stomach and duodenum, but the liver rarely is involved. Only nine cases of hepatic pancreatic heterotopia are reported in the literature, two of which exhibited malignant transformation (islet cell carcinoma and adenocarcinoma).

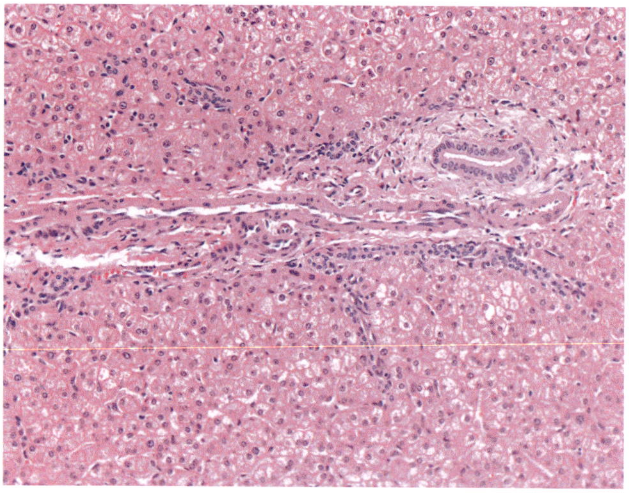

Fig. 3.32 Congenital intrahepatic portosystemic venous shunt. An aberrant hepatic arteriole is seen here in a portal tract with the absence of a portal vein. Intrahepatic portosystemic shunts may be congenital or acquired. Acquired forms are much more common than congenital ones, and may be associated with cirrhosis, portal hypertension, trauma, or iatrogenic causes (surgery or liver biopsy). Congenital intrahepatic portosystemic shunts are rare and believed to represent persistent venous communication between the cranial and caudal hepatic sinusoids formed by the vitelline veins and umbilical vein. Pathologic manifestations include aberrant hepatic arterioles, hepatic atrophy, mild steatosis, and focal nodular hyperplasia.

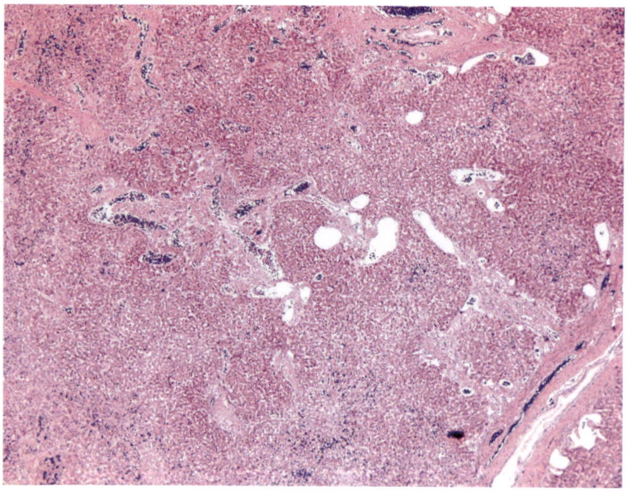

Fig. 3.33 Hereditary haemorrhagic telangiectasia (HHT). Many dilated sinusoids with loose fibrous stroma are distributed haphazardly in the liver. HHT, also known as Osler-Weber-Rendu disease, is an autosomal dominant vascular disorder associated with mutations of the *ENG*, *ACRLR-1*, or *SMAD4* gene. *SMAD4* gene mutation is associated with an overlap with juvenile polyposis syndrome. HHT is characterised by the presence of multiple small telangiectases on the skin and mucous membranes, and arteriovenous malformations in internal organs. Hepatic involvement usually is asymptomatic but may be manifest as portal hypertension, ischaemic cholangiopathy, or high-output cardiac failure.

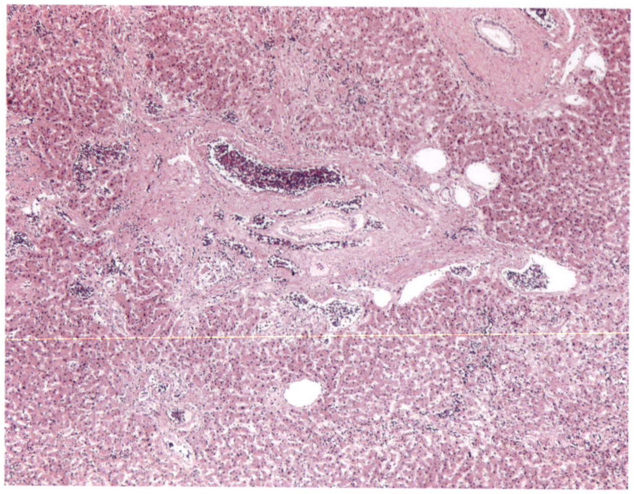

Fig. 3.34 Hereditary haemorrhagic telangiectasia. A fibrotic portal tract contains many dilated vessels. Some distended vessels connect to dilated sinusoids with loose fibrous stroma. HHT has three histological patterns: (1) a haphazardly distributed honeycomb meshwork of dilated sinusoidal channels lined by endothelial cells with or without loose fibrous stroma, (2) aberrant tortuous portal veins and hepatic arteries traversing through hepatic parenchyma with loose fibrous tissue, and (3) multiple dilated portal veins, hepatic arteries, and lymphatics in fibrotic portal tracts. Large regenerative nodules, focal nodular hyperplasia, and ischaemic cholangiopathy may be found.

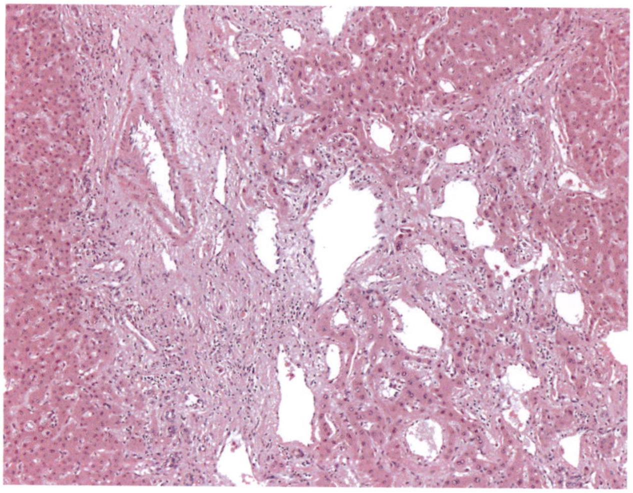

Fig. 3.35 Ataxia telangiectasia. In this case, there are numerous dilated sinusoids accompanied by periportal fibrosis. Ataxia telangiectasia is an autosomal recessive disease characterised by cerebellar ataxia, oculocutaneous telangiectases, recurrent infection due to deficiencies of immunoglobulin A and E, and increased cancer risk. Hepatic manifestations are uncommon and include telangiectases, chronic hepatitis with fibrosis and cirrhosis, sinusoidal obstruction syndrome, and hepatocellular carcinoma.

4 Metabolic Liver Disease

The liver has complex metabolic functions with a central role in various aspects of protein, lipid and carbohydrate metabolism, homeostasis, and detoxification. It is not surprising, therefore, that the liver is involved in many metabolic disorders, either directly when a specific mutation affects the function of a specific enzymatic pathway or secondarily (e.g. metabolic syndrome). Indications for liver biopsy may vary from assessment of the severity of liver damage in patients with a known metabolic condition, to a more diagnostic intent in patients with a liver disorder of unknown aetiology. In some cases, liver histology may be suggestive of a metabolic disorder in patients with a clinical diagnosis of liver disease of other aetiology or cryptogenic.

The classification of metabolic disorders is complex, and usually based on a systematic grouping according to metabolic pathways and function. However, knowledge of the incidence and clinical manifestation of the various metabolic conditions in relation to age and their main histological patterns may be more practical. In this chapter we provide the reader with examples of the common and of some of the rare conditions as a quick image reference.

A.W.H. Chan et al., *Atlas of Liver Pathology*, Atlas of Anatomic Pathology,
DOI 10.1007/978-1-4614-9114-9_4, © Springer Science+Business Media New York 2014

4.1 Disorders of Iron Metabolism

DISEASE	PROTEIN DEFECT	LOCUS
Hereditary haemochromatosis type 1	Haemochromatosis	*HFE* (6q22.2)
Hereditary haemochromatosis type 2A (Juvenile haemochromatosis)	Haemojuvelin	*HJV* (1q21.1)
Hereditary haemochromatosis type 2B (Juvenile haemochromatosis)	Hepcidin	*HAMP* (19q13.12)
Hereditary haemochromatosis type 3	Transferrin receptor 2	*TFR2* (7q22.1)
Hereditary haemochromatosis type 4A/B (Ferroportin disease)	Ferroportin	*HFE4* (2q32.2)
DMT1 deficiency	Divalent metal transporter 1	*SLC11A2* (12q13.12)
Atransferrinaemia	Transferrin	*TF* (3q22.1)
Acaeruloplasminaemia	Caeruloplasmin	*CP* (3q24-25)

Fig. 4.1 Hereditary iron overload. The table summarises genetic diseases associated with hepatic iron overload. Type 1 hereditary haemochromatosis (HH) is the commonest genetic disease associated with hepatic iron overload and has a prevalence rate between 1:200 and 1:500 in Caucasian populations; all the other genetic diseases are rare. Type 4 HH is an autosomal dominant disease, whereas all others are autosomal recessive disorders. Type 2 HH, divalent metal transporter 1 (DMT1) deficiency, and atransferrinaemia present during childhood or adolescence, whereas all others occur in adulthood. Type 4A HH (ferritin loss-of-function mutation), atransferrinaemia, and acaeruloplasminaemia are associated primarily with hepatic mesenchymal haemosiderosis, whereas all others are characterised primarily by hepatic parenchymal haemosiderosis.

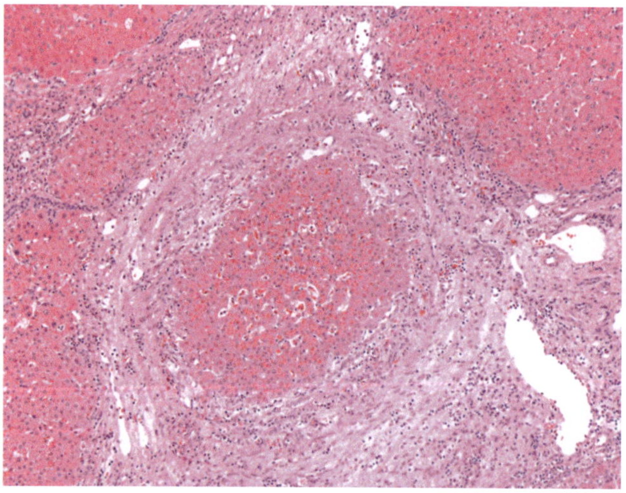

Fig. 4.2 Hereditary haemochromatosis. Cirrhosis is present with regenerative nodules separated by broad fibrous septa. HH, or genetic haemochromatosis, is characterised by inappropriately increased intestinal iron absorption, with consequent accumulation in various organs, notably the liver, pancreas, heart, joints, pituitary gland, and skin, with resultant organ damage. Men are affected by HH two to three times more often than women. Cirrhosis, hepatocellular carcinoma (HCC), and, less commonly, cholangiocarcinoma are important liver complications in HH. HCC accounts for up to 45% of deaths in HH. The risk of HCC is >200 times greater in people with HH than in the general population and seems not to be altered by venesection. Up to 20% of HCCs in HH occur within a noncirrhotic liver.

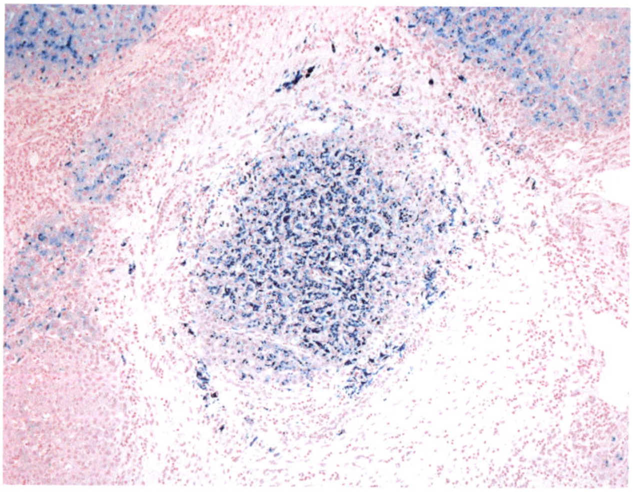

Fig. 4.3 Hereditary haemochromatosis (Perls stain). There is marked (grade 4) haemosiderosis in regenerative nodules, with the exception of the left lower nodule (an iron-free focus). Type 1 HH is characterised by mutations in the *HFE* gene. C282Y and H63D mutations are the two most common allelic variants of *HFE* genes. The frequencies of C282Y homozygosity and heterozygosity in Europe are 0.4% and 9.2%, respectively. In the Asian, African, Middle Eastern, and Australasian populations, C282Y homozygotes are not found and C282Y heterozygotes are uncommon (up to 0.5%). The prevalence of both C282Y/H63D compound heterozygosity and H63D homozygosity in Europe is 2%. The carrier rate of H63D mutation is 22% in Europe.

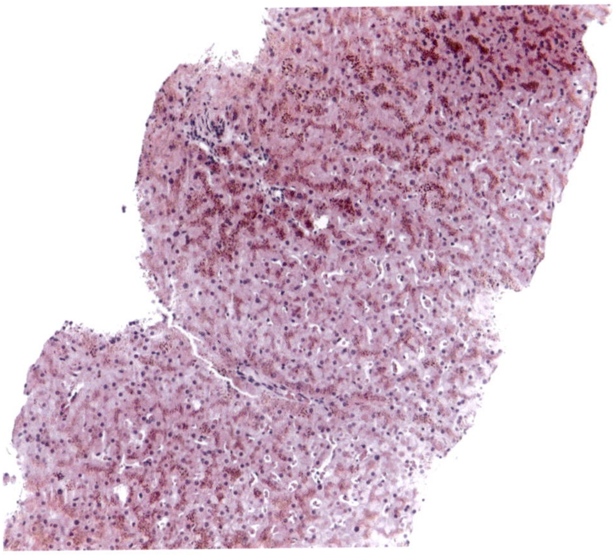

Fig. 4.4 Hereditary haemochromatosis. Marked (grade 4) haemosiderosis with pericanalicular accentuation is noted in hepatocytes. Excessive iron is deposited in hepatocytes and characteristically concentrated in the cytoplasm around bile canaliculi (parenchymal haemosiderosis). The haemosiderin deposition spreads from periportal to perivenular regions, initially with a decreasing gradient, but eventually there is a homogenous appearance. Apoptosis or spotty necrosis (so-called sideronecrosis) occurs as haemosiderin accumulates. Engulfment of the necrotic haemosiderin-laden hepatocytes by Kupffer cells may result in a mixed mesenchymal and parenchymal haemosiderosis. A small amount of haemosiderin also may be seen in portal macrophages and biliary epithelial cells. Progressive portal-based fibrosis may evolve to bridging fibrosis and cirrhosis with an apparent biliary-type pattern.

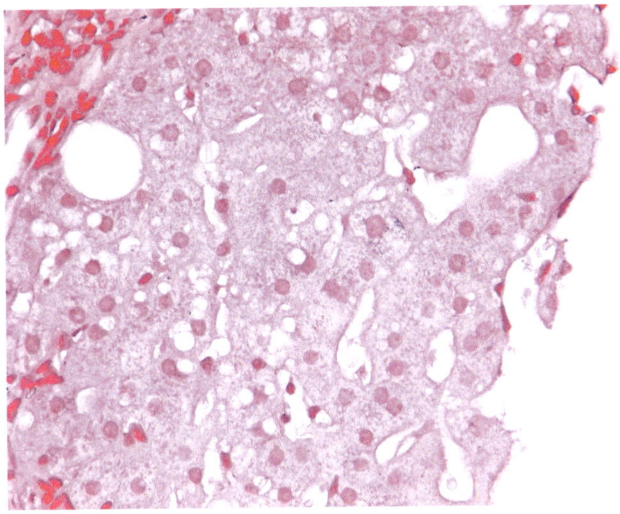

Fig. 4.6 Hereditary haemochromatosis following treatment with venesection. A single hepatocyte contains scanty residual haemosiderin. Regular venesection is the mainstay of treatment for HH; removing excessive iron prevents disease progression and most complications. The life expectancy of treated patients without cirrhosis or diabetes is similar to that of the general population. In livers of patients with successful venesection, the amount of stainable iron is markedly reduced and hepatic fibrosis (and even cirrhosis) may regress.

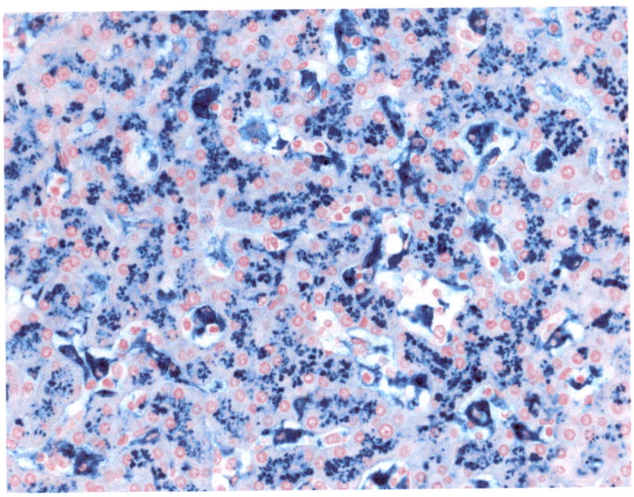

Fig. 4.5 Hereditary haemochromatosis (Perls stain). Marked (grade 4) haemosiderosis with pericanalicular accentuation is noted in hepatocytes. Kupffer cells also contain haemosiderin. All forms of HH, except type 4A, are characterised by predominantly hepatic parenchymal haemosiderosis. However, a mixed parenchymal and mesenchymal pattern commonly is found in later stages of HH with "sideronecrosis," bridging fibrosis, or cirrhosis.

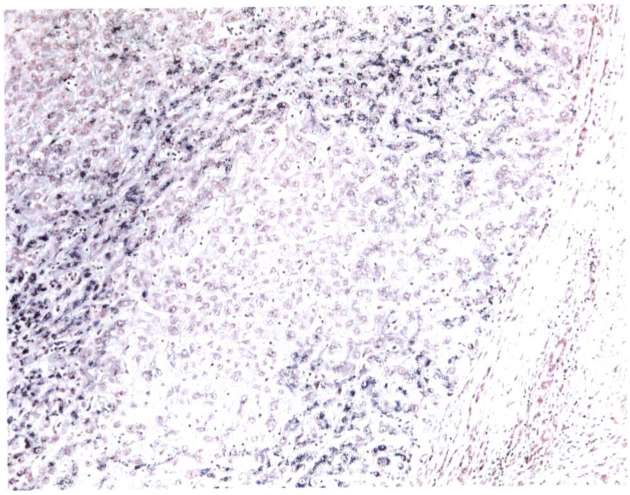

Fig. 4.7 Hereditary haemochromatosis with an iron-free focus. This focus is characterised by the absence of haemosiderin in hepatocytes. These cells are smaller, with a high nucleocytoplasmic ratio, features of concurrent small cell change. Iron-free foci in HH are more frequent in livers with HCC (50.0%) than those without (8.3%), and have a high proliferative index and coexisting large cell change/small cell change (71.4%). HCCs in HH are not uncommonly iron-free, and the sequential development from iron-free nodules to iron-free HCC in a recent rat model further supports the notion that iron-free foci are premalignant lesions. However, the underlying mechanisms of iron resistance in these foci and subsequent malignant transformation remain unknown.

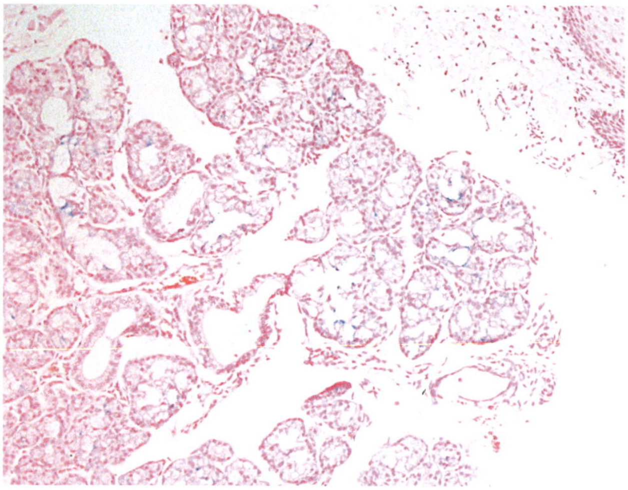

Fig. 4.8 Neonatal haemochromatosis (NH; Perls stain). Haemosiderosis is present in salivary gland epithelium. NH, or perinatal haemochromatosis, is an iron overload disorder with deposition of excessive iron in the liver and other organs, with a distribution similar to that found in HH. It presents with stillbirth or acute liver failure in the perinatal period. Its aetiology is uncertain. Despite a high recurrence rate in subsequent pregnancies and clustering in consanguineous families, suggesting that NH is a genetic disease, no candidate gene has been identified. NH currently is postulated to be a gestational alloimmune disorder. The diagnosis of NH is confirmed by the demonstration of excessive iron in the buccal salivary glands by biopsy, or in the liver, pancreas, and heart by MRI.

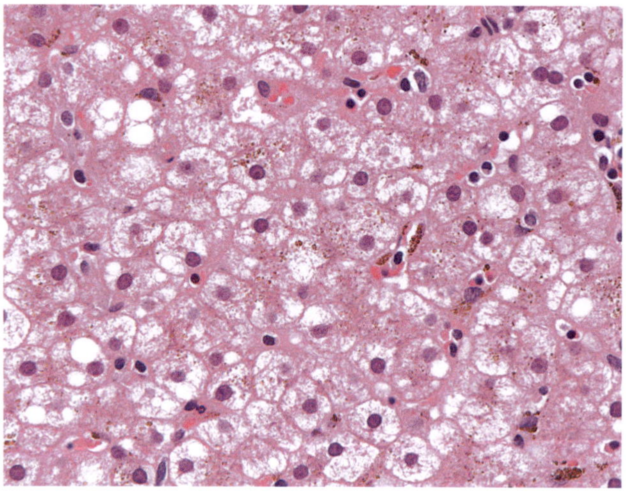

Fig. 4.9 Secondary iron overload. Brownish refractile, granular haemosiderin pigment is present in the hepatocytes and Kupffer cells in a patient with haemoglobin E disease. Secondary iron overload is associated with blood disorders (e.g., ineffective erythropoiesis, haemolysis, and sickle cell anaemia), transfusion, inflammatory syndromes, and various chronic liver diseases (e.g., chronic viral hepatitis, alcoholic liver disease, nonalcoholic steatohepatitis, Wilson disease, and porphyria cutanea tarda [PCT]).

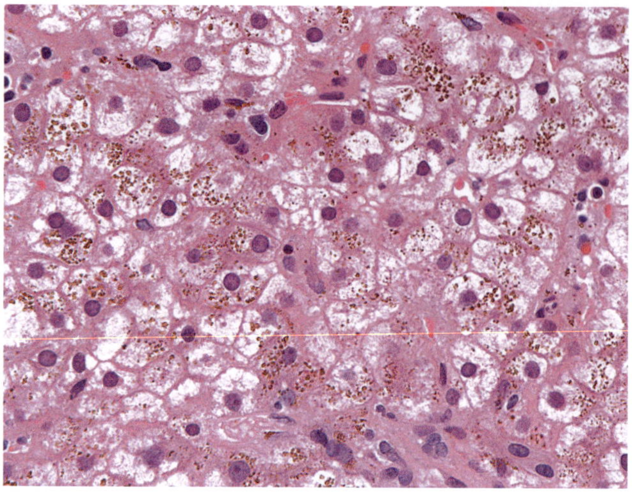

Fig. 4.10 Secondary iron overload. Here, the haemosiderin granules appear coarse and in many hepatocytes, are dispersed within the cytoplasm. Ineffective erythropoiesis is associated with a predominantly parenchymal pattern of iron overload. By contrast, multiple blood transfusions, haemolysis, and sickle cell anaemia lead to a primarily mesenchymal pattern of iron overload. In many cases of longstanding injury, there may be a mixed pattern.

4.2 Disorders of Copper Metabolism

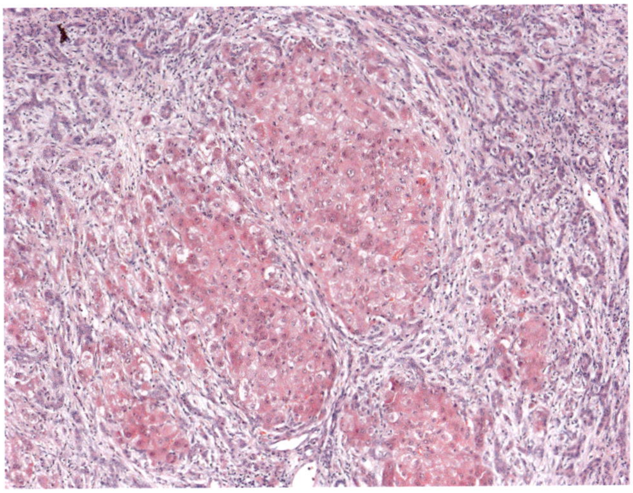

Fig. 4.11 Wilson disease. Regenerative nodules are seen, accompanied by a marked ductular reaction in a cirrhotic liver. Wilson disease is an autosomal recessive disorder of copper metabolism, with an incidence of 1:30,000. It is associated with mutations in the *ATP7B* gene on chromosome 13q14.3, which encodes a transmembrane transporter of copper in hepatocytes. It affects both sexes equally. Hepatic and neuropsychiatric manifestations are the commonest clinical presentations. Hepatic manifestations include asymptomatic liver function test abnormalities, fulminant hepatitis, chronic hepatitis, and cirrhosis, and may present in the second decade of life. Neuropsychiatric manifestations include parkinsonian symptoms and behavioural changes and occur 10 years later.

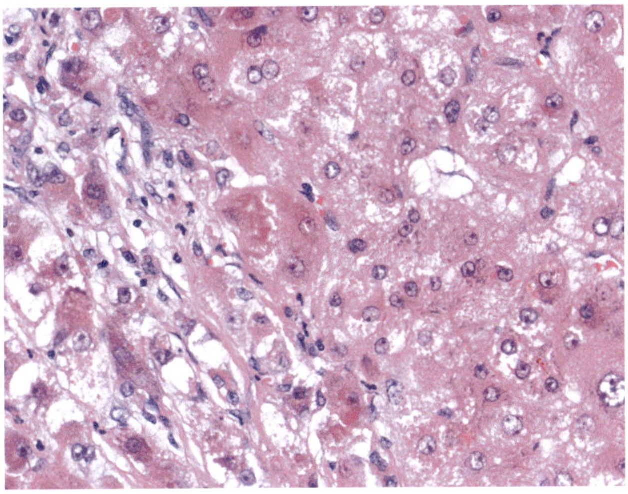

Fig. 4.13 Wilson disease. Hepatocytes at the periphery of a regenerative nodule exhibit ballooning degeneration and contain Mallory-Denk bodies. In later stages, a chronic hepatitic pattern becomes more prominent, with increased portal inflammation, mild interface hepatitis, and portal fibrosis. Periportal fibrosis, bridging fibrosis, and macronodular cirrhosis may occur as the disease progresses. In cirrhotic livers, periseptal hepatocytes may show prominent ballooning degeneration and contain Mallory-Denk bodies. Copper deposition may be demonstrated by histochemical stains directly (rhodanine and rubeanic acid) or indirectly (orcein or Victoria blue stain), but its distribution is heterogeneous, particularly in cirrhosis. Wilson disease with fulminant hepatitis is characterised pathologically by panacinar and multiacinar necrosis, indistinguishable from other causes of fulminant hepatitis.

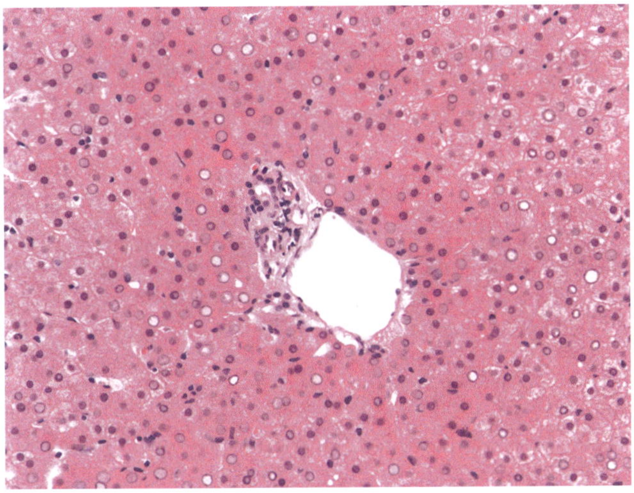

Fig. 4.12 Wilson disease. Periportal hepatocytes contain many glycogenated nuclei. Wilson disease is characterised biochemically by low serum caeruloplasmin, elevated urinary copper excretions, and an elevated hepatic copper concentration (>250 μg/g dry weight). Pathologic changes in early-stage Wilson disease include nonspecific hepatitic changes with spotty necrosis, apoptosis, and a mild portal lymphocytic infiltrate. Mild macrovesicular steatosis throughout the lobules and glycogenated nuclei in periportal hepatocytes often are found. Copper deposition typically is not demonstrable in the early stages. Note, however, that hepatic nuclear glycogenation is nonspecific and a common physiologic phenomenon in children and young adults.

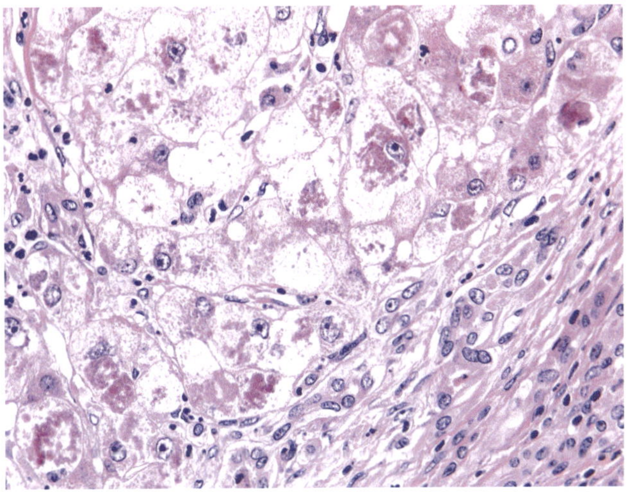

Fig. 4.14 Wilson disease. Periseptal hepatocytes in this case contain exuberant Mallory-Denk bodies. There are other rare disorders associated with copper overload. Collectively, they may be termed *non–Wilson disease copper toxicosis*, and they include Indian childhood cirrhosis, endemic Tyrolean infantile cirrhosis, and idiopathic copper toxicosis. These differ from Wilson disease by having normal/elevated serum caeruloplasmin levels and an absence of neuropsychiatric symptoms and Kayser-Fleischer rings.

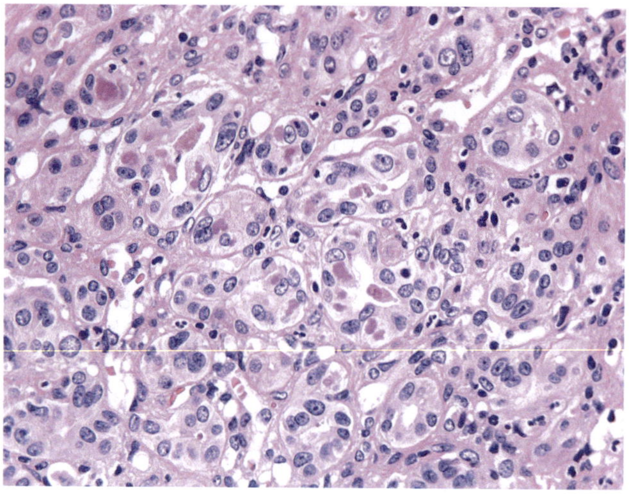

Fig. 4.15 Wilson disease. Mallory-Denk bodies also are present here, within the bile ductules. Periportal changes may be similar in Wilson disease and chronic cholestatic disease. Identification of distinctive biliary lesions (florid duct lesions in primary biliary cirrhosis and fibro-obliterative lesions in primary sclerosing cholangitis) and ductopaenia, together with clinical correlation, helps make the differentiation. Steatosis, glycogenated nuclei, and Mallory-Denk bodies may be present in both Wilson disease and steatohepatitis. The chronic hepatitic pattern of Wilson disease may mimic viral hepatitis and autoimmune hepatitis.

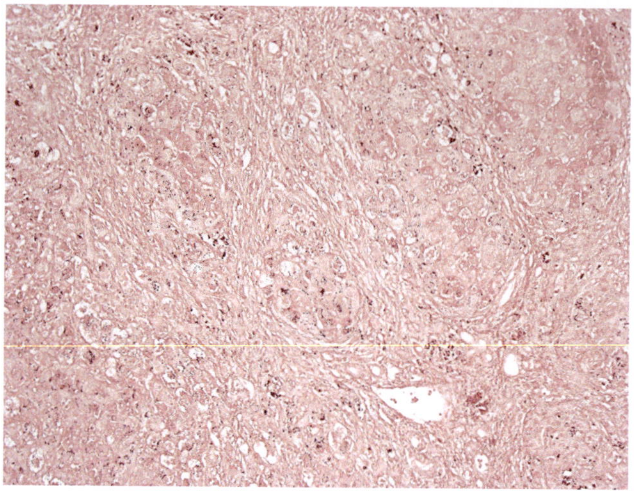

Fig. 4.16 Wilson disease (orcein stain). Numerous tiny deposits of copper-associated protein are seen in the hepatocytes. Negative staining for copper or copper-associated protein does not exclude the diagnosis of Wilson disease, because copper deposition typically is absent in the early stages and is heterogeneously distributed in the later stages. Clinical, biochemical, and genetic correlations are essential to establish the diagnosis. Dry weight measurement of copper also may help, but it must be noted that elevated levels also may be seen in chronic cholestatic diseases.

4.3 Disorders of Carbohydrate Metabolism

TYPE	EPONYM	PROTEIN DEFECT	LOCUS
0	-	Glycogen synthase	*GYS2* (12p12.1)
Ia	Von Gierke disease	Glucose-6-phosphatase	*G6PC* (17q21.31)
Ib	-	Glucose-6-phosphatase translocase	*SLC37A4* (11q23.3)
II	Pompe disease	Acid maltase	*GAA* (17q25.3)
III	Cori disease/ Forbe disease	Debranching enzyme	*AGL* (1p21.2)
IV	Andersen disease	Branching enzyme	*GBE1* (3p12.2)
VI	Hers disease	Liver phosphorylase E	*PYGL* (14q22.1)
IX	-	Liver phosphorylase kinase	*PHKA2* (Xp22.13) *PHKB* (16q12.1) *PHKG2* (16p11.2)
XI	Fanconi-Bickel syndrome	GLUT2 transporter	*SLC2A2* (3q26.2)

Fig. 4.17 Glycogen storage disease (GSD). This table summarises defective enzymes and gene loci of different types of GSDs that have hepatic manifestations. GSD, also known as glycogenosis, comprises a group of inherited disorders of glycogen metabolism leading to accumulation of excessive and abnormal glycogen. All forms, except some subtypes of GSD type IX (X-linked), are autosomal recessive. The clinical presentation and prognosis vary. The definitive diagnosis requires biochemical characterisation of the defective enzyme. Liver is the commonest organ involved in GSD, because it normally contains abundant glycogen.

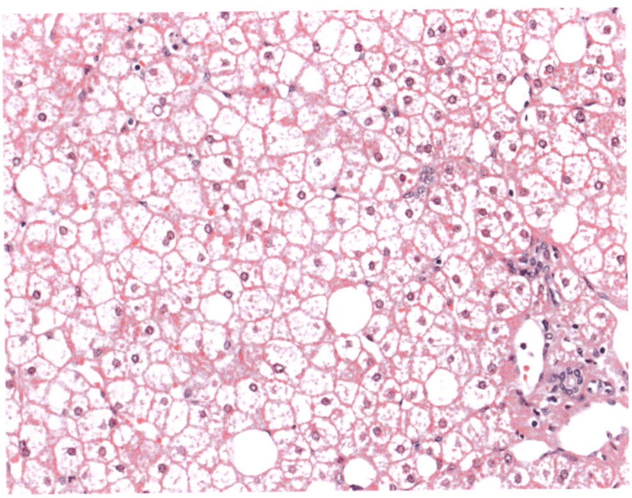

Fig. 4.18 Glycogen storage disease, type I. Glycogenic hepatocyte distension (GHD) is accompanied by the presence of glycogenated nuclei and mild macrovesicular steatosis. Prominent hepatocyte cell membranes and markedly compressed sinusoids produce a mosaic or plant-like morphology. Type I GSD is the commonest GSD, with an incidence of 1:100,000. It is associated with defects of glucose-6-phosphatsase (G6P; type Ia) and G6P translocase (type Ib). Hepatic pathologic changes include GHD, nuclear glycogenation, steatosis, peliosis, hepatocellular adenoma(–tosis), and carcinoma. GHD is characterised by marked enlargement of hepatocytes with cytoplasmic clearing by excessive accumulation of cytoplasmic glycogen.

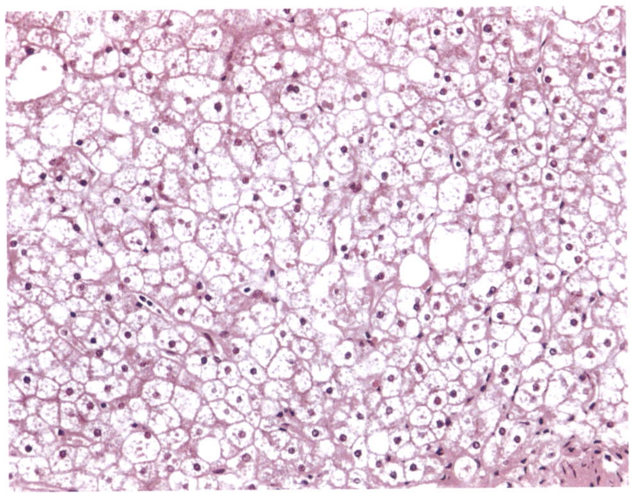

Fig. 4.19 Glycogen storage disease, type I. GHD is accompanied by mild macrovesicular steatosis. GHD with a mosaic pattern typically is uniform in type Ia and III GSDs but nonuniform in type Ib, VI, IX, and XI GSDs. As type II GSD is characterised by lysosomal accumulation of glycogen and lipid, hepatocytes are enlarged only slightly with pale, finely vacuolated cytoplasm. Hence, sinusoidal compression and a mosaic pattern typically are absent in type II GSD. However, glycogen-rich hepatocytes are not unique to GSD; they also are found in urea cycle defect and glycogenic hepatopathy in poorly controlled type 1 diabetes mellitus (Mauriac syndrome). Nuclear glycogenation and macrovesicular steatosis are more common in type I and III GSDs than other forms.

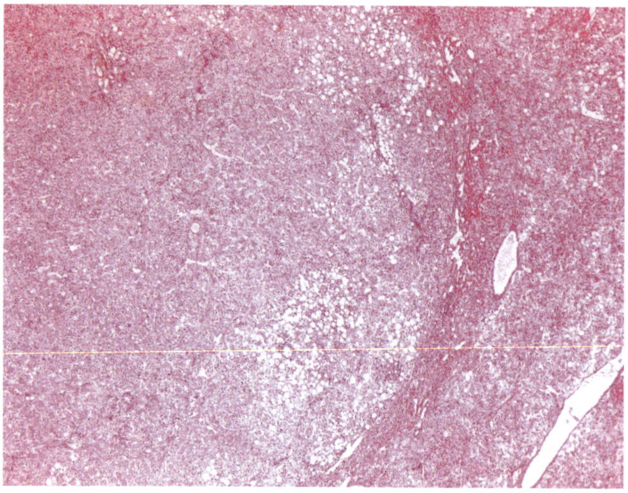

Fig. 4.20 Hepatocellular adenoma in type I glycogen storage disease. The development of hepatocellular adenomas is a feature of type Ia and III GSDs. It usually affects young patients, with a male-to-female ratio of 2:1, in contrast to the marked female predominance otherwise seen with hepatocellular adenoma. Most cases present in the second decade. Adenomatosis (10 or more adenomas) may occur. GSD-associated hepatocellular adenoma commonly is of the inflammatory sub-type, and is considered to be at risk of malignant transformation.

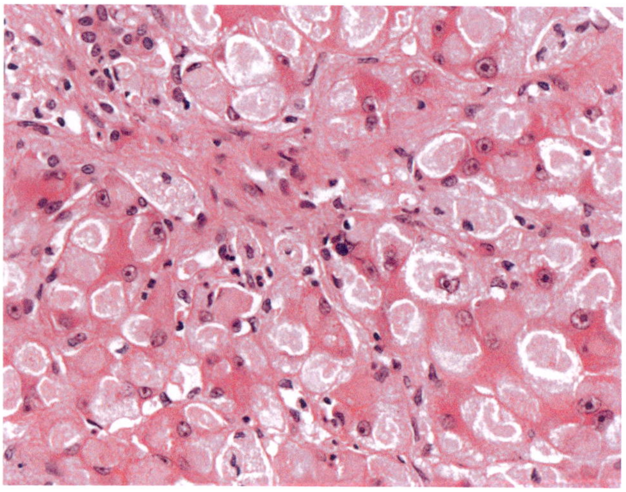

Fig. 4.21 Glycogen storage disease, type IV. Hepatocytes are enlarged and contain pale eosinophilic ground-glass–like intracytoplasmic inclusions with an occasional surrounding clear halo. Type IV GSD is rare and associated with a defective branching enzyme (amylo-1,4 glycan 6-glycosyltransferase). Its pathologic feature is completely different from that of other GSDs and is characterised by the presence of unusual intracytoplasmic inclusions. These are periodic acid-Schiff (PAS) positive and diastase resistant.

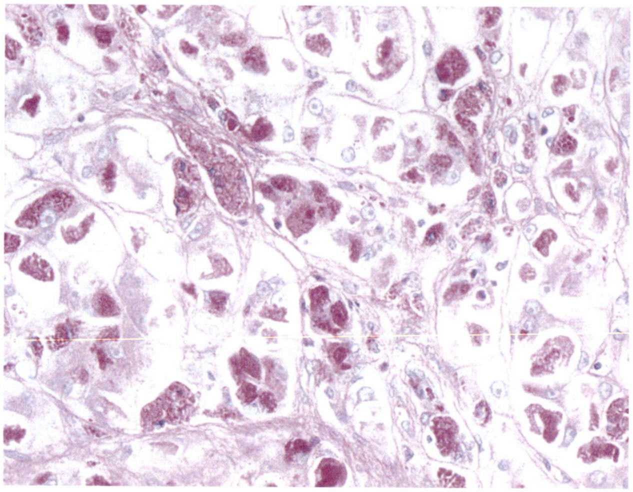

Fig. 4.22 Glycogen storage disease, type IV (PAS stain with diastase [PASD]). The ground-glass–like intracytoplasmic inclusions are seen here to be PAS positive and diastase resistant. These characteristic inclusions should be differentiated from inclusions in chronic hepatitis B, Lafora disease, cyanamide-induced injury, and immunocompromised patients on multiple medications. Ground-glass hepatocytes in chronic hepatitis B typically are reactive with orcein, Victoria blue, and immunostaining for hepatitis B surface antigen. Inclusions in Lafora disease are PAS positive but diastase sensitive.

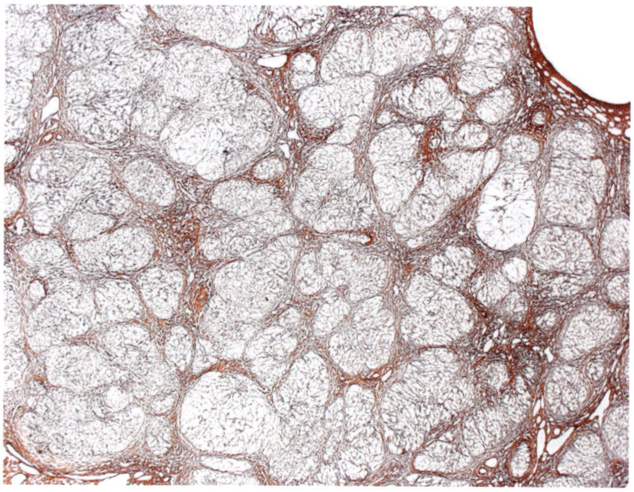

Fig. 4.23 Glycogen storage disease, type IV (Gordon-Sweets reticulin stain). Cirrhosis is evident by multiple regenerative nodules separated by fibrous septa. Portal fibrosis with progression to bridging fibrosis and cirrhosis frequently is present in type IV GSD, but is seen less commonly in types III and IX and is absent in other types.

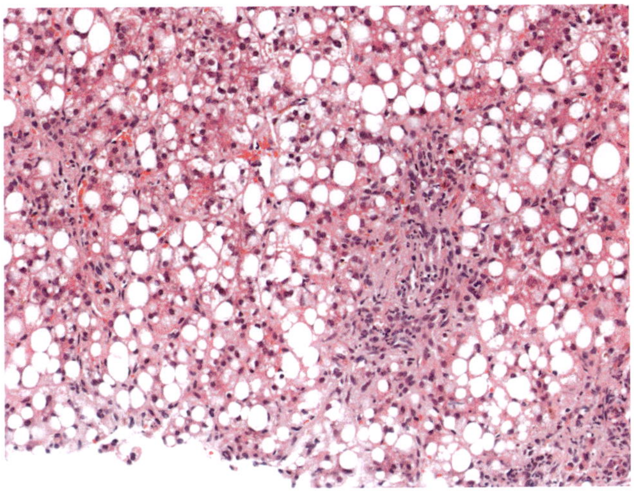

Fig. 4.24 Galactosaemia. Severe macrovesicular steatosis is present. A mild ductular reaction is found in the portal tracts. Galactosaemia is an autosomal recessive disorder of galactose metabolism with an incidence of 1:45,000. It is associated with mutation in the *GALT* gene on chromosome 9p13, encoding galactose-1-phosphate uridyl transferase. It affects both sexes equally and usually presents in the neonatal period. Failure to thrive, vomiting, diarrhoea, jaundice, liver dysfunction, hepatosplenomegaly, hypoglycaemia, sepsis, cataract, renal tubular dysfunction, and muscle hypotonia may be early clinical manifestations after ingestion of galactose. Late complications include mental retardation, dyspraxia, motor abnormality, and hypogonadism. The definitive diagnosis requires biochemical enzyme assay or genetic testing.

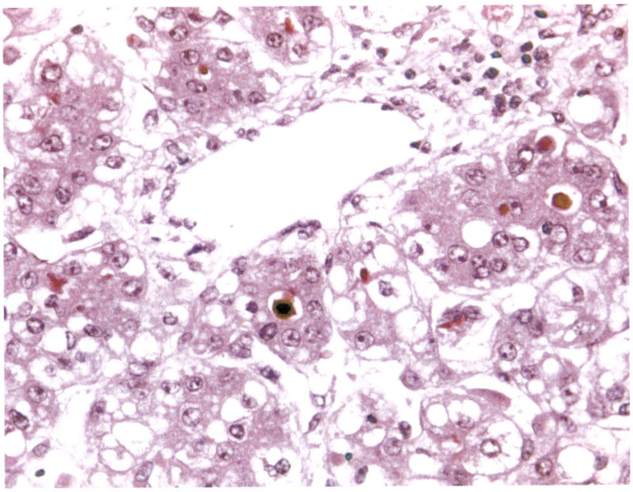

Fig. 4.25 Galactosaemia. Hepatocyte rosettes are accompanied by canalicular bilirubinostasis and steatosis, seen here in a perivenular region. Pathologic features of galactosaemia in the liver are quite distinctive but not entirely specific. Marked steatosis, ductular reaction, and ductular cholestasis occur within 2 weeks after birth. Prominent formation of hepatocyte rosettes with or without canalicular bilirubinostasis occurs from 2 weeks of age and is fully developed by 6 weeks. Portal and periportal fibrosis may occur from as early as 2 weeks and progresses to cirrhosis by 3 to 6 months in untreated cases. Giant cell transformation also may be found. The differential diagnosis of galactosaemia includes hereditary fructose intolerance and hereditary tyrosinaemia.

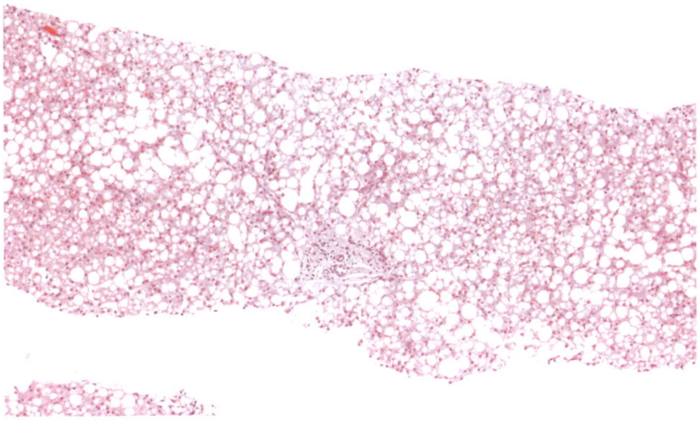

Fig. 4.26 Hereditary fructose intolerance. Marked steatosis is present throughout this core liver biopsy. Hereditary fructose intolerance is an autosomal recessive disorder of fructose metabolism with an incidence of 1:26,000. It is associated with a mutation in the *ALDOB* gene on chromosome 9q21.3-22.2, encoding aldolase B (fructose-1,6-biphosphatase). It affects both sexes equally and usually presents in infancy at the time of milk weaning. Hypoglycaemia, vomiting, and abdominal pain after fructose ingestion are common. Long-term exposure to fructose leads to hepatosplenomegaly, liver failure, cirrhosis, renal tubular dysfunction, and growth retardation. Patients who survive beyond infancy develop an aversion to sweets and fruits. The definitive diagnosis requires biochemical enzyme assay or genetic testing.

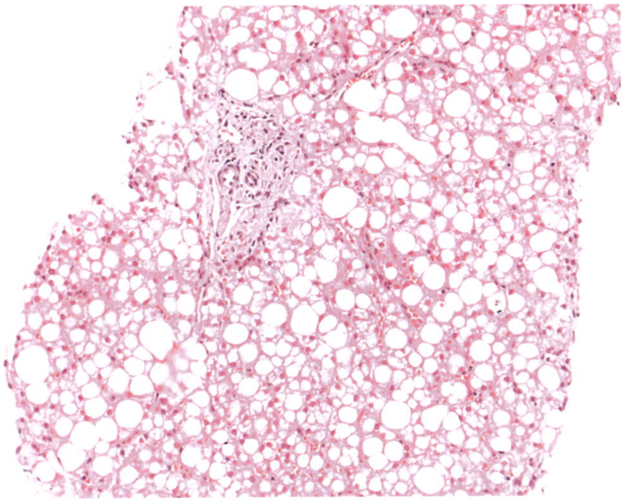

Fig. 4.27 Hereditary fructose intolerance. Pathologic features of hereditary fructose intolerance in the liver are nonspecific and include neonatal hepatitis with giant cell transformation, steatosis, canalicular bilirubinostasis, and ductular reaction. Portal and pericellular fibrosis may occur, but progression to cirrhosis is rare. Differential diagnoses of hereditary fructose intolerance are galactosaemia and other metabolic disorders manifesting with steatosis.

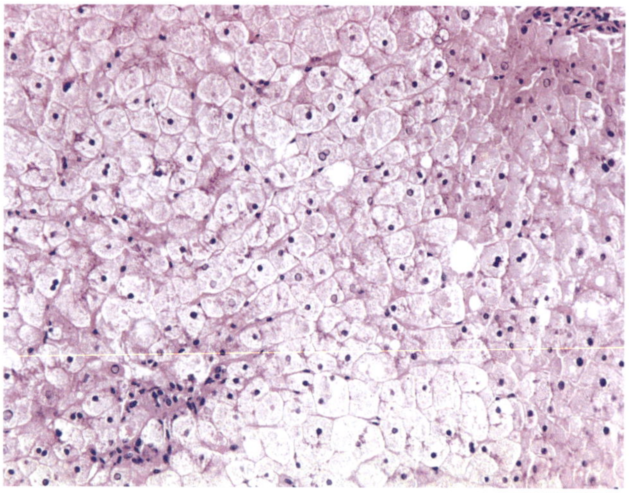

Fig. 4.28 Mauriac syndrome. GHD is noted, with marked enlargement of hepatocytes, which have a pale cytoplasm due to excessive accumulation of glycogen. Few glycogenated nuclei are seen. Mauriac syndrome is a rare complication in some paediatric patients with poorly controlled type 1 diabetes mellitus and is characterised by hepatomegaly, growth retardation, and cushingoid features. In contrast to type 2 diabetes mellitus, which is associated with nonalcoholic fatty liver disease, poorly controlled diabetes mellitus leads to glycogenic hepatopathy.

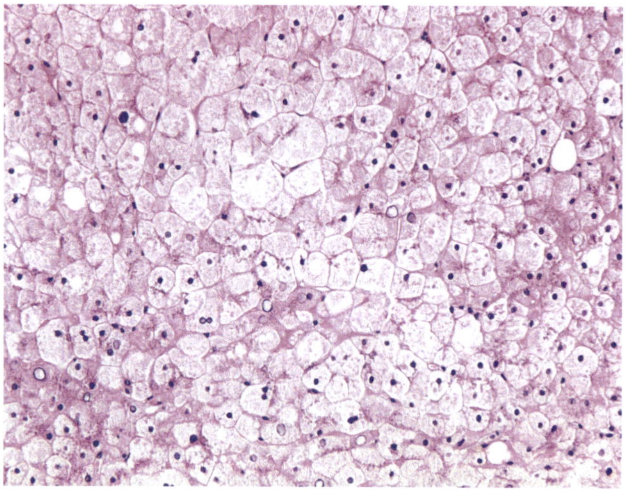

Fig. 4.29 Mauriac syndrome. GHD is marked by enlargement of hepatocytes with pale cytoplasm by excessive accumulation of cytoplasmic glycogen. A few glycogenated nuclei are found. GHD is not specific to glycogenic hepatopathy in Mauriac syndrome; it also is present in GSD and urea cycle defect.

4.4 Endoplasmic Reticulum Storage Disorders

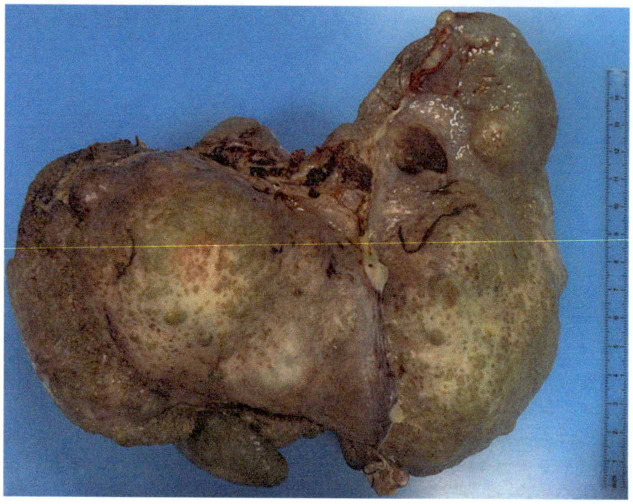

Fig. 4.30 α_1-Antitrypsin (A1AT) deficiency. A cirrhotic liver is markedly distorted by multiple large regenerative nodules. A1AT deficiency is an autosomal recessive disorder associated with mutations of the *SERPINA1* gene on chromosome 14q32.1, encoding A1AT. A1AT, the commonest serum protease inhibitor (Pi), is crucial in controlling protease-mediated tissue degradation. More than 100 allelic variants of A1AT have been described. PiM is the commonest allele, and homozygous PiMM status is found in 95% of the world's population. Two common deficiency alleles are PiZ and PiS. Patients with homozygous PiZZ and PiSS and heterozygous PiMZ and PiSZ status may develop pulmonary emphysema and liver disease. Hepatic manifestations include neonatal cholestasis, chronic hepatitis, and cirrhosis. HCC develops in up to 15% of cases.

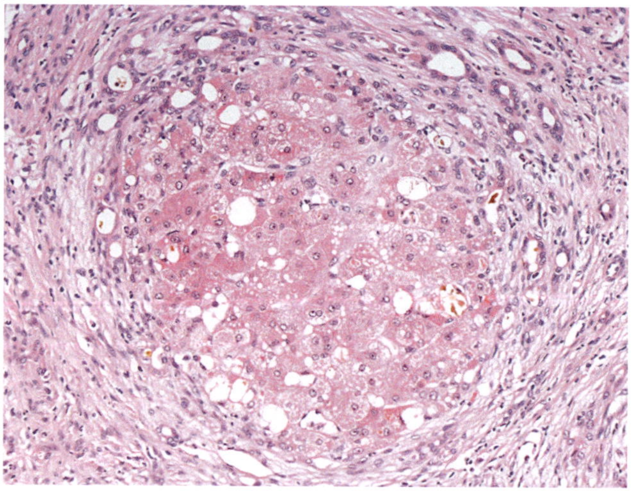

Fig. 4.31 α_1-Antitrypsin deficiency. Steatosis and bilirubinostasis are present in a regenerative nodule. A moderate ductular reaction surrounds the regenerative nodule. A1AT deficiency shows marked racial differences in incidence, with 1:2,000 to 5,000 in the Caucasian population, but it is virtually absent in Asian and African populations. It affects both sexes equally. The serum A1AT level typically is low but may be normal in infection or inflammatory conditions, as A1AT is an acute-phase protein. Demonstration of an abnormal allelic variant by electrophoresis or genetic testing is confirmatory.

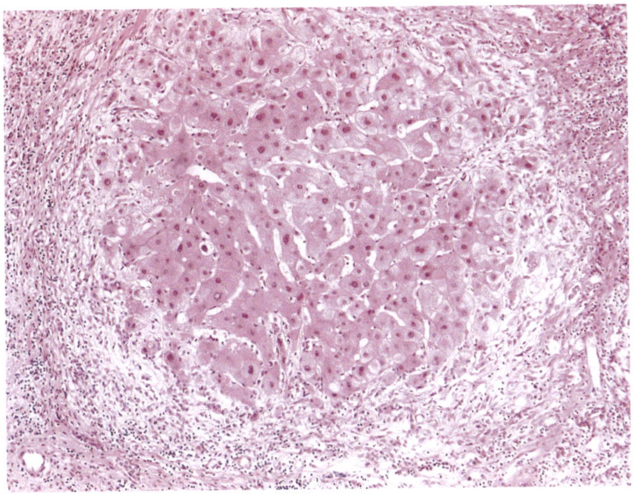

Fig. 4.32 α_1-Antitrypsin deficiency. In a regenerative nodule, some periseptal hepatocytes appear pale. These pale hepatocytes contain eosinophilic globular intracytoplasmic inclusions, which are visualized at higher magnification. Accumulation of A1AT globules, particularly in periportal or periseptal hepatocytes, is characteristic of A1AT deficiency. On haematoxylin and eosin (H&E) section, these globules are eosinophilic globular intracytoplasmic inclusions, which are intensely positive on PAS and diastase resistant. Immunohistochemistry is more specific and helps highlight small inconspicuous globules. These globules are variably sized, but their amount and size increase with age. Absence of A1AT globules in infants younger than 3 months does not exclude the diagnosis of A1AT deficiency, because these globules may not be sufficiently well-developed to be demonstrated, even by immunostaining.

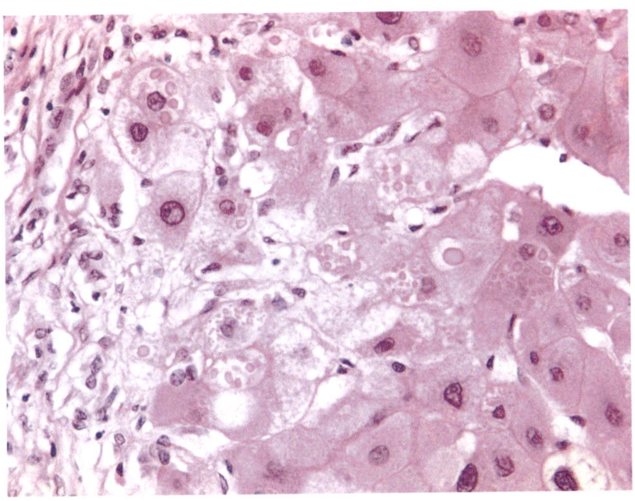

Fig. 4.33 α_1-Antitrypsin deficiency. Periseptal hepatocytes contain eosinophilic globular intracytoplasmic inclusions of variable size. The presence of small amounts of A1AT in hepatocytes is not highly specific and may be found in cirrhosis of other causes and in critically ill elderly patients with high serum A1AT levels. A1AT inclusions should be differentiated from other eosinophilic intracytoplasmic inclusions. α_1-Antichromotrypsin (A1ACT) appears finely granular rather than discretely globular in H&E sections, weakly positive on PASD stain, and immunoreactive to A1ACT. So-called pale bodies vary from lightly to deeply eosinophilic on H&E section and are immunoreactive to fibrinogen.

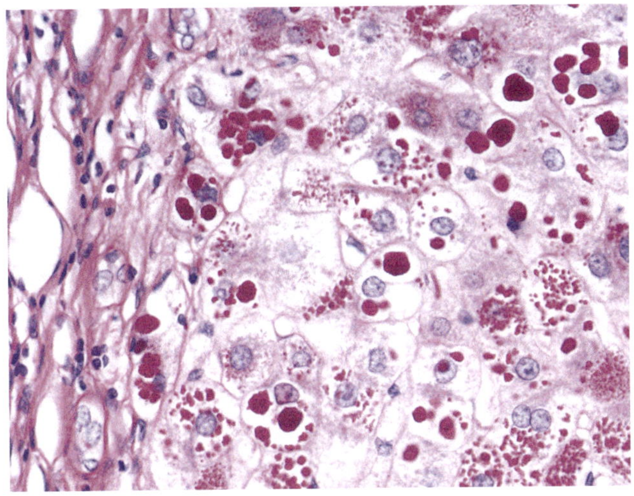

Fig. 4.34 α_1-Antitrypsin deficiency (PASD stain). A1AT inclusions are intensively positive on PAS and diastase resistant, but this depends on the variant, as globules are not seen in the PiSS or PiMS variants. In patients who present early with neonatal jaundice or hepatitis, there are different pathologic manifestations, including a parenchymal hepatitic pattern (bilirubinostasis, mild lobular disarray, hepatocyte rosettes with or without giant cell transformation), a biliary atresia–like pattern (bilirubinostasis and ductular reaction) with a paucity of intrahepatic bile ducts (ductopaenia and chronic cholate stasis may occur in up to 10% of cases), or a combination of these patterns. Mild periportal steatosis and varying degrees of fibrosis usually are present. In patients who present later in childhood or in adulthood, the pathologic manifestation usually is a chronic hepatitic pattern or cirrhosis.

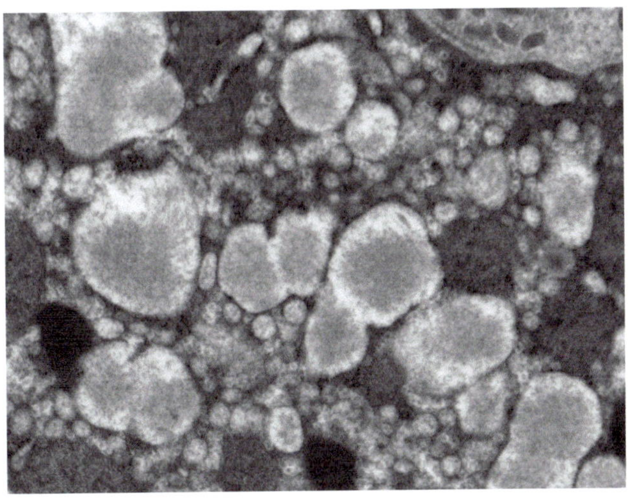

Fig. 4.35 α_1-Antitrypsin deficiency (transmission electron microscopy). The lumina of the endoplasmic reticulum are distended by aggregates of electron-dense amorphous material. A1AT deficiency is one of the hepatic endoplasmic reticulum storage diseases, which also include A1ACT deficiency, afibrinogenaemia, and hypofibrinogenaemia. All are characterised by their intracytoplasmic inclusions. A1ACT inclusions appear finely granular rather than discretely globular on H&E section, weakly positive on PASD stain, and immunoreactive to A1ACT.

4.5 Disorders of Amino Acid Metabolism

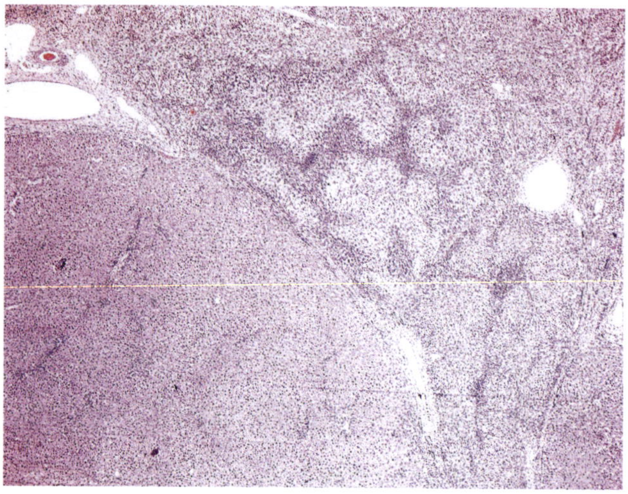

Fig. 4.36 Hereditary tyrosinaemia. A low-grade dysplastic nodule (*lower left*) is present. Hereditary tyrosinaemia, also known as tyrosinaemia type I, is an autosomal recessive disorder of tyrosine metabolism. The worldwide incidence is 1:120,000, whereas the incidence in Quebec is 1:17,000. It is associated with mutation of the *FAH* gene on chromosome 15q23-25, encoding fumarylacetoacetate hydrolase. It affects both sexes equally. The clinical presentation is heterogeneous, even within the same family, and varies from failure to thrive, to acute liver failure, cirrhosis, HCC, renal tubular dysfunction, hypophosphataemic rickets, and peripheral neuropathy. Liver and neurologic crises often are precipitated by sepsis. Demonstration of succinylacetone, a metabolite of tyrosine, in urine and serum is diagnostic.

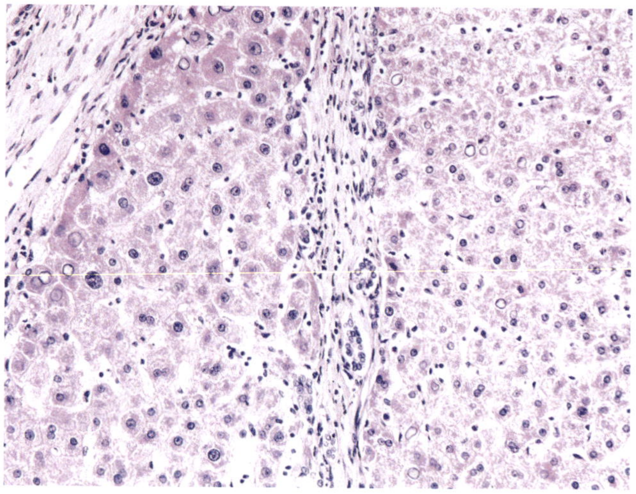

Fig. 4.38 Hereditary tyrosinaemia. Large cell change (*left*) is seen with cellular and nuclear enlargement, nuclear pleomorphism and hyperchromasia, and prominent nucleoli, but a preserved nucleocytoplasmic ratio. Seen elsewhere in this specimen was a well-differentiated HCC.

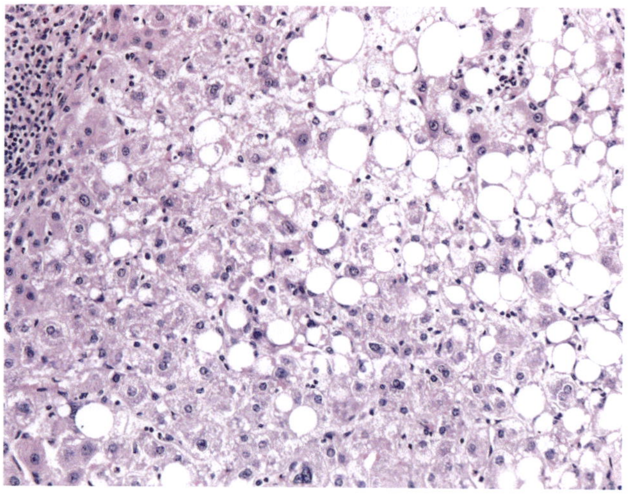

Fig. 4.37 Hereditary tyrosinaemia. Moderate macrovesicular steatosis is accompanied by a mild sinusoidal inflammatory infiltrate and moderate septal inflammation. Pathologic features in infants with hereditary tyrosinaemia include steatosis, lobular disarray, formation of hepatocyte rosettes with or without canalicular bilirubinostasis, giant cell transformation, and parenchymal haemosiderosis. Portal and periportal fibrosis is present early, even in the intrauterine period, and progresses rapidly to cirrhosis. Large cell change, small cell change, and dysplastic nodules are common. Malignant transformation to HCC occurs in 10% to 37% of cases. Differential diagnoses of hereditary tyrosinaemia include galactosaemia and neonatal hepatitis of other causes.

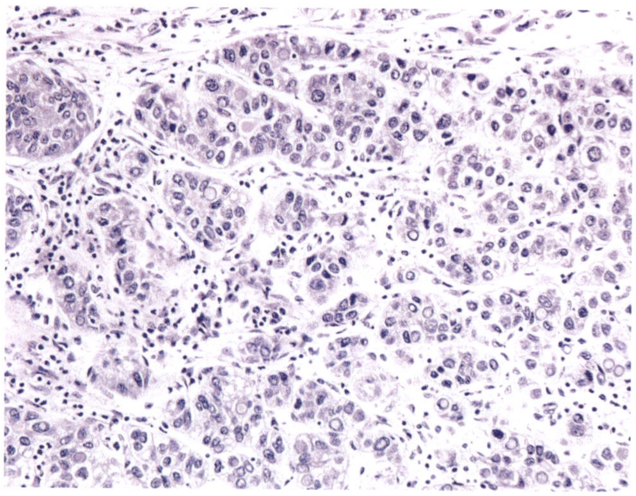

Fig. 4.39 Hereditary tyrosinaemia. Malignant transformation to HCC is evident with thickened trabeculae and nests of malignant tumour cells. HCC is known to be associated with certain metabolic diseases, including hereditary tyrosinaemia, HH, and A1AT deficiency. Malignant transformation from hepatocellular adenomatosis in type I and III GSDs is well documented. Rare cases of HCC arising in porphyria, cystinosis, hereditary fructose intolerance, Wilson disease, and type 1 progressive familial intrahepatic cholestasis (PFIC) also have been reported.

DISEASE	PROTEIN DEFECT	LOCUS
Carbamoylphosphate synthetase I deficiency	Carbamoylphosphate synthetase I	*CPS1* (2q34)
Ornithine transcarbamylase deficiency	Ornithine transcarbamylase	*OTC* (Xp11.4)
Citrullinaemia type I	Argininosuccinic acid synthetase	*ASS1* (9q34.11)
Argininosuccinic aciduria	Argininosuccinate lyase	*ASL* (7q11.21)
Argininaemia	Arginase	*ARG1* (6q23.2)
N-acetylglutamate synthetase deficiency	N-acetylglutamate synthetase	*NAGS* (17q21.31)
Hyperornithinaemia-hyperammonaemia-homocitrullinuria syndrome	Ornithine transporter	*SLC25A15* (13q14.11)
Citrullinaemia type II	Citrin	*SLC25A13* (7q21.3)

Fig. 4.40 Urea cycle defects and related diseases. This table summarizes defective enzymes/transporters and gene loci of different forms of urea cycle defect and related diseases. Urea cycle defects are inherited disorders associated with defective enzymes of urea cycle metabolism leading to hyperammonaemia and encephalopathy. There are two closely related inherited disorders associated with defective transporters (ornithine transporter and citrin) in the urea cycle. Ornithine transcarbamylase deficiency is X-linked, whereas all others are autosomal recessive. Early presentation in the neonatal period is common and presents initially with irritability, vomiting, lethargy, and respiratory distress. Muscle hypotonia, seizures, coma, and respiratory arrest may occur.

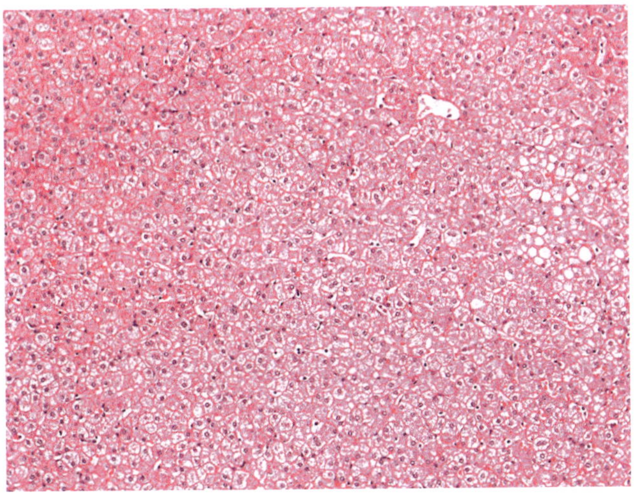

Fig. 4.41 Urea cycle defect. Mild macrovesicular steatosis is present. Microscopic appearances of the liver in urea cycle defect depend on the clinical condition of the patient (e.g., hyperammonaemic crisis) rather than on the particular enzyme defect. It may be normal or show varying degrees of steatosis, glycogen-rich hepatocytes, lobular disarray, portal inflammation, interface hepatitis, and portal fibrosis. Glycogen-rich hepatocytes may be focal or diffuse, the latter resembling nonlysosomal GSDs. Necroinflammation usually is minimal, but portal fibrosis may progress to bridging fibrosis and cirrhosis.

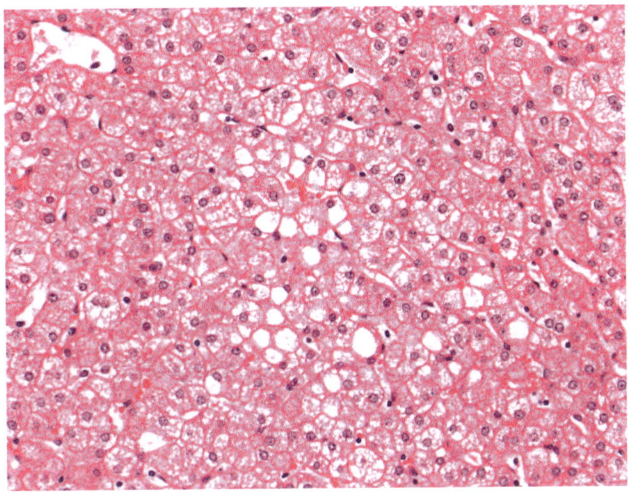

Fig. 4.42 Urea cycle defects. Mild macrovesicular steatosis is accompanied by some hepatocytes with pale or clear cytoplasm.

4.6 Lysosomal Storage Disorders

DISEASE	PROTEIN DEFECT & LOCUS	STORAGE MATERIAL
SPHINGOLIPIDOSIS		
Gaucher disease	Acid beta-glucosidase (*GBA*, 1q22)	Glucosylceramide
Niemann-Pick A & B	Sphingomyelin phosphodiesterase 1 (*SMPD1*, 11p15.4)	Sphingomyelin
Farber lipogranulomatosis	Acid ceramidase (*ASAH1*, 8p22)	Ceramide
GM1 gangliosidosis	Acid beta-galactosidase (GLB1, 3p22.3)	GM1 ganglioside
CHOLESTEROL TRANSPORT DEFECT		
Niemann-Pick C	Niemann-Pick proteins (*NPC1*, 18q11.2; *NPC2*, 14q24.3)	Cholesterol & lipid
CHOLESTEROL ESTER STORAGE DISEASE		
Wolman disease/ Cholesterol ester storage disease	Acid lipase (*LIPA*, 10q23.31)	Cholesterol ester & triglyceride
GLYCOGEN STORAGE DISEASE		
Pompe disease	Acid maltase (*GAA*, 17q25.3)	Glycogen
GLYCOPROTEIN STORAGE DISEASE		
Galactosialidosis	Cathespin A (*CTSA*, 20q13.12)	Ganglioside & sialic acid-rich Oligosaccharide, glycolipid & glycoprotein
MUCOLIPIDIOSIS		
Mucolipidosis, types II (I-cell disease) & III (Pseudo-Hurler polydystrophy)	N-acetylglucosamine-1-phosphate transferase (*GNPTAB*, 12q23.2)	Oligosaccharide, glycosaminoglycan & lipid

Fig. 4.43 Lysosomal storage diseases. This table summarises the lysosomal storage diseases in which there is significant hepatic involvement. Lysosomal storage diseases comprise a heterologous group of more than 40 inherited diseases associated with defective lysosomal proteins responsible for the metabolism of lipid, glycoprotein, or mucopolysaccharide. Although the incidence of the entire group is about 1:5,000 to 1:10,000, individual disease generally is rare, with an incidence of fewer than 1:100,000. Most of these diseases are autosomal recessive, but a few of them are X-linked (e.g., Hurler disease and Fabry disease). There are other lysosomal storage diseases with less significant hepatic involvement, such as various mucopolysaccharidoses, Fabry disease (defective α-galactosidase A; *GLA* on Xq22.1), fucosidosis (defective α-L-fucosidase; *FUC1A* on 1p36.11), α-mannosidosis (defective α-mannosidase; *MAN2B1* on 19p13.2), and neuraminidase deficiency (defective neuraminidase; *NEU1* on 6p21.33).

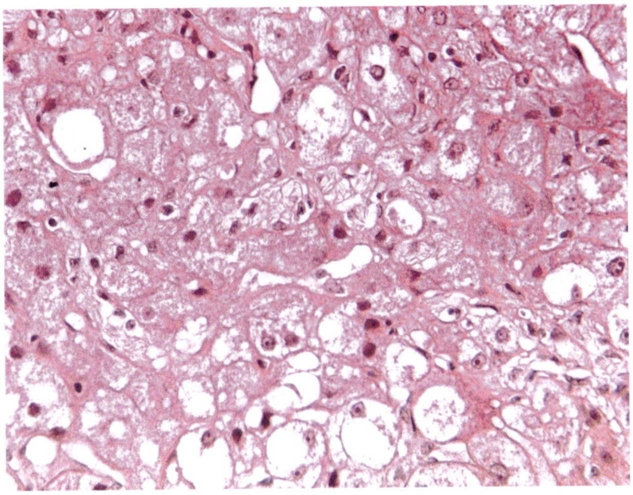

Fig. 4.44 Gaucher disease. Hypertrophied Kupffer cells show a characteristic striated or wrinkled cytoplasm. Gaucher disease is the commonest lysosomal storage disease and is related to lysosomal accumulation of glucosylceramide (glucocerebroside), mainly in macrophages. It is an autosomal recessive disease associated with the mutation of the *GBA* gene on chromosome 1q22, encoding acid β-glucosidase. There are three major clinical phenotypes with different racial predilections, onsets, clinical manifestations, and prognoses. Hepatomegaly is present in all three types, whereas neurodegeneration is confined to types 2 and 3. The confirmatory diagnosis requires biochemical enzyme assay of acid β-glucosidase.

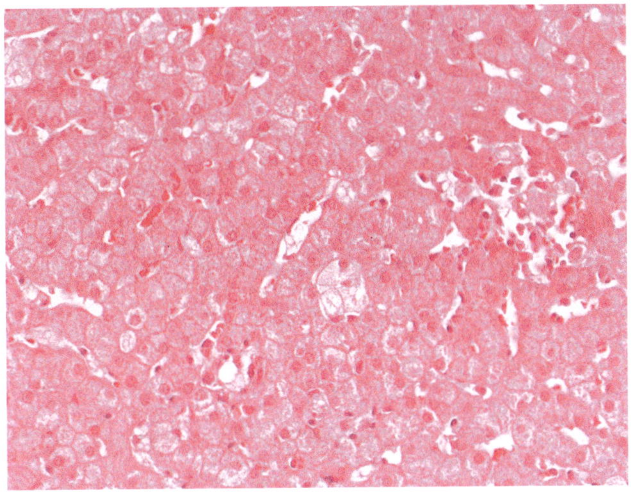

Fig. 4.46 Niemann-Pick disease, type C. Occasional foamy macrophage cells are present. Niemann-Pick disease comprises a group of autosomal recessive diseases and may be classified into types A, B, and C. Types A and B are associated with the mutation of the *SMPD1* gene on chromosome 11p15.4, encoding sphingomyelin phosphodiesterase 1. Type A begins in utero and presents soon after birth with hepatosplenomegaly, lymphadenopathy, and macular cherry-red spots. Progressive neurodegeneration with seizures is typical. It usually is fatal before the age of 5. Type B is characterised by hepatosplenomegaly and deteriorating pulmonary function. Type C is linked to the mutation of the *NPC1* or *NPC2* gene on chromosome 18q11.2 or 14q24.3, leading to lysosomal accumulation of cholesterol and lipid. It may present at any age with milder degrees of hepatosplenomegaly and neurodegeneration.

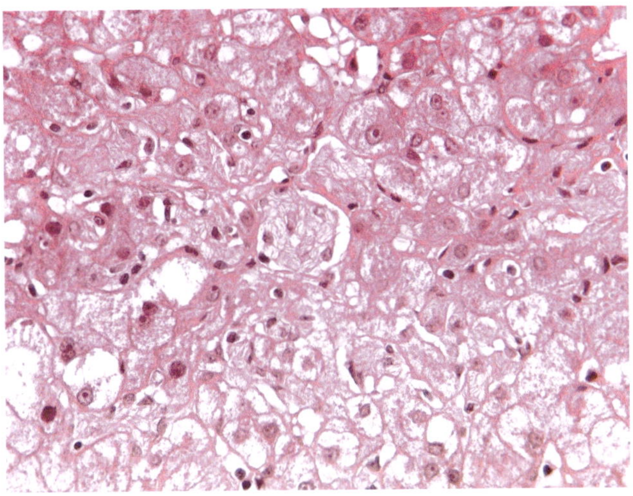

Fig. 4.45 Gaucher disease. The diagnostic hallmark of Gaucher disease is the presence of macrophages filled with glucosylceramide, imparting a striated or wrinkled cytoplasm, and pyknotic nuclei. The striations are better visualized on Masson trichrome or PAS stain. Hepatic sinusoids generally are distended by these so-called Gaucher cells and often accompanied by varying degrees of pericellular fibrosis and hepatocyte atrophy. The pericellular fibrosis may progress to bridging fibrosis and cirrhosis. Pseudo-Gaucher cells are found in many haematologic diseases, including leukaemia, Hodgkin and non-Hodgkin lymphoma, multiple myeloma, myelodysplastic syndrome, and thalassemia; these may not always be readily distinguished from Gaucher cells in H&E sections.

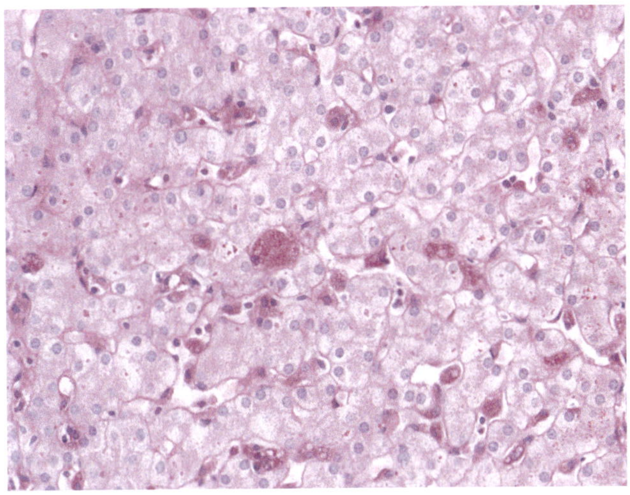

Fig. 4.47 Niemann-Pick disease, type C (PASD stain). Scattered hypertrophied Kupffer cells with lipid vacuoles are present. The accumulation of hypertrophied Kupffer cells with foamy, microvesicular cytoplasm is characteristic of Niemann-Pick disease but may be less obvious in type C disease. Hepatocytes with fine cytoplasmic vacuolation may be found in type A and B disease. As with Gaucher disease, varying degrees of pericellular fibrosis and hepatocyte atrophy may occur, with possible progression to bridging fibrosis and cirrhosis.

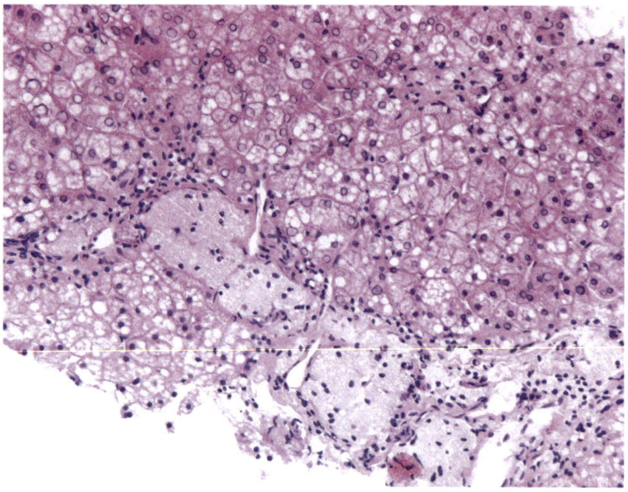

Fig. 4.48 Cholesterol ester storage disease (CESD). Microvesicular steatosis is seen here associated with hypertrophied sinusoidal and portal macrophages, which have an amphophilic foamy cytoplasm. Wolman disease and CESD are caused by lysosomal accumulation of cholesterol ester and triglyceride, mainly in macrophages. They are autosomal recessive disorders associated with mutations of the *LIPA* gene on chromosome 10q23.31, encoding lysosomal acid lipase. Wolman disease is an infantile-onset disorder with multiple organ involvement and normally is fatal in the first year of life. CESD is a milder, later-onset form with primarily hepatic involvement. It usually presents with hepatosplenomegaly, liver dysfunction, and premature atherosclerosis.

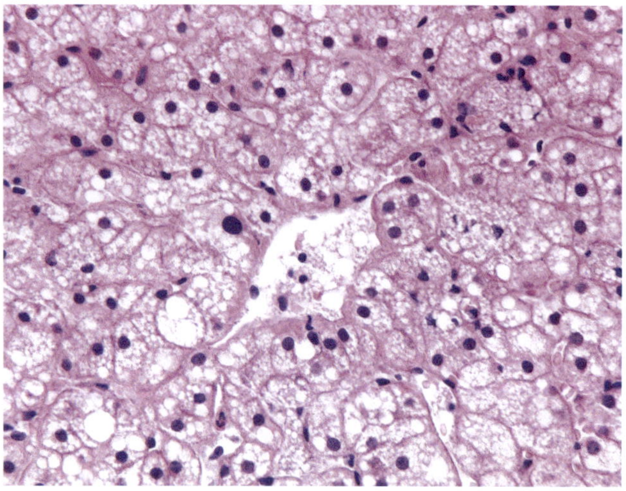

Fig. 4.49 Cholesterol ester storage disease. Diffuse microvesicular steatosis is present. The characteristic pathologic feature of CESD and Wolman disease is the presence of hypertrophied Kupffer cells and portal macrophages with amphophilic foamy cytoplasm. These Kupffer cells and portal macrophages are distended by cholesterol esters, which may appear as silvery birefringent crystals under polarized light. Marked steatosis and varying degrees of portal and periportal fibrosis usually are present. Progression to cirrhosis is rare.

4.7 Primary Mitochondrial Hepatopathy

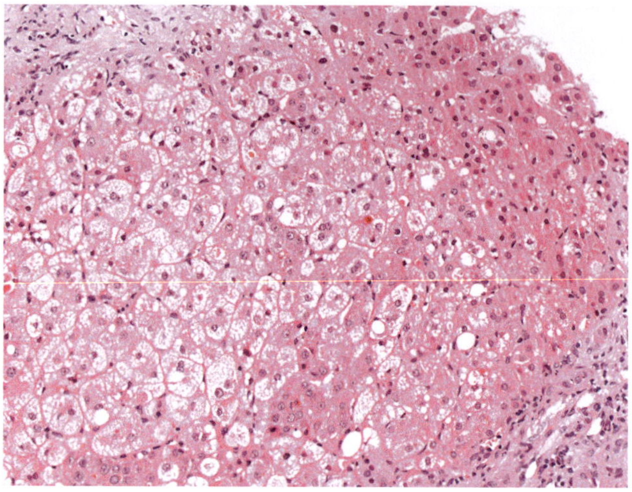

Fig. 4.50 Primary mitochondrial hepatopathy. Extensive, predominantly microvesicular steatosis is present. *Mitochondriopathy* is a term applied to a group of heterogeneous diseases with a range of clinical manifestations from single-organ involvement to multiorgan systemic disease. Hepatic manifestations also are heterogeneous, including acute liver failure, lactic acidosis, steatosis, cholestasis, and chronic hepatitis. Mitochondriopathy with predominant hepatic involvement may be classified as primary or secondary, depending on whether the mitochondrial defect is the principle cause of the liver disease. Examples of secondary mitochondrial hepatopathies are effects of certain drugs (e.g., valproate, nucleoside analogue, and amiodarone), hepatic copper/iron overload, and cholestasis.

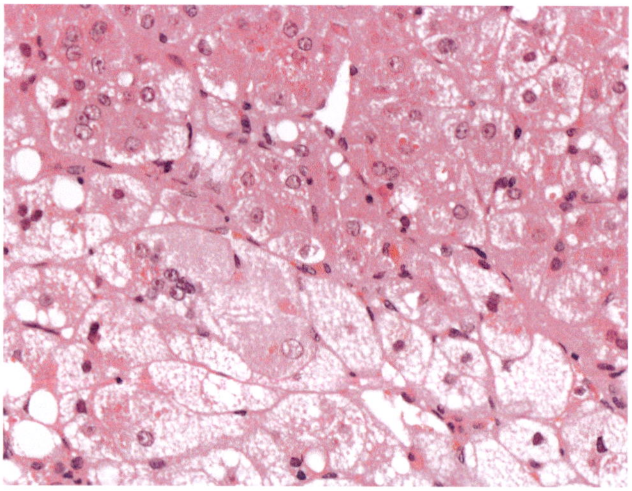

Fig. 4.51 Primary mitochondrial hepatopathy. Extensive, predominantly microvesicular steatosis is present, as are some giant mitochondria. Primary mitochondrial hepatopathy may be classified into respiratory chain defects, fatty acid oxidation and transport defects, disorders of mitochondrial translation process, urea cycle defects, and mitochondrial phosphoenolpyruvate carboxykinase deficiency. Respiratory chain defects in primary mitochondrial hepatopathy include neonatal liver failure (mutations of *SCO1* and *BCS1L*), mitochondrial DNA depletion syndrome (mutations of *POLG*, *DGUOK*, and *MPV17*), Alpers-Huttenlocher syndrome (mutation of *POLG*), Navajo neurohepatopathy (mutation of *MPV17*), Pearson syndrome (mitochondrial DNA deletion), and villous atrophy syndrome (mitochondrial DNA rearrangement).

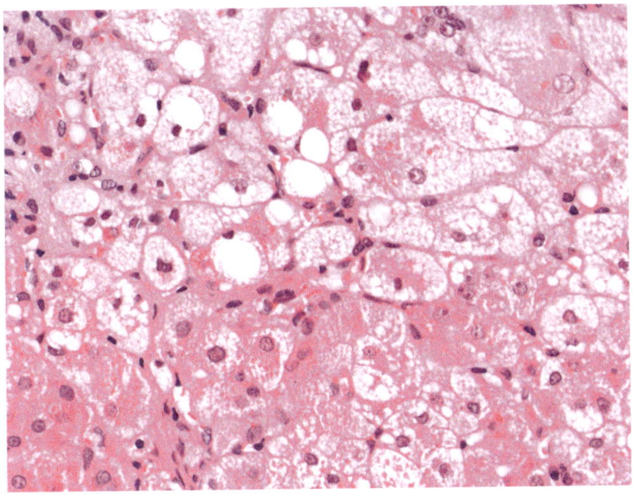

Fig. 4.52 Primary mitochondrial hepatopathy. There is extensive microvesicular steatosis. Histologic features of primary mitochondrial hepatopathy include patchy or extensive microvesicular and macrovesicular steatosis, cholestasis, hepatocellular degeneration and swelling, and mixed portal and lobular inflammation. Progressive portal fibrosis to cirrhosis is found. Parenchymal haemosiderosis is present in Pearson syndrome and mitochondrial DNA depletion syndrome. Prominent pseudo-acinar formation is found in neonates with Navajo neurohepatopathy.

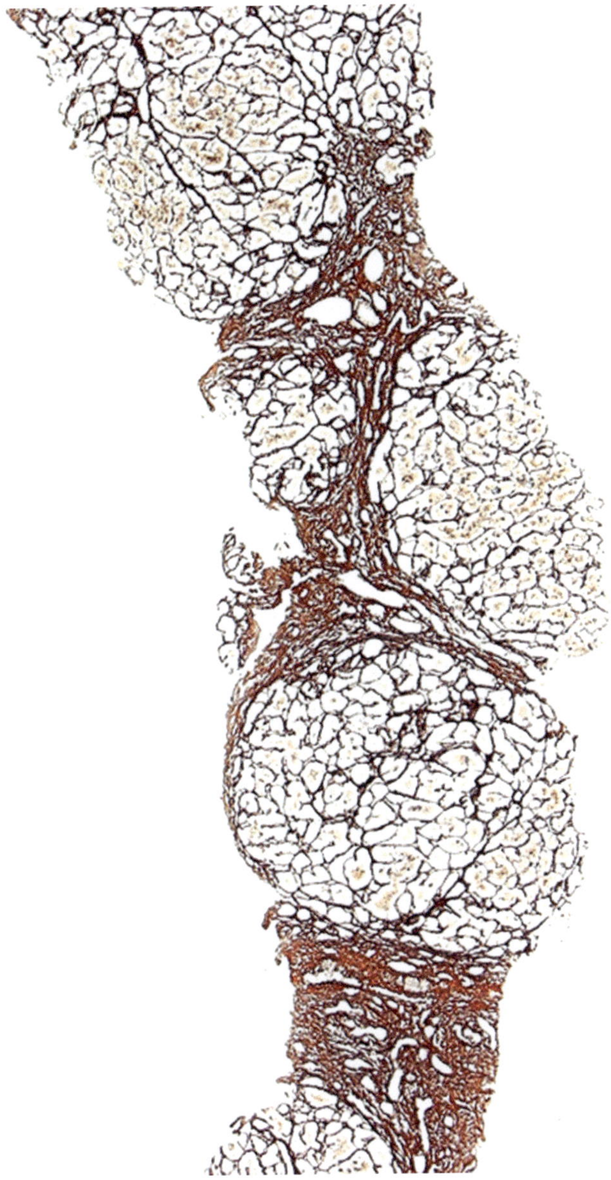

Fig. 4.53 Primary mitochondrial hepatopathy. (Gordon-Sweets reticulin stain). Cirrhosis is evident with the presence of multiple regenerative nodules separated by fibrous septa. A high index of suspicion is crucial in the diagnosis of primary mitochondrial hepatopathy. Primary mitochondrial hepatopathy should be considered in patients with (1) liver dysfunction with concomitant neuromuscular symptoms, (2) acute or chronic liver disease with multisystem involvement, or (3) hepatic steatosis with lactic acidosis or ketonaemia, and in (4) neonates with rapidly deteriorating liver disease. The definitive diagnosis is made by biochemical assay or genetic testing.

4.8 Disorders of Bile Acid and Bilirubin Metabolism

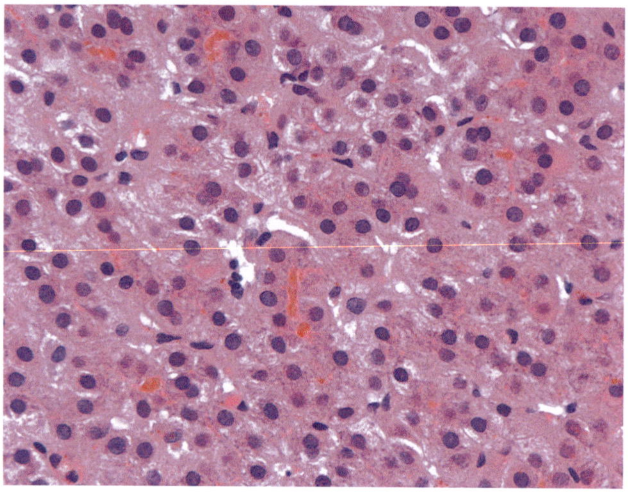

Fig. 4.54 Genetic disorders of intrahepatic cholestasis. Canalicular bilirubinostasis is present in the absence of significant necroinflammation or fibrosis (bland cholestasis). The manifestations of autosomal recessive disease associated with mutations of the *ATP8B1* or *ABCB11* gene on chromosome 18q21.31 or 2q31.1, encoding familial intrahepatic cholestasis 1 (FIC1) or bile salt export pump (BSEP) protein, are part of a spectrum ranging from intermittent episodes of conjugated hyperbilirubinaemia and pruritus, which may be precipitated by infection, pregnancy, and hormone intake (BRIC), to rapid progression to end-stage liver disease (PFIC). Liver histology ranges from bland cholestasis (BRIC) to neonatal giant cell hepatitis, or advanced fibrosis (PFIC).

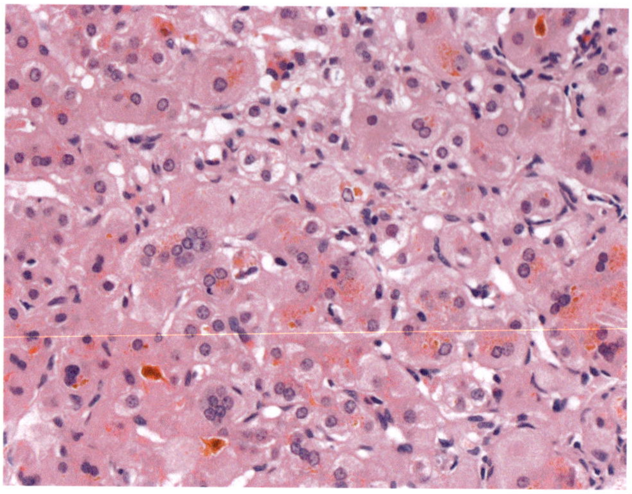

Fig. 4.56 Progressive familial intrahepatic cholestasis, type 2. Canalicular and hepatocellular bilirubinostasis is seen here together with giant cell transformation. Type 2 PFIC, also known as BSEP deficiency, is associated with mutation of the *ABCB11* gene on chromosome 2q31.1, encoding BSEP. It presents as jaundice and severe pruritus with normal/low serum GGT and very high serum bile acid levels. Extrahepatic manifestations are not a feature. Histologic changes include bilirubinostasis and a neonatal hepatitis with giant cell transformation. Pericellular and periportal fibrosis may develop and progress to cirrhosis. Absence of canalicular BSEP immunoreactivity is diagnostic.

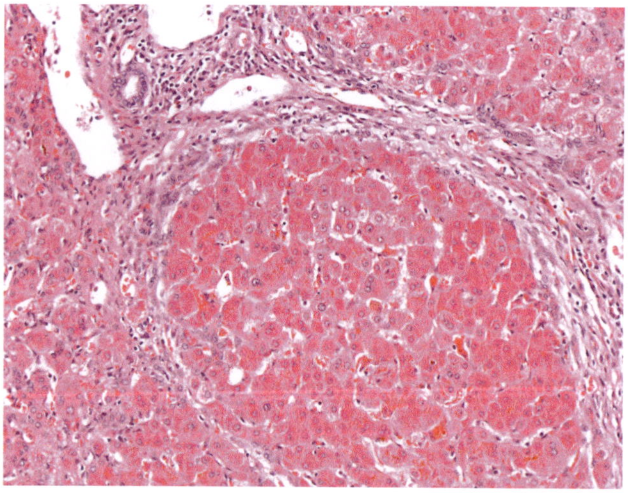

Fig. 4.55 Progressive familial intrahepatic cholestasis (PFIC), type 1. Bilirubinostasis in hepatocyte canaliculi and Kupffer cell bilirubinostasis are present in a cirrhotic liver. PFIC is a group of autosomal recessive diseases related to defective canalicular proteins and characterized by intrahepatic cholestasis and progression to liver failure and cirrhosis. Type 1 PFIC, also known as Byler disease and FIC1 deficiency, is associated with mutation of the *ATP8B1* gene on chromosome 18q21.31, encoding FIC1. It presents as jaundice and severe pruritus with normal/low serum γ-glutamyl transpeptidase (GGT) and very high serum levels of bile acid. Extrahepatic manifestations include pancreatitis, diarrhoea, and growth and mental retardation. Liver histology shows bland cholestasis. Pericellular and periportal fibrosis may develop and progress to bridging fibrosis and cirrhosis. Immunostaining for FIC1 is of limited use. Coarsely granular intracanalicular bile may be demonstrated by electron microscopy.

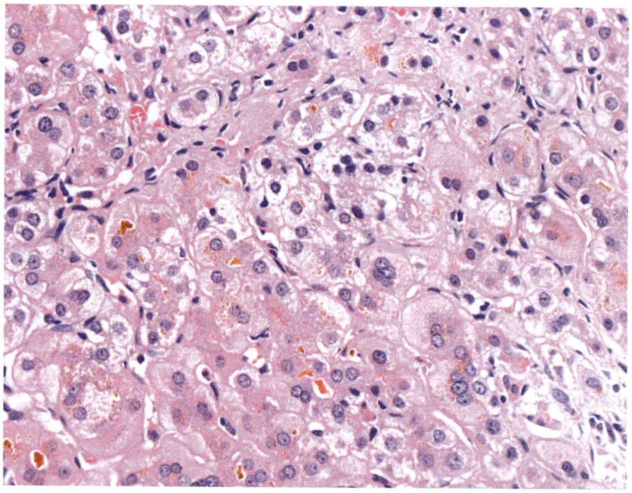

Fig. 4.57 Progressive familial intrahepatic cholestasis, type 3. Canalicular and hepatocellular bilirubinostasis is associated with giant cell transformation. Type 3 PFIC, also known as MDR3 (multidrug resistance p-glycoprotein 3) deficiency, is associated with mutation of the *ABCB4* gene on chromosome 7q21.12, encoding MDR3. It presents as jaundice and moderate pruritus with high serum GGT and high serum bile acid levels. Liver histology is characterised by bilirubinostasis, ductular reaction, bile plugs, and cholesterol clefts in bile duct lumina. Giant cell transformation may occur, but lobular necroinflammatory activity typically is mild. Chronic cholate stasis may be present. Absence of canalicular MDR3 immunoreactivity is diagnostic.

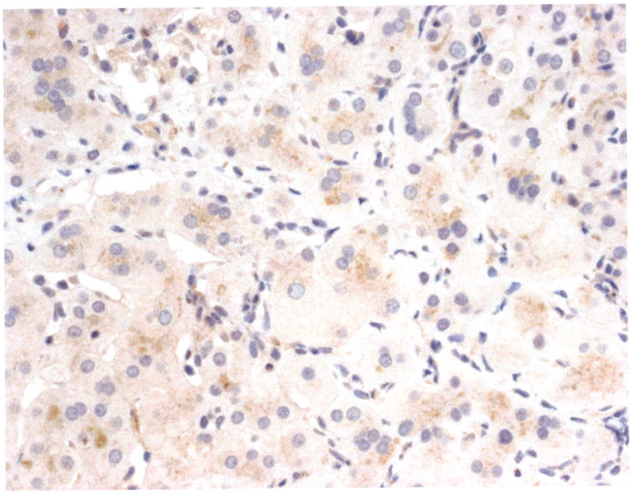

Fig. 4.58 Progressive familial intrahepatic cholestasis, type 2 (BSEP stain). The absence of canalicular expression of BSEP support BSEP deficiency (courtesy of Dr. Alex Knisely).

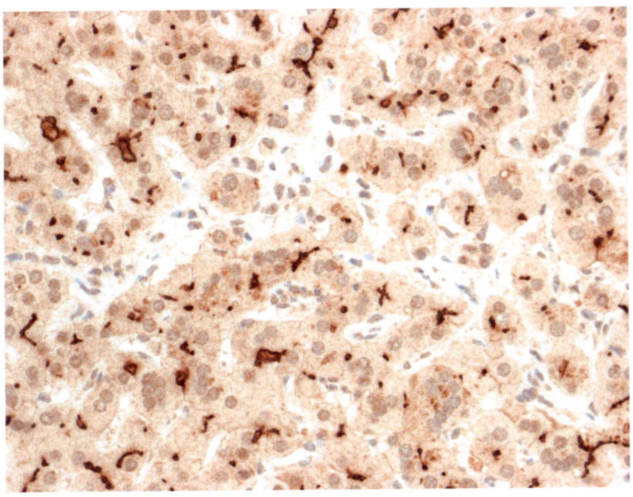

Fig. 4.59 Progressive familial intrahepatic cholestasis, type 2 (MDR3 stain). Retained canalicular expression of MDR3 is demonstrated here.

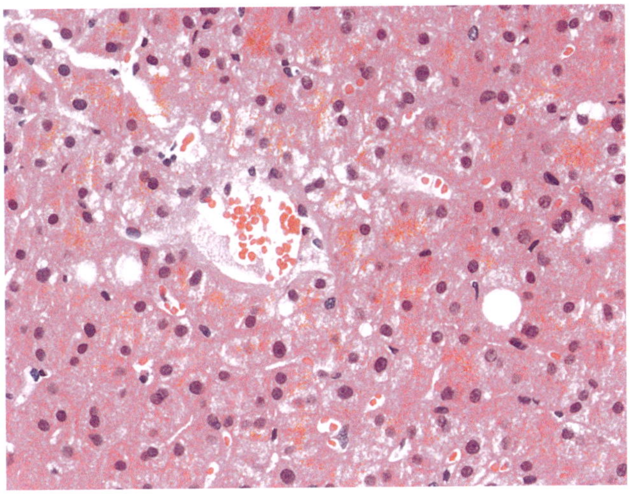

Fig. 4.60 Gilbert syndrome. There are abundant golden-yellow, finely granular lipofuscin pigments in the pericanalicular cytoplasm of perivenular hepatocytes in this case. Gilbert syndrome is an autosomal dominant or recessive disease associated with mutation or polymorphism of the *UGT1A1* gene on chromosome 2q37.1, resulting in mild reduction of activity or expression of uridine diphosphate (UDP)-glucuronosyltransferase. It is the commonest familial disorder of bilirubin metabolism, affecting up to 6% of the general population. Intermittent unconjugated hyperbilirubinaemia, usually during concurrent disease or fasting, is the typical clinical presentation. It follows a benign course without any significant morbidity or mortality.

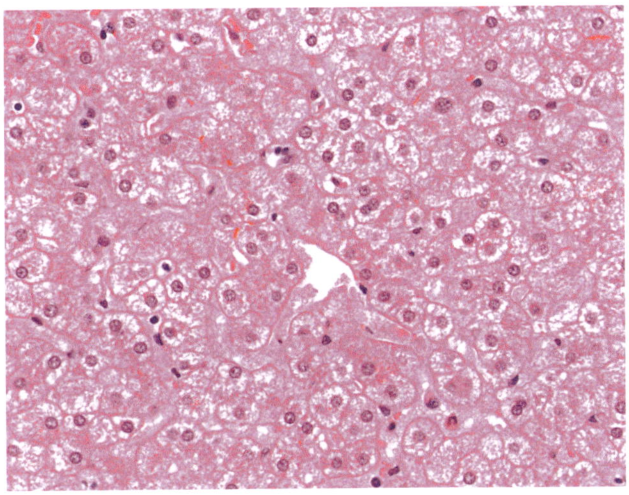

Fig. 4.61 Crigler-Najjar disease. Mild canalicular bilirubinostasis is present, with no significant necroinflammation or fibrosis. Crigler-Najjar syndrome is an autosomal recessive (type 1) or dominant (type 2) disease associated with mutation of the *UGT1A1* gene on chromosome 2q37.1, resulting in absence (type 1) or markedly reduced (type 2) expression of UDP-glucuronosyltransferase. Type 1 is associated with fatal unconjugated hyperbilirubinaemia in the neonatal period, whereas type 2 is associated with nonfatal unconjugated hyperbilirubinaemia in older children. The main histopathologic finding is bland cholestasis, but the liver may be normal.

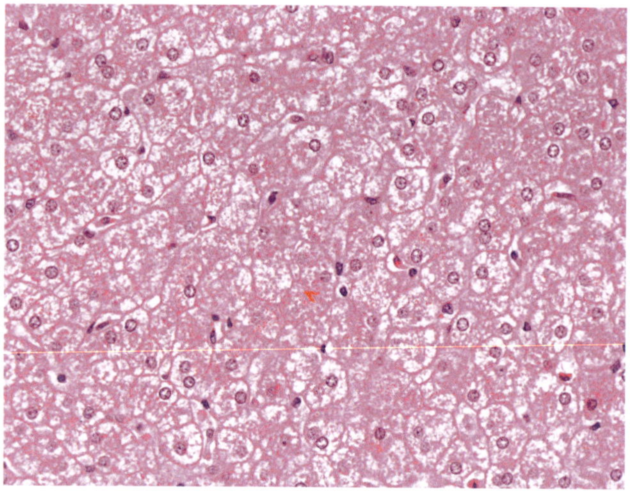

Fig. 4.62 Crigler-Najjar disease. Mild canalicular bilirubinostasis is seen with minimal necroinflammation. Dubin-Johnson syndrome and Rotor syndrome are two other familial disorders of bilirubin metabolism. Dubin-Johnson syndrome is an autosomal recessive disorder associated with mutation of the *ABCC2* gene on chromosome 10q24.2, encoding multidrug resistance-associated protein 2 (MRP2). Rotor syndrome is an autosomal recessive disorder with an unknown genetic defect. Both syndromes present with asymptomatic conjugated hyperbilirubinaemia without any significant morbidity or mortality. Gross greyish to blackish liver pigmentation and microscopic deposition of brown, coarsely granular pigments in hepatocytes are characteristic for Dubin-Johnson syndrome but not Rotor syndrome. Absence of immunostaining for MRP2 is diagnostic for Dubin-Johnson syndrome.

4.9 Miscellaneous Metabolic Disorders

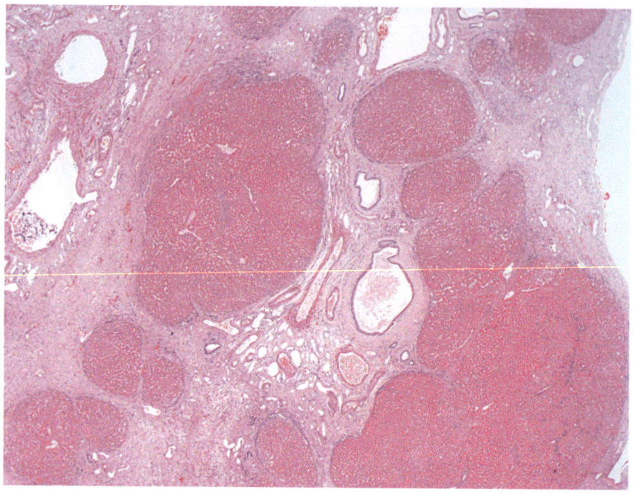

Fig. 4.63 Cystic fibrosis. Biliary cirrhosis is evident with regenerative nodules of varying sizes and shapes surrounded by thick fibrous septa and a rim of ductular reaction. Dilated bile ducts contain pink amorphous material. Cystic fibrosis, also known as mucoviscidosis, is an autosomal recessive disease associated with mutation of the *CFTR* gene on chromosome 7q31.2, encoding cystic fibrosis conductance regulator. The worldwide incidence varies from 1:3,000 (European and white American), 1:4,000 to 1:10,000 (Latin American), 1:15,000 to 1:20,000 (African American), to less than 1:100,000 (Africa and Asia). Multiple organs generally are involved in cystic fibrosis. Sinopulmonary disease and pancreatic insufficiency are two major manifestations of greatest clinical significance.

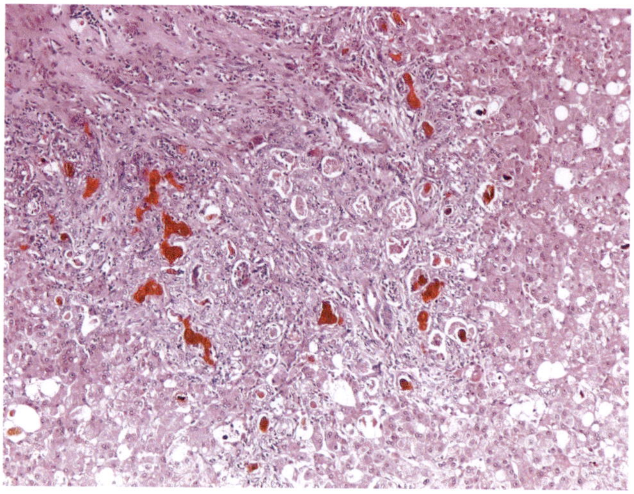

Fig. 4.64 Cystic fibrosis. Focal biliary fibrosis is evident with expanded portal tracts containing multiple dilated bile ductules filled with bile concretions and pink amorphous material. The exact prevalence of hepatic involvement in cystic fibrosis is uncertain. Clinically significant hepatic involvement with portal hypertension occurs in only 4% to 6% of patients. However, liver function derangement and hepatomegaly are detected incidentally in up to 50% and 30% of asymptomatic patients, respectively.

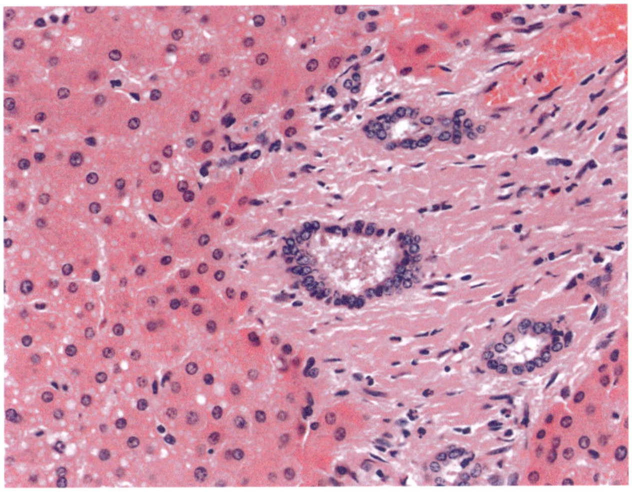

Fig. 4.65 Cystic fibrosis. Amorphous pink secretions are present in the bile duct lumina. Pathologic features of cystic fibrosis in the liver include steatosis, focal biliary fibrosis, and multinodular biliary cirrhosis. Steatosis is reported in 20% to 60% of cases. Macrovesicular steatosis with predilection in the periportal region is common and shows no correlation with the general nutritional status of patients. Focal biliary fibrosis is documented in 10% to 72% of cases and is the most characteristic lesion of cystic fibrosis. It is characterised by expansion of portal tracts by varying degrees of portal and periportal fibrosis, ductular reaction, and chronic inflammation. Bile ductules are irregularly dilated and contain bile plugs, orange concretions, and pink amorphous material, which typically are PAS positive and diastase resistant. Rupture of ductules with extravasation of luminal contents leads to acute inflammation.

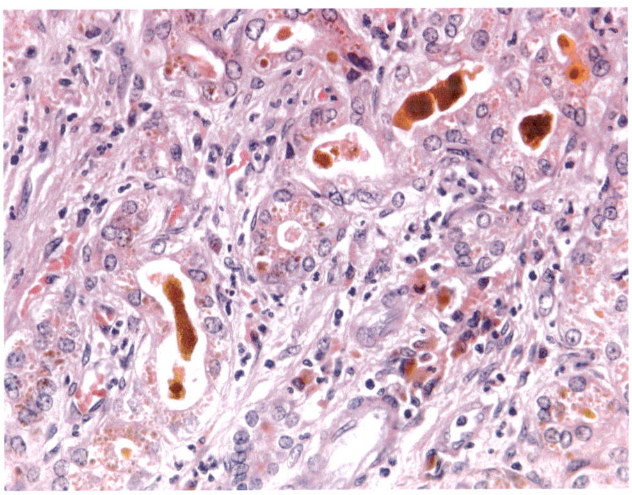

Fig. 4.66 Cystic fibrosis. Dilated bile ductules are filled by bile concretions. Multilobular biliary cirrhosis is reported in 7% to 20% of cases and results from coalescence of focal biliary fibrosis with progressive fibrosis, atrophy of the intervening parenchyma, and entrapment of adjacent hepatic lobules. In neonates with cystic fibrosis, neonatal hepatitis with giant cell transformation and prominent bilirubinostasis may be seen. Pathologic differential diagnoses include large duct obstruction, biliary cirrhosis of any cause, and congenital hepatic fibrosis. Characteristic PAS-positive and diastase-resistant concretions and amorphous material are found only in cystic fibrosis.

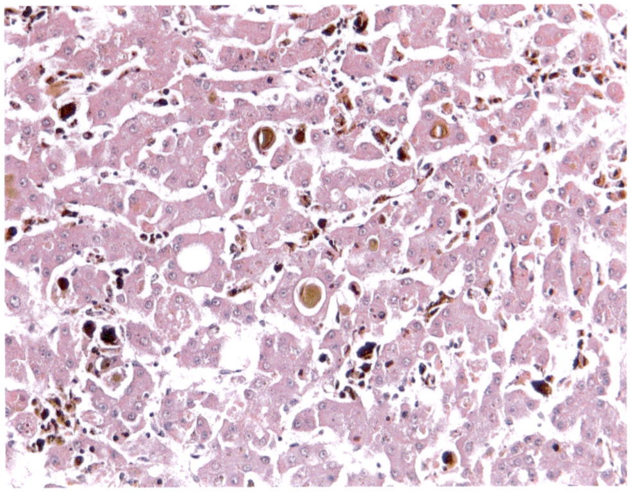

Fig. 4.67 Erythropoietic protoporphyria (EPP). There is extensive accumulation of dark brown pigments in canaliculi and Kupffer cells. The porphyrias are a group of inherited disorders of haem and porphyrin biosynthesis leading to excessive accumulation and excretion of porphyrin and its precursor. EPP is an autosomal dominant disease with incomplete penetrance and is associated with mutation of the *FECH* gene on chromosome 18q21.31, encoding ferrochelatase. The incidence is between 1:75,000 and 1:200,000. Skin photosensitivity with burning pain, erythema, and swelling usually begins before the age of 6. A small portion of cases develop hepatic complications and present commonly after the age of 30. Cirrhosis is found in 1% to 10% of cases.

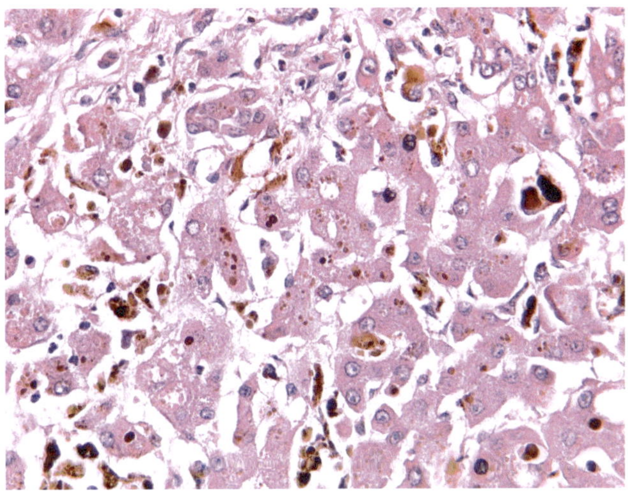

Fig. 4.68 Erythropoietic protoporphyria. There is extensive accumulation of dark brown pigments in hepatocytes and Kupffer cells. The principal histologic manifestation of EPP in the liver is the presence of dark brown protoporphyrin pigments in hepatocytes, canaliculi, Kupffer cells, and biliary epithelial cells. These pigments demonstrate bright red birefringence with an occasional Maltese cross configuration.

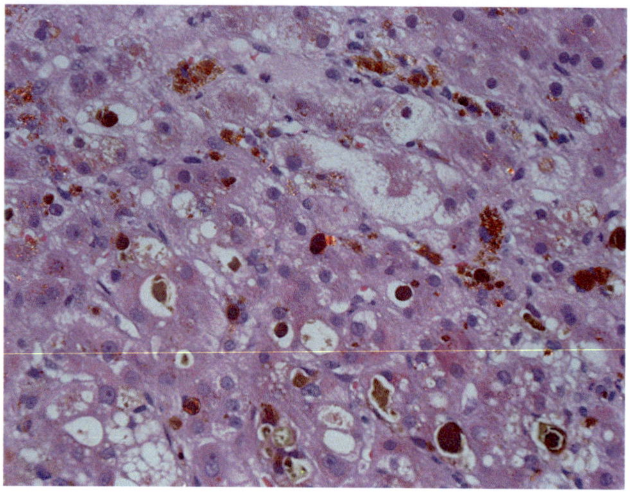

Fig. 4.69 Erythropoietic protoporphyria. Bright red birefringence is noted in some brown pigments under polarized light. Other forms of porphyria, notably acute intermittent porphyria (AIP) and porphyria cutanea tarda (PCT), also may involve the liver. AIP is an autosomal dominant disease associated with mutation of *HMBS* on chromosome 11q23.3, encoding hydroxymethylbilane synthase. It is the commonest form of porphyria, with an incidence of 1:20,000. Its hepatic pathology is characterised by nonspecific steatosis and parenchymal and mesenchymal haemosiderosis. PCT is an autosomal dominant disease with low penetration and is associated with mutation of *UROD* on chromosome 1p34.1, encoding uroporphyrinogen decarboxylase. Its hepatic pathology is characterised by deposition of birefringent needle-shaped crystals of variable length in hepatocytes, with steatosis, parenchymal haemosiderosis, and fibrosis.

5 Fatty Liver Disease

Steatosis is very common and is associated with numerous conditions, the most common of which are alcoholism and the metabolic syndrome. Others include drugs, viruses, disorders of nutrition, and endocrine, metabolic, and systemic diseases. Steatosis manifests histologically as the accumulation of droplets of triglycerides inside the cytoplasm of hepatocytes. The size of these droplets varies from a single large one (macrovesicular steatosis) occupying the cytoplasm almost completely and pushing the nucleus to the periphery, to one or more of medium size (mediovesicular steatosis). The term *microvesicular* should be used when steatosis manifests as an accumulation of very fine vesicular material, without nuclear displacement, which cannot be differentiated from other accumulations (e.g., glycogen) or cytoplasmic changes (e.g., hydropic degeneration) without the use of special techniques. Microvesicular steatosis usually is associated with a congenital or acquired defect in β-oxidation and severe hepatic dysfunction.

Another important distinction is between steatosis and steatohepatitis. The latter is characterised by a constellation of changes (inflammation, degenerative hepatocellular changes, and fibrosis), in addition to steatosis, that delineate the risk of progressive liver injury. Distinction between alcoholic and nonalcoholic steatohepatitis is not straightforward because of a considerable overlap at both the morphologic and clinical levels. Paediatric fatty liver disease is a serious emerging problem in developed countries. The particular pattern of fibrosis progression in steatohepatitis has warranted the design and validation of specific semiquantitative methods of grading and staging.

5.1 Alcoholic Liver Disease

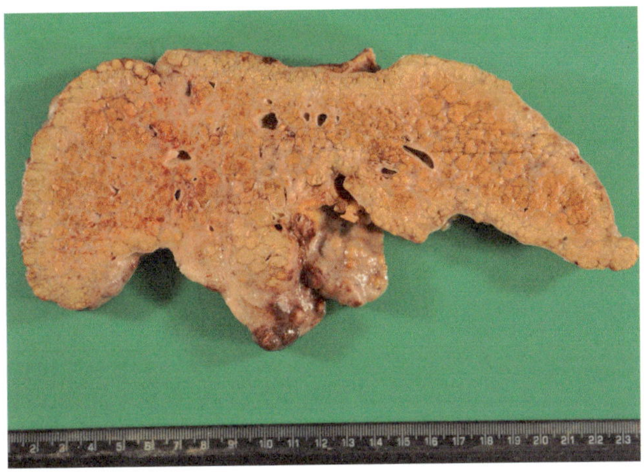

Fig. 5.1 Alcoholic liver disease. This liver explant was removed from a patient with established alcoholic cirrhosis. The cut surface shows a macronodular cirrhosis and an orange-yellowish greasy appearance. Alcohol is the most used and abused agent worldwide and leads to a wide range of physical, psychological, and social problems. There is a full spectrum of alcoholic liver disease, including simple steatosis, alcoholic foamy degeneration, alcoholic hepatitis, cirrhosis, and hepatocellular carcinoma. Simple steatosis is present in at least 90% of people with excessive alcohol consumption. About 20% to 40% and 10% to 20% of these people will progress to alcoholic hepatitis and cirrhosis, respectively. Classically, alcoholic cirrhosis is micronodular in gross appearance. However, micronodular cirrhosis in alcoholic liver disease transforms to macronodular following abstinence.

A.W.H. Chan et al., *Atlas of Liver Pathology*, Atlas of Anatomic Pathology,
DOI 10.1007/978-1-4614-9114-9_5, © Springer Science+Business Media New York 2014

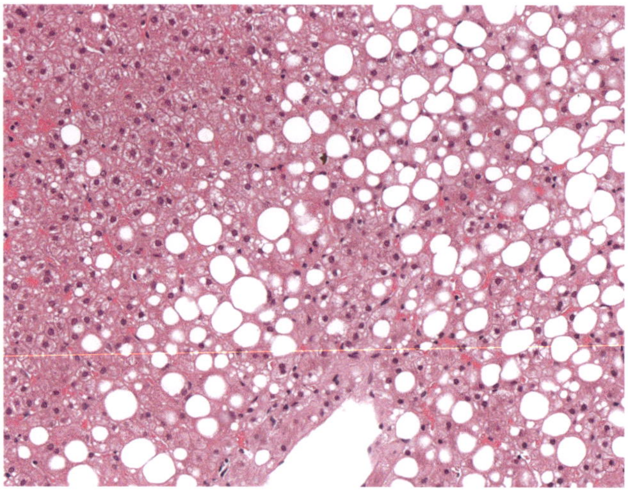

Fig. 5.2 Alcoholic steatosis. Macrovesicular steatosis is located predominantly in the perivenular region. Steatosis is the commonest and earliest pathologic feature of alcoholic liver disease. It first appears in zone 3 and spreads to other zones as alcohol liver injury persists. It may disappear within a month after cessation of alcohol consumption. Simple steatosis generally is believed to be a relatively benign condition, although this notion has been challenged by several recent studies. The presence of severe steatosis is significantly associated with premature death in alcoholic liver disease. However, the association between degree of steatosis and disease progression to cirrhosis is controversial.

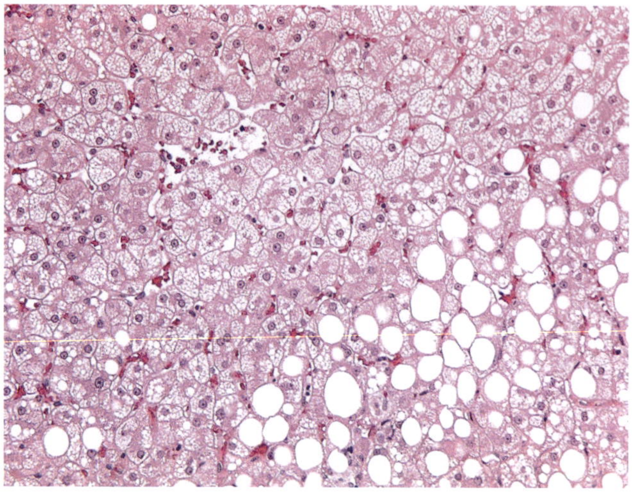

Fig. 5.4 Alcoholic foamy degeneration. Shown here is a predominantly microvesicular steatosis without any significant necroinflammatory activity, which is characteristic of alcoholic foamy degeneration. Mild macrovesicular steatosis, perivenular bilirubinostasis, and mild pericellular fibrosis also may be present. The typical clinical presentation is one of jaundice, abdominal pain, and hepatomegaly and characteristically resolves rapidly after withdrawal of alcohol.

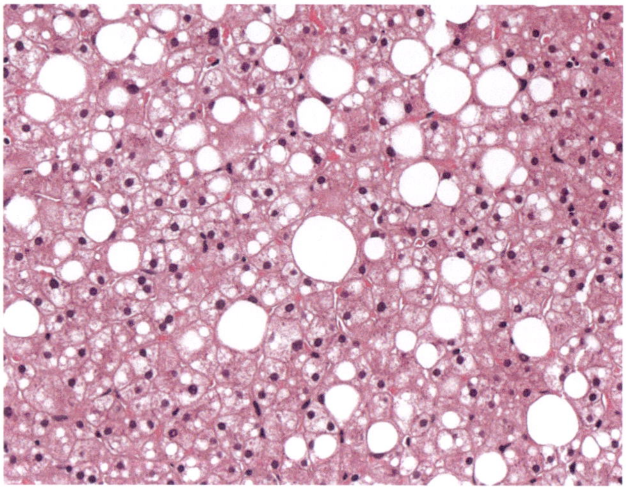

Fig. 5.3 Alcoholic steatosis. In this case, there is a mixed pattern of macrovesicular/"mediovesicular" steatosis. The formation of a single large fat droplet in macrovesicular steatosis arises by fusion of multiple small fat droplets, which was demonstrated elegantly in several animal models. Mediovesicular steatosis may represent the intermediate step in such a conversion. It is not uncommon to find mediovesicular steatosis admixed with macrovesicular steatosis. The association of a mixed pattern of steatosis in alcoholic liver disease and progression to cirrhosis is controversial.

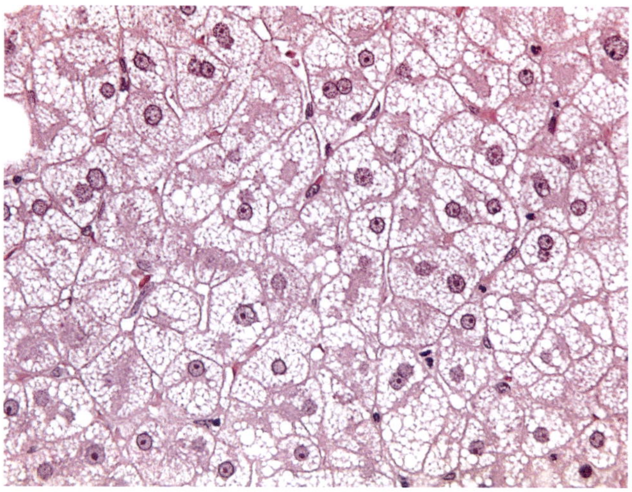

Fig. 5.5 Alcoholic foamy degeneration. Here, there is extensive microvesicular steatosis, characterised by multiple minute fat droplets in hepatocytes without displacement of the nucleus. Diffuse microvesicular steatosis is uncommon and associated with serious mitochondriopathies with fatty acid oxidation defects. Apart from alcoholic foamy degeneration, it also is associated with acute fatty liver of pregnancy, drug/toxin-induced liver injury, and various primary mitochondrial hepatopathies.

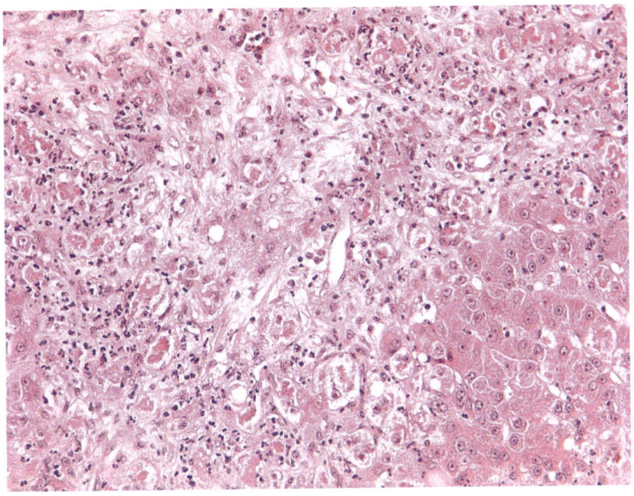

Fig. 5.6 Alcoholic hepatitis. In this case, there are numerous ballooned hepatocytes in the perivenular zone. Most of the ballooned hepatocytes contain Mallory-Denk bodies. Ballooning degeneration of hepatocytes is a hallmark feature of steatohepatitis and is characterised by cellular swelling, rarefaction of cytoplasm, and clumped strands of intermediate filaments. Some clumped intermediate filaments may form Mallory-Denk bodies. However, one should note that Mallory-Denk bodies are not always found in ballooned hepatocytes; furthermore, ballooned hepatocytes do not necessarily contain Mallory-Denk bodies. Ballooning degeneration is regarded as the most important feature for distinguishing steatohepatitis from simple steatosis.

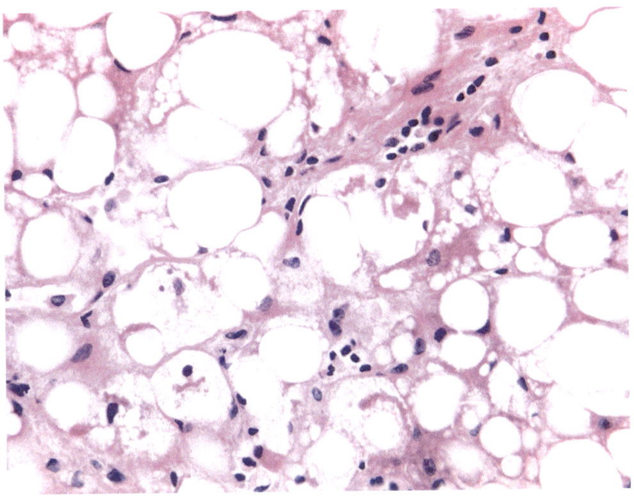

Fig. 5.7 Alcoholic hepatitis. Many ballooned hepatocytes with Mallory-Denk bodies are noted with macrovesicular steatosis. Although ballooning degeneration typically is found in alcoholic and nonalcoholic steatohepatitis, it may be observed in acute viral hepatitis, chronic hepatitis C with concurrent steatohepatitic features, autoimmune hepatitis, neonatal giant cell hepatitis, drug-induced liver injury, and ischaemia/reperfusion injury in liver allografts. Steatosis usually is present in alcoholic hepatitis, but is not necessarily a diagnostic criterion. Its severity may vary, and it may disappear within a month after cessation of alcohol consumption.

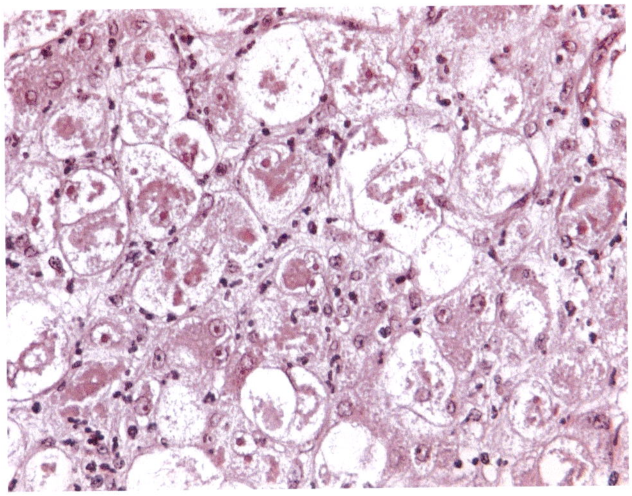

Fig. 5.8 Alcoholic hepatitis. Most ballooned hepatocytes contain deeply eosinophilic ropey Mallory-Denk bodies. Many neutrophils are found close to these ballooned hepatocytes (satellitosis). Mallory-Denk bodies represent misfolded and aggregated intermediate filaments combined with other different classes of proteins, including p62 and ubiquitin. Compared with the situation in nonalcoholic fatty liver disease, Mallory-Denk bodies in alcoholic liver diseases tend to be more well-formed and thickly ropey and more commonly are associated with satellitosis. They persist within hepatocytes for several months after abstinence from alcohol. Extensive formation of Mallory-Denk bodies is a poor prognostic factor associated with increased risk of progression to cirrhosis.

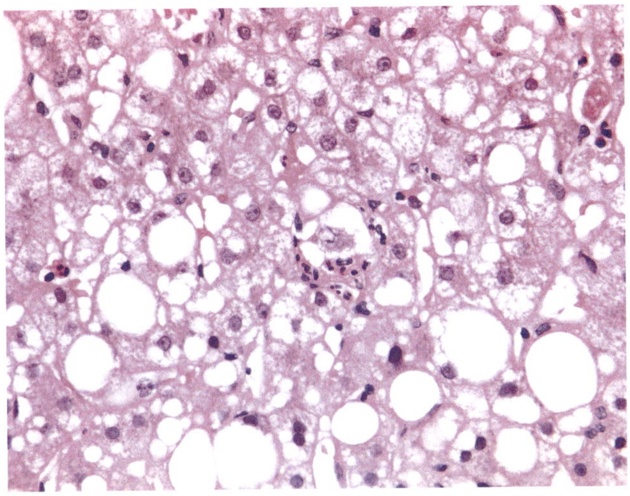

Fig. 5.9 Alcoholic hepatitis. A ballooned hepatocyte is surrounded by neutrophils (satellitosis). An apoptotic body (*upper right*) also is present. Lobular inflammation in alcoholic hepatitis typically is composed of a neutrophil-predominant inflammatory infiltrate and, less frequently, a mononuclear cell-rich inflammatory infiltrate. The neutrophils may surround ballooned hepatocytes with Mallory-Denk bodies (satellitosis). Satellitosis is observed much more commonly in alcoholic steatohepatitis than in nonalcoholic steatohepatitis and is thought to a result of the chemotactic effect of Mallory-Denk bodies and/or local production of chemokines. Lipogranulomas and microgranulomas also are components of lobular inflammation. Apoptosis is less prominent in alcoholic hepatitis than other diseases with significant lobular inflammation, such as acute viral hepatitis, drug-induced liver injury, and autoimmune hepatitis.

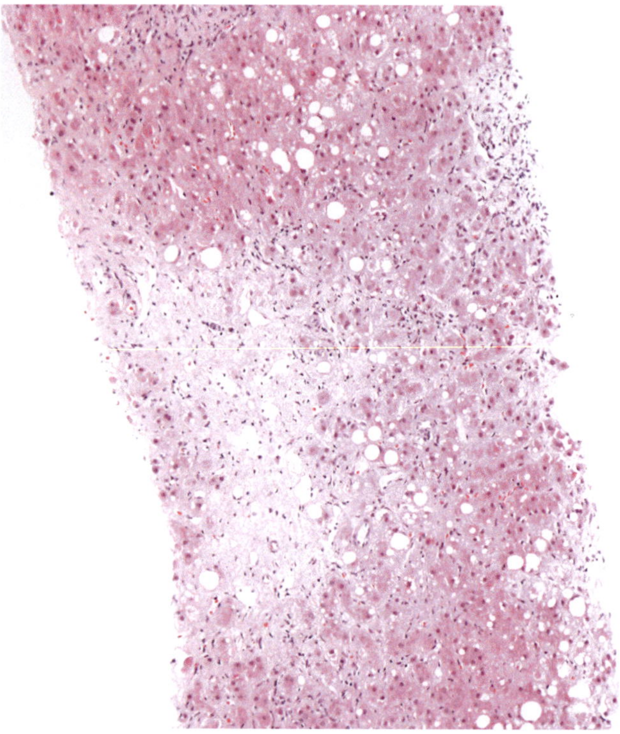

Fig. 5.10 Sclerosing hyaline necrosis. Fibrous occlusion of terminal hepatic venules is associated with perivenular necrosis and fibrosis. Sclerosing hyaline necrosis represents a severe form of alcoholic hepatitis and is associated with development of noncirrhotic portal hypertension. It is not seen in nonalcoholic steatohepatitis.

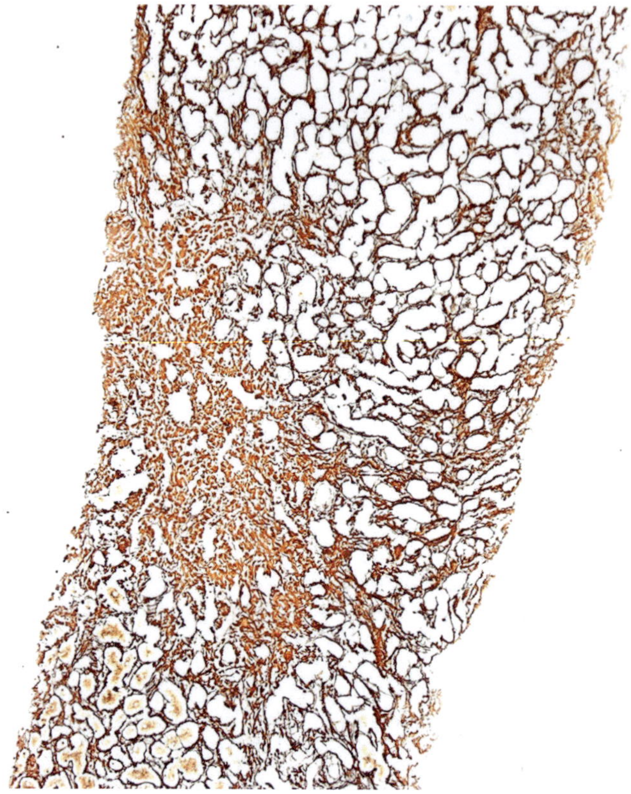

Fig. 5.11 Sclerosing hyaline necrosis (Gordon-Sweet reticulin stain). Fibrous occlusion of terminal hepatic venules is associated with dense perivenular fibrosis. Fibrous occlusion of terminal hepatic venules due to perivenular fibrosis (phlebosclerosis) is present in virtually all cases of alcoholic hepatitis and cirrhosis. Lymphocytic phlebitis and veno-occlusive lesion are other vascular lesions that may be seen in alcoholic liver disease and are present in 4% and 10% of biopsy material, respectively. These lesions typically are not found in nonalcoholic fatty liver disease.

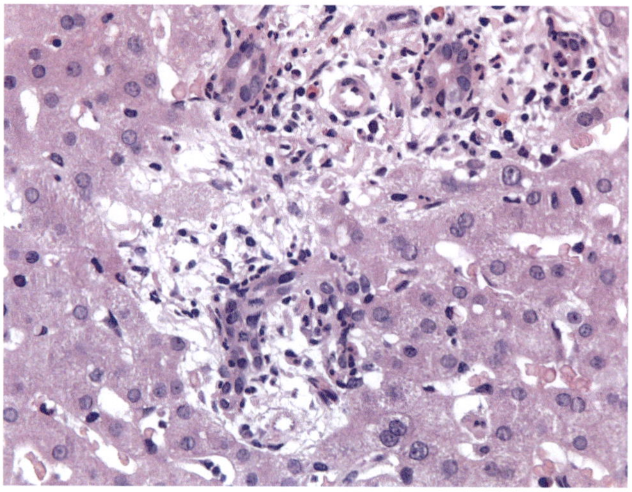

Fig. 5.12 Alcoholic liver disease. This portal tract is oedematous and contains a ductular reaction. Neutrophils are intimately associated with proliferating bile ductules. Portal lymphocytic inflammatory infiltrate, mild interface hepatitis, and ductular reaction are portal tract pathologic manifestations in alcoholic liver disease. These portal inflammatory changes may contribute to the development of portal and periportal fibrosis in alcoholic liver disease. When prominent, it is important to consider a concomitant cholestatic disorder, such as biliary obstruction, or pancreatitis.

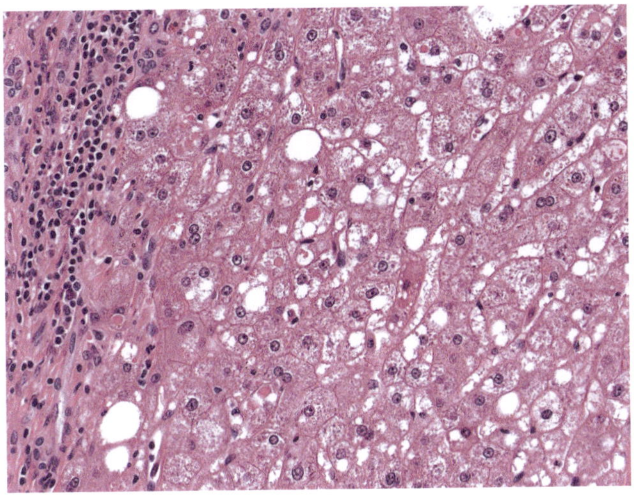

Fig. 5.13 Alcoholic liver disease. Several giant mitochondria are present in hepatocytes. Giant mitochondria, also called megamitochondria, are eosinophilic oval or needle-shaped intracytoplasmic inclusions. Their presence in alcoholic liver disease is associated with recent heavy alcoholic intake and disease progression. Although they typically are found in alcoholic and nonalcoholic fatty liver diseases, they may be associated with a wide variety of physiologic and pathologic conditions, such as aging, acute fatty liver of pregnancy, glycogen storage disease, urea cycle defect, and glycogenic hepatopathy. Giant mitochondria should be distinguished from other eosinophilic globular intracytoplasmic inclusions, particularly α_1-antitrypsin globules. The latter are periodic acid-Schiff positive, diastase resistant, and immunoreactive to α_1-antitrypsin, whereas the former are not.

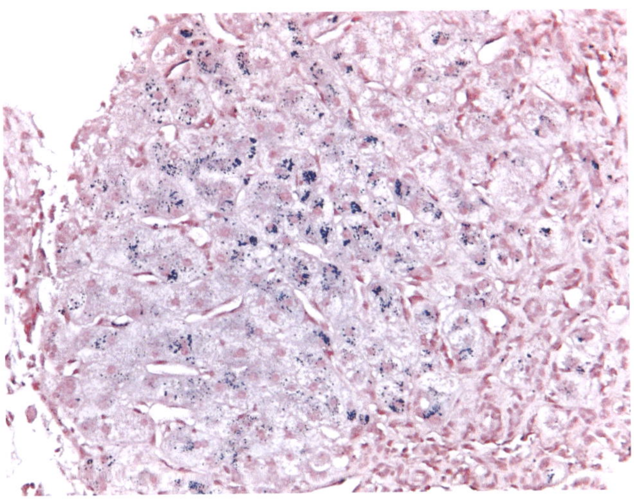

Fig. 5.14 Alcoholic siderosis (Perls stain). Grade 2 parenchymal siderosis is evident by the presence of a moderate deposition of iron in hepatocytes. Some Kupffer cells also contain iron deposits. Alcoholic siderosis usually is mild (grade 1–2) and found mainly in hepatocytes and occasionally Kupffer cells. Accumulation of iron is associated with increased small bowel iron absorption by a direct effect of alcohol and with chronic haemolysis, high iron content in some beverages, down-regulation of hepcidin, and up-regulation of transferrin receptor. In cases of severe (grade 3–4) parenchymal siderosis, coexisting hereditary haemochromatosis should be excluded.

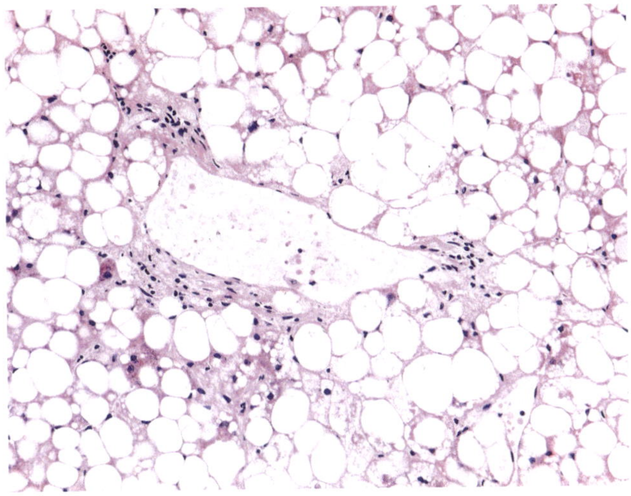

Fig. 5.15 Alcoholic liver disease with perivenular fibrosis. A thick rim of fibrous tissue surrounds the terminal hepatic venule against a background of marked macrovesicular steatosis. Perivenular fibrosis is defined as fibrosis surrounding at least two-thirds of the perimeter of terminal hepatic venules, with a minimum thickness of 4 μm. It is characteristic of alcoholic liver disease and usually is accompanied by zone 3 pericellular fibrosis. In contrast to pericellular fibrosis, perivenular fibrosis is found less frequently in nonalcoholic fatty liver disease. Progression of perivenular fibrosis may lead to fibrous occlusion of terminal hepatic venules (phlebosclerosis) and sclerosing hyaline necrosis.

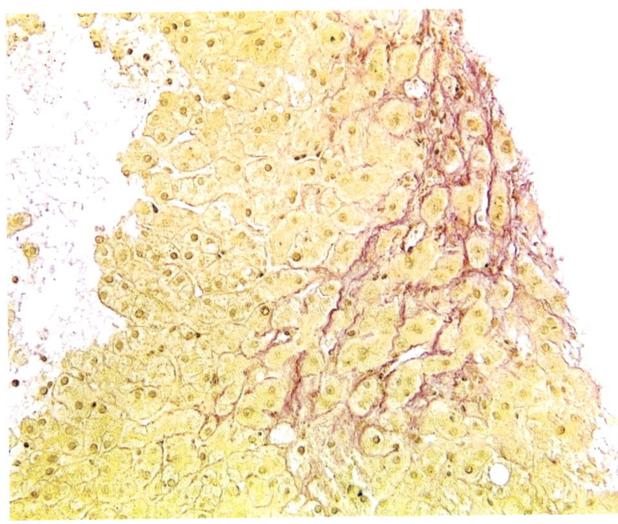

Fig. 5.16 Alcoholic liver disease with pericellular fibrosis (van Gieson stain). Thick fibrous strands are deposited around hepatocytes. Pericellular (perisinusoidal) fibrosis is deposition of fibrous tissue in the space of Disse and is related to the activation of stellate cells. It usually is accompanied by perivenular fibrosis in alcoholic liver disease. It occurs in both alcoholic and nonalcoholic fatty liver diseases but tends to be thicker and more diffuse in the former. During disease progression to cirrhosis, this pattern of pericellular fibrosis may persist, and its presence is a helpful marker of an underlying steatohepatitis, as both steatosis and ballooning degeneration may burn out in the later stages of the disease when there is advanced fibrosis or cirrhosis.

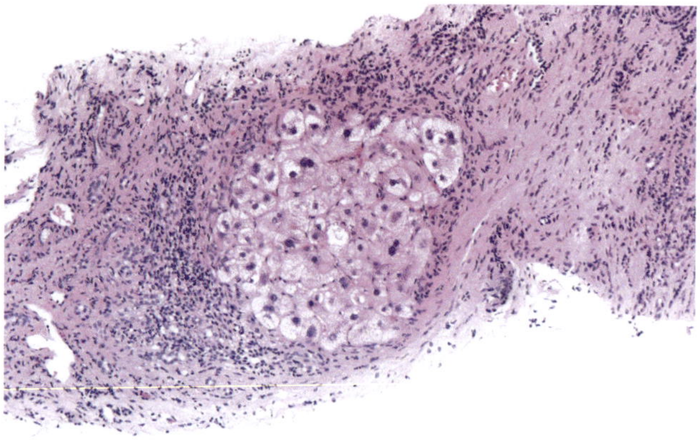

Fig. 5.17 Alcoholic cirrhosis. A residual island of ballooned hepatocytes is surrounded by thick fibrous septa. The presence of steatosis and/or ballooning degeneration in cirrhosis indicates active drinking or coexisting nonalcoholic fatty liver disease. However, steatosis and ballooning degeneration may burn out in advanced fibrosis or cirrhosis, even if alcohol consumption has not ceased. This phenomenon may be associated with impaired alcohol or lipid transport to hepatocytes due to altered sinusoidal blood flow or permeability.

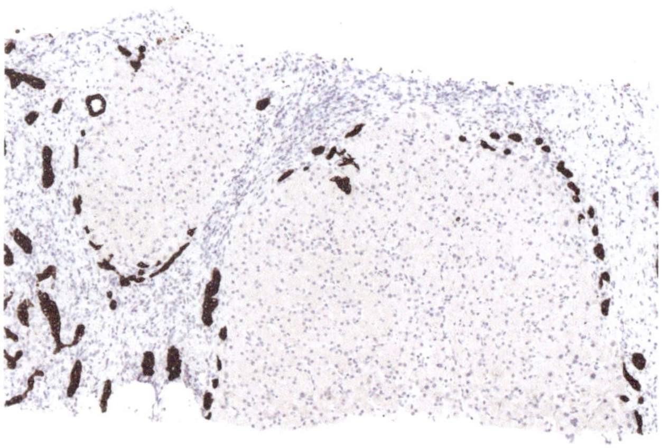

Fig. 5.18 Alcoholic cirrhosis (cytokeratin 19 [CK19] stain). A prominent ductular reaction is present at the periphery of regenerative nodules. Ductular reaction is a common but nonspecific finding in alcoholic liver disease, particularly in the setting of cirrhosis after alcohol abstinence. It formerly was known as ductular proliferation and may represent a stem or progenitor cell response to the injury of hepatocytes and/or bile ducts. As noted in other chapters, ductular reaction is seen more commonly in chronic cholestatic diseases, but it also is associated with acute hepatitis with bridging/panacinar necrosis, chronic hepatitis with bridging fibrosis/cirrhosis, acute ascending cholangitis, focal nodular hyperplasia, and inflammatory hepatocellular adenoma.

5.2 Nonalcoholic Fatty Liver Disease

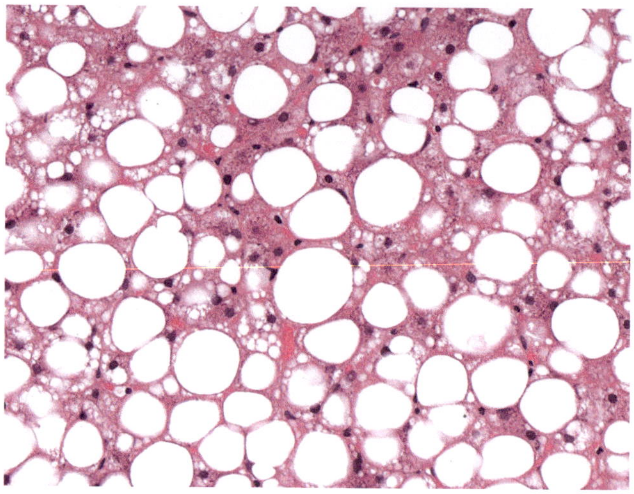

Fig. 5.19 Nonalcoholic fatty liver disease. A predominantly macrovesicular steatosis is present. Hepatic steatosis is the accumulation of lipids in hepatocytes. Triglycerides are the major form of stored lipids, whereas free fatty acids, cholesterols, and phospholipids are other, minor forms of accumulated lipids. The accumulation of triglycerides, in fact, may be a protective mechanism against lipotoxicity.

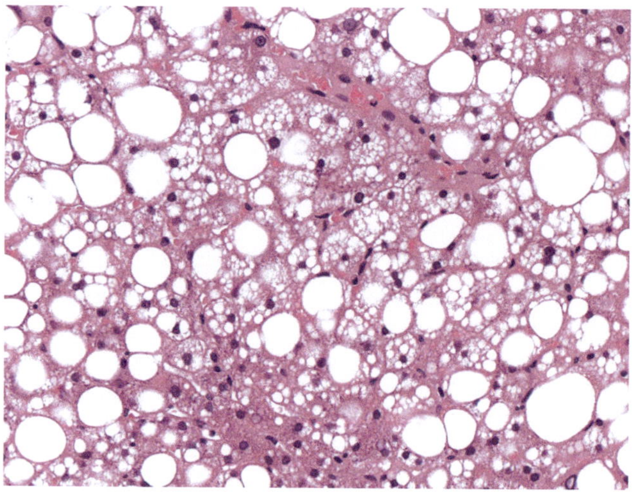

Fig. 5.20 Nonalcoholic fatty liver disease. There is mixed macrovesicular/mediovesicular steatosis. Steatosis is the hallmark feature of nonalcoholic fatty liver disease. The cutoff value between physiologic and pathologic steatosis is 5% of affected hepatocytes, but this is based on studies by lipid content measurement and imaging. The distribution of steatosis is predominantly zone 3 in adults, which is similar to alcoholic steatosis, but mainly zone 1 in children. Steatosis may disappear in nonalcoholic fatty liver disease when there is advanced fibrosis or cirrhosis. Disappearance of steatosis may be associated with decreased hepatocyte exposure to insulin and impaired lipoprotein transport secondary to extrahepatic and intrahepatic portosystemic shunts. Some cases of cryptogenic cirrhosis may be the result of unrecognised and burned-out nonalcoholic fatty liver disease.

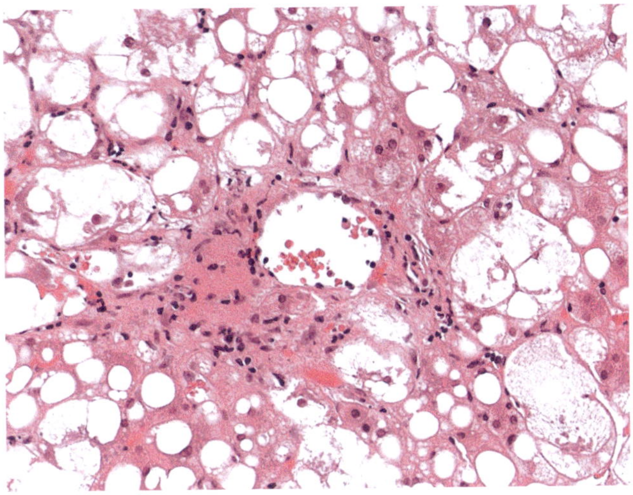

Fig. 5.21 Nonalcoholic steatohepatitis. There are numerous ballooned hepatocytes in acinar zone 3. Ballooning degeneration is the hallmark of hepatocellular injury in steatohepatitis and is characterised by cellular swelling, rarefaction of the hepatocytic cytoplasm, and clumped strands of intermediate filaments. It is considered the lesion critical to differentiating steatohepatitis from steatosis. The degree of ballooning degeneration is one of the parameters assessing the activity/grading of nonalcoholic steatohepatitis. However, ballooning degeneration is seldom found in paediatric nonalcoholic steatohepatitis.

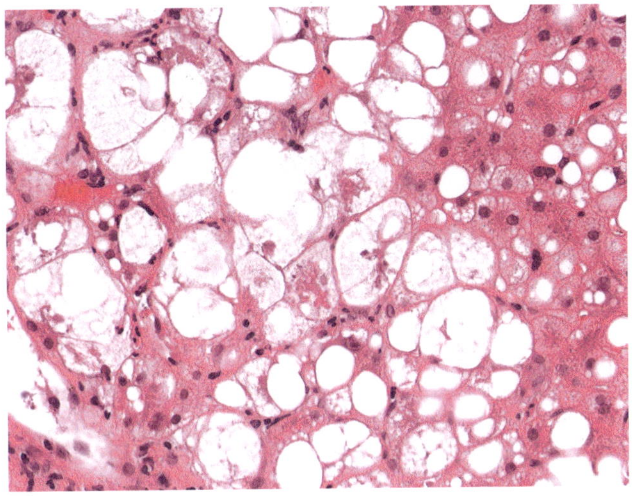

Fig. 5.23 Nonalcoholic steatohepatitis. A few Mallory-Denk bodies are present within ballooned hepatocytes. Mallory-Denk bodies are misfolded and aggregated intermediate filaments combined with other different classes of proteins, including p62 and ubiquitin. It is a deeply eosinophilic, ropey intracytoplasmic inclusion and often but not always found in ballooned hepatocytes. Compared with Mallory-Denk bodies in alcoholic liver disease, those in nonalcoholic fatty liver diseases tend to be more poorly formed, thin and wispy, and much less commonly associated with satellitosis. Mallory-Denk bodies also may be observed in chronic cholestatic disease, Wilson disease and other copper overload disorders, α_1-antitrypsin deficiency, drug-induced liver injury, focal nodular hyperplasia, and benign and malignant hepatocellular neoplasm.

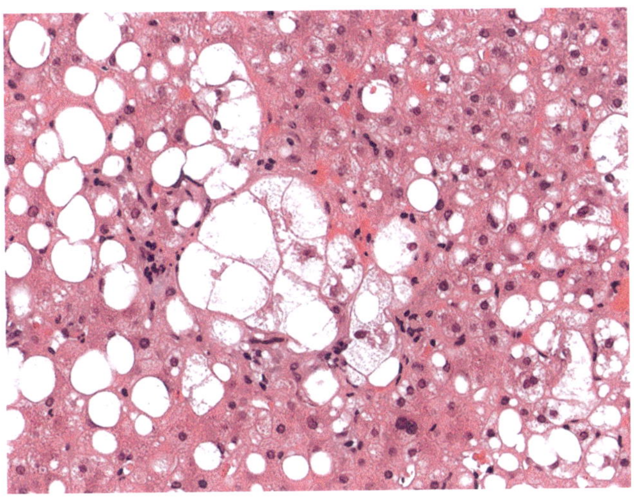

Fig. 5.22 Nonalcoholic steatohepatitis. Many ballooned hepatocytes are seen within a background of moderate macrovesicular steatosis. The mimickers of ballooning degeneration are feathery degeneration, steatosis (in particular the microvesicular form), and glycogen-rich hepatocytes. Feathery degeneration per se is almost indistinguishable from ballooning degeneration but one can differentiate them by the presence of histologic features of cholestasis and/or cholate stasis in the former. Glycogen-rich hepatocytes in glycogen storage disease or glycogenic hepatopathy show diffuse cytoplasmic enlargement and clearing, and sometimes contain glycogenated nuclei and giant mitochondria without any significant steatosis.

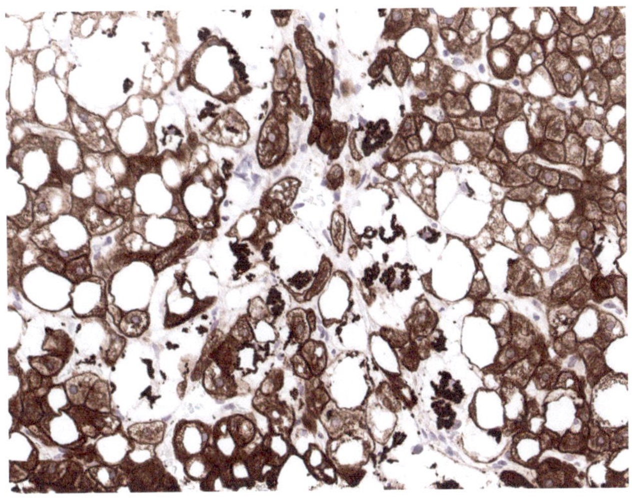

Fig. 5.24 Nonalcoholic steatohepatitis (cytokeratin 8/18 [CK8/18] stain). Ballooned hepatocytes lose cytoplasmic expression of CK8/18, whereas residual immunoreactivity is confined to their Mallory-Denk bodies. Diminished expression of CK8/18 in ballooned hepatocytes is characteristic of both alcoholic and nonalcoholic steatohepatitis. However, ballooned hepatocytes show similar patterns in chronic hepatitis C with concurrent steatohepatitic features, and in ischaemia/reperfusion injury in liver allografts. On the other hand, ballooned cells in acute viral hepatitis, autoimmune hepatitis, neonatal giant cell hepatitis, and drug-induced liver injury retain normal cytoplasmic expression of CK8/18.

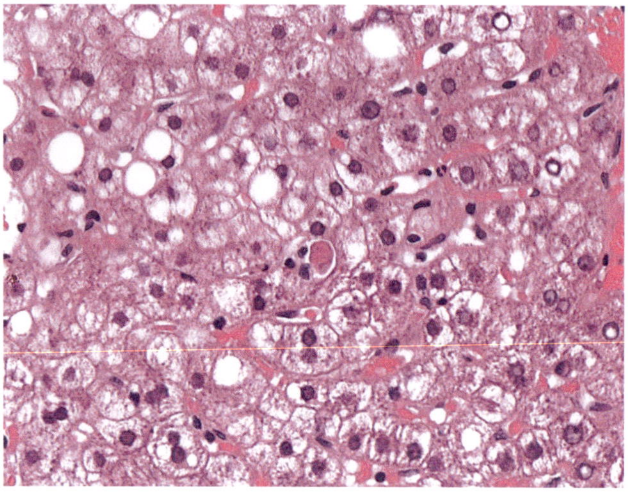

Fig. 5.25 Nonalcoholic steatohepatitis. An apoptotic body is present. Apoptosis is another manifestation of hepatocellular injury in nonalcoholic steatohepatitis and may be responsible in part for disease progression. Apoptotic pathways may be activated by saturated free fatty acids and free cholesterol, key mediators of lipotoxicity. Serum markers of hepatocyte apoptosis (CK18 fragment and soluble Fas) are used as noninvasive diagnostic markers of nonalcoholic steatohepatitis.

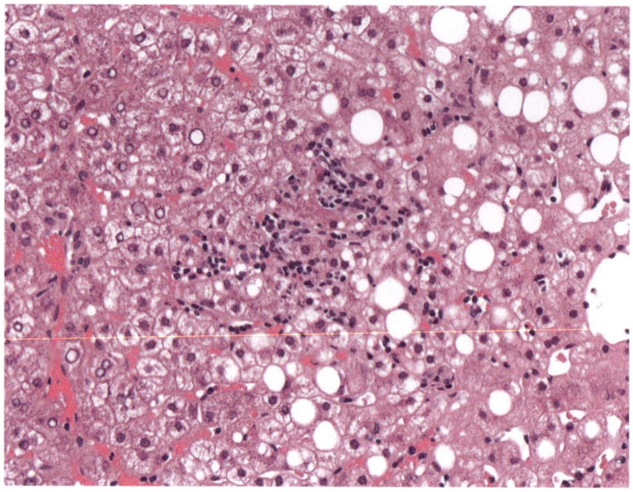

Fig. 5.27 Nonalcoholic fatty liver disease. A moderate sinusoidal lymphohistiocytic infiltrate is noted. Lobular inflammation in nonalcoholic steatohepatitis usually is mild and composed of sinusoidal mixed inflammatory infiltrate of mainly lymphocytes with some eosinophils and a few neutrophils. Lipogranulomas and microgranulomas also may be present. However, the presence of lobular inflammation and steatosis alone, without ballooning degeneration and perivenular/pericellular fibrosis, is insufficient to establish the diagnosis of steatohepatitis. Such cases may be diagnosed as steatosis with nonspecific inflammation.

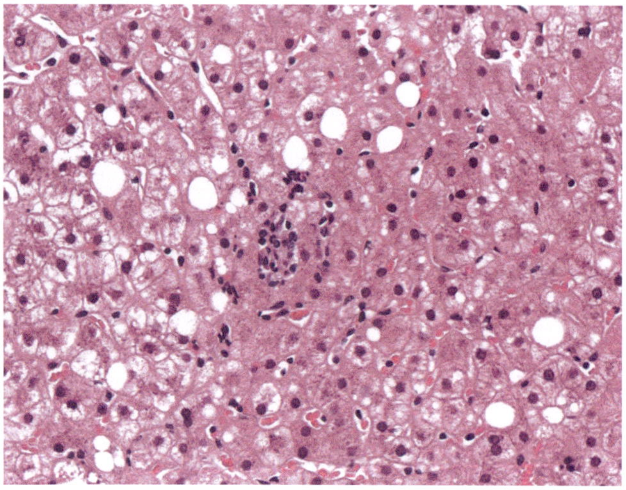

Fig. 5.26 Nonalcoholic steatohepatitis. There is a focus of spotty necrosis characterised by an aggregate of lymphocytes and activated Kupffer cells/macrophages "filling" the gap of dropped-out hepatocytes. A mild sinusoidal lymphocytic infiltrate also is noted. Spotty necrosis is another form of hepatocellular injury sometimes found in nonalcoholic steatohepatitis. However, confluent necrosis and bridging necrosis are rare whereas panacinar necrosis typically is absent.

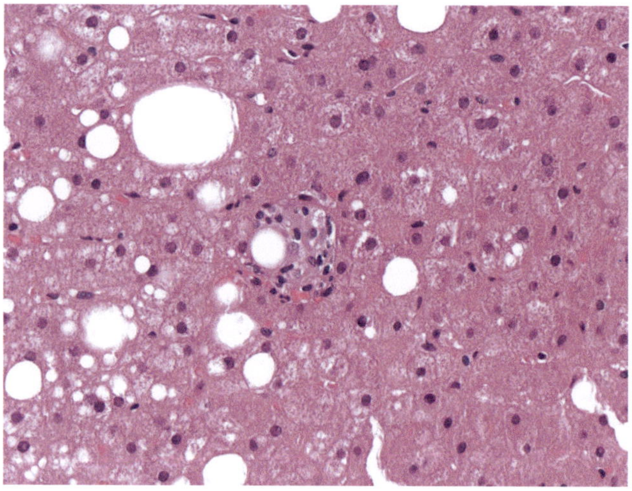

Fig. 5.28 Nonalcoholic fatty liver disease. Here, we see a lipogranuloma consisting of a loose aggregate of lymphocytes and macrophages surrounding a central fat globule. Lipogranulomas are one of the components of lobular inflammation in nonalcoholic fatty liver disease. They also are a feature of alcoholic liver disease, as well as of ingestion of mineral oil in food and medication. They may be distinguished from fibrin ring granulomas, which have a characteristic fibrin ring highlighted by phosphotungstic acid-haematoxylin stain, Martius scarlet blue stain, or immunostaining for fibrin.

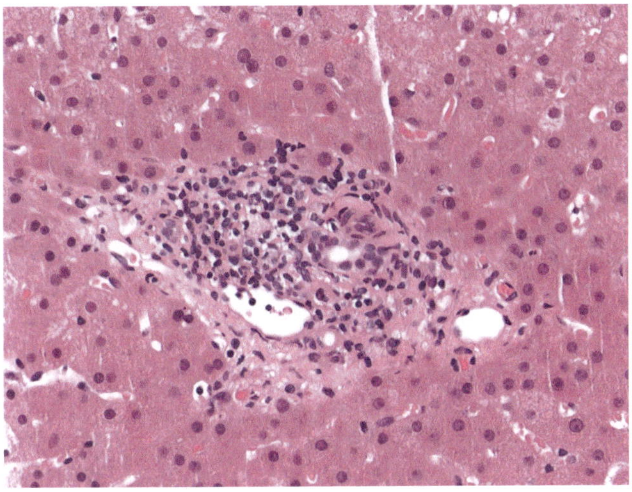

Fig. 5.29 Nonalcoholic fatty liver disease. This portal tract is infiltrated by a mild lymphocytic infiltrate. Portal inflammation is common in nonalcoholic fatty liver disease. It usually is mild and composed mainly of lymphocytes, with some eosinophils and macrophages. Ductular reaction and portal neutrophils raise the possibility of concurrent alcoholic intake or pancreatitis. A disproportionately dense portal inflammation may be observed in paediatric nonalcoholic fatty liver disease, advanced nonalcoholic fatty liver disease, and posttreatment nonalcoholic fatty liver disease, and when there is concomitant chronic liver disease (e.g., chronic viral hepatitis, autoimmune hepatitis, and chronic cholestatic disease).

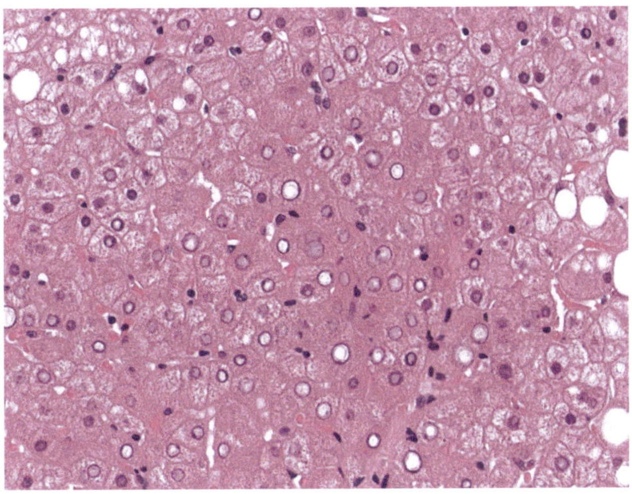

Fig. 5.30 Nonalcoholic fatty liver disease. Many hepatocytes exhibit nuclear clear vacuolation due to the accumulation of glycogen. Glycogenated nuclei are found much more commonly in nonalcoholic fatty liver disease than in alcoholic liver disease. They may be considered evidence of impaired glucose tolerance or insulin resistance. However, they may occur physiologically in children and young adults (11% and 4% in the 20s and early 30s, respectively) or pathologically in other diseases, including chronic hepatitis C with steatohepatitic features, glycogen storage disease, Wilson disease, and other copper overload disorders.

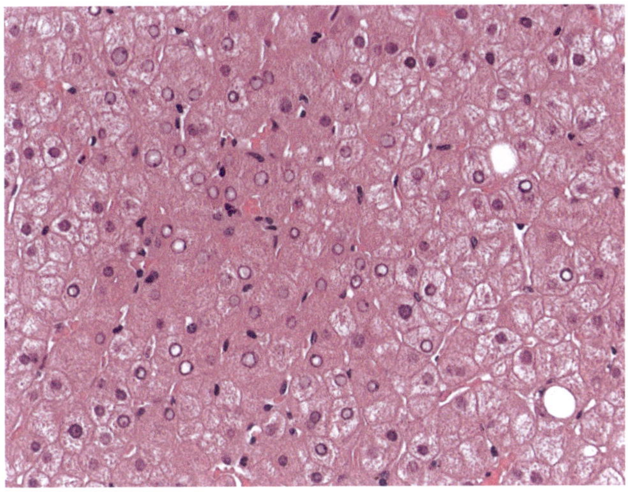

Fig. 5.31 Nonalcoholic fatty liver disease. Many hepatocytes exhibit nuclear clear vacuolation due to glycogen accumulation. Glycogenated nuclei must be distinguished from sanded nuclei in chronic hepatitis B, which are palely eosinophilic and finely granular intranuclear inclusions immunoreactive to hepatitis B core antigen.

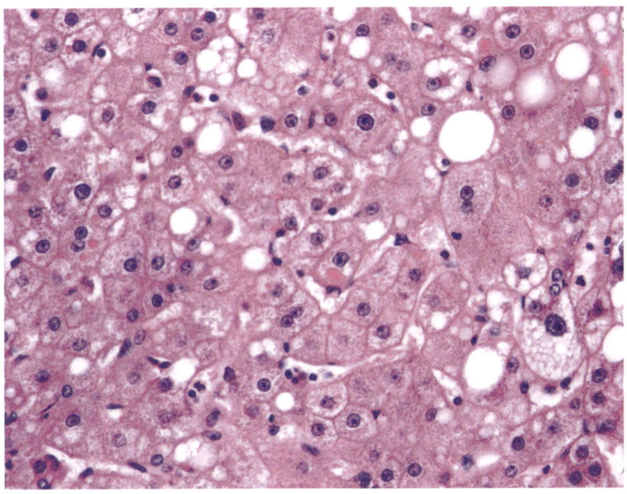

Fig. 5.32 Nonalcoholic fatty liver disease. Occasional giant mitochondria are present in the hepatocytes. Giant mitochondria, also called megamitochondria, are eosinophilic oval or needle-shaped intracytoplasmic inclusions. Although they typically are found in alcoholic and nonalcoholic fatty liver diseases, they may be associated with a wide variety of physiologic and pathologic conditions, such as aging, acute fatty liver of pregnancy, glycogen storage disease, urea cycle defects, and glycogenic hepatopathy.

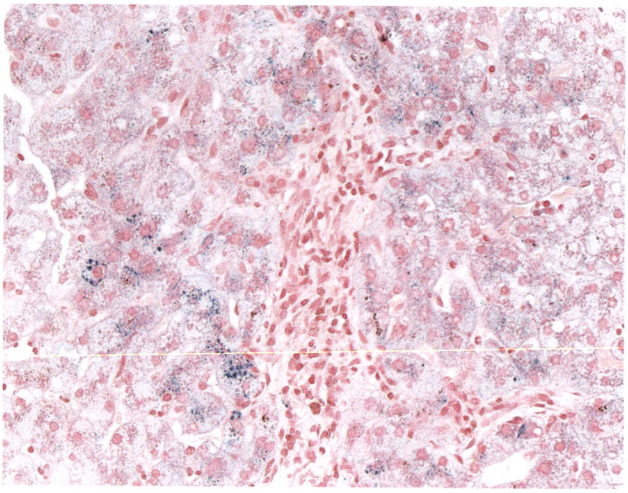

Fig. 5.33 Nonalcoholic fatty liver disease (Perls stain). Mild parenchymal siderosis is noted in periportal hepatocytes. Nonalcoholic fatty liver disease commonly is associated with hyperferritinaemia, but the use of serum ferritin as a biomarker in assessing the stage of nonalcoholic fatty liver disease is controversial. Nonalcoholic fatty liver disease frequently is associated with siderosis histologically. Hepatic siderosis, however, usually is mild (grade 1–2) and located mainly in hepatocytes. As in alcoholic liver disease, the presence of severe (grade 3–4) parenchymal siderosis should raise the possibility of coexisting hereditary haemochromatosis.

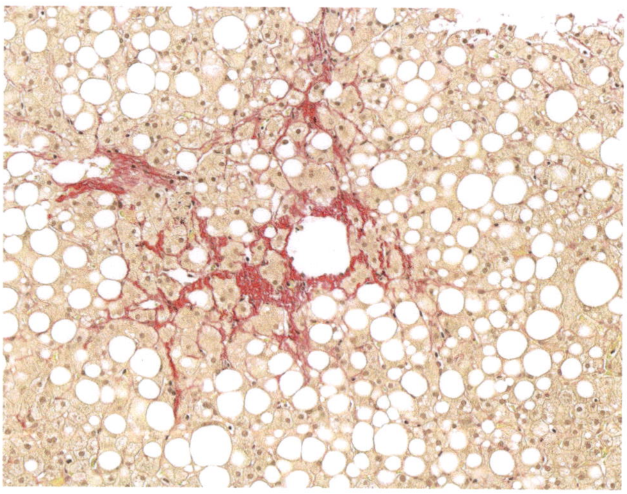

Fig. 5.34 Nonalcoholic fatty liver disease with zone 3 pericellular fibrosis (picrosirius red stain). Thick and thin fibrous strands are deposited around hepatocytes in the perivenular region. Zone 3 pericellular (perisinusoidal) fibrosis is deposition of fibrous tissue in the space of Disse and is related to activation of stellate cells. It is typical in the early stages of fibrosis in nonalcoholic fatty liver disease in adults, similar to that in alcoholic fatty liver. However, the fibres tend to be thinner and less marked in nonalcoholic fatty liver disease. Moreover, the characteristic perivenular fibrosis with phlebosclerosis of alcoholic liver disease is unusual in nonalcoholic fatty liver disease.

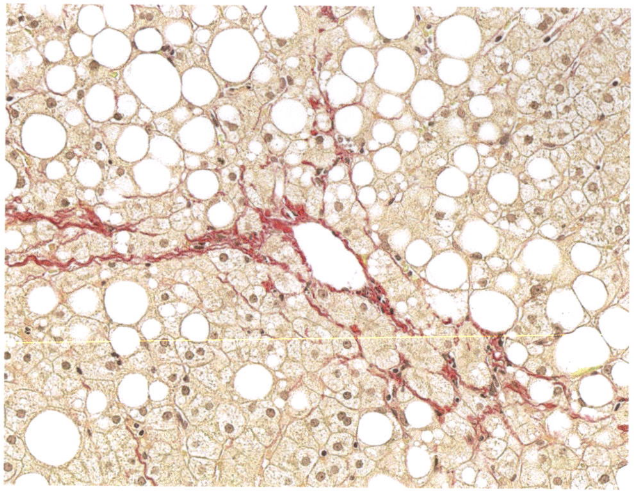

Fig. 5.35 Nonalcoholic fatty liver disease with zone 3 pericellular fibrosis (picrosirius red stain). Delicate fibrous strands are deposited around hepatocytes in the perivenular region. Zone 3 pericellular fibrosis corresponds to stage 1 disease of the Non-alcoholic Steatohepatitis Clinical Research Network (NASH CRN) system. Subclassification into stage 1a and 1b disease depends on whether the fibrous strands are delicate (visible on connective tissue stain only) or dense (recognizable on haematoxylin and eosin [H&E] stain). The NASH CRN has applied a term, *borderline steatohepatitis*, for cases with steatosis and zone 3 pericellular fibrosis in the absence of ballooning degeneration. However, this practice is controversial and not yet accepted universally. Many pathologists prefer to describe this as steatosis with fibrosis or steatofibrosis in such cases.

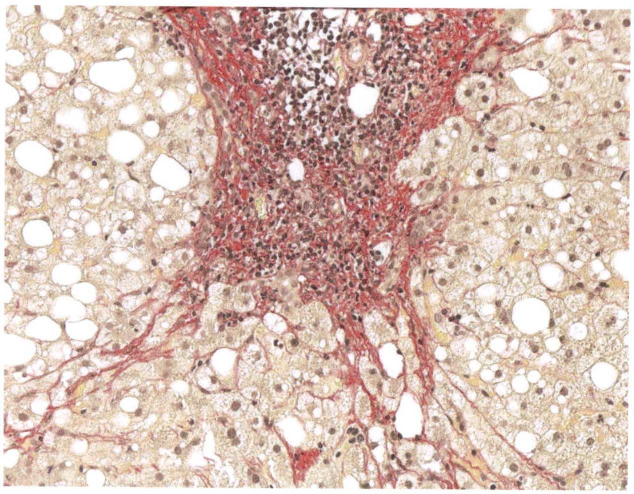

Fig. 5.36 Nonalcoholic fatty liver disease with portal and periportal fibrosis (picrosirius red stain). A portal tract is expanded by portal and periportal fibrous tissue and moderate portal lymphocytic infiltrate. Portal fibrosis without zone 3 pericellular fibrosis is typical in children with fatty liver disease and in morbidly obese adults, and is designated stage 1c disease by the NASH CRN system. Periportal fibrosis, together with zone 3 pericellular fibrosis, corresponds to stage 2 disease of the NASH CRN system.

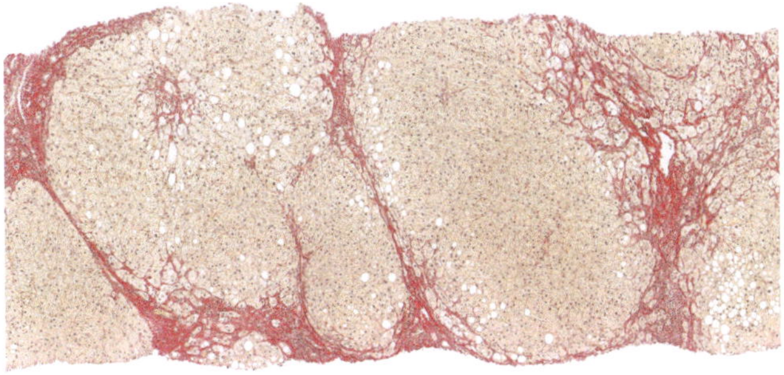

Fig. 5.37 Nonalcoholic fatty liver disease with cirrhosis (picrosirius red). Here, we see regenerative nodules surrounded by bridging fibrous septa. Pericellular fibrosis also is prominent. Cirrhosis represents stage 4 disease in the NASH CRN system.

SCORE	STEATOSIS	LOBULAR INFLAMMATION	BALLOONING
0	<5%	None	None
1	5 to 33%	<2foci/200x field	Few
2	>33% to 66%	2-4 foci/200x field	Many
3	>66%	<4 foci/200x field	

Fig. 5.38 Non-alcoholic Steatohepatitis Clinical Research Network system. The nonalcoholic fatty liver disease activity score (0–8) is the sum of scores of all three components: steatosis (0–3), lobular inflammation (0–3), and ballooning degeneration (0–2). This score is used to assess the disease activity (grading) of histologically evident steatohepatitis. It should not be applied as diagnostic criteria for establishing the diagnosis of steatohepatitis.

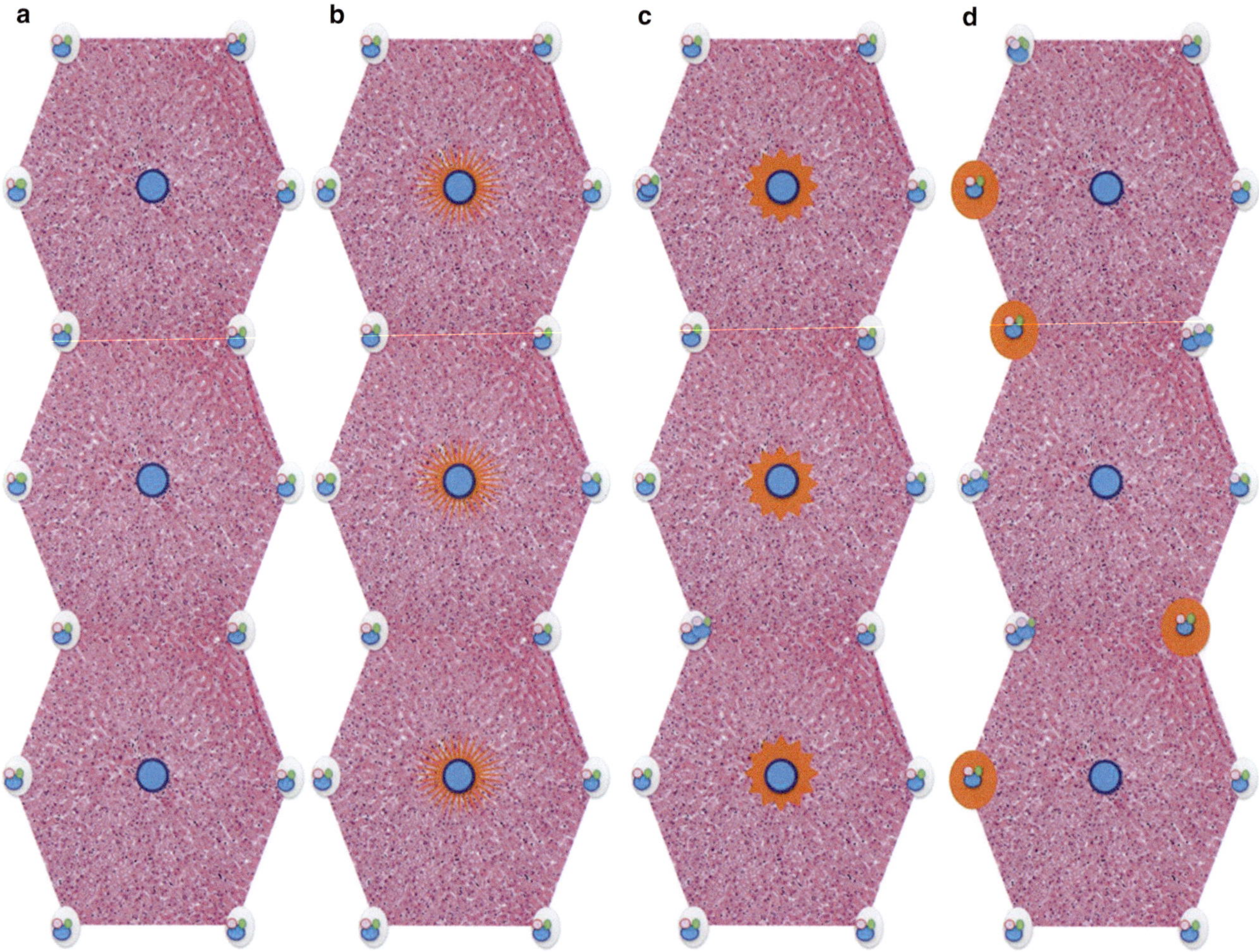

Fig. 5.39 Staging of the Non-alcoholic Steatohepatitis Clinical Research Network system (orange region represents fibrosis). (**A**) Stage 0: normal liver without any fibrosis. (**B**) Stage 1a: mild zone 3 pericellular fibrosis, visualized only on trichrome stain. (**C**) Stage 1b: moderate zone 3 pericellular fibrosis, readily visualized on H&E stain. (**D**) Stage 1c: portal fibrosis only.

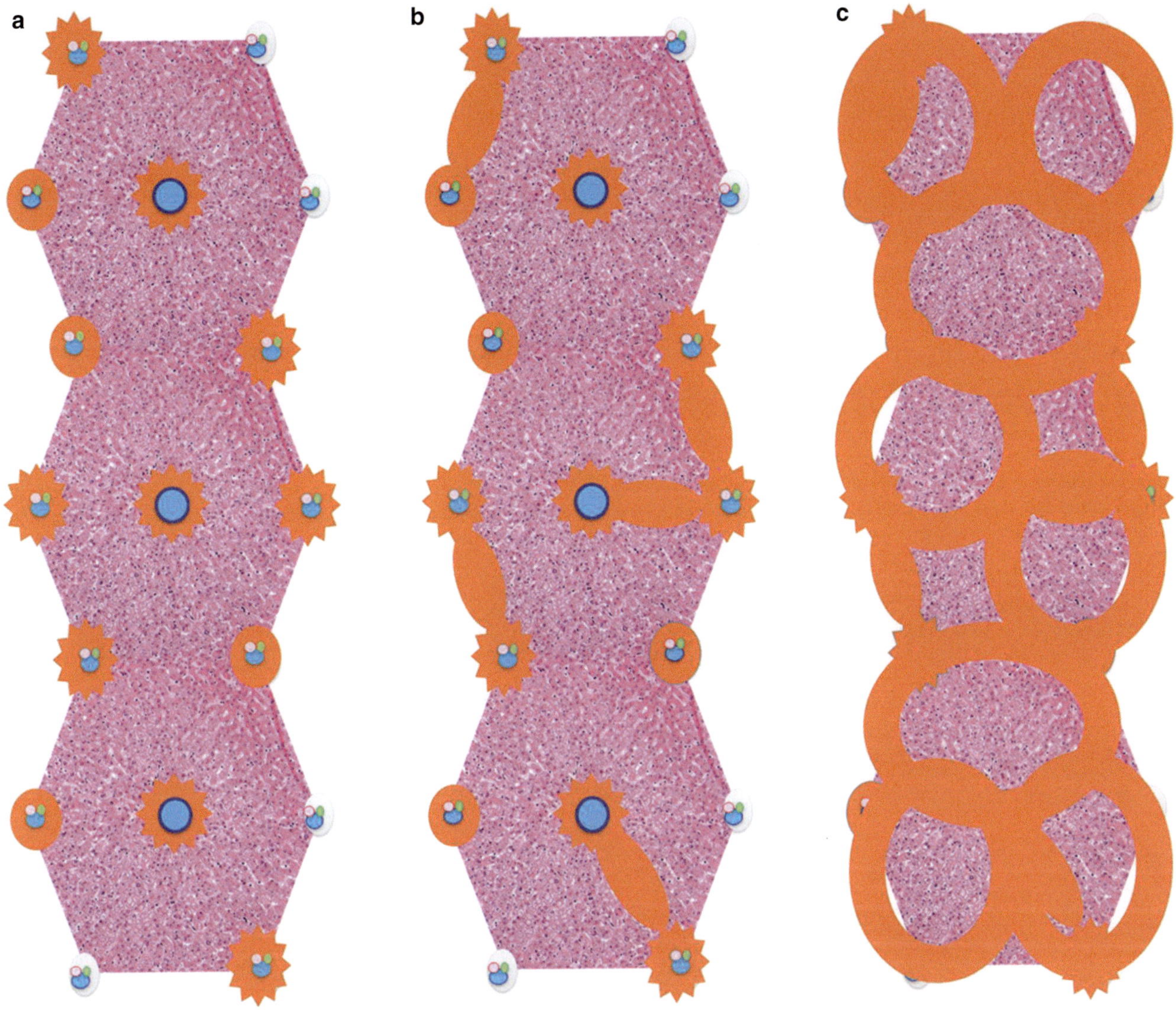

Fig. 5.40 Staging of the Non-alcoholic Steatohepatitis Clinical Research Network system (orange region represents fibrosis). (**A**) Stage 2: zone 3 pericellular fibrosis and periportal fibrosis. (**B**) Stage 3: bridging fibrosis. (**C**) Stage 4: probable or definite cirrhosis.

5.3 Focal Fatty Change

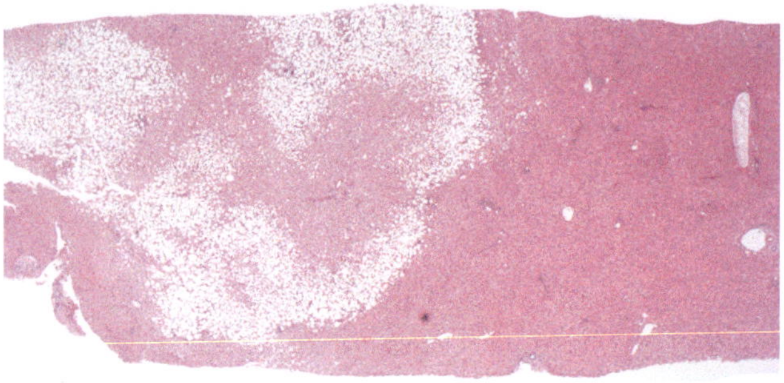

Fig. 5.41 Focal fatty change. A steatotic nodule is seen against a background of nonsteatotic liver. Focal fatty change may be found in about 10% to 20% of livers. It typically is asymptomatic and discovered incidentally on imaging studies. It is characterized by single or multiple localized regions of marked macrovesicular steatosis. The liver architecture within and adjacent to focal fatty liver is preserved without any distortion. The possible pathogenesis may be related to focal ischaemia or aberrant localized (endogenous or exogenous) insulin effects. The differential diagnoses of focal fatty change include steatotic hepatocellular adenoma and carcinoma, angiomyolipoma, rarely lipoma, myelolipoma, and coelomic fat ectopia.

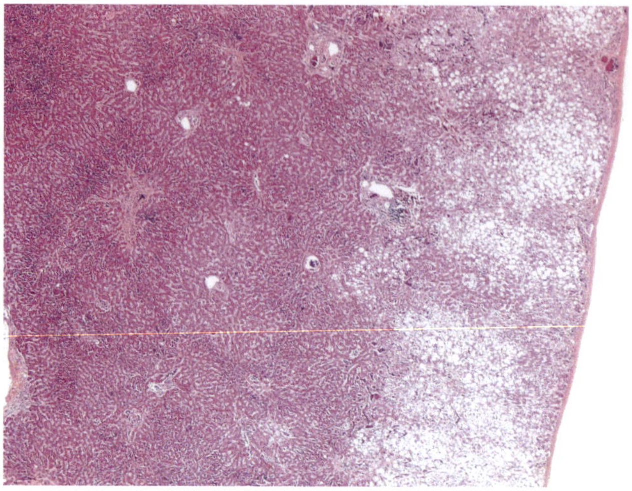

Fig. 5.42 Focal fatty change. Accumulation of macrovesicular steatosis is concentrated in the subcapsular liver of a patient receiving intraperitoneal insulin injections.

6 Viral Liver Disease

Hepatotropic viruses (A–E) may cause a wide range of injuries to the hepatic parenchyma, from mild acute subclinical to acute liver failure requiring liver transplantation, from "healthy carrier" state to advanced chronic liver disease and hepatocellular carcinoma. The pattern of injury depends on several factors, including the type of virus, host immune response, and coexistence with other viruses or pathologies. Liver biopsy now is performed rarely in the context of acute hepatitis, as its histologic pattern usually is nonspecific for an aetiologic diagnosis. Its use to gauge the severity of liver injury also is very limited because of sampling error. The role of liver biopsy in staging and grading chronic viral hepatitis has been challenged by the introduction of noninvasive markers of fibrosis and new imaging modalities. Nevertheless, liver histology still is considered the gold standard and semiquantitative methods of histologic grading and staging still are in use worldwide. Other, nonhepatotropic viruses, such as adenovirus, herpes cytomegalovirus (CMV), and Epstein-Barr virus (EBV), may cause liver injury, usually in immunocompromised patients. Parvovirus may cause acute hepatitis in children.

6.1 Hepatotropic Viral Hepatitis

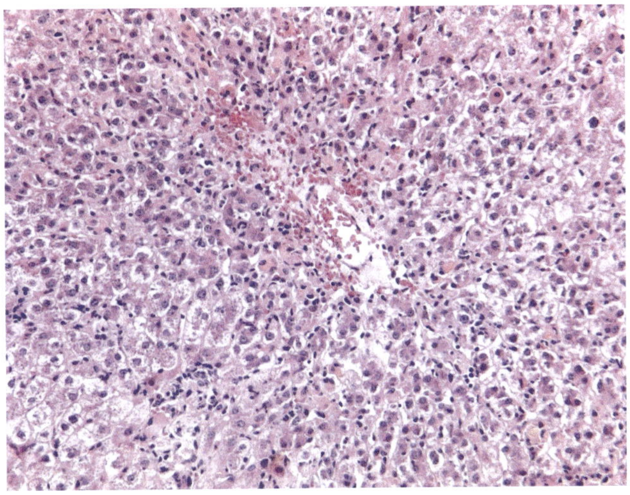

Fig. 6.1 Acute hepatitis A. Perivenular confluent necrosis is present, together with large numbers of ballooned hepatocytes and a mild sinusoidal lymphocytic infiltrate. Primary infection by hepatotropic viruses may vary from asymptomatic subclinical infection, to acute hepatitis, to fulminant hepatitis. Acute hepatitis usually presents as fever, right upper quadrant pain, jaundice, anorexia, malaise, and deranged liver enzymes with a duration arbitrarily defined as less than 6 months. Fulminant hepatitis is a severe form of acute hepatitis rapidly progressing to liver failure and encephalopathy within a few days/weeks and carrying mortality rates of 25% to 90%.

A.W.H. Chan et al., *Atlas of Liver Pathology*, Atlas of Anatomic Pathology,
DOI 10.1007/978-1-4614-9114-9_6, © Springer Science+Business Media New York 2014

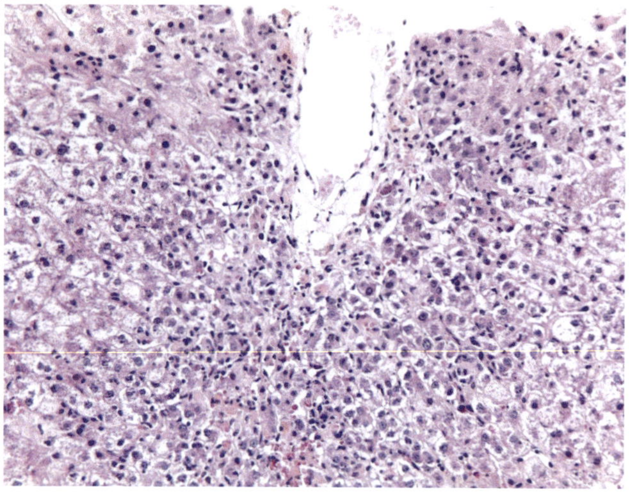

Fig. 6.2 Acute hepatitis A. Perivenular confluent necrosis is present, and there is marked lobular disarray together with lobular inflammation. Liver biopsy rarely is required to confirm the diagnosis of acute viral hepatitis, because serologic tests are more informative and confirmatory. Nevertheless, several histopathologic patterns of acute hepatitis are recognized. The classic or prototypical pattern is lobular necroinflammation characterised by numerous swollen or ballooned hepatocytes; scattered apoptotic hepatocytes and a varying degree of spotty necrosis; resultant collapse of reticulin framework; a lobular inflammatory cell infiltrate of varying combinations of lymphocytes, plasma cells, and macrophages; hypertrophied ceroid-laden Kupffer cells; and variable bilirubinostasis.

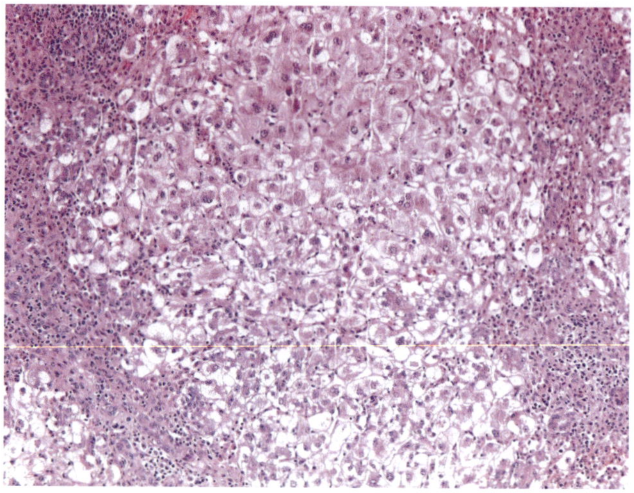

Fig. 6.4 Acute hepatitis A. Extensive bridging necrosis is seen in this case, in which there was acute liver failure. Most pathologic features of acute hepatotropic viral hepatitis are essentially nonspecific and common to different causes of acute hepatitis. Periportal necrosis, prominent portal plasmacytic infiltrate, and perivenular bilirubinostasis with minimal lobular necrosis are found most commonly in acute hepatitis A. A lobular mixed neutrophilic and lymphocytic infiltrate, together with acute cholangitis, is characteristic of acute hepatitis E. The acute phase of hepatitis C usually is clinically silent and not observed histologically, although reported cases show the histological picture is nonspecific. Ground-glass hepatocytes, sanded nuclei, and even immunoreactivity to hepatitis B surface antigen (HBsAg) and hepatitis B core antigen (HBcAg) typically are absent in acute hepatitis B but are characteristic in chronic disease.

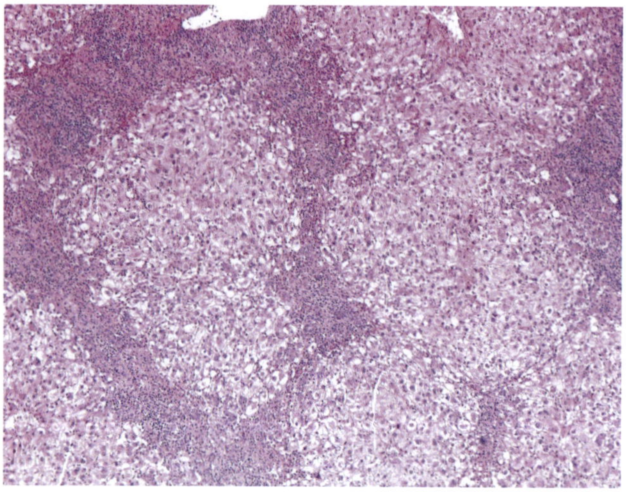

Fig. 6.3 Acute hepatitis A. Extensive bridging necrosis is seen together with islands of residual ballooned hepatocytes. In more severe forms of acute viral hepatitis, confluent necrosis, bridging necrosis, and even panacinar necrosis may be present and generally are accompanied by regenerative changes and a ductular reaction. An uncommon pattern of acute viral hepatitis is the presence of periportal necrosis with variable degrees of ductular reaction, in addition to lobular necroinflammation. Such a pattern can mimic that of interface hepatitis in chronic hepatitis. Absence of entrapped hepatocytes among the periportal inflammatory infiltrate, the presence of prominent lobular necroinflammation, and, more importantly, serologic evidence of acute viral hepatitis may help in making the distinction.

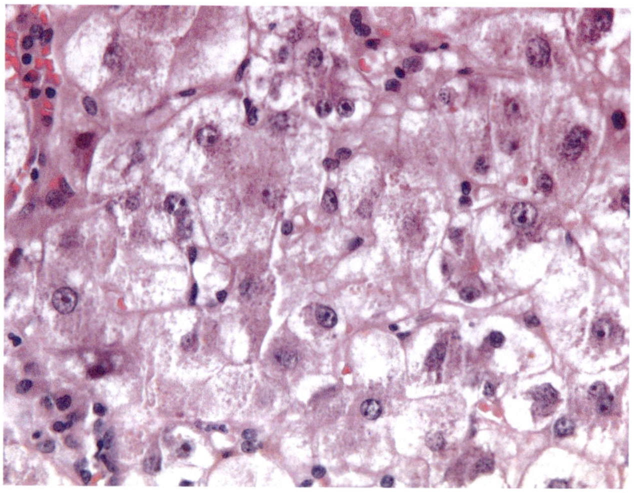

Fig. 6.5 Acute hepatitis A. These ballooned hepatocytes are characterised by cellular swelling, rarefaction of their cytoplasm, and clumped strands of intermediate filaments. Focal hepatocyte rosettes and canalicular bilirubinostasis are noted. Acute hepatitis-like clinical and pathologic pictures also may be caused by acute nonhepatotropic viral infections, drug/toxin-induced hepatitis, acute alcoholic hepatitis, autoimmune hepatitis, and Wilson disease. Clinical, biochemical, serologic, and pathologic correlations are essential to establish the definitive diagnosis.

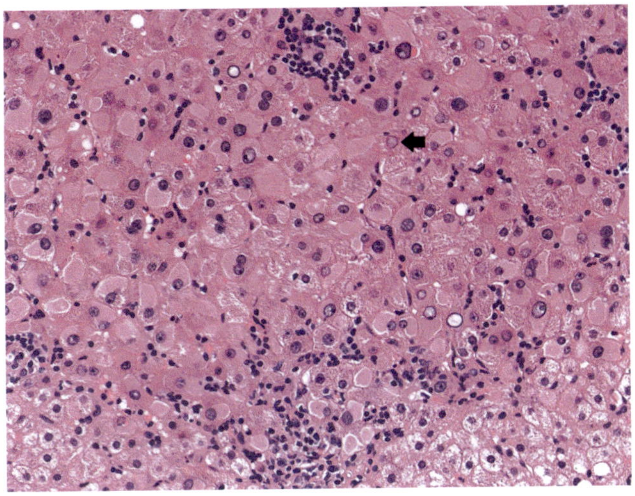

Fig. 6.6 Chronic hepatitis B. Large numbers of ground-glass hepatocytes are present; these are characterised by their eosinophilic, finely granular intracytoplasmic inclusions with an occasional surrounding clear halo. A sanded nucleus (*arrow*) also is seen. Ground-glass inclusions represent endoplasmic reticulum filled with HBsAg and are one of the hallmark pathologic features of chronic hepatitis B. So-called sanded nuclei represent pale pink, finely granular intranuclear inclusions containing HBcAg and also are characteristic of chronic hepatitis B. Other pathologic features of chronic hepatitis B are nonspecific and similar to all types of chronic hepatitis, including variable portal inflammation, interface hepatitis, lobular necroinflammation, and fibrosis.

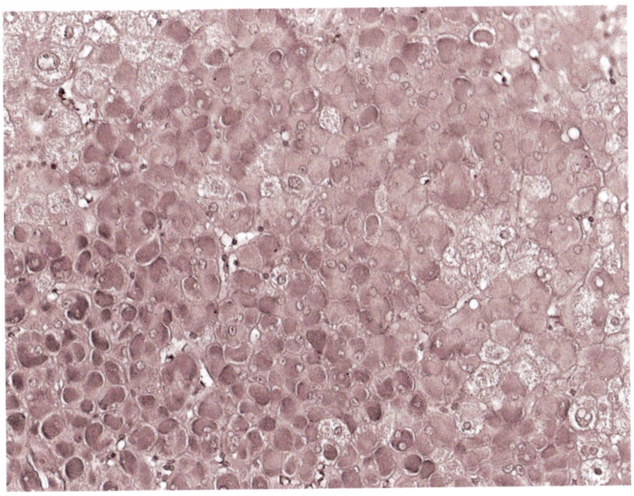

Fig. 6.7 Chronic hepatitis B (orcein stain). Extensive ground-glass hepatocyte change is highlighted. Orcein or Victoria blue stain confirms the nature of ground-glass inclusions and helps differentiate them from pseudo–ground-glass inclusions, pale bodies, oncocytic hepatocytic change, and hepatocyte with enzyme induction. Pseudo–ground-glass inclusions may be found in glycogen storage disease type IV, Lafora disease, cyanamide-induced injury, and immunocompromised patients on multiple medications.

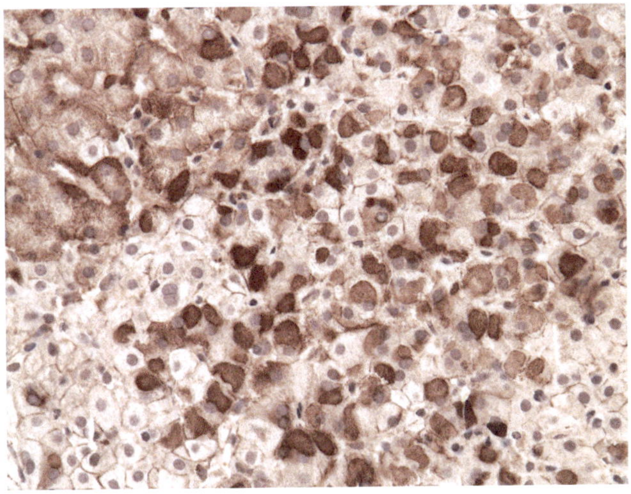

Fig. 6.8 Chronic hepatitis B (HBsAg stain). Extensive ground-glass hepatocytes are highlighted and exhibit both membranous and intracytoplasmic staining patterns. Immunostaining for HBsAg confirms the diagnosis of chronic hepatitis B. Extensive membranous staining indicates a high viral replicative rate, whereas diffuse intracytoplasmic staining suggests a low replicative state. By contrast, immunostaining for HBcAg shows mainly nuclear staining and, less commonly, cytoplasmic or membranous staining. The presence of immunoreactivity to core antigen signifies high viral replication, which correlates with the serum hepatitis B DNA level.

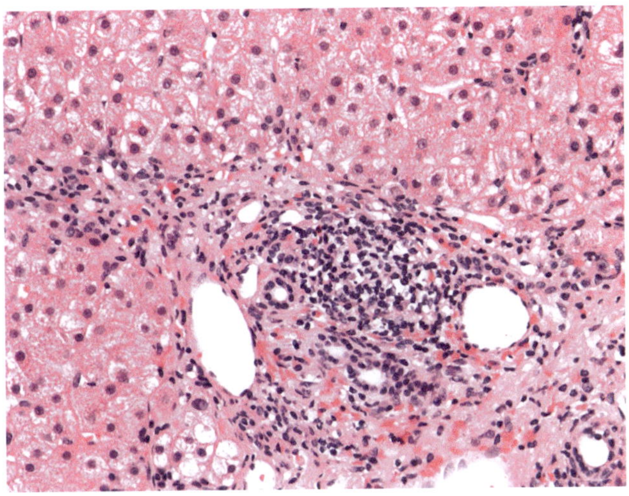

Fig. 6.9 Chronic hepatitis B. This portal tract shows a moderate chronic inflammatory infiltrate and mild interface hepatitis. Portal inflammation is the hallmark feature of chronic hepatitis of any cause. A lymphocyte-predominant infiltrate is common in chronic viral hepatitis. Lymphoid aggregates or follicles, although seen more commonly in chronic hepatitis C, also may be found in chronic hepatitis B.

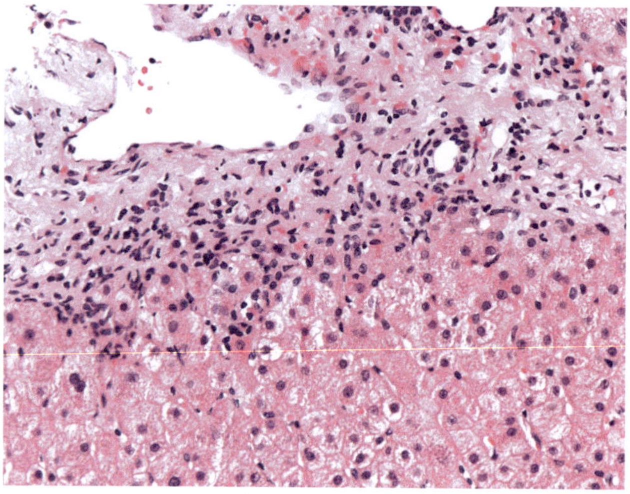

Fig. 6.10 Chronic hepatitis B. Moderate interface hepatitis is seen at the circumference of a portal tract. Interface hepatitis, previously referred to as piecemeal necrosis, is characterised by portal inflammatory cells eroding through the interface between portal tracts and the liver parenchyma and surrounding individual and small groups of periportal hepatocytes. It differs from the simple spillover of inflammatory cells in acute hepatitis by the presence of periportal hepatocellular liver cell apoptosis and drop-out.

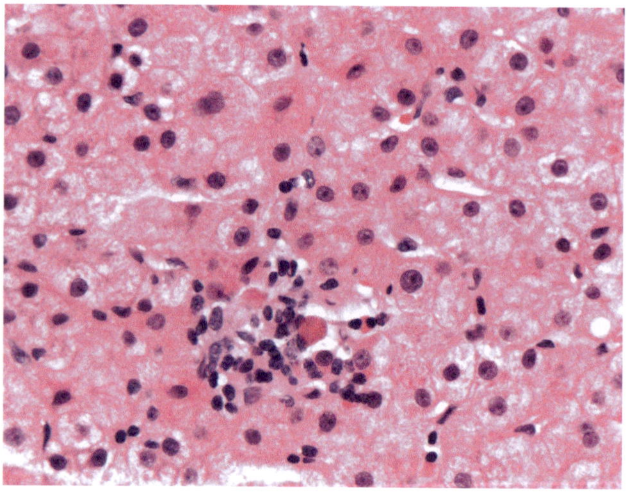

Fig. 6.11 Chronic hepatitis B. Shown is a focus of spotty necrosis comprising an apoptotic body and associated lymphocytes. Lobular necroinflammatory activity in chronic hepatitis B usually is mild and composed of scattered foci of spotty necrosis and apoptotic bodies. More marked lobular necroinflammation with the presence of multiple foci of spotty necrosis, confluent necrosis, or bridging necrosis in chronic hepatitis B indicates possible hepatitis B e antigen (HBeAg) seroconversion (loss of serum HBeAg and development of anti-HBe antibody), superinfection of hepatitis D, reactivation of hepatitis B under immunosuppression, or concomitant drug/toxin-induced injury.

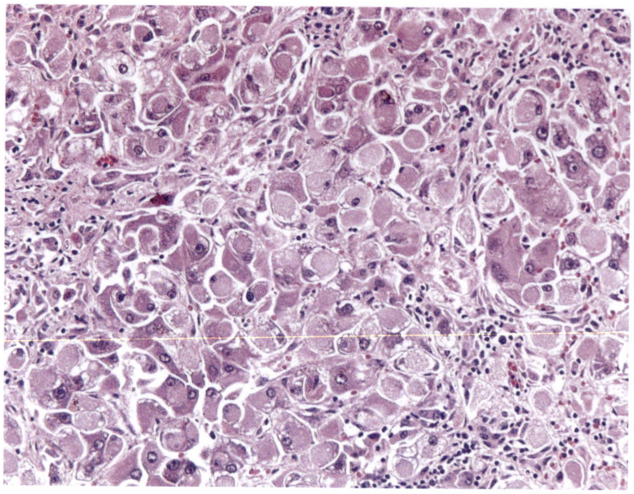

Fig. 6.12 Fibrosing cholestatic hepatitis B. The hepatocytes exhibit extensive ground-glass cytoplasmic inclusions. Delicate pericellular fibrous strands also are noted. Fibrosing cholestatic hepatitis is a distinct variant of chronic hepatitis B affecting immunocompromised patients resulting in cholestatic liver function derangement and rapid progression to hepatic failure and encephalopathy over several weeks. Pathologically, it is characterised by variable combinations of portal, periportal, and pericellular fibrosis, ductular reaction, ballooning degeneration, bilirubinostasis, and steatosis. In fibrosing cholestatic hepatitis, prominent expression of HBsAg and HBcAg is typical.

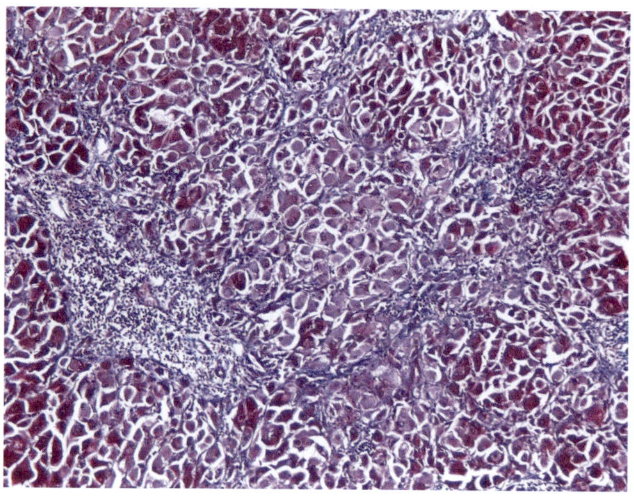

Fig. 6.13 Fibrosing cholestatic hepatitis B (Masson trichrome stain). Portal and periportal fibrosis is accompanied by delicate pericellular fibrosis.

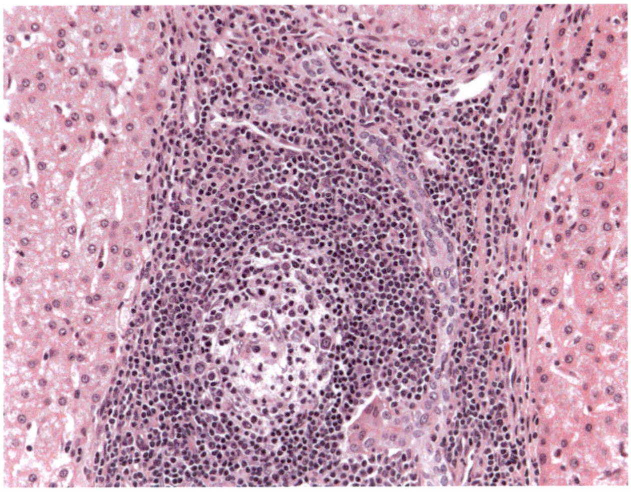

Fig. 6.14 Chronic hepatitis C. This portal tract contains a dense lymphocyte-predominant inflammatory infiltrate and a reactive lymphoid follicle. Portal lymphoid follicles are a characteristic feature in chronic hepatitis C but may be found in many other liver diseases, such as chronic hepatitis B, autoimmune hepatitis, and primary biliary cirrhosis. Portal lymphoid follicles, bile duct damage, and steatosis are three pathologic features characteristic of chronic hepatitis C. Other pathologic features are nonspecific and similar to all types of chronic hepatitis; these include variable portal inflammation, interface hepatitis, lobular necroinflammation, and fibrosis.

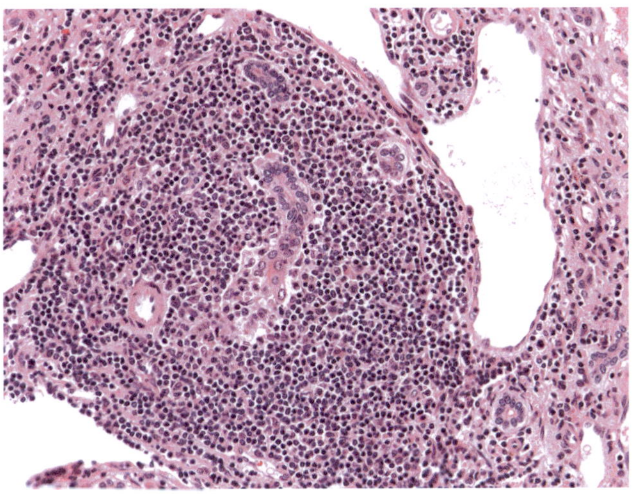

Fig. 6.15 Chronic hepatitis C. An interlobular bile duct shows focal epithelial disarray, and there is an intraepithelial lymphocytic infiltrate. The portal tract contains a dense lymphocyte-predominant inflammatory infiltrate. Bile duct damage frequently is found in chronic hepatitis C. Mild ductular reaction and even ductopaenia occasionally are present. Such biliary features make the distinction between chronic hepatitis and chronic biliary disease difficult in a minority of cases. More prominent bile duct damage, ductular reaction, and ductopaenia with chronic cholate stasis all favour a diagnosis of chronic biliary disease.

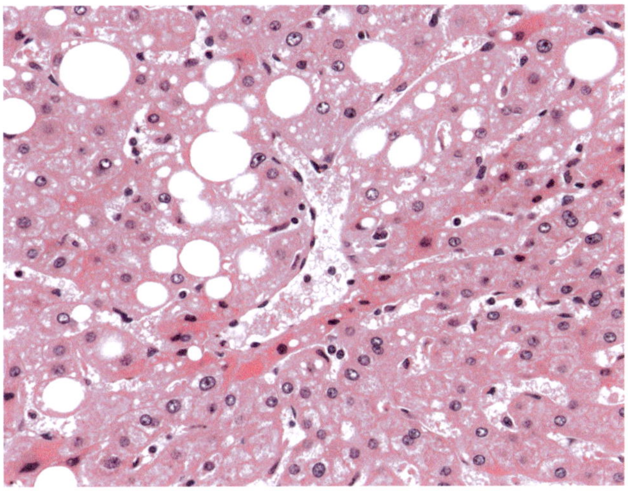

Fig. 6.16 Chronic hepatitis C. Macrovesicular and mediovesicular steatosis is noted. Mild macrovesicular and mediovesicular steatosis without any zonal predilection is present in 40% to 80% of cases of chronic hepatitis C as a result of either direct viral effect (particularly genotype 3) or indirect virally induced insulin resistance (particularly with genotypes 1 and 4). The presence of ballooning degeneration, Mallory-Denk bodies, neutrophilic infiltrate, and pericellular fibrosis raises the possibility of coexisting alcoholic or nonalcoholic steatohepatitis and requires clinical correlation with alcoholic intake and risk factors for the metabolic syndrome.

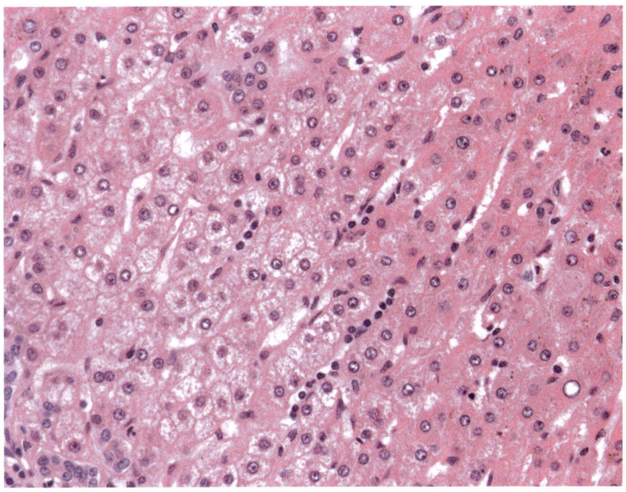

Fig. 6.17 Chronic hepatitis C. Sinusoidal lymphocytes are arranged in a linear, bead-like configuration. Sinusoidal lymphocytosis is another typical feature of chronic hepatitis C. However, it is not entirely specific and may be found in EBV hepatitis, CMV hepatitis in immunocompetent patients, autoimmune hepatitis, and drug-induced liver injury.

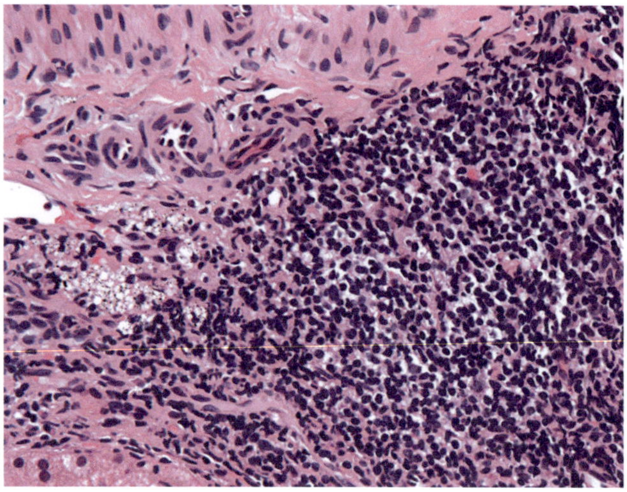

Fig. 6.18 Chronic hepatitis C. Collections of macrophages containing refractile foreign bodies are noted within a moderately inflamed portal tract. These refractile foreign bodies contain talc or titanium and are a frequent finding in liver biopsy samples from intravenous drug abusers.

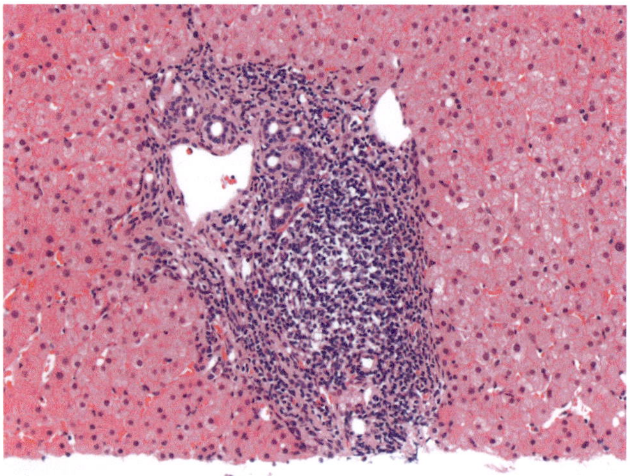

Fig. 6.19 Chronic hepatitis C. This portal tract contains a dense lymphocyte-predominant inflammatory infiltrate with focal mild interface hepatitis. The biopsy sample is from a patient with elevated serum anti–liver kidney microsomal (LKM) antibody. Elevation of autoantibodies such as anti–smooth muscle antigen and anti-LKM in low titres is found in 20% to 40% of cases of chronic hepatitis C (as well as chronic hepatitis B). It implies activation of virally driven autoimmune mechanisms, which may explain the pathogenesis of some extrahepatic manifestations of chronic hepatitis C, such as mixed cryoglobulinaemia, autoimmune thyroiditis, mesangiocapillary glomerulonephritis, lichen planus, and polyarteritis nodosa.

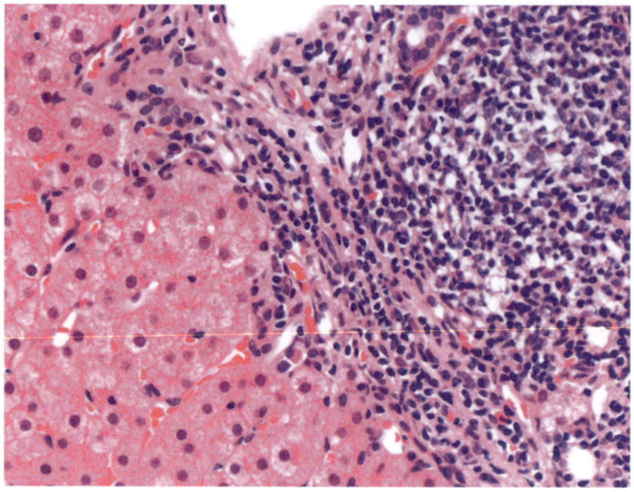

Fig. 6.20 Chronic hepatitis C in a patient with elevated serum anti-LKM antibody. Chronic hepatitis C may be associated with circulating autoantibodies and mimic autoimmune hepatitis. On the other hand, autoimmune hepatitis may be associated with false positive anti–hepatitis C virus serology and confused with chronic hepatitis C. However, chronic hepatitis C with elevated autoantibodies should be distinguished from autoimmune hepatitis because of the therapeutic implications. The use of a clinical scoring system for the diagnosis of autoimmune hepatitis is helpful in excluding chronic hepatitis C with elevated autoantibodies.

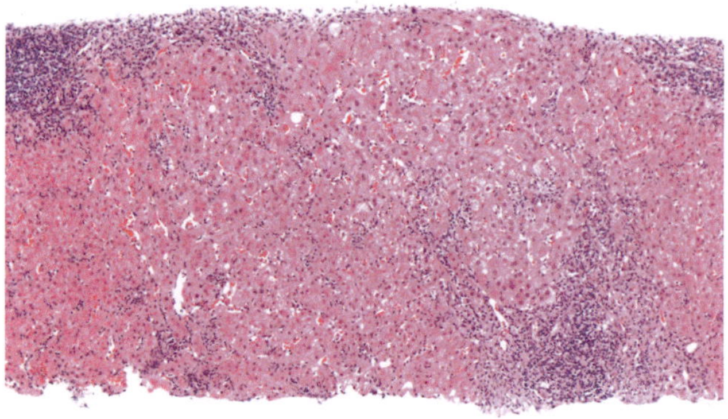

Fig. 6.21 Chronic hepatitis D. Prominent lobular necroinflammation with bridging necrosis is present, in addition to a dense portal chronic inflammatory infiltrate and significant interface hepatitis. Hepatitis D virus is a defective RNA virus requiring coinfection or superinfection with hepatitis B virus for propagation. Chronic hepatitis D typically is associated with prominent lobular necroinflammatory activity and interface hepatitis. Sanded nuclei with immunoreactivity to delta antigen are diagnostic for chronic hepatitis D. Morula-like hepatocytes, which are ballooned hepatocytes with large nuclei, prominent nucleoli, and microvesicular steatosis, also are considered characteristic for chronic hepatitis D.

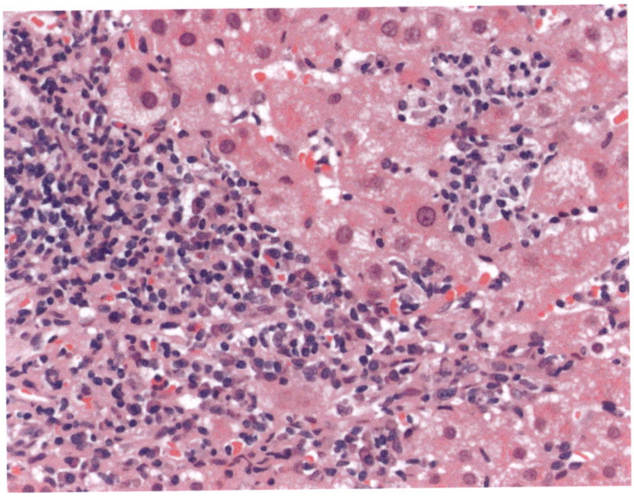

Fig. 6.22 Chronic hepatitis D. Significant interface hepatitis is present, with periportal hepatocytic injuries and a dense portal lymphoplasmacytic infiltrate.

6.2 Grading and Staging of Chronic Viral Hepatitis

Several semiquantitative scoring systems have been developed to assess the degree of necroinflammatory activity (grading) and fibrosis (staging) in chronic viral hepatitis. Such an assessment is one of the key indications for liver biopsy and essential in both routine medical practices and clinical trials for therapeutic decision making, prognostic predictions, and disease monitoring. Commonly used scoring systems include the Scheuer, METAVIR, and Ishak (modified histologic activity index) systems.

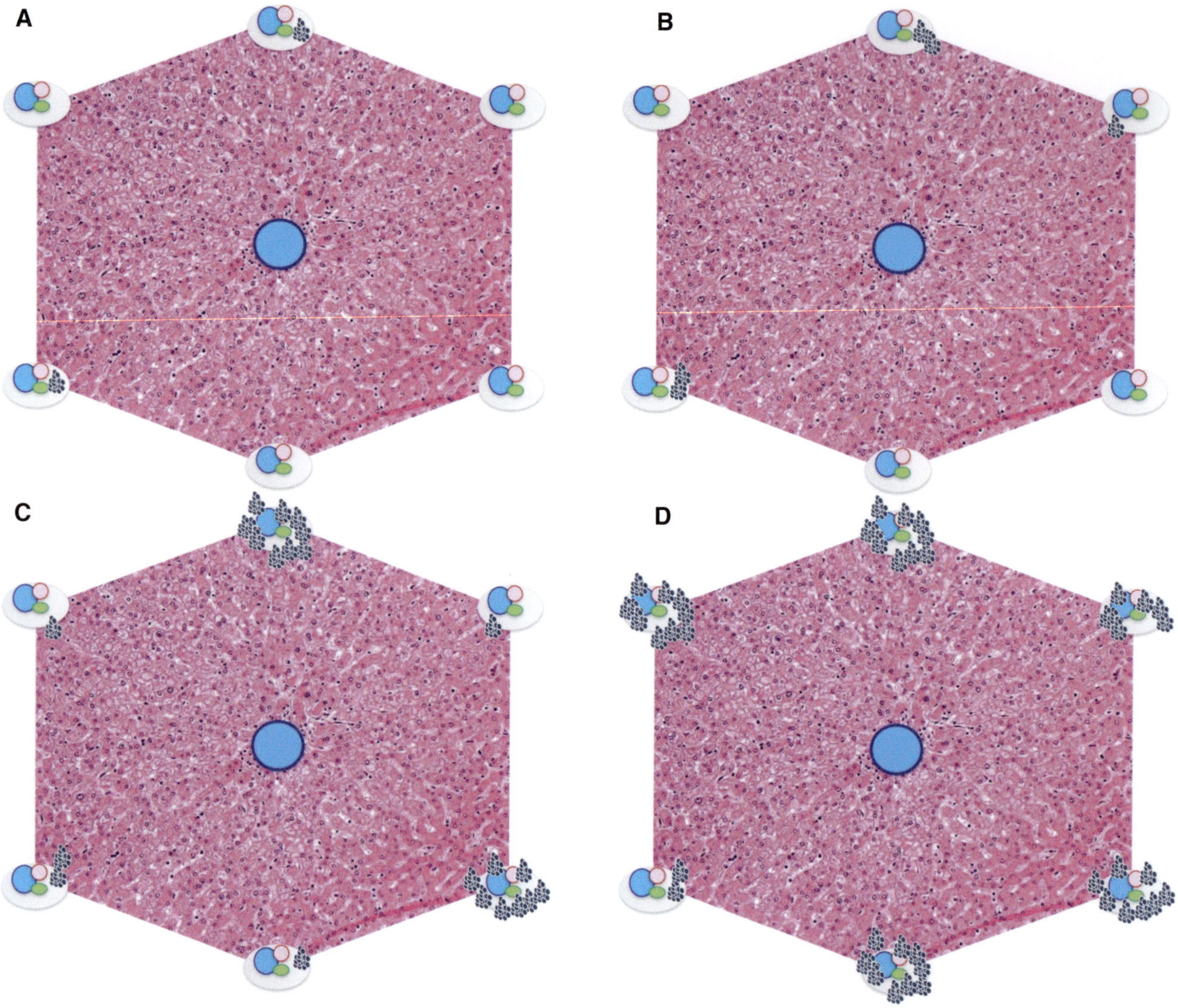

Fig. 6.23 Scheuer's grading of portal–periportal activity (*blue dots* represent inflammatory cells). (**A**) Grade 1: portal inflammation only. (**B**) Grade 2: mild interface hepatitis. (**C**) Grade 3: moderate interface hepatitis. (**D**) Grade 4: severe interface hepatitis. The final Scheuer grade is determined by the higher grade of portal–periportal and lobular activities.

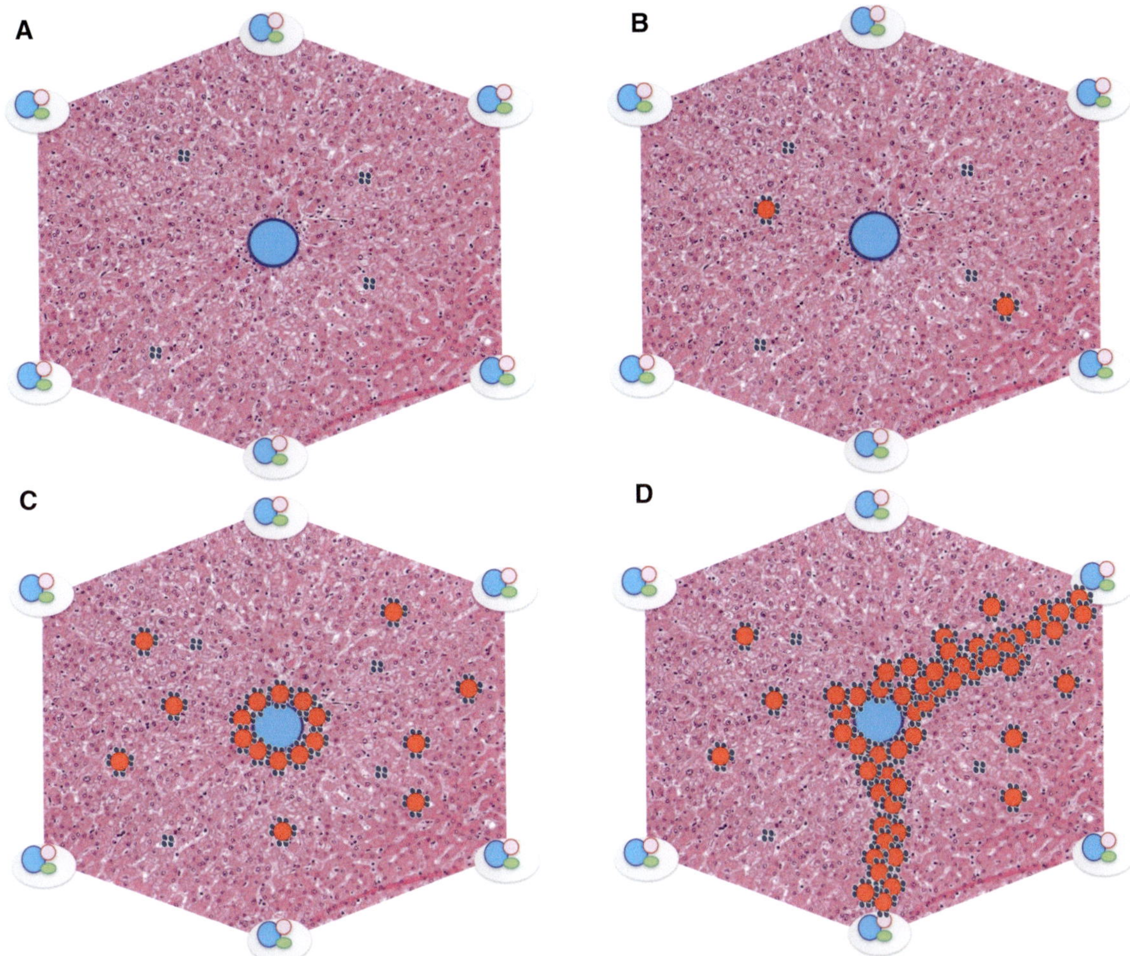

Fig. 6.24 Scheuer's grading of lobular activity (*blue dots* and *red dots* represent inflammatory cells and hepatic necrosis, respectively). (**A**) Grade 1: inflammatory cells only, without any hepatocellular death. (**B**) Grade 2: focal necrosis or apoptotic bodies. (**C**) Grade 3: severe focal cell damage. (**D**) Grade 4: bridging necrosis. The final Scheuer grade is determined by the higher grade of portal–periportal and lobular activities.

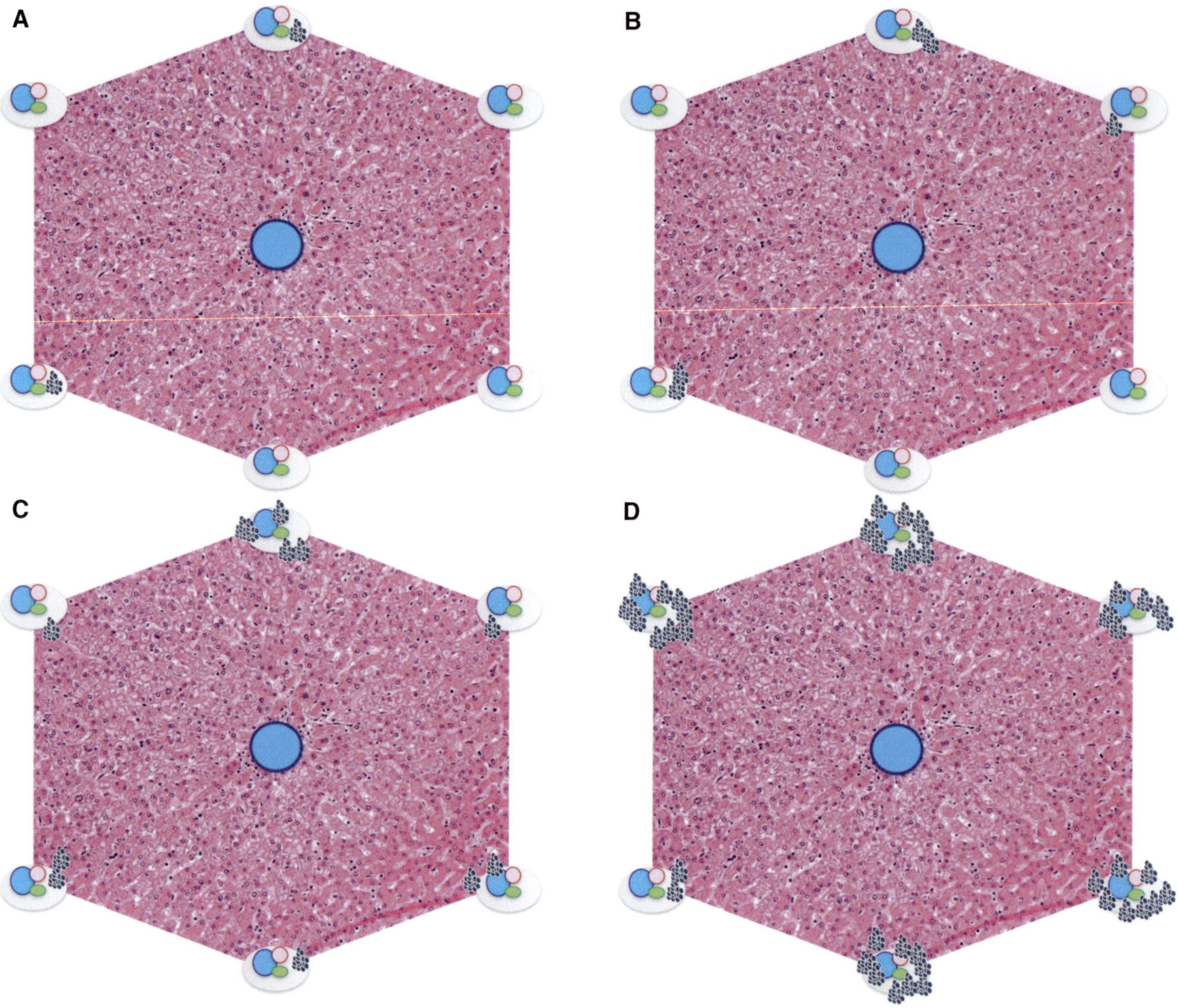

Fig. 6.25 METAVIR score of piecemeal necrosis (PMN; interface hepatitis) (*blue dots* represent inflammatory cells). (**A**) PMN 0: absent. (**B**) PMN 1: focal alteration of periportal plate in some portal tracts. (**C**) PMN 2: focal alteration of periportal plate in all portal tracts. (**D**) PMN 3: diffuse alteration of periportal plate in all portal tracts.

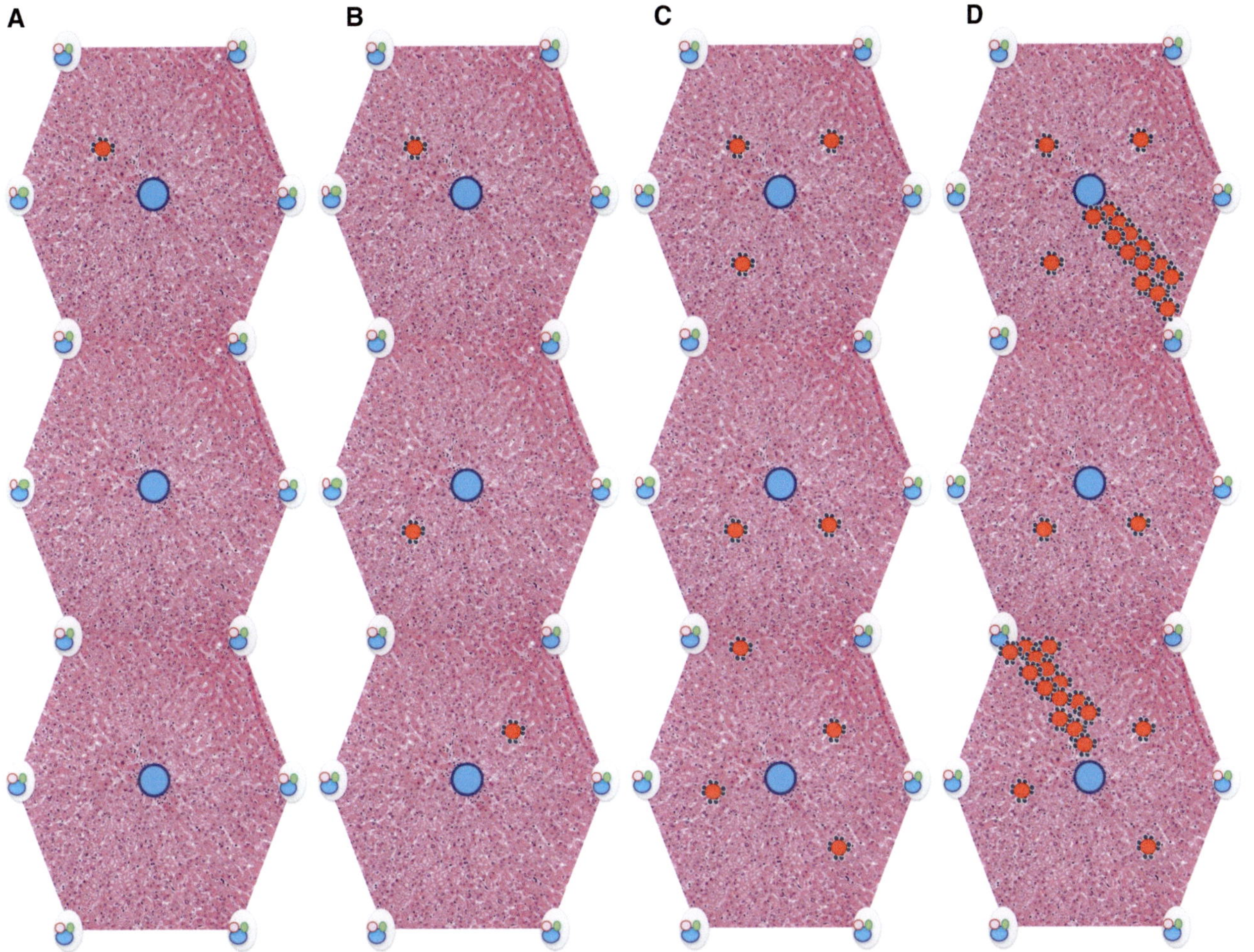

Fig. 6.26 Schematic diagram of METAVIR score of lobular necrosis (LN) (*blue dots* and *red dots* represent inflammatory cells and hepatic necrosis, respectively). (**A**) LN0: fewer than one necroinflammatory focus per lobule. (**B**) LN 1: at least one necroinflammatory focus per lobule. (**C**) LN 2: several necroinflammatory foci per lobule. (**D**) LN 3: bridging necrosis.

PIECEMEAL NECROSIS	LOBULAR NECROSIS	METAVIR GRADE
PMN = 0	LN = 0	A = 0
	LN = 1	A = 1
	LN = 2	A = 2
PMN = 1	LN = 0,1	A = 1
	LN = 2	A = 2
PMN = 2	LN = 0,1	A = 2
	LN = 2	A = 3
PMN = 3	LN = 0,1,2	A = 3

Fig. 6.27 METAVIR grade is a composite of the scores of piecemeal necrosis (interface hepatitis) and lobular necrosis.

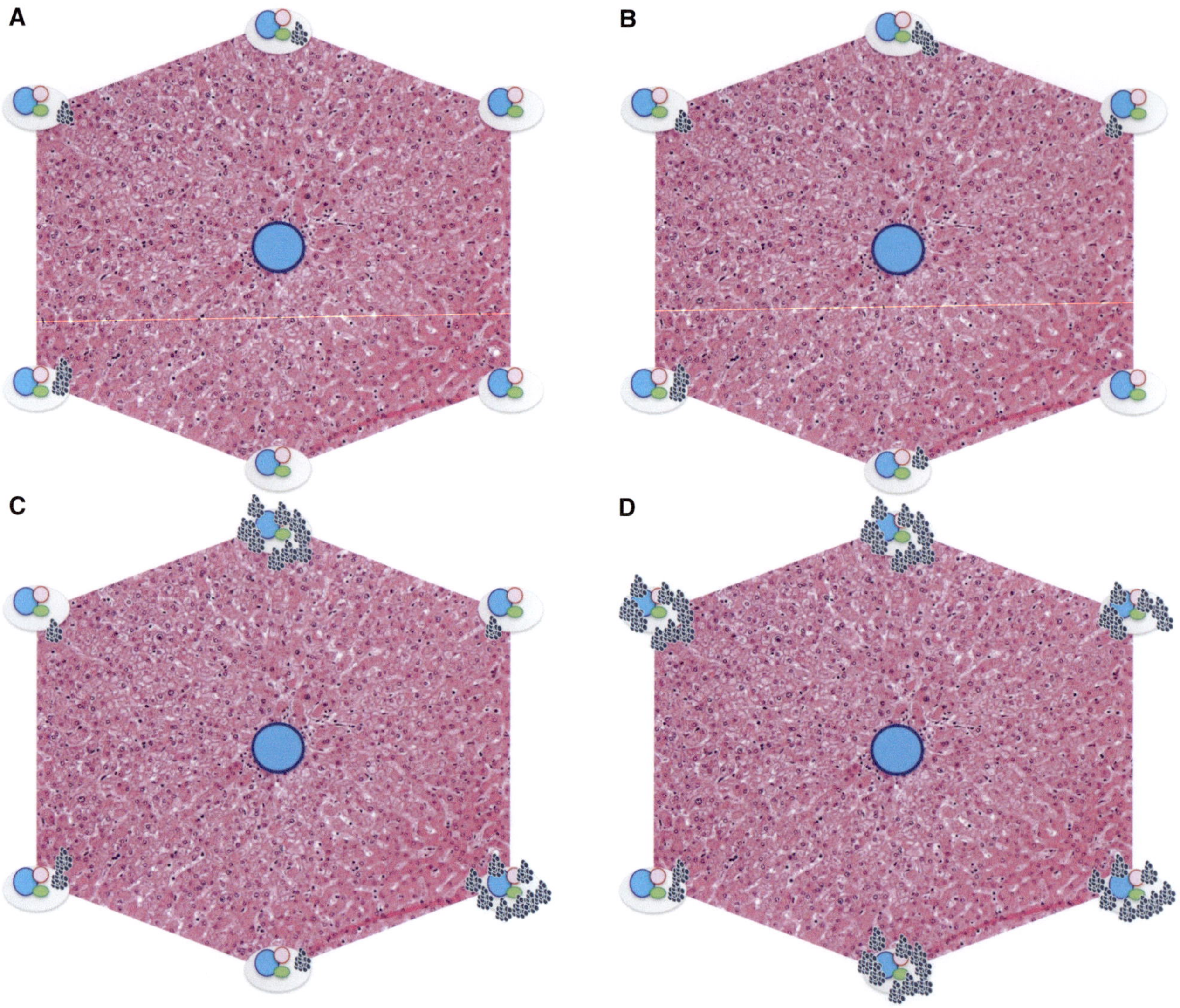

Fig. 6.28 Ishak score of interface hepatitis (*blue dots* represent inflammatory cells). (**A**) Score 1: mild (focal, few portal areas). (**B**) Score 2: mild/moderate (focal, most portal areas). (**C**) Score 3: moderate (continuous around <50% of tracts or septa). (**D**) Score 4: severe (continuous around ≥50% of tracts or septa). The Ishak score for grading (modified histological activity index, 0–18) is the sum of scores of interface hepatitis (0–4), confluent necrosis (0–6), spotty necrosis (0–4), and portal inflammation (0–4).

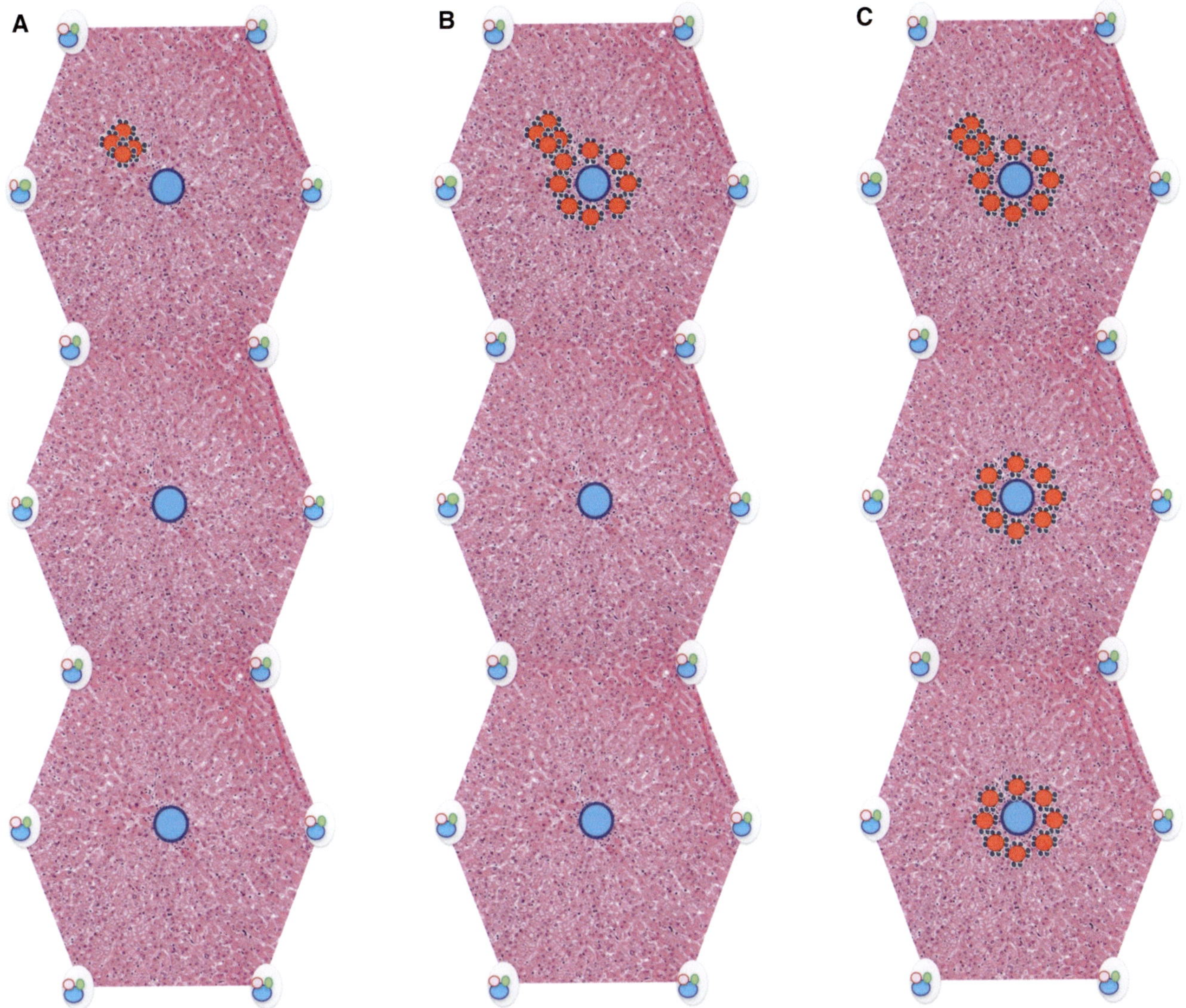

Fig. 6.29 Ishak score of confluent necrosis (*blue dots* and *red dots* represent inflammatory cells and hepatic necrosis, respectively). (**A**) Score 1: focal confluent necrosis. (**B**) Score 2: zone 3 necrosis in some areas. (**C**) Score 3: zone 3 necrosis in most areas. The Ishak score for grading (modified histological activity index, 0–18) is the sum of scores of interface hepatitis (0–4), confluent necrosis (0–6), spotty necrosis (0–4), and portal inflammation (0–4).

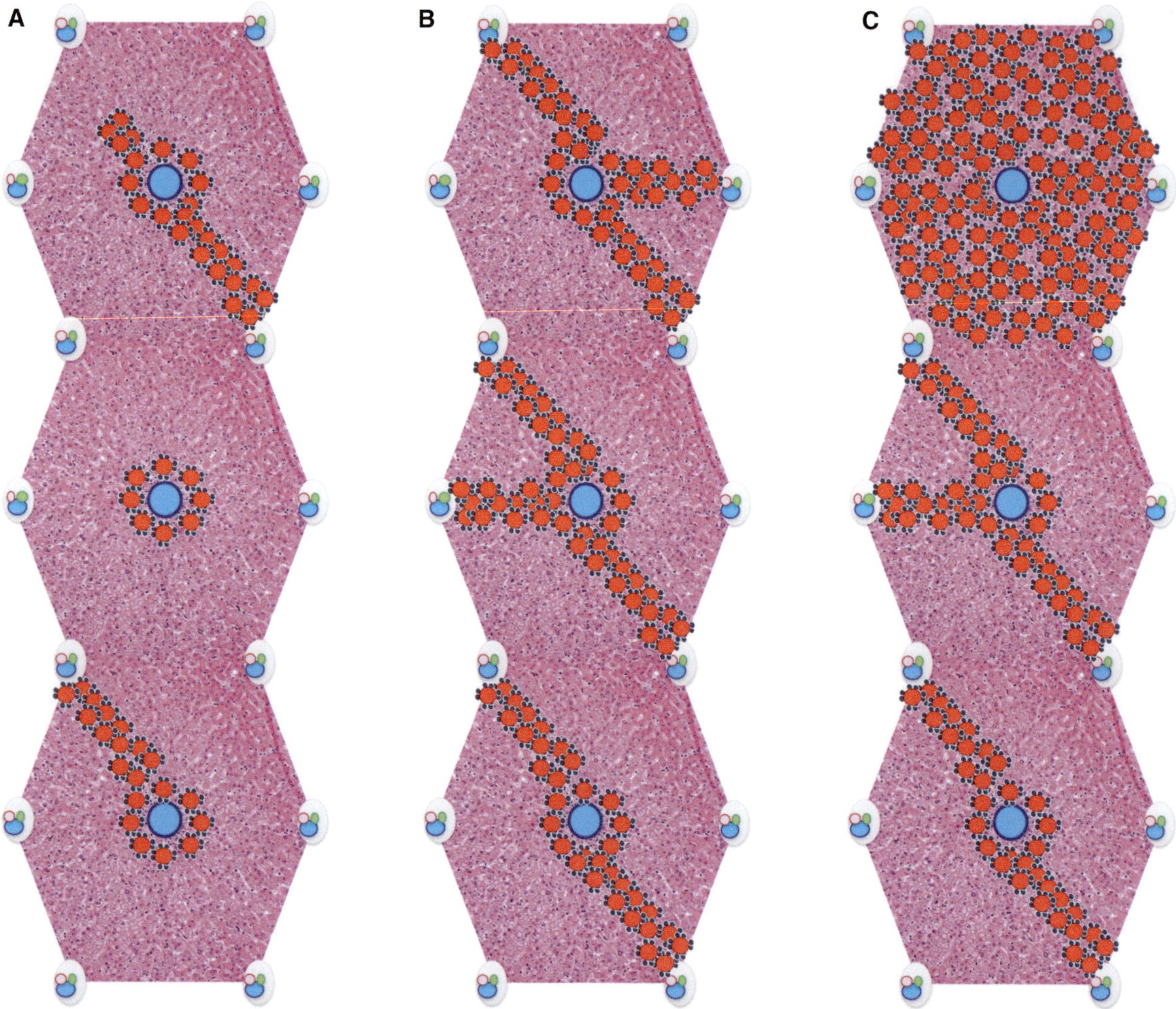

Fig. 6.30 Ishak score of confluent necrosis (*blue dots* and *red dots* represent inflammatory cells and hepatic necrosis, respectively). (**A**) Score 4: zone 3 necrosis and occasional portal–central bridging necrosis. (**B**) Score 5: zone 3 necrosis and multiple portal–central bridging necrosis. (**C**) Score 6: panacinar or multiacinar necrosis. The Ishak score for grading (modified histological activity index, 0–18) is the sum of scores of interface hepatitis (0–4), confluent necrosis (0–6), spotty necrosis (0–4), and portal inflammation (0–4).

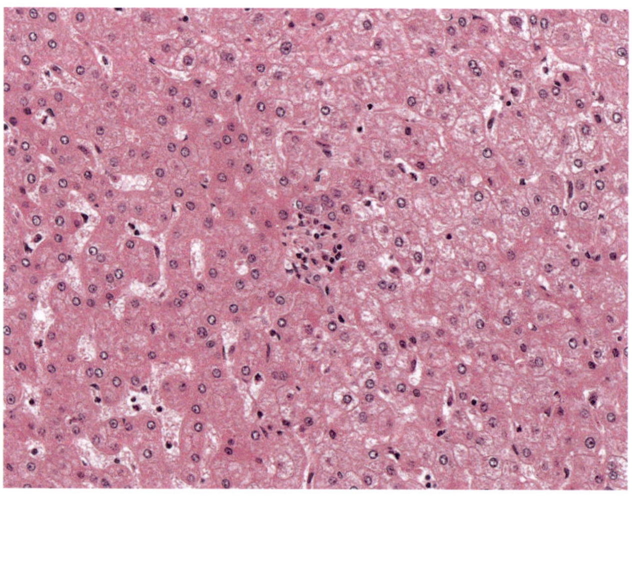

Fig. 6.31 Ishak score for spotty necrosis. Score 1: ≤1 focus per 10× objective. Score 2: 2–4 foci per 10× objective. Score 3: 5–10 foci per 10× objective. Score 4 : >10 foci per 10× objective. The Ishak score for grading (modified histological activity index, 0–18) is the sum of scores of interface hepatitis (0–4), confluent necrosis (0–6), spotty necrosis (0–4), and portal inflammation (0–4).

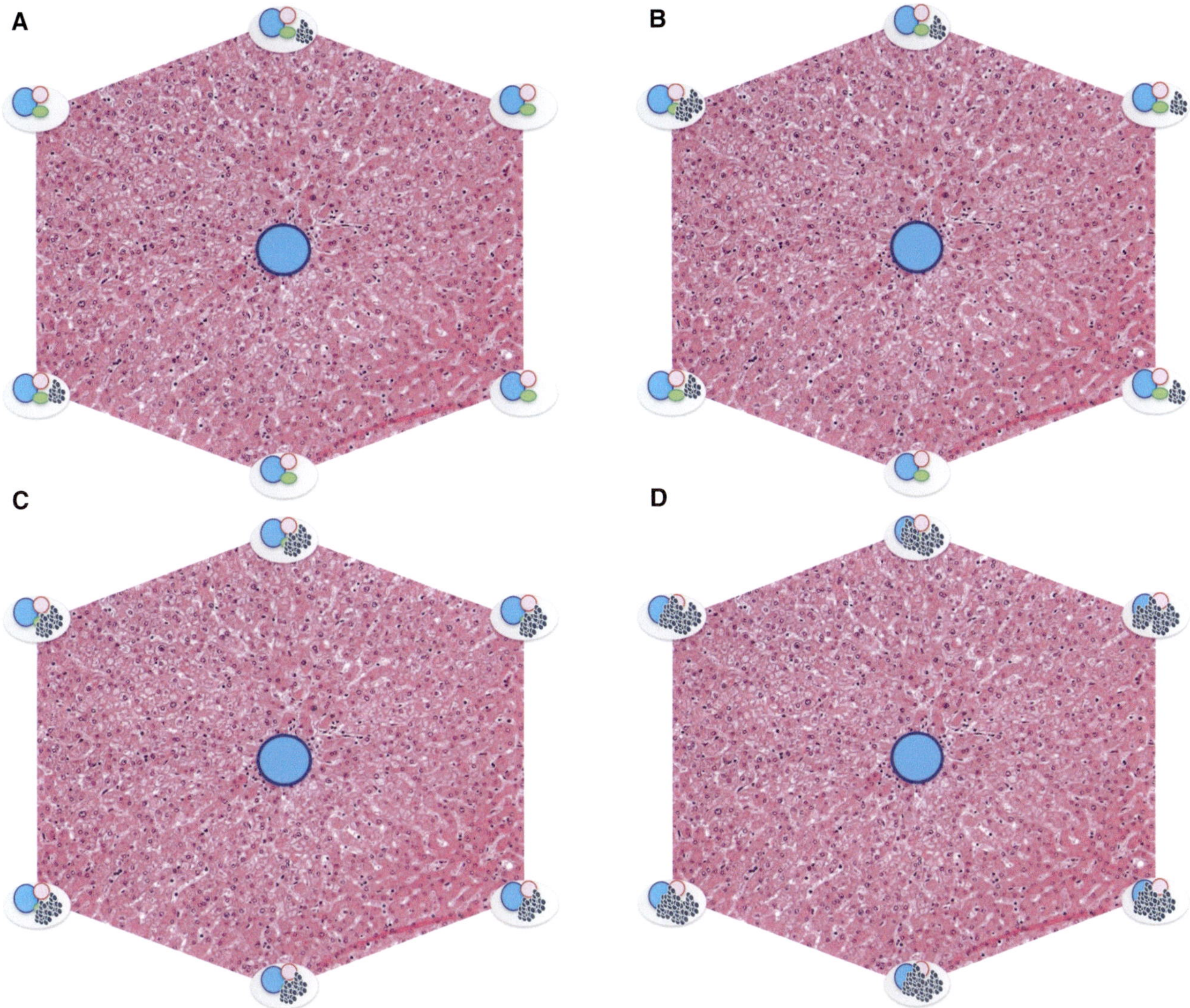

Fig. 6.32 Ishak score for portal inflammation (*blue dots* represent inflammatory cells). (**A**) Score 1: mild (some or all portal areas). (**B**) Score 2: moderate (some or all portal areas). (**C**) Score 3: moderate/marked (all portal areas). (**D**) Score 4: marked (all portal areas). The Ishak score for grading (modified histological activity index, 0–18) is the sum of scores of interface hepatitis (0–4), confluent necrosis (0–6), spotty necrosis (0–4), and portal inflammation (0–4).

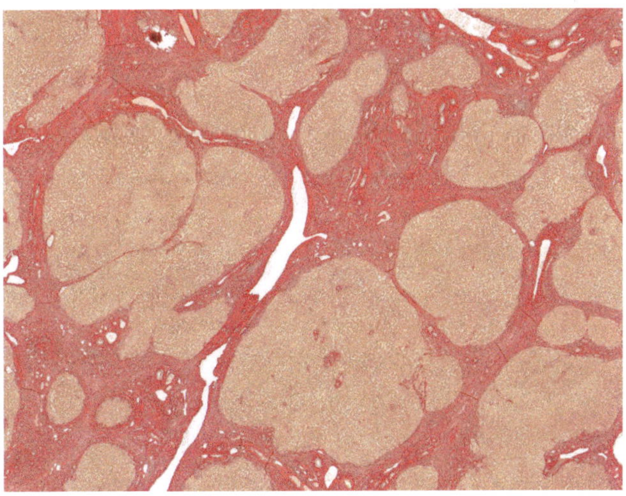

Fig. 6.33 Staging (picrosirius red stain). Multiple cirrhotic regenerative nodules are surrounded by thick fibrous septa. When chronic persistent liver injury exceeds the regenerative capacity of the liver, deposition of fibrous connective tissue occurs, replacing the damaged tissue. Fibrosis is a dynamic and bidirectional process resulting from the balance between fibrogenesis and fibrolysis. The degree of fibrosis indicates the chronicity (or "stage") of the liver disease. The use of connective tissue stains, such as Masson trichrome, Gordon-Sweets reticulin, and picrosirius red, is essential for proper assessment of the degree of fibrosis.

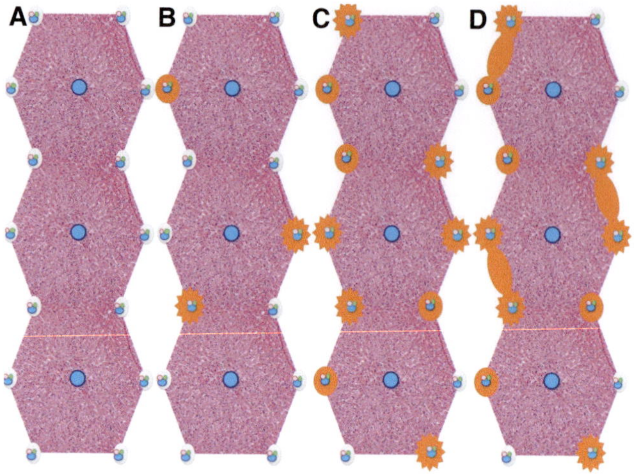

Fig. 6.34 Staging (orange region represents fibrosis). (**A**) Normal liver with no fibrosis (Scheuer stage 0, METAVIR stage 0, Ishak stage 0). (**B**) Fibrous expansion of some portal tracts with or without short septa (Scheuer stage 1, METAVIR stage 1, Ishak stage 2). (**C**) Fibrous expansion of most portal tracts with or without short septa (Scheuer stage 1, METAVIR stage 1, Ishak stage 1). (**D**) Fibrous expansion of most portal tracts with occasional portal–portal bridging (Scheuer stage 2, METAVIR stage 2, Ishak stage 3).

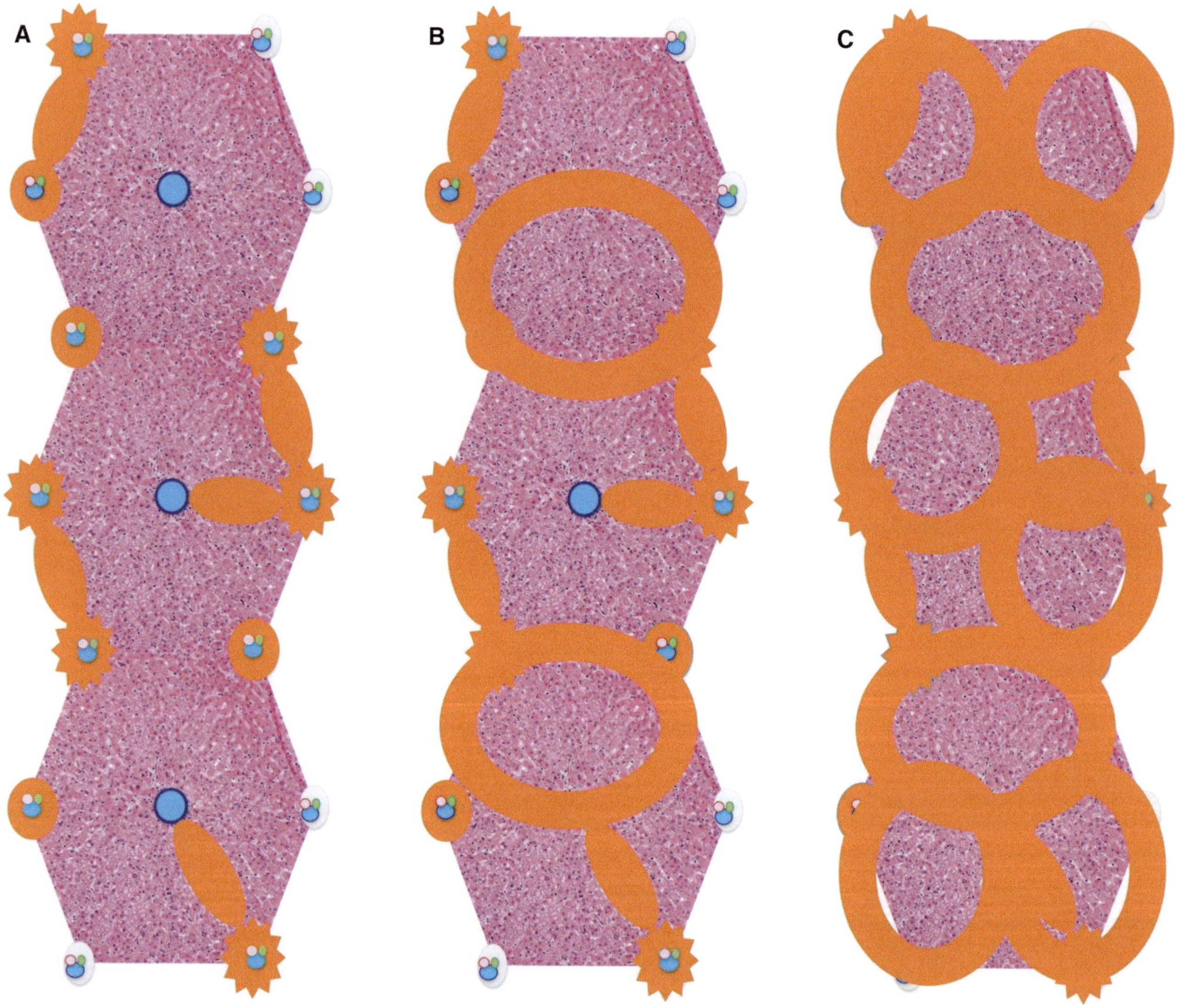

Fig. 6.35 Staging (orange region represents fibrosis). (**A**) Fibrous expansion of most portal tracts with marked portal–portal and portal–central bridging (Scheuer stage 2, METAVIR stage 2, Ishak stage 4). (**B**) Incomplete cirrhosis with marked bridging and occasional nodules (Scheuer stage 3, METAVIR stage 3, Ishak stage 5). (**C**) Cirrhosis, probable or definite (Scheuer stage 4, METAVIR stage 4, Ishak stage 6).

6.3 Nonhepatotropic Viral Hepatitis

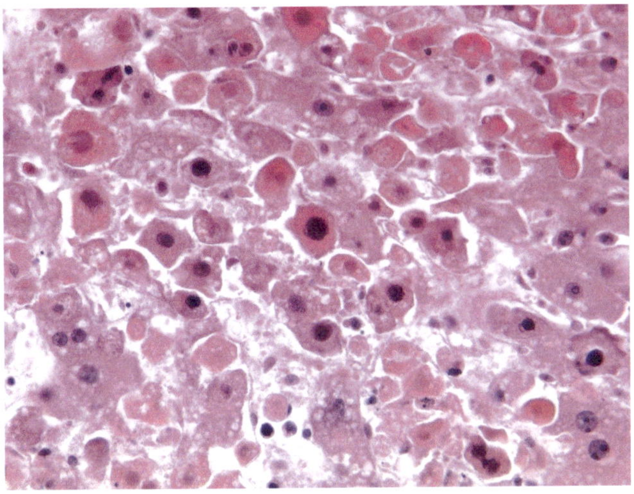

Fig. 6.36 Adenovirus hepatitis. Several hepatocytes contain a large basophilic intranuclear inclusion, imparting a smudgy appearance. Some necrotic cells are noted in the background without any significant inflammatory infiltrate. Adenovirus is a nonenveloped double-stranded DNA virus causing upper/lower respiratory tract infection, lymphadenopathy, and conjunctivitis. It occasionally leads to acute hepatitis, particularly in immunocompromised patients. Adenovirus hepatitis is characterised by geographic areas of haemorrhagic necrosis. The necrotic centre is composed of debris and mixed inflammatory cells. At the periphery of the necrotic area, hepatocytes containing a large angulated basophilic intranuclear inclusion are found and are accompanied by typically minimal inflammation. Immunostaining for adenovirus confirms the diagnosis.

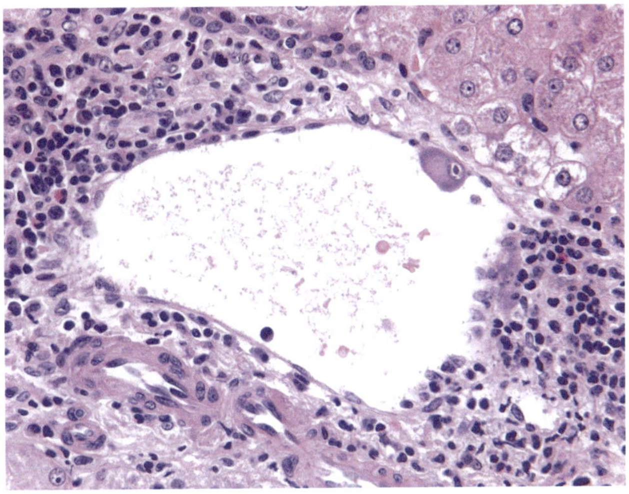

Fig. 6.38 Cytomegalovirus hepatitis. An endothelial cell in a portal vein shows cytomegaly with a large eosinophilic intranuclear inclusion surrounded by a clear halo. The portal tract contains a moderate chronic inflammatory infiltrate composed mainly of small lymphocytes with a few plasma cells and eosinophils. CMV is an enveloped double-stranded DNA virus and belongs to the Herpesviridae family. It is one of the common opportunistic infective agents in immunocompromised patients and affects 50% to 70% of all liver transplant patients with or without overt clinical disease. Coinfection of hepatic cryptosporidiosis is common in HIV-associated cholangiopathy.

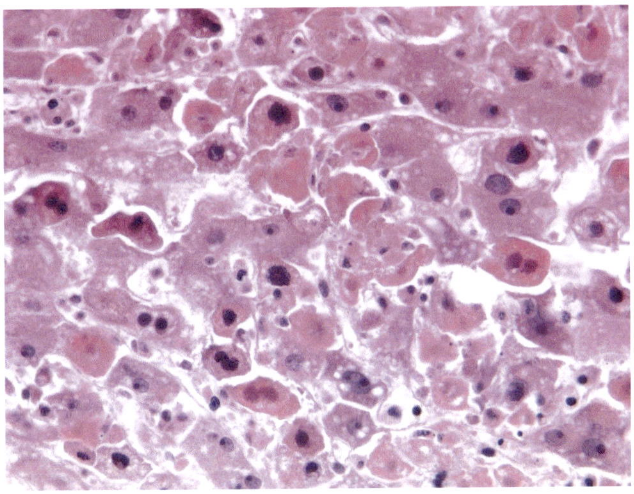

Fig. 6.37 Adenovirus hepatitis. Several hepatocytes contain a large angulated basophilic intranuclear inclusion. Herpes simplex virus (HSV) hepatitis resembles adenovirus hepatitis morphologically, but it is distinguished by the presence of characteristic Cowdry A and B viral inclusions and immunostaining for HSV. Uncommon viruses causing viral haemorrhagic fever, such as yellow fever, dengue fever, and Ebola fever, are other possible differential diagnoses. Apart from acute nonhepatotropic viral hepatitis, dose-dependent drug-induced liver injury and vascular disorders (e.g., acute ischaemia and Budd-Chiari syndrome) also may be associated with multiacinar necrosis with minimal inflammation.

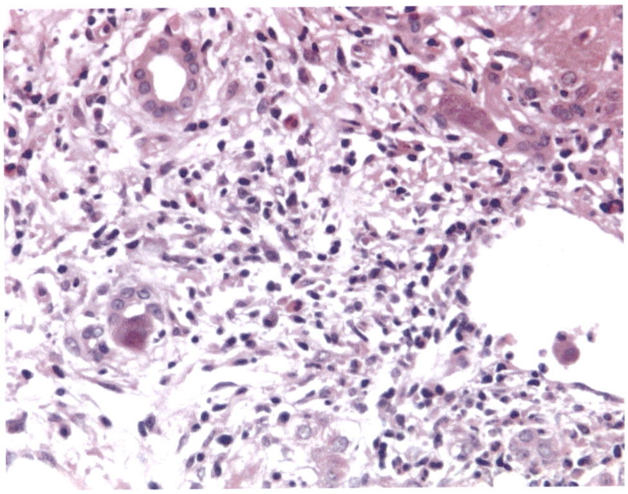

Fig. 6.39 Cytomegalovirus hepatitis. A biliary epithelial cell is markedly enlarged and contain a large eosinophilic intranuclear inclusion and several basophilic intracytoplasmic inclusions. The characteristic viral inclusion is pathognomonic for CMV and may be found in endothelial cells, bile duct epithelial cells, and hepatocytes. The affected cells show cytomegaly with a large eosinophilic intranuclear inclusion surrounded by a clear halo. Basophilic cytoplasmic inclusions also may be found. Immunostaining for CMV is confirmatory. Other pathologic features of CMV hepatitis include the presence of a variable portal and lobular mononuclear infiltrate, lobular microabscesses, and microgranulomas. Viral inclusions and microabscesses typically are absent in immunocompetent patients.

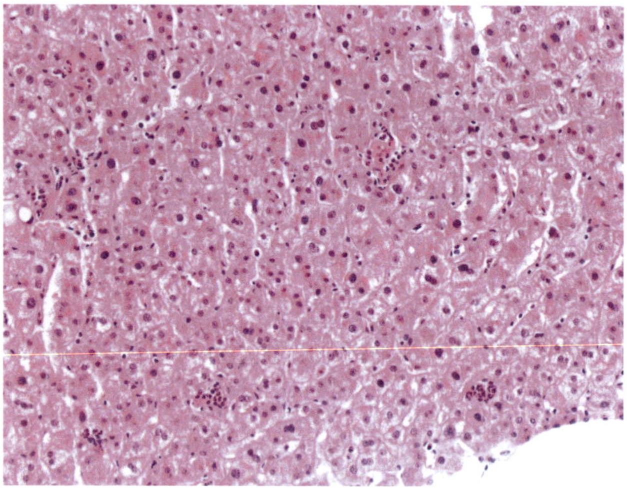

Fig. 6.40 Cytomegalovirus hepatitis. Several microabscesses are scattered within the lobule. A histopathologic diagnosis of CMV hepatitis usually is straightforward in immunocompromised patients. However, CMV hepatitis in immunocompetent patients resembles Epstein-Barr hepatitis. Correlation with serologic tests is helpful in the latter situation.

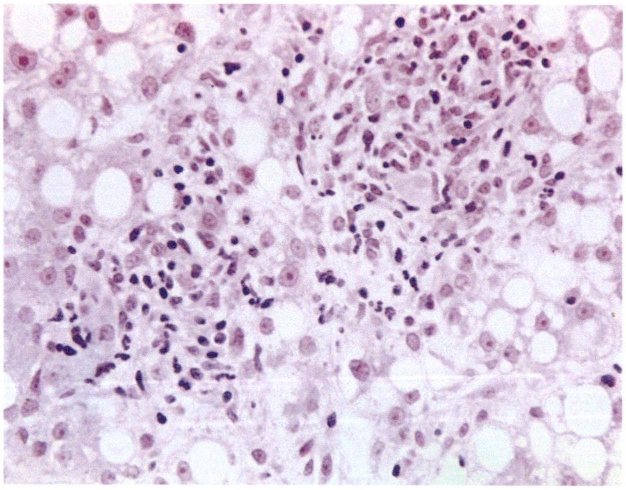

Fig. 6.41 Epstein-Barr virus hepatitis. Aggregates of epithelioid histiocytes admixed with small lymphocytes (noncaseating epithelioid granulomas) are noted in the lobule. EBV is an enveloped double-stranded DNA virus and belongs to the Herpesviridae family. Primary EBV infection may be asymptomatic in children or may lead to infectious mononucleosis in adolescents and adults. EBV infection also is associated with other hepatic diseases, including posttransplant lymphoproliferative disease, lymphoepithelioma-like cholangiocarcinoma, inflammatory pseudotumour-like follicular dendritic cell tumour, EBV-associated smooth muscle tumour, and haemophagocytic syndrome.

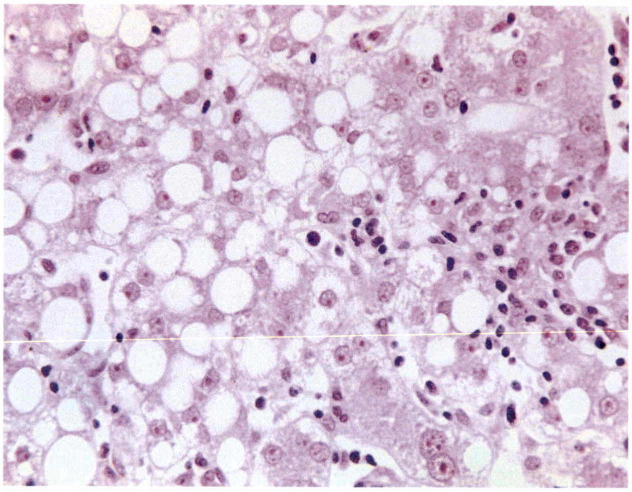

Fig. 6.42 Epstein-Barr virus hepatitis. Several atypical lymphocytes are noted among the sinusoidal mononuclear infiltrate. EBV hepatitis is characterized by the presence of a diffuse sinusoidal lymphocytic infiltrate with occasional atypical activated lymphoid cells. Apoptotic hepatocytes, steatosis, noncaseating epithelioid granulomas, and portal atypical lymphoid infiltrate also are present. Demonstration of EBV within infiltrating lymphoid cells by immunostaining for EBV latent membrane protein (EBV-LMP) or by in situ hybridization for EBV-encoded RNA (EBER) is diagnostic. A positive Monospot test (Meridian Bioscience, Cincinnati, OH) or serum IgM to Epstein-Barr viral capsid antigen (EBV-VCA) is confirmatory.

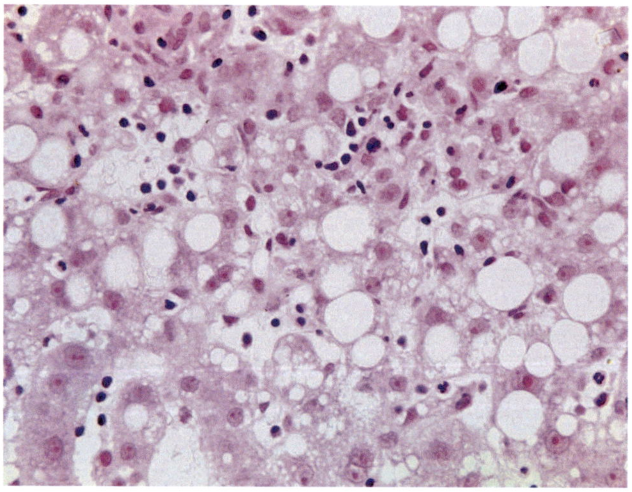

Fig. 6.43 Epstein-Barr virus hepatitis. A few atypical lymphocytes are noted within the parenchyma. The principal differential diagnoses here are diseases with a prominent sinusoidal mononuclear infiltrate, including CMV hepatitis in immunocompetent patients, viral hepatitis C, drug-induced liver injury, extramedullary haematopoiesis, chronic lymphoid leukaemia, and non-Hodgkin lymphoma.

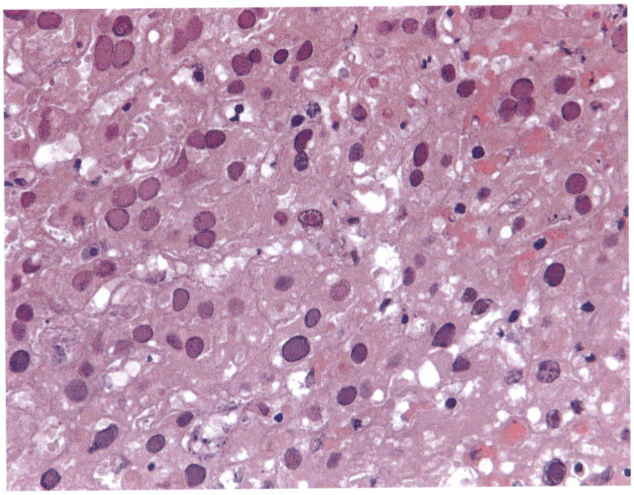

Fig. 6.44 Herpes simplex virus hepatitis. Almost all hepatocytes contain a ground-glass intranuclear viral inclusion (Cowdry B) with chromatin margination. One of the hepatocytes (*c*) possesses a large eosinophilic intranuclear inclusion surrounded by a clear halo (Cowdry A). HSV is an enveloped double-stranded DNA virus and belongs to the Herpesviridae family. HSV hepatitis is associated with disseminated systemic infection affecting immunocompromised patients, malnourished children, and, rarely, immunocompetent adults. HSV hepatitis is characterized by "punched-out" haemorrhagic necrosis with minimal inflammation. At the periphery of the necrotic area, hepatocytes containing a large eosinophilic intranuclear inclusion (Cowdry A) or ground-glass intranuclear inclusion (Cowdry B) are observed. Syncytial multinucleated hepatocytes also are found. Immunostaining for HSV confirms the diagnosis.

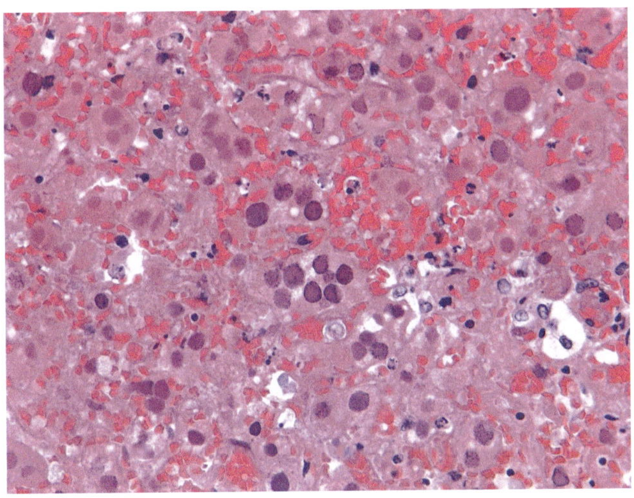

Fig. 6.45 Herpes simplex virus hepatitis. Almost all hepatocytes contain a ground-glass intranuclear viral inclusion (Cowdry B) with chromatin margination. Marked sinusoidal congestion and haemorrhage are noted in the background. Adenovirus hepatitis resembles HSV hepatitis morphologically, but it is distinguished by the smudgy intranuclear viral inclusions and immunostaining for adenovirus. Uncommon viruses causing viral haemorrhagic fever, such as yellow fever, dengue fever, and Ebola fever, are other possible differential diagnoses.

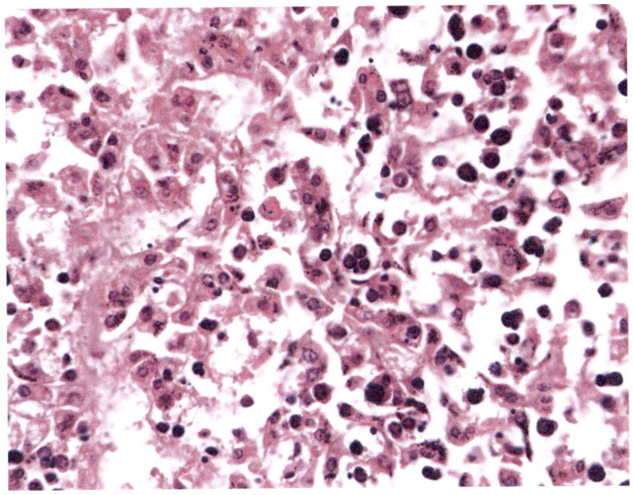

Fig. 6.46 Parvovirus B19 infection. Many ground-glass intranuclear inclusions are found within extramedullary haematopoietic cells lying between degenerating hepatocytes in a fetal liver. Parvovirus B19 is a nonenveloped single-strand DNA virus and well-known to cause fifth disease (erythema infectiosum). Maternofetal transmission from an infected pregnant woman leads to hydropic fetalis with involvement of multiple fetal organs, including the liver.

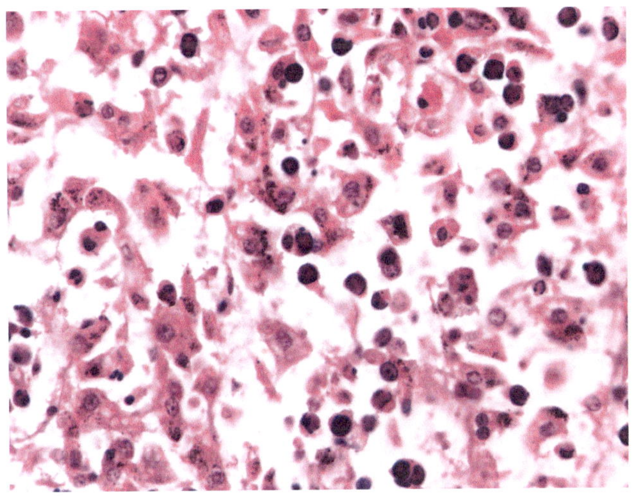

Fig. 6.47 Parvovirus B19 hepatitis. Many ground-glass intranuclear inclusions are found within extramedullary haematopoietic cells in this fetal liver. Congenital parvovirus B19 infection in the liver is featured by the presence of ground-glass intranuclear inclusions in erythroblasts and hepatocytes, prominent extramedullary haematopoiesis, and hepatic necrosis. Confirmation is made by immunostaining for parvovirus B19.

7 Nonviral Infectious Liver Disease

As an essential component of the mononuclear phagocytic system and a natural large blood filter, the liver constantly comes into contact with circulating pathogens, particularly those entering the portal circulation. The biliary tree is protected from infections by tight hepatocellular junctions at the parenchymal/vascular interface, bile flow and bile constituents, and the sphincter of Oddi at the ampulla of Vater.

Nonviral infections can manifest histologically in various ways, including minimal and nonspecific hepatitic changes, granulomas, deposition of pigments such as haemozoin, abscess formation, and the presence of ova or parasites. Cholestasis, particularly the presence of cholangiolar bile casts, is a histologic sign of sepsis.

Although some of these infective agents are more common in certain parts of the world, geographic boundaries now are reduced, and disorders once limited to specific areas may be seen potentially everywhere. Primary or acquired immunodeficiencies are predisposing factors to infections by various agents.

7.1 Bacterial Infection

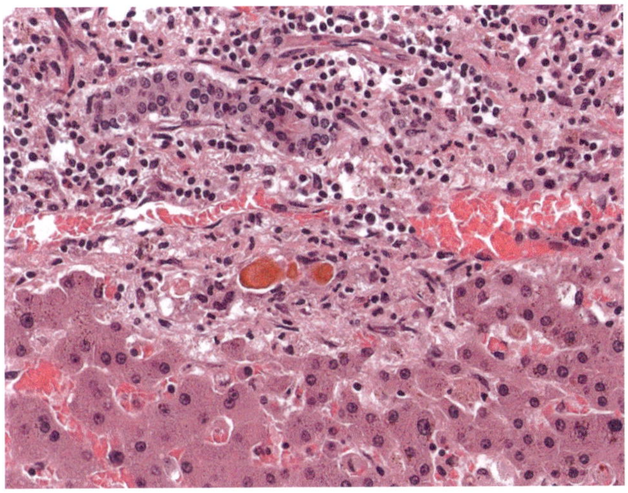

Fig. 7.1 Sepsis. A bile ductule is distended by inspissated bile concretions (ductular cholestasis). Ductular cholestasis, sometimes referred to as cholangitis lenta, is a pathognomonic feature of sepsis. This lesion typically is not associated with uncomplicated large duct obstruction or other acute and chronic cholestatic conditions. Although it is seen uncommonly in other situations—for example, post massive necrosis—its presence should flag the need for urgent investigation and appropriate treatment for septic complications. The spread of bacteria and associated (endo)toxins to the liver may originate from the bile duct (acute ascending cholangitis complicating large duct obstruction), the hepatic artery (systemic septicaemia), or the portal vein (intra-abdominal infection).

A.W.H. Chan et al., *Atlas of Liver Pathology*, Atlas of Anatomic Pathology,
DOI 10.1007/978-1-4614-9114-9_7, © Springer Science+Business Media New York 2014

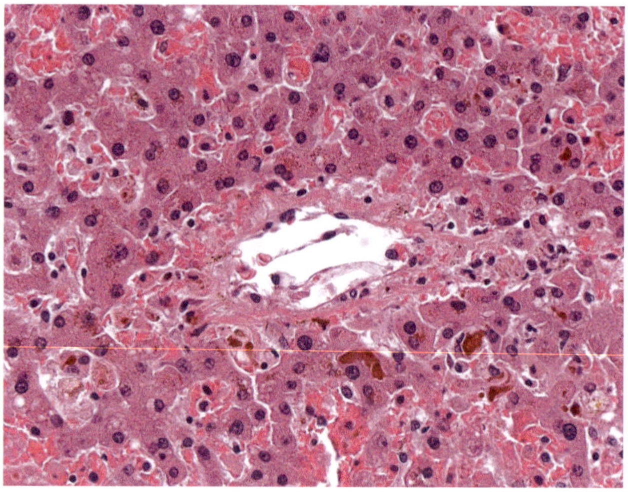

Fig. 7.2 Sepsis. Prominent bilirubinostasis is seen with many bile plugs in dilated bile canaliculi, together with the presence of cytoplasmic bile pigments in Kupffer cells and hepatocytes. Bland cholestasis is another common but nonspecific pathologic feature of sepsis. Perivenular ischaemic necrosis (secondary to septic shock) and mild steatosis are other nonspecific findings in sepsis.

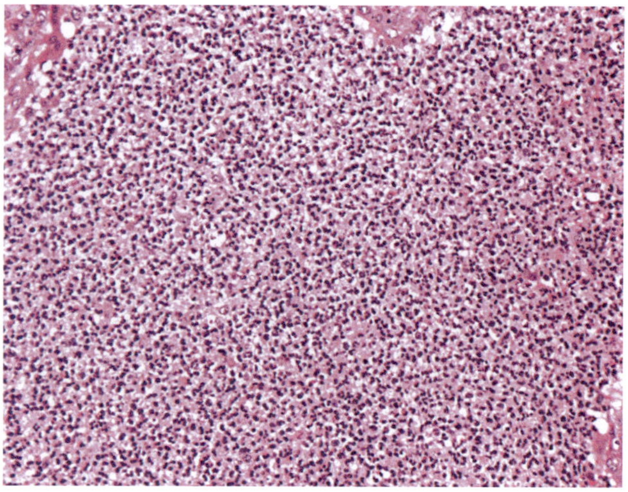

Fig. 7.3 Pyogenic abscess. A large collection of neutrophils is present. Pyogenic abscess usually is solitary (70%) with right lobe predominance (66%). The route of infection most frequently is the biliary tree, followed by the portal vein and hepatic artery. However, 10% to 20% of cases are cryptogenic, without an identifiable source of primary infection. *Escherichia coli*, *Streptococcus milleri*, *Klebsiella pneumoniae*, and *Bacteroides* are the most common causative organisms. An amoebic abscess is the principal differential diagnosis; these abscesses contain eosinophilic granular necrotic debris with some lymphocytes and plasma cells. Neutrophils tend to be very scanty unless secondary bacterial superinfection occurs. The trophozoites are characterised by round to oval-shaped organisms of 20 to 50 μm, a single eccentric nucleus, eosinophilic granular cytoplasm, and phagocytosed red cells, and are highlighted sharply by periodic acid-Schiff (PAS) stain.

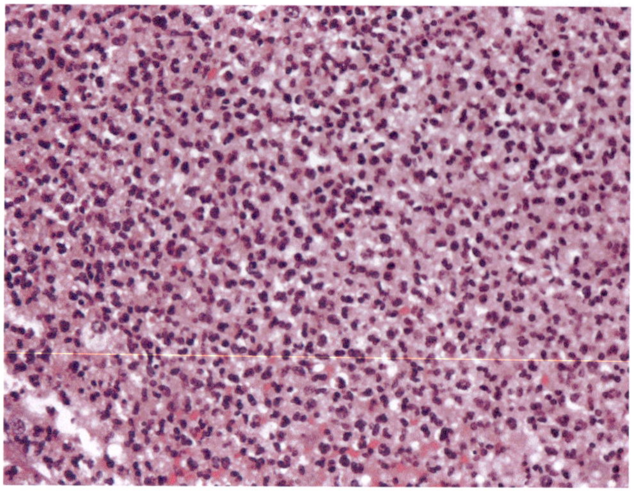

Fig. 7.4 Pyogenic abscess. Preexisting liver diseases associated with pyogenic abscess formation include helminth infections of the biliary tree, predisposing to bacterial cholangitis, and recurrent pyogenic cholangitis. Helminth infections involved include clonorchiasis, opisthorchiasis, ascariasis, and fascioliasis. Identification of adult worms and/or ova is essential to establish the diagnosis, but tissue eosinophilia and suppurative granulomatous inflammation provide histologic clues. Recurrent pyogenic cholangitis should be considered in the presence of acute and chronic cholangitis, pigmented calculi, bile duct dilatation, and periductal and portal fibrosis.

7.2 Mycobacterial Infection

Mycobacterium tuberculosis and *Mycobacterium leprae* are the two commonest mycobacterial pathogens in man and are not uncommonly associated with hepatic infection. *Mycobacterium avium* intracellulare is the most frequent atypical mycobacterium affecting immunocompromised patient with disseminated mycobacterioses. Other less common atypical mycobacteria with liver involvement include *Mycobacterium kansasii*, *Mycobacterium fortuitum*, *Mycobacterium scrofulaceum*, *Mycobacterium xenopi*.

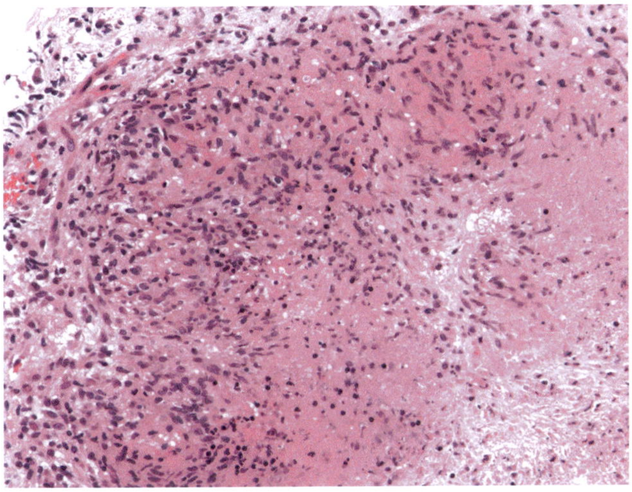

Fig. 7.5 *Mycobacterium tuberculosis*. Necrotizing epithelioid granulomatous inflammation is present. Hepatic tuberculosis is not a common clinical problem but is reported to occur in 50% to 80% of patients dying from tuberculosis. It is divided broadly into (1) hepatic miliary tuberculosis, which manifests as diffuse granulomatous hepatitis and results from the spread of mycobacteria from the systemic circulation through the hepatic artery, and (2) hepatic tuberculoma, which presents as a space-occupying lesion and originates from the spread of intestinal mycobacteria through the portal vein.

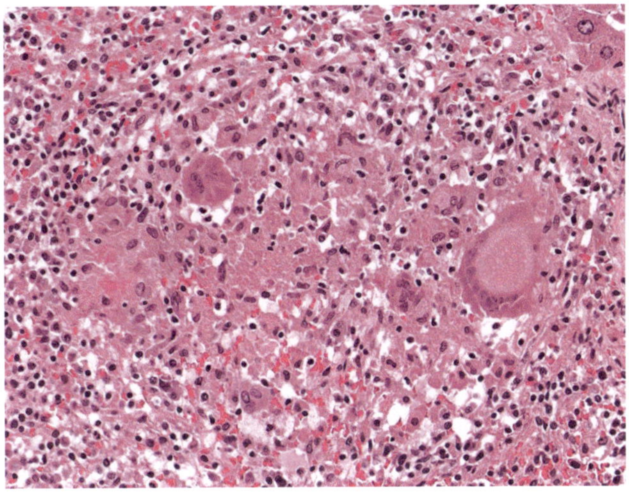

Fig. 7.6 *M. tuberculosis*. Necrotizing epithelioid granulomatous inflammation with a Langhans-type multinucleated giant cell is shown. Necrotizing epithelioid granulomas are the hallmark histologic feature and are situated in both portal tracts and lobules. Foamy macrophage aggregates, more typically found in *Mycobacterium avium* complex, also are seen in hepatic tuberculosis in immunocompromised patients (anergic or nonreactive tuberculosis). The differential diagnoses of necrotizing epithelioid granulomas include other mycobacterial infections, tertiary syphilis, brucellosis, parasitic infestation, fungal infection, and, rarely, viral infection. Special stains for various organisms and microbiologic investigations normally are required to establish the definitive diagnosis.

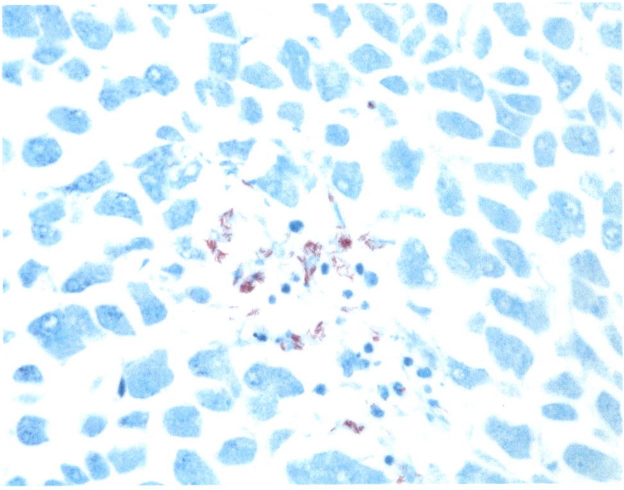

Fig. 7.7 *M. tuberculosis* (Ziehl-Neelsen stain). Numerous acid-fast bacilli are highlighted in this liver biopsy sample from a renal transplant patient with disseminated tuberculosis. In immunocompetent patients with hepatic tuberculosis, the Ziehl-Neelsen stain may show only scanty or even no acid-fast bacilli within the granulomatous inflammation. By contrast, in immunocompromised patients, numerous acid-fast bacilli readily are found. Polymerase chain reaction (PCR) for *M. tuberculosis* on tissue sections is helpful in diagnosing tuberculosis in cases of necrotizing granulomatous inflammation with negative results on multiple Ziehl-Neelsen and other infective stains. It also is useful in differentiating tuberculosis from atypical mycobacteria. However, a negative Ziehl-Neelsen stain and PCR assay do not entirely exclude the possibility of tuberculosis.

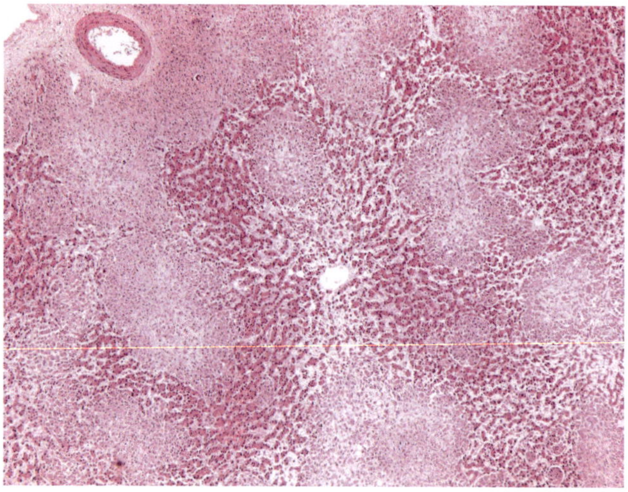

Fig. 7.8 *Mycobacterium avium-intracellulare* (MAI). Numerous aggregates of foamy macrophages are widely distributed with a geographic pattern. There is no significant necrosis or inflammatory infiltrate present. MAI is a pulmonary pathogen primarily in immunocompromised patients, although it occurs rarely in immunocompetent individuals with underlying lung disease and in young children. Disseminated disease with hepatic involvement is common in immunocompromised patients. MAI is the commonest atypical mycobacterium affecting HIV/AIDS patients.

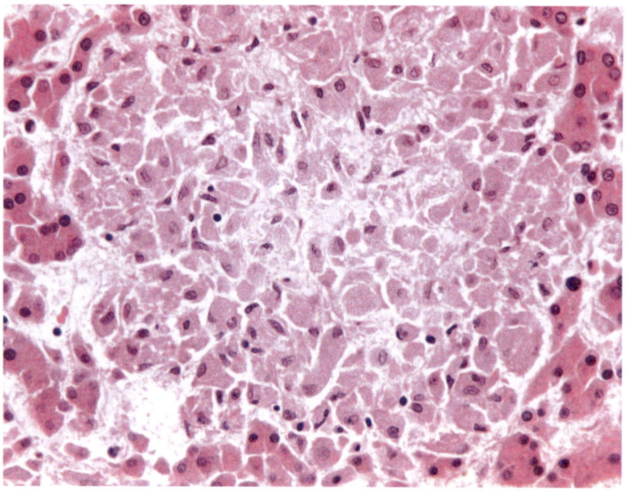

Fig. 7.9 *M. avium-intracellulare*. An aggregate of foamy macrophages is noted in the lobule, without any significant necrosis or inflammatory infiltrate. Anergic tuberculosis, lepromatous leprosy, other atypical mycobacteria, and Whipple disease may exhibit similar histologic appearances. Ziehl-Neelsen, Wade-Fite, PAS, and Gram stains are helpful in differentiating these conditions: (1) MAI is positive on Ziehl-Neelsen, Wade-Fite, and PAS; (2) *M. tuberculosis* is positive on Ziehl-Neelsen and Wade-Fite; (3) *Mycobacterium leprae* is positive on Wade-Fite; and (4) *Tropheryma whippelii* is positive on PAS and Gram stains.

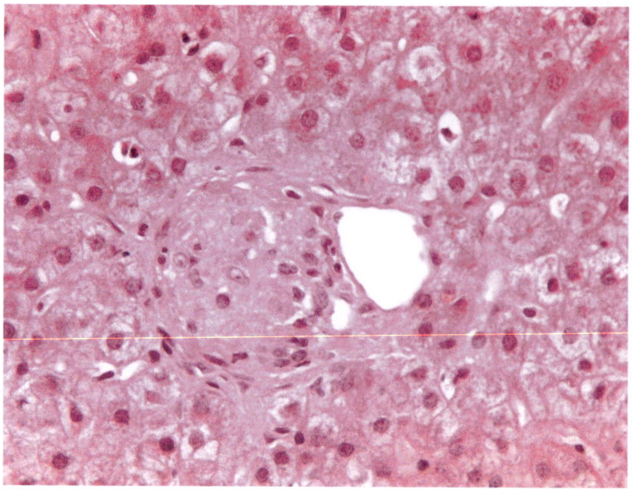

Fig. 7.10 *Bacillus Calmette-Guérin* (BCG). A small noncaseating epithelioid granuloma is noted in a portal tract. BCG contains an attenuated strain of *Mycobacterium bovis* and is used as a prophylactic vaccine for tuberculosis and in intravesicular therapy for superficial urinary bladder carcinoma. Hepatic involvement as a complication of BCG administration is uncommon, with a reported incidence between 0.7% and 3%.

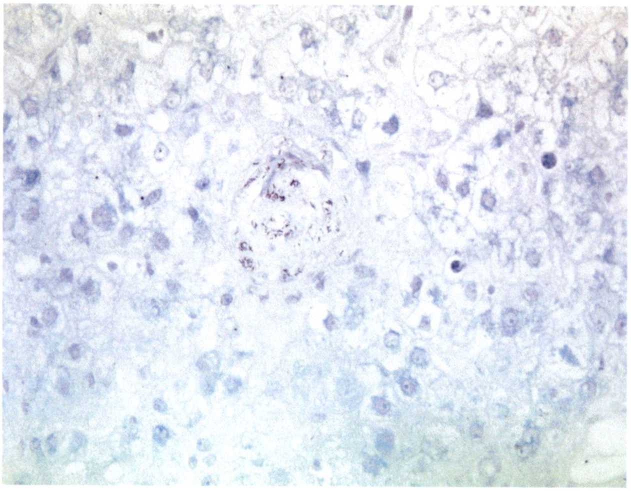

Fig. 7.11 *Bacillus Calmette-Guérin* (Ziehl-Neelsen stain). Many acid-fast bacilli are present in a noncaseating epithelioid granuloma. There are two major hypotheses for the pathogenesis of BCG-associated systemic complications: disseminated active infection with *M. bovis* and a hypersensitivity reaction. Demonstration of acid-fast bacilli in tissue sections and the positive culture and molecular assay support the former. However, most cases do not have any laboratory evidence of *Mycobacterium*, and as some cases contain a striking amount of eosinophilic infiltration, it raises the possibility of a hypersensitivity reaction. Rapid clinical improvement by coadministration of steroids in addition to antituberculosis medications further supports a hypersensitivity reaction.

7.3 Rickettsial Infection

Rickettsial diseases are caused by a group of gram-negative, obligately intracellular coccobacilli. Most of them are transmitted by an arthropod vector. Sudden-onset fever with severe headache, malaise, and often skin rash is a typical clinical presentation. All rickettsial infections may be associated with mild liver function abnormalities, but several forms of rickettsial and closely related infections lead to clinically significant liver disease, namely Q fever (*Coxiella burnetii*), Rocky Mountain spotted fever (*Rickettsia rickettsii*), Boutonneuse fever (*Rickettsia conorii*), ehrlichiosis (*Ehrlichia chaffeensis*), and chlamydiasis (*Chlamydia psittaci* and *Chlamydia trachomatis*).

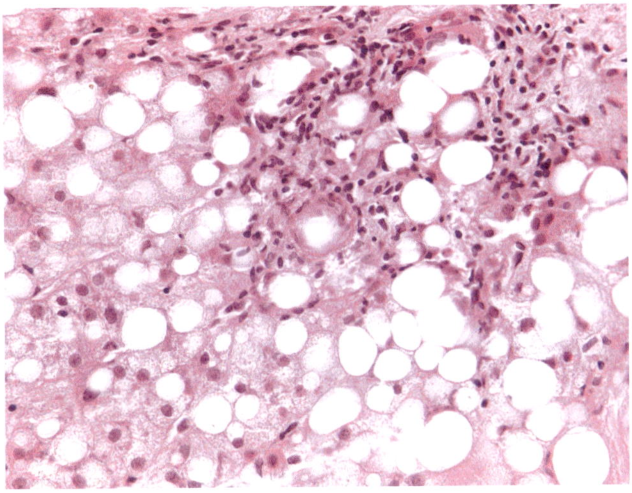

Fig. 7.12 Q fever. This image shows a fibrin-ring granuloma with a central fat globule or clear space surrounded by a circumferential rim of fibrin. Q fever is a worldwide zoonosis caused by *Coxiella burnetii* transmitted by inhalation of infected aerosols and, less commonly, ingestion of contaminated dairy products from domestic ruminants. About 12% to 20% of cases of acute Q fever are associated with deranged liver function, acute hepatitis, and even, rarely, fatal fulminant hepatitis, whereas only <1% of chronic Q fever cases are complicated by chronic hepatitis.

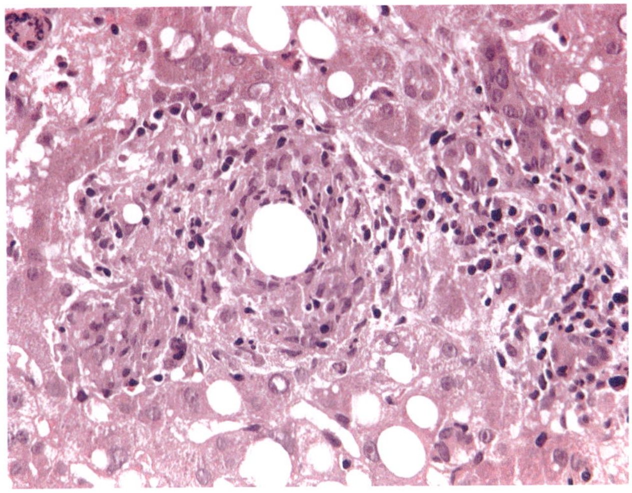

Fig. 7.13 Q fever. A fibrin-ring granuloma with a large central clear space is present. Fibrin rings may not always be obvious but may be highlighted by phosphotungstic acid-haematoxylin stain, Martius scarlet blue stain, or immunostaining for fibrin. A variable degree of macrovesicular steatosis, spotty necrosis, and lymphohistiocytic infiltrate are other histologic features of the hepatic response to Q fever. Although fibrin-ring granulomas are classically associated with Q fever, they now are known to be rather nonspecific. Other associations include mycobacterial infection, staphylococcal bacteraemia, leishmaniasis, toxoplasmosis, cytomegalovirus infection, Epstein-Barr virus infection, acute hepatitis A, systemic lupus erythematosus, giant cell arteritis, allopurinol toxicity, and lymphoma.

7.4 Fungal Infection

Hepatic fungal infection occasionally results from haematogenous dissemination of fungal infection in immunocompromised patients. Identification of fungal yeasts and/or hyphae with attention to their size and morphology provides diagnostic clues to particular fungal infections. Grocott and PAS (with/without diastase) stains are useful for highlighting fungal elements. Immunostains for specific species are also very helpful but not widely available. Candidiasis, aspergillosis, and cryptococcosis are the three most frequent fungal infections. Other less common fungal infections include histoplasmosis, blastomycosis (*Blastomyces dermatitidis*), coccidioidomycosis (*Coccidioides immitis*), paracoccidioidomycosis (*Paracoccidioides brasiliensis*), penicilliosis (*Penicillium marneffei*), zygomycosis, and *Pneumocystis jiroveci* infection.

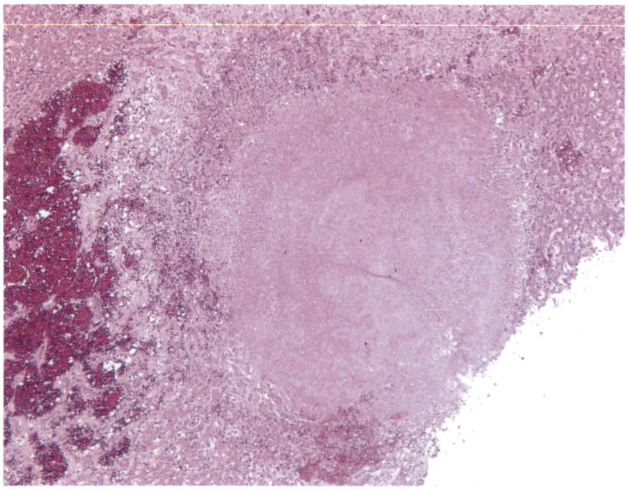

Fig. 7.14 Aspergillosis. An eosinophilic fungal mass is surrounded by haemorrhagic necrosis. *Aspergillus* species are ubiquitous fungi found in the environment. Disseminated aspergillosis with hepatic involvement occurs in immunocompromised patients and patients with acute liver failure and end-stage cirrhosis. It is the second commonest fungal infection in immunosuppressed patients behind candidiasis. *Aspergillus fumigatus* and *Aspergillus* flavus are the most common species isolated in such patients.

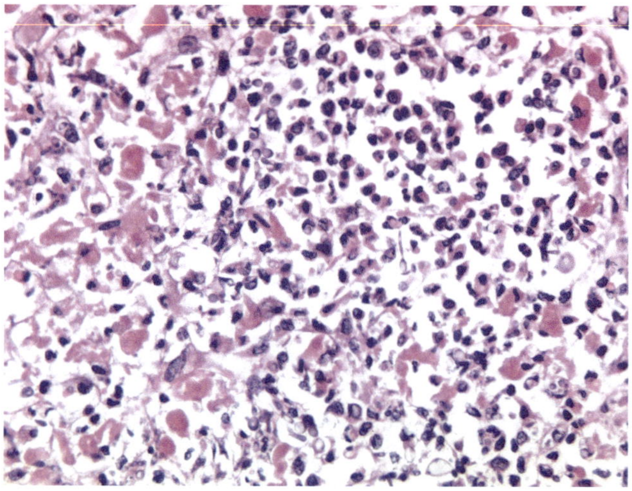

Fig. 7.16 Candidiasis. Fungal yeasts and pseudohyphae are found among necrotic cells and neutrophils. More than 20 species of *Candida* are human pathogens. The commonest is *Candida albicans*, which is a commensal organism of the oral cavity and intestine in healthy individuals. Hepatic candidiasis usually affects premature newborns and immunocompromised patients, particularly those with acute leukaemia (reported incidence up to 6.8%). It occasionally arises in pregnant women and patients receiving total parenteral nutrition.

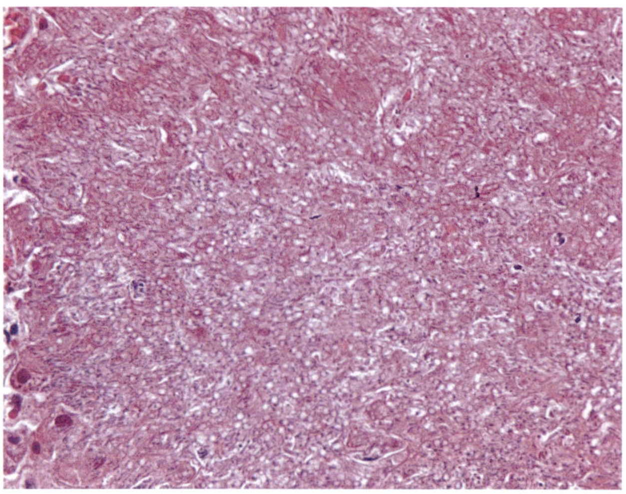

Fig. 7.15 Aspergillosis. Abundant degenerate fungal hyphae are present. Hepatic aspergillosis is characterised by the presence of 3- to 6-μm septated fungal hyphae branching at acute angles of 45°, commonly accompanied by thrombosis and haemorrhagic necrosis resulting from fungal angioinvasion. In less severe cases, suppurative granulomas with scanty fungal hyphae are observed. Hepatic zygomycosis may elicit similar pathologic features. Identification of broad-branching fungal hyphae with few or no septa differentiates zygomycosis from aspergillosis.

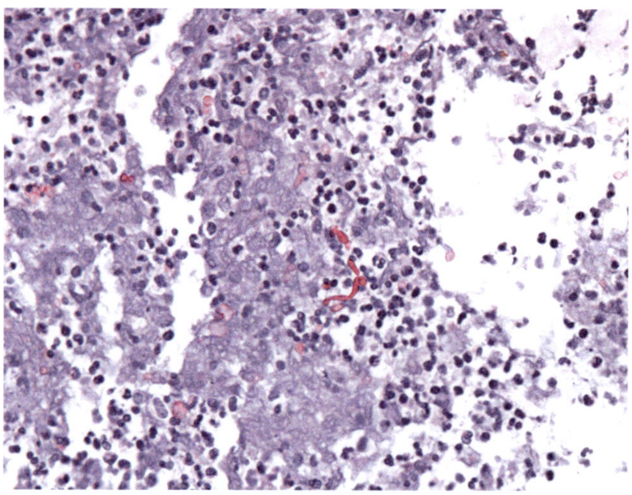

Fig. 7.17 Candidiasis (PAS with diastase [PASD] stain). Fungal yeasts and pseudohyphae are seen among necrotic cells and neutrophils. Hepatic candidiasis is characterised by the presence of budding yeasts and pseudohyphae, associated with suppurative granulomatous inflammation and varying degrees of necrosis. Fungal yeasts and pseudohyphae typically are found within necrotic debris.

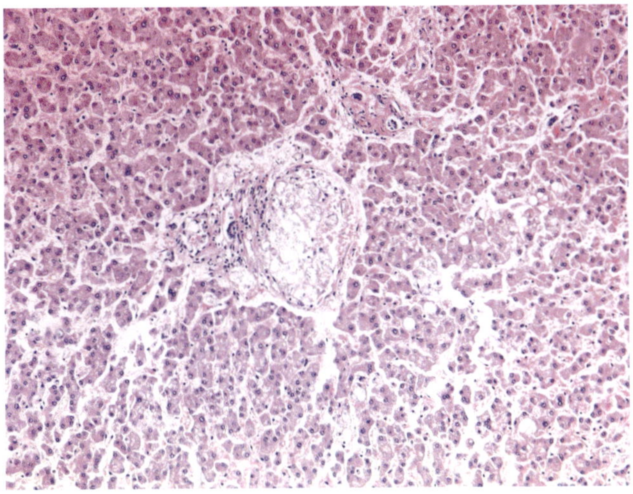

Fig. 7.18 Cryptococcosis. A group of variably sized yeasts with a thick empty rim is seen in a portal tract. *Cryptococcus neoformans* is a ubiquitous fungus in the soil enriched by bird droppings. Hepatic involvement in disseminated disease is commonly associated with immunosuppression. Cryptococcosis is the third commonest fungal infection in immunocompromised patients, following candidiasis and aspergillosis.

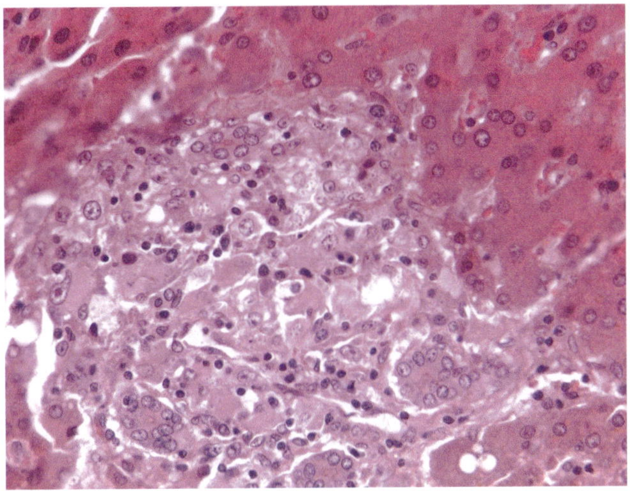

Fig. 7.20 Histoplasmosis. Small refractile yeasts with an (artefactual) retracted clear space are seen here engulfed by portal macrophages. Histoplasmosis is caused by *Histoplasma capsulatum* and *Histoplasma duboisii*. *H. capsulatum* is a budding refractile yeast of 2 to 5 μm. The fungal wall is invisible in H&E-stained sections but is highlighted by PASD and Grocott stains. A portal lymphohistiocytic infiltrate and Kupffer cell hyperplasia with yeasts engulfed by macrophages and Kupffer cells are common histologic patterns. Less commonly, discrete small epithelioid granulomas, large histoplasmomas, and fibrotic calcified granulomas also are found.

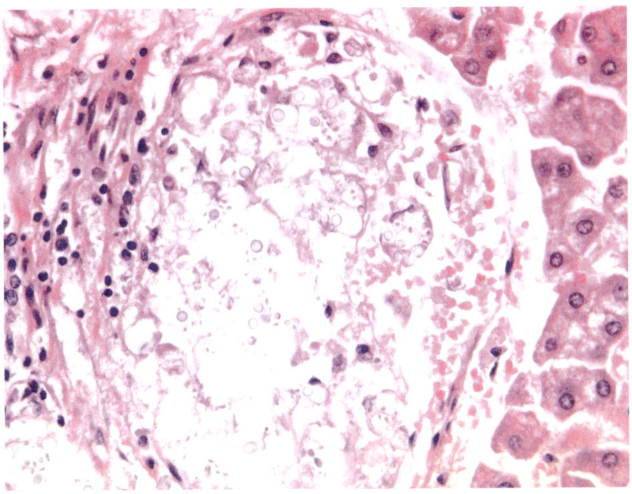

Fig. 7.19 Cryptococcal infection. Cryptococcal infection is characterised by the presence of budding yeasts of 5 to 20 μm with a thin wall and thick mucoid capsule, which appears as an empty rim on haematoxylin and eosin (H&E), PASD, and Grocott stains, and is highlighted by mucicarmine stain. These yeasts commonly are engulfed within portal macrophages and Kupffer cells. Epithelioid granulomatous inflammation and a nonspecific mild portal lymphocytic infiltrate occasionally are seen. Small-sized or capsule-deficient *Cryptococcus* sometimes may be difficult to differentiate from other fungal yeasts, particularly *Histoplasma* and *Blastomyces*, but immunostaining for *Cryptococcus* is helpful in this situation.

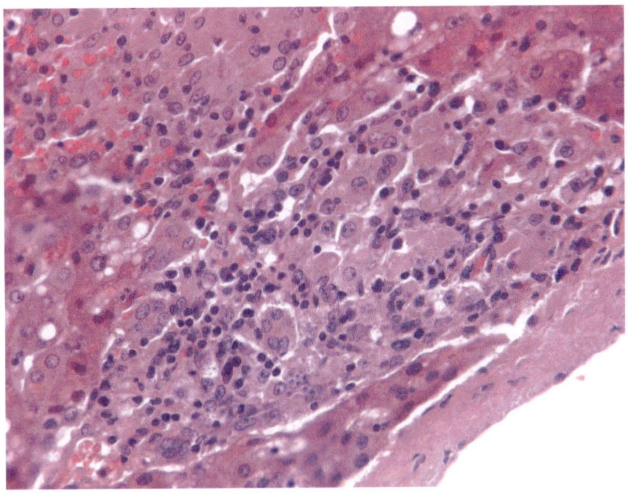

Fig. 7.21 Histoplasmosis. Small refractile yeasts with an artefactual retracted clear space are present, engulfed by portal macrophages. *Histoplasma* resembles other intracellular organisms in H&E-stained sections, including small-sized *Cryptococcus*, *Penicillium*, and *Leishmania*. *Cryptococcus* possesses a mucicarmine-positive capsule. *Penicillium marneffei* is a nonbudding yeast of 5 × 2 μm with a characteristic transverse septum. *Leishmania* contains a kinetoplast and is negative on PASD and Grocott stains. *Histoplasma* mimics *Pneumocystis* on Grocott stain, but *Pneumocystis* appears as an extracellular frothy pink exudate on H&E.

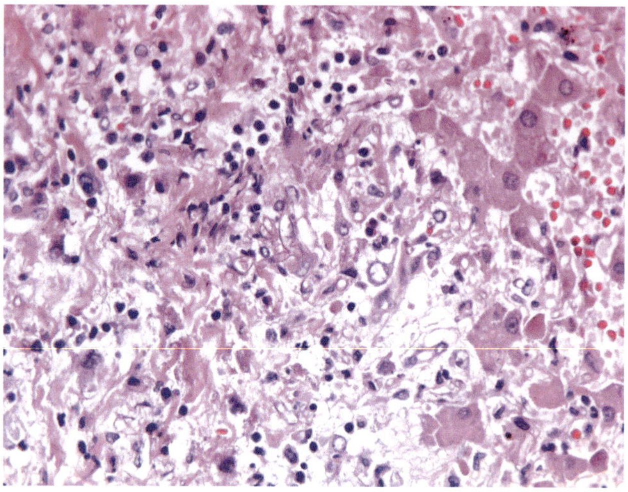

Fig. 7.22 Zygomycosis. Broad-branching fungal hyphae with some septation are found among necroinflammatory debris. Zygomycosis is caused by a group of opportunistic fungal species that includes *Rhizopus*, *Mucor*, and *Absidia*, sharing similar a characteristic morphology. They tend to present as multiple necrotic nodules up to 1 cm in diameter, accompanied by thrombosis and haemorrhagic necrosis as a consequence of fungal angioinvasion, with or without suppurative granulomatous inflammation. Broad-branching fungal hyphae of 6 to 25 μm with few septa are characteristic for zygomycosis. Hepatic aspergillosis, however, may elicit similar features. Identification of septated aspergillus hyphae branching at acute angles of 45° differentiates aspergillosis from zygomycosis.

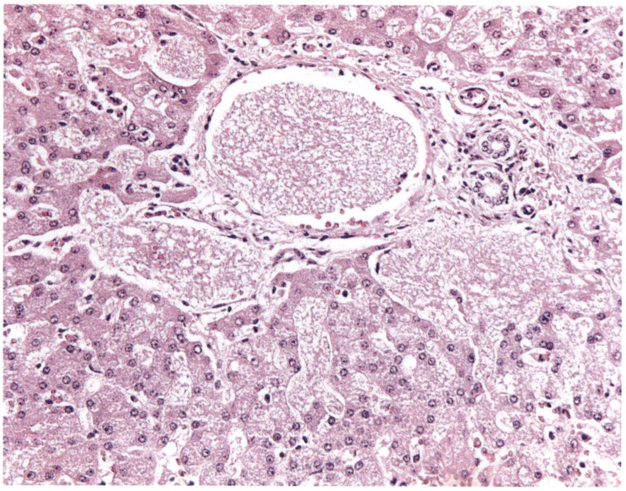

Fig. 7.23 *Pneumocystis jiroveci* (ex *carinii*). Several pools of extracellular "frothy" pink exudate are present in a portal venule and dilated sinusoids. *P. jiroveci*, formerly referred to as *P. carinii*, is now classified as a fungus. It is a worldwide ubiquitous fungus in soil or air. A minority (<3%) of patients with *Pneumocystis* pneumonia develop extrapulmonary pneumocystosis, commonly involving the lymph nodes, liver, spleen, and bone marrow. *P. jiroveci* in the liver is characterized by an extracellular frothy pink exudate in dilated sinusoids, associated with patchy hepatocellular necrosis with an inconspicuous inflammatory infiltrate. Pale cysts containing a few basophilic dots may be seen in H&E sections. A Grocott stain demonstrates characteristic cup-shaped or helmet-shaped cysts of 4 to 6 μm. Immunostaining for *Pneumocystis* is available for confirming the diagnosis.

7.5 Protozoal Infection

Malaria and amoebiasis are the two commonest and important protozoal infections in the liver. Visceral leishmaniasis, cryptosporidiosis, microsporidiosis (*Enterocytozoon bieneusi* and *Encephalitozoon intestinalis*), isosporiasis (*Isospora belli*), giardiasis (*Giardia lamblia*), toxoplasmosis (*Toxoplasma gondii*), babesiosis (*Babesia divergens*), and balantidiasis (*Balantidium coli*) are other protozoal infections affecting hepatobiliary system.

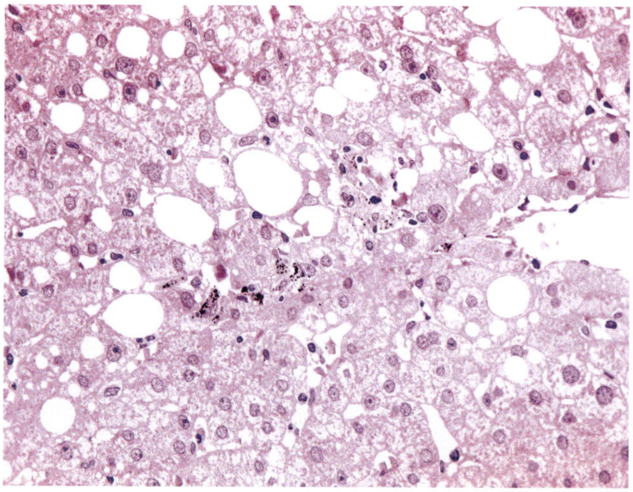

Fig. 7.24 Malaria. Hyperplastic Kupffer cells contain dark-brownish refractile haemozoin pigments. The hallmark pathologic feature of malaria is the accumulation of dark-brownish malarial haemozoin pigments in hyperplastic Kupffer cells and, in the later stage, portal macrophages. Ring forms of *Plasmodium falciparum*, which appear as faint, clear rings with a basophilic dot, may be found within red cells but frequently are obscured by haemozoin pigments. Sinusoidal congestion, mild macrovesicular steatosis, a mild portal lymphoplasmacytic infiltrate, and a variable degree of haemosiderosis also may be observed.

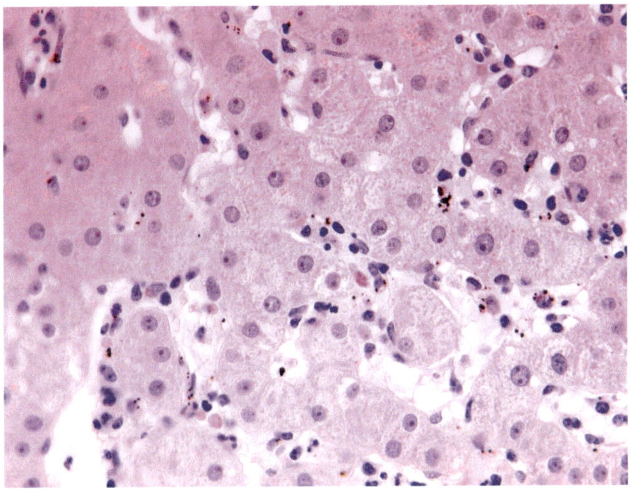

Fig. 7.25 Malaria. Hyperplastic Kupffer cells are present and contain dark-brownish refractile haemozoin pigments. Malarial pigment may mimic schistosomal haemozoin pigment, haemosiderin, and protoporphyrin. The presence of schistosomal ova, granulomata, portal fibrosis, and calcification helps differentiate schistosomiasis from malaria. Negativity of malarial pigment on Perls stain distinguishes malarial pigment from haemosiderin in mesenchymal iron overload. Protoporphyrin in erythropoietic protoporphyria is deposited in hepatocytes and bile canaliculi in addition to Kupffer cells and demonstrates a red-to-yellow birefringence with a Maltese cross configuration under polarized light.

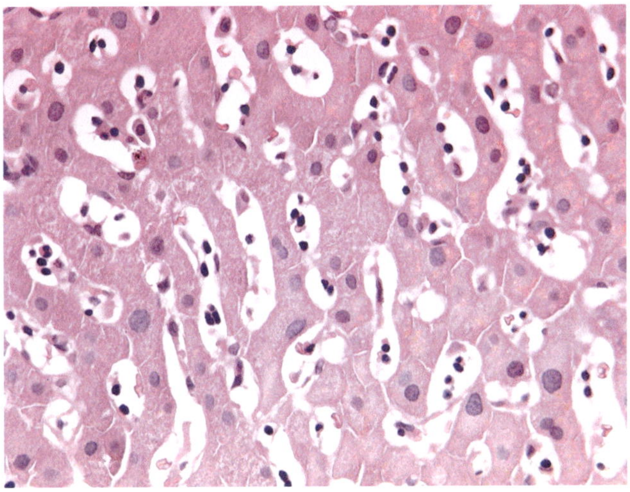

Fig. 7.26 Tropical splenomegaly syndrome. Abundant lymphocytes infiltrate the sinusoids and are accompanied by hyperplastic Kupffer cells. No haemozoin pigment is identified. Tropical splenomegaly syndrome, properly named hyperreactive malarial splenomegaly, is an idiosyncratic response to a low-grade chronic *P. falciparum* infection. Histopathologically, it is characterised by sinusoidal lymphocytosis with Kupffer cell hyperplasia and variable portal lymphocytic infiltration. Haemozoin pigment typically is absent. Differential diagnoses include other causes of sinusoidal lymphocytosis, including viral hepatitis C, Epstein-Barr virus infection, cytomegalovirus infection, drug-induced liver injury, nonspecific reactive hepatitis, extramedullary haematopoiesis, leukaemia, and non-Hodgkin lymphoma. The definitive diagnosis depends on clinical and serologic correlation.

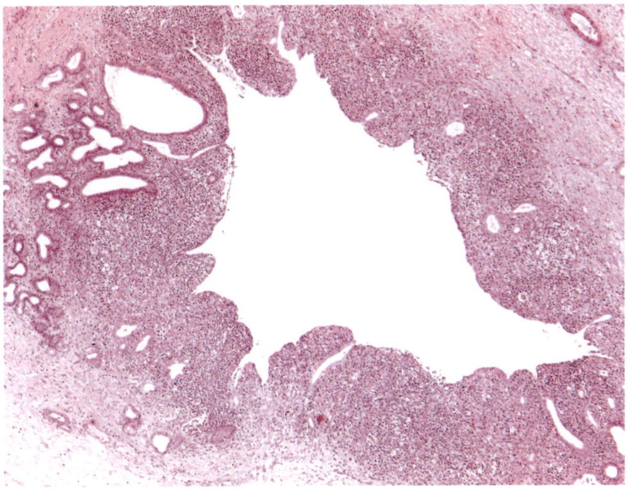

Fig. 7.27 Cryptosporidiosis. A large bile duct shows surface erosion with regenerative activity, a dense inflammatory infiltrate, and periductal fibrosis. *Cryptosporidium parvum*, a protozoan found in the intestine of humans and animals and excreted in their stools, accounts for 2.2% and 6.1% of diarrhoea in immunocompetent individuals in developed and developing countries, respectively. In immunocompromised patients, the biliary system also may be involved, leading to secondary sclerosing cholangitis, acalculous cholecystitis, and papillary stenosis. About 20% to 32% of HIV-associated cholangiopathy is associated with cryptosporidiosis.

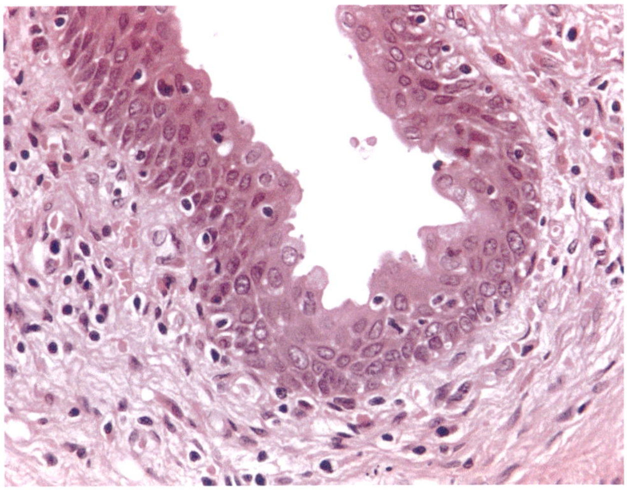

Fig. 7.28 Cryptosporidiosis. Small dots of cryptosporidial organisms are seen here attached to the luminal surface of hyperplastic biliary epithelial cells. Hepatic cryptosporidiosis is characterised by secondary sclerosing cholangitis, mainly affecting large to medium-sized extrahepatic and intrahepatic bile ducts with a variable degree of mucosal damage, epithelial hyperplastic change, inflammation, and periductal fibrosis. Adhesion of 1- to 2-μm organisms onto the luminal surface of involved bile duct is the characteristic feature. Smaller intrahepatic bile ducts are affected much less commonly. Coinfection with cytomegalovirus is a frequent phenomenon, and viral inclusions are found more readily in the extrahepatic than in the intrahepatic ducts.

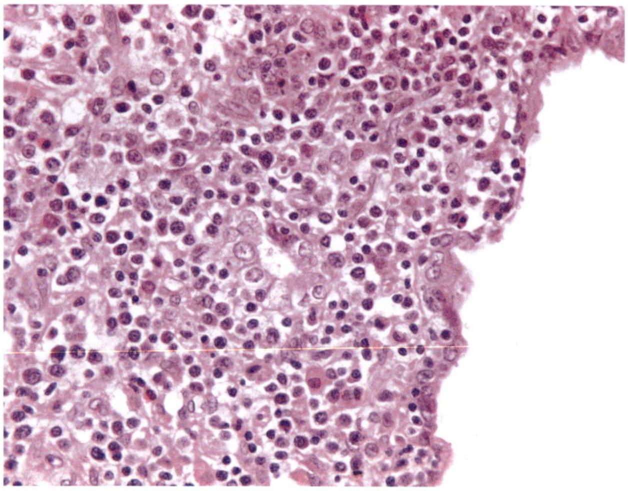

Fig. 7.29 Cryptosporidiosis. Primary and other secondary sclerosing cholangitides are part of the list of differential diagnoses. In immunocompromised patients, unusual infectious cholangitis, such as microsporidiosis, isosporiasis, and giardiasis, may need to be considered.

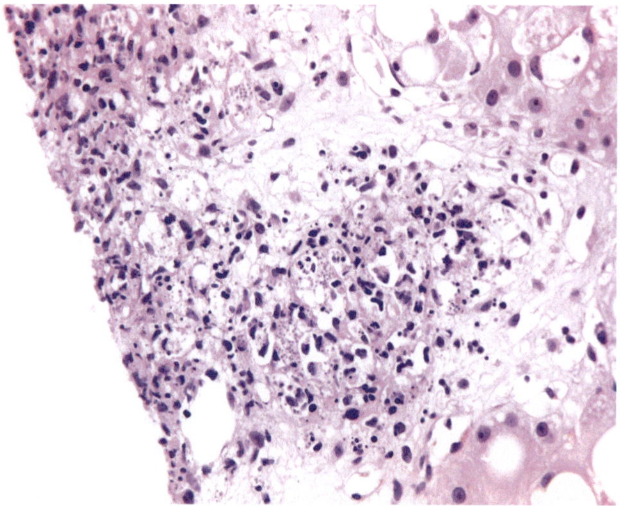

Fig. 7.30 Visceral leishmaniasis. There is a large cluster of Kupffer cells containing intracellular amastigotes with a small basophilic nucleus surrounded by a clear rim; this is accompanied by a mild lymphoplasmacytic infiltrate and epithelioid histiocytes. Visceral leishmaniasis, also known as kala azar, is transmitted by the bite of an infected sandfly and usually caused by *Leishmania donovani* or *Leishmania infantum*. The classic pathologic pattern of acute leishmaniasis is characterised by Kupffer cell hyperplasia, a portal lymphoplasmacytic inflammation, and a diffuse sinusoidal lymphoplasmacytic infiltrate. The intracellular parasites in amastigote form are 2 to 5 µm and oval shaped and contain a basophilic nucleus with a hallmark paranuclear rod-shaped kinetoplast phagocytised by Kupffer cells, portal macrophages, and, rarely, hepatocytes.

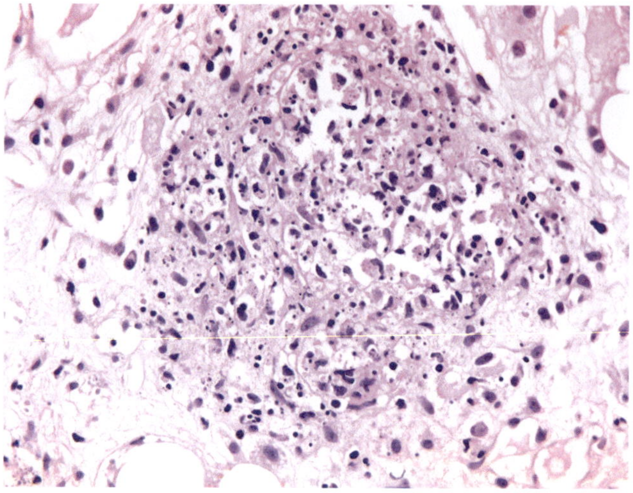

Fig. 7.31 Visceral leishmaniasis. There is a large cluster of Kupffer cells containing intracellular amastigotes with a small basophilic nucleus surrounded by a clear rim, which is accompanied by mild lymphoplasmacytic infiltrate and epithelioid histiocytes. Another histologic pattern of acute leishmaniasis is the presence of multiple aggregates of Kupffer cells containing scanty parasites. Other, less common features include epithelioid granulomas, fibrin-ring granulomas, necrosis, necrotizing granuloma, and mild macrovesicular steatosis. In chronic leishmaniasis, so-called Rogers cirrhosis, associated with diffuse pericellular fibrosis preserving portal tracts, occasionally may be found.

7.6 Helminth Infection

Helminths are metazoan parasites which can be further classified into cestodes (tapeworms), trematodes (flukes), and nematodes (roundworm). Cestodes causing hepatic diseases include echinococcosis, rarely sparganosis (*Sparganum proliferum*) and cysticercosis (*Taenia solium*). Trematodes leading to liver infestation include schistosomiasis, clonorchiasis, opisthorchiasis, fascioliasis (*Fasciola hepatica*) and pentastomiasis (*Armillifer armillatus*). Nematodes associated with hepatic involvement comprise toxocariasis, ascariasis (*Ascaris lumbricoides*), enterobiasis (*Enterobius vermicularis*), strongyloidiasis (*Strongyloides stercoralis*), and capillariasis (*Capillaria hepatica*).

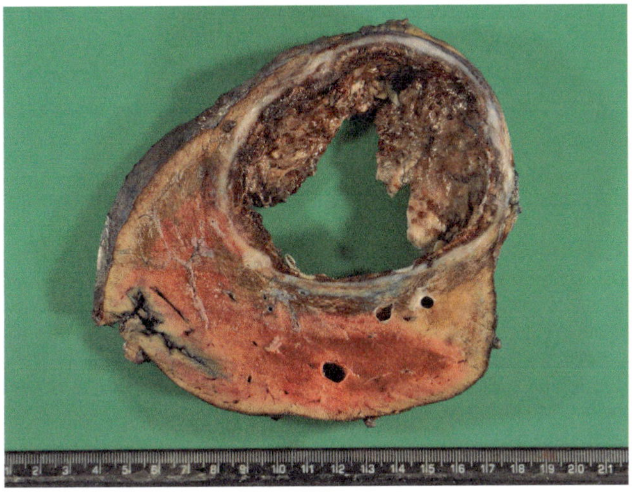

Fig. 7.32 Echinococcosis. A treated unilocular hydatid cyst is seen here with a well-circumscribed unilocular cyst accompanied by a fibrous wall and necrotic content. Echinococcosis is caused by infestation of *Echinococcus* cestodes. The two major forms are cystic (unilocular) echinococcosis and alveolar (multilocular) echinococcosis, caused by *Echinococcus granulosus* and *Echinococcus multilocularis*, respectively.

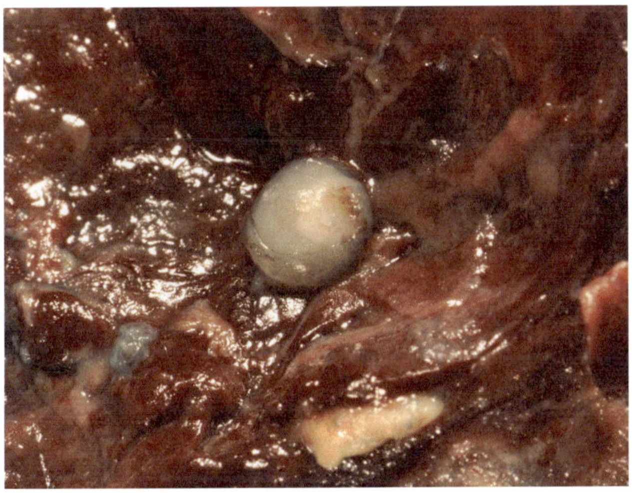

Fig. 7.33 Echinococcosis. A white daughter cyst is found within the unilocular hydatid cyst. Unilocular hydatidosis is characterised by a hydatid cyst of up to 30 cm that may be of single unilocular form or may contain multiple daughter cysts within a mother cyst, with a fibrous rim. The cyst wall is composed of an outer 1-mm–thick acellular laminated membrane, a thin nucleated germinal membrane, and attached protoscolices with suckers and hooklets. Host reaction is minimal, with only a thin fibrous wall and a granulation tissue response. When the cyst ruptures or becomes necrotic, granulomatous inflammation with giant cells and eosinophils may result.

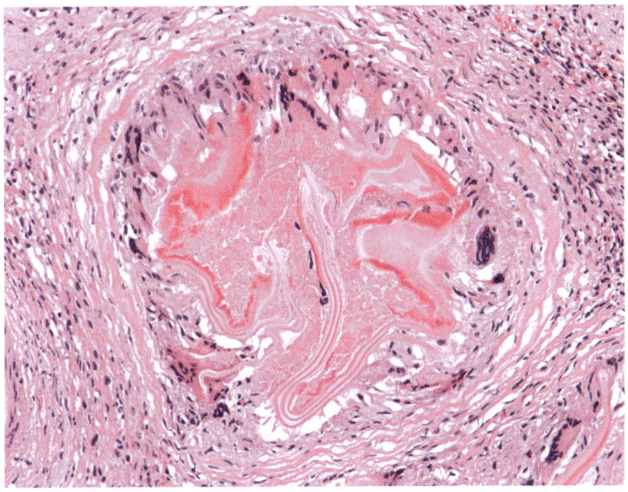

Fig. 7.34 Echinococcosis. Shown is a ruptured hydatid cyst with an acellular laminated membrane in the absence of protoscolices, surrounded by epithelioid histiocytes, multinucleated giant cells, and fibrosis. Multilocular hydatidosis is characterised by multiloculated necrotic cysts composed of a direct extension of the budding and proliferating cyst wall into the liver parenchyma, resulting in necrosis, prominent granulomatous inflammation, eosinophilic infiltrate, and fibrous tissue reaction. The cyst wall is composed of an irregular, fragmented, laminated membrane only, without a germinal membrane or protoscolices.

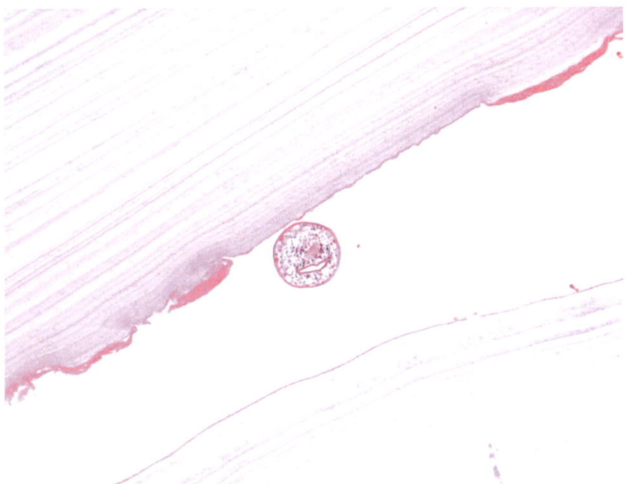

Fig. 7.35 Echinococcosis. A protoscolex and acellular laminated membranes are shown. Differential diagnoses include other cystic hepatic lesions, such as solitary bile duct cyst, ciliated foregut cyst, mucinous cystic neoplasm, biliary intraductal papillary neoplasm, cystic haematoma, amoebic abscess, pyogenic abscess, and necrotizing eosinophilic granuloma. Identification of the characteristic laminated membrane with or without a germinal membrane and protoscolices distinguishes hydatid cyst from other hepatic cystic lesions.

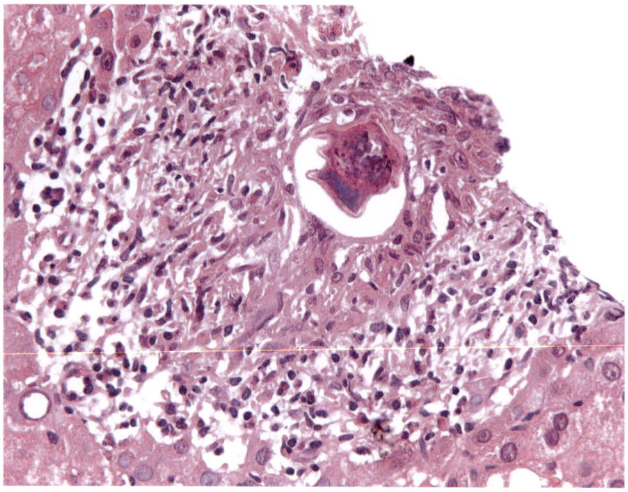

Fig. 7.36 Schistosomiasis. A schistosomal ovum is seen here surrounded by epithelioid granulomatous inflammation. Schistosomiasis, sometimes referred to as bilharzia, results from direct skin contact or ingestion of water contaminated by infected freshwater snails. *Schistosoma mansoni*, *Schistosoma japonicum*, and *Schistosoma mekongi* are the three main blood flukes (trematodes) causing clinically significant liver diseases. Chronic hepatosplenic schistosomiasis is the commonest cause of portal hypertension worldwide. The morphology of parasitic ova depends on the species: an *S. mansoni* ovum is 140 × 60 µm with a lateral spine, an *S. japonicum* ovum is 85 × 60 µm with a small lateral knob, and an *S. mekongi* ovum is 60 × 50 µm with a small lateral knob. All three species are acid-fast on Ziehl-Neelsen stain.

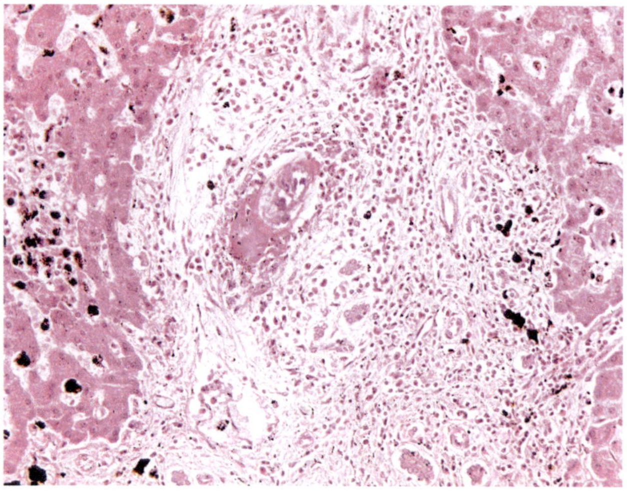

Fig. 7.37 Schistosomiasis. A schistosomal ovum is associated with a prominent inflammatory infiltrate and portal oedema. Portal macrophages and Kupffer cells contain schistosomal haemozoin pigment. The early phase of schistosomiasis is characterised by the presence of live ova in portal venous radicles associated with an eosinophilic infiltrate and abscess formation, granulomatous inflammation, haemozoin pigment-laden portal macrophages, and Kupffer cells. The late phase of schistosomiasis is characterised by degenerated and calcified ova in portal venous radicles associated with portal and periportal fibrosis (pipestem fibrosis), portal vein obliteration and thrombosis, and hepatic arteriolar proliferation. Schistosomal haemozoin pigment is similar to malarial haemozoin pigment as products of haemoglobin breakdown, and both are negative on Perls stain.

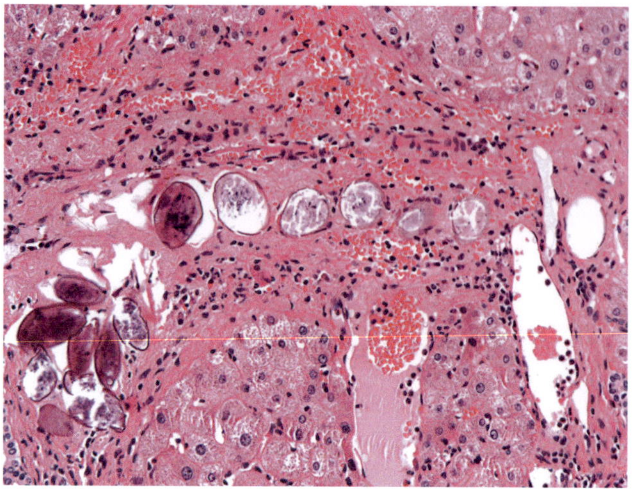

Fig. 7.38 Schistosomiasis. Partially calcified and dead schistosomal ova are present in a fibrotic portal tract. Granulomatous inflammation and an eosinophilic reaction seen in the early phase of schistosomiasis also may be found in other infections. Identification of schistosomal ova is diagnostic, whereas schistosomal haemozoin pigments and portal-based inflammation provide additional histologic clues. Schistosomal haemozoin pigment per se may resemble malarial haemozoin pigment, haemosiderin, and protoporphyrin, but the associated histologic features in schistosomiasis usually make differentiation straightforward.

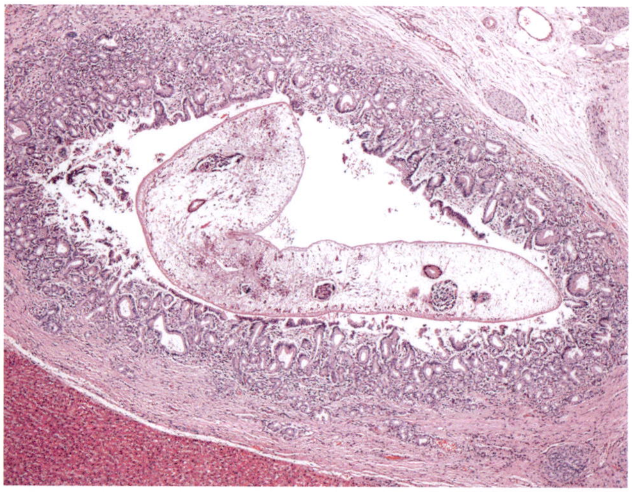

Fig. 7.39 Clonorchiasis and opisthorchiasis. A liver fluke (*Clonorchis sinensis*) is present within a large bile duct with prominent peribiliary gland hyperplasia. *C. sinensis*, *Opisthorchis viverrini*, and *Opisthorchis felineus* are common liver flukes (trematodes). Clonorchiasis and opisthorchiasis are caused by ingestion of infected uncooked freshwater fish, crab, or crayfish, and exhibit similar clinical and pathologic manifestations. *C. sinensis* is detected in 30% to 40% of recurrent pyogenic cholangitis. Cholangiocarcinoma is a rare but important complication in endemic areas, with an increased risk of 20- to 40-fold.

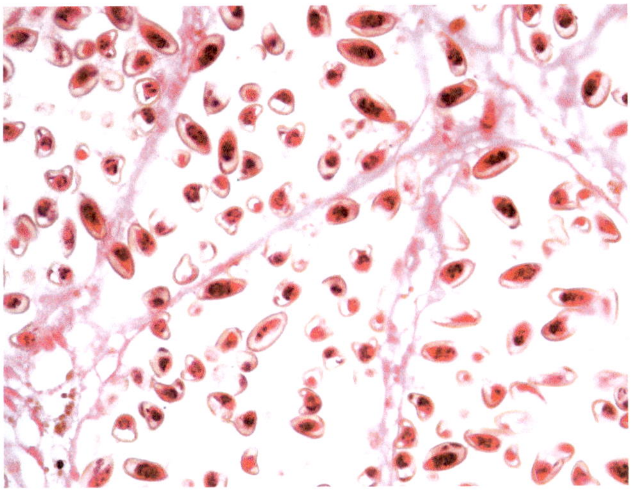

Fig. 7.40 Clonorchiasis and opisthorchiasis. Numerous ova up to 30 μm in length are shown. Clonorchiasis and opisthorchiasis mainly involve the extrahepatic and large intrahepatic bile ducts. *C. sinensis* measures 8 to 25 mm × 2 to 5 mm and contains many ova of 30 × 15 μm, whereas *O. viverrini* is 11 to 20 mm × 3 mm. The left hepatic lobe is preferentially involved. A prominent reactive hyperplasia of peribiliary glands ("adenomatous hyperplasia"), often with intestinal metaplasia, a variable eosinophil-rich inflammatory infiltrate, and periductal fibrosis, frequently is associated with the infected bile ducts. Necrotizing eosinophilic granulomas occasionally are found. Other pathologic manifestations are complications including acute cholangitis, pyogenic abscess, intrahepatic choledocholithiasis, and, rarely, multicentric, mucin-secreting intrahepatic cholangiocarcinoma.

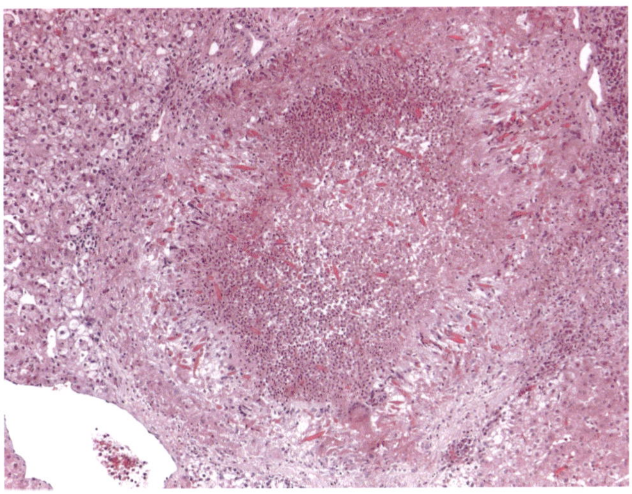

Fig. 7.41 Visceral larva migrans (toxocariasis). A large necrotizing eosinophilic granuloma is seen with abundant Charcot-Leyden crystals. Toxocariasis is a zoonosis caused by ingestion of nematodes from faeces of infected dogs (*Toxocara canis*) and cats (*Toxocara cati*). Visceral larva migrans usually is ascribed to toxocariasis but also may be seen with other parasitic infestations, such as baylisascariasis, ascariasis, strongyloidiasis, and capillariasis. Visceral larva migrans is characterized histopathologically by multifocal granulomatous inflammation with central fibrinoid necrosis containing degenerating eosinophils and neutrophils and surrounded by palisading fibroblasts, a striking amount of eosinophils, and occasional multinucleated giant cells. Charcot-Leyden crystals formed by degranulated eosinophils also are present. Rarely, a larval segment of 300 × 20 μm is found within the granulomas.

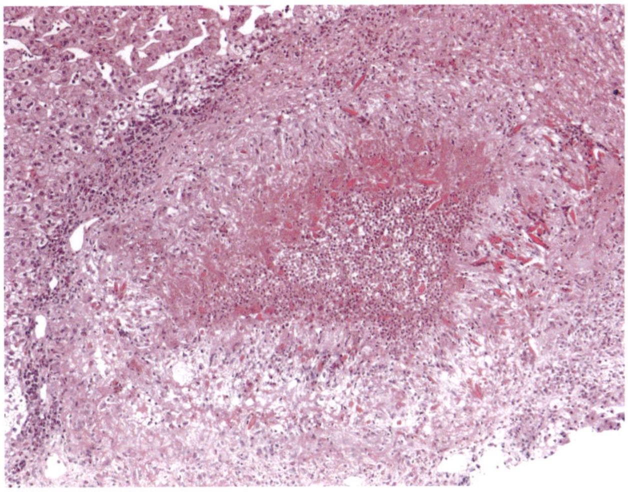

Fig. 7.42 Visceral larva migrans (toxocariasis). A large necrotizing eosinophilic granuloma with some Charcot-Leyden crystals is present. Other aetiologies of necrotizing eosinophilic granuloma in the liver include other parasitic infestations (enterobiasis, capillariasis, fasciolia-sis, and schistosomiasis), drug-induced liver injury, Langerhans cell histiocytosis, Hodgkin lymphoma, T-cell lymphoma, and Churg-Strauss syndrome. Multiple levelling of the histologic sections with or without ancillary special stains is required to look for parasites or diagnostic lesions. Correlation with clinical and travel history and microbiologic investigation also are essential.

8 Drug-Induced Liver Injury

Drug- and toxin-induced liver injury is responsible for a significant amount of morbidity and mortality. A very wide range of clinical and pathologic presentations may result. The time of onset after drug exposure varies from hours to months. The clinical manifestations range from asymptomatic deranged liver function to fulminant hepatic failure and death. Drug- or toxin-induced liver injuries can mimic all forms of acute, chronic, vascular, or neoplastic liver diseases that are caused by other aetiologies; hence, they always are included in the differential diagnosis of virtually any form of liver disease.

Drug/toxin reactions may be intrinsic or predictable, in cases in which they are dose dependent (e.g., paracetamol, carbon tetrachloride), or idiosyncratic and unpredictable, when they are dose independent (e.g., isoniazid, halothane). The underlying mechanisms include direct/indirect toxicity, aberrant metabolism producing toxic metabolites, and immune-mediated hypersensitivity.

The diagnosis of drug- or toxin-induced liver injuries requires clinical, biochemical, and pathologic correlation. Recognition of the overall morphologic pattern in the pathologic examination is essential in the diagnostic process. The morphologic patterns may be categorized as those associated with (1) necroinflammatory injury, (2) cholestatic injury, (3) steatosis and steatohepatitis, (4) vascular lesions, (5) neoplasm and neoplasm-like lesions, and (6) adaptive change.

8.1 Necroinflammatory Injury

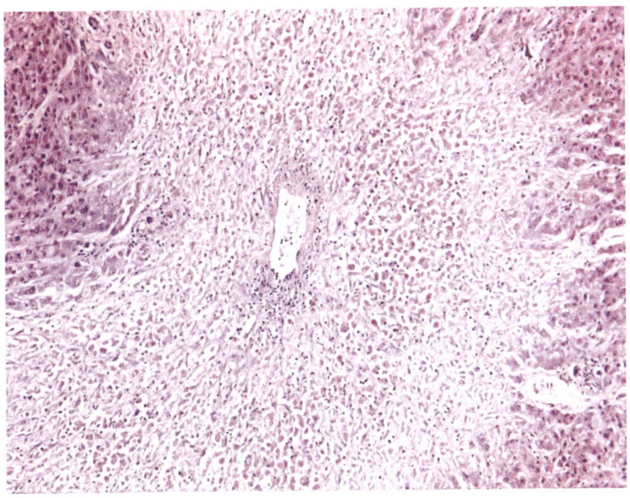

Fig. 8.1 Acute hepatic necrosis induced by paracetamol. Extensive zone 3 necrosis is accompanied by a mild inflammatory infiltrate. Drug/toxin-induced acute hepatic necrosis typically has an abrupt onset, with latency within 2 weeks. Patients usually present with malaise, nausea, and abdominal pain. Hepatic encephalopathy may occur early. Dysfunction or failure of other organs (kidney, lung, and bone marrow) and sepsis related to immunoparesis may complicate the clinical picture. Markedly elevated (>20× upper normal limit) serum aminotransferase levels with normal or modestly elevated (<2× upper normal limit) serum bilirubin and alkaline phosphatase levels are the usual biochemical profile. Although a proportion of patients may recover, other die or are saved by liver transplantation.

A.W.H. Chan et al., *Atlas of Liver Pathology*, Atlas of Anatomic Pathology,
DOI 10.1007/978-1-4614-9114-9_8, © Springer Science+Business Media New York 2014

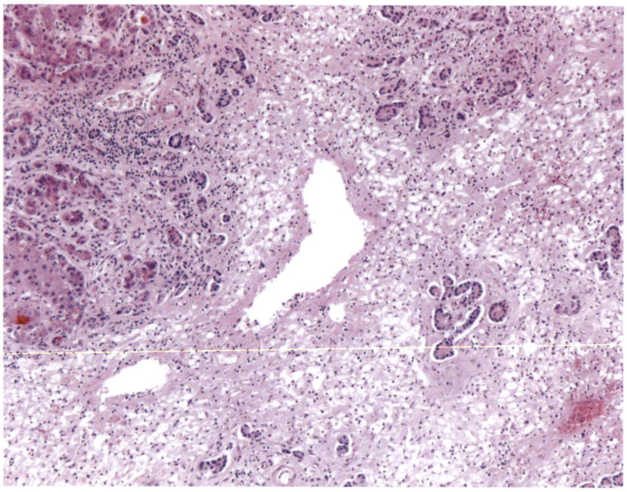

Fig. 8.2 Acute hepatic necrosis induced by rifampicin. Panacinar necrosis is accompanied by a ductular reaction with minimal inflammatory infiltrate. A few residual hepatocytes are noted in the zone 1 regions. It would not be possible to identify the cause of this injury on histological grounds alone and clinico-pathological correlation is essential.

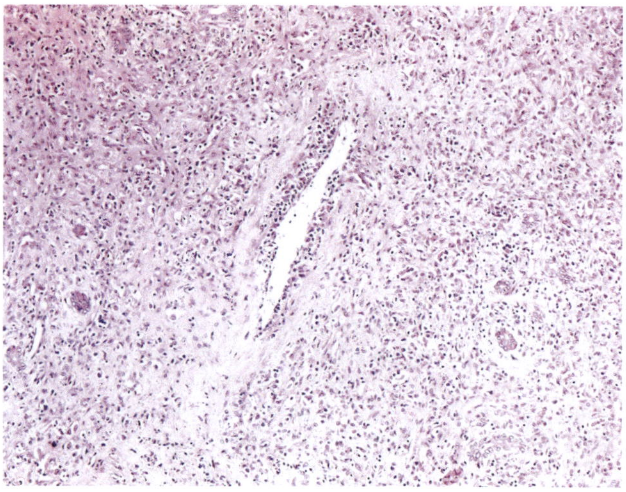

Fig. 8.3 Acute hepatic necrosis induced by halothane. Panacinar necrosis is accompanied by a ductular reaction and a moderate inflammatory infiltrate. There may be some overlapping clinical, biochemical, and histologic features between drug/toxin-induced acute hepatic necrosis and drug/toxin-induced acute hepatitis. The latter is characterised by a more insidious onset, less rapid recovery, a lower level of serum aminotransferase, more inflammatory infiltrate, and less hepatic necrosis on histology.

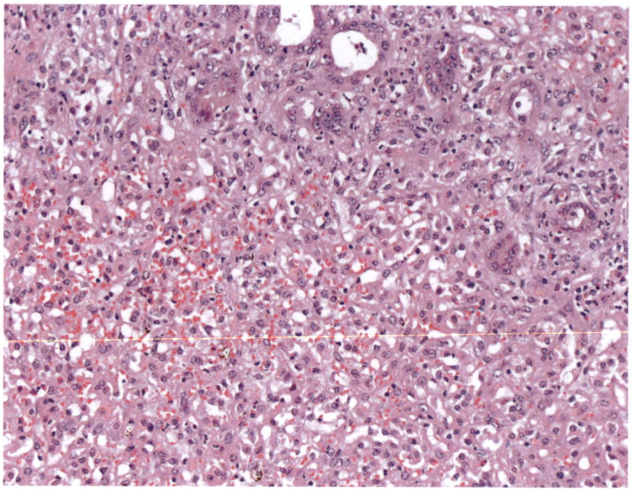

Fig. 8.4 Acute hepatic necrosis induced by ferrous sulphate. Extensive zone 1 necrosis is accompanied by ductular reaction and sinusoidal congestion. Most forms of drug/toxin-induced hepatic necrosis produce zone 3 or panacinar necrosis, whereas a small proportion lead to zone 1 or zone 2 necrosis. The zonal localisation of necrosis may be related to the underlying mechanism of injury.

Table 8.1 Drugs and toxins associated with acute hepatic necrosis

2-Chloropropane (zone 3)	Ebrotidine (zone 3)	Norfloxacin (zone 3)
2-Nitropropane (diffuse)	Enflurane (zone 3)	Paracetamol (zone 3)
Aflatoxins (zone 1, zone 3)	Ethionamide (zone 3)	Paraquat (zone 3)
Albitocin (zone 1)	Ethylene dibromide (zone 3)	Phalloidin (zone 3)
Alloxan (zone 1)	Ethylene dichloride (zone 3)	Phosphorus (zone 1)
Allyl compounds (zone 1)	Ferrous sulphate (zone 1)	Piroxicam (diffuse)
Amanitin (zone 3)	Fluroxene (zone 3)	Propylthiouracil (zone 3)
Amodiaquine (zone 3)	Galactosamine (diffuse)	Proteus vulgaris endotoxin (zone 1)
Anastrozole (zone 3)	Halogenated hydrocarbons (zone 3, diffuse)	Quetiapine (zone 3)
Aniline (diffuse)	Halothane (zone 3)	Quinidine (zonal)
Arsenic compounds (zone 3, diffuse)	Imatinib mesylate (zone 3)	Rifampin (zonal)
Bacillus cereus toxin (zone 2)	Imipramine (zonal)	Roxithromycin (zone 3)
Benorylate (zonal)	Indomethacin (zonal)	Rubratoxin (zone 3)
Beryllium (zone 2)	Iodoform (zone 3)	Selenium (diffuse)
Bromobenzene (zone 3)	Iproniazid (zone 3)	Sporidesmin (zone 1)
Carbon tetrachloride (zone 3)	Isoflurane (zone 3)	Sulindac (zonal)
Chlorinated benzenes (zone 3, diffuse)	Isoniazid (zonal)	Sulphasalazine (zonal)
Chlorinated diphenyls (diffuse)	Ketoconazole (zone 3)	Synthaline (zone 1)
Chlorinated naphthalene (diffuse)	Labetalol (zone 3)	Tacrolimus (zone 3)
Chloroform (zone 3)	Lamotrigine (zone 1, zone 3)	Telithromycin (zone 3)
Chloroprene (zone 3)	Levetiracetam (zone 3)	Tetrachloroethane (zone 3, diffuse)
Chlorzoxazone (zone 3)	Levofloxacin (zone 3)	Tetrachloroethylene (zone 3)
Ciprofloxacin (zone 3)	Lovastatin (zone 3)	Thioacetamide (zone 3)
Citalopram (zone 3)	Luteoskyrin (zone 3)	Ticrynafen (tienilic acid) (zone 3)
Cocaine (zone 1, zone 3)	Manganese compounds (zone 1)	Tolazamide (zonal)
Copper sulphate (zone 3)	Mesalamine (mesalazine) (zone 1)	Toloxatone (zone 3)
DDT (zone 3)	Methoxyflurane (zonal)	Trichloroethylene (zone 3)
Desipramine (zonal)	Methyldopa (zone 3)	Trinitrotoluene (zone 3, diffuse)
Dichloropropane (zone 3)	Metoprolol (zone 3)	Troglitazone (zone 3)
Dimethylnitrosamine (zone 3)	Mithramycin (plicamycin) (zone 3)	Trovafloxacin (zone 3)
Dinitrobenzene (zone 3, diffuse)	Mushrooms (zone 3, diffuse)	Urethane (ethyl carbamate) (zone 3)
Dinitrotoluene (zone 3, diffuse)	Naphthalene (zone 3)	Valproic acid (zone 3)
Dioxane (zone 2, diffuse)	Nefazodone (zone 3)	Venlafaxine (zone 3)
Diphtheria toxin (zone 3)	Nevirapine (zone 3)	
Duloxetine (zone 3)	Ngaione (zone 2)	

Adapted from Lewis JH, Kleiner DE. Hepatic injury due to drugs, herbal compounds, chemicals and toxins. In: Burt AD, Portmann BC, Ferrell LD, editors. MacSween's Pathology of the liver. 6th ed. London: Churchill-Livingstone; 2012 with permission.

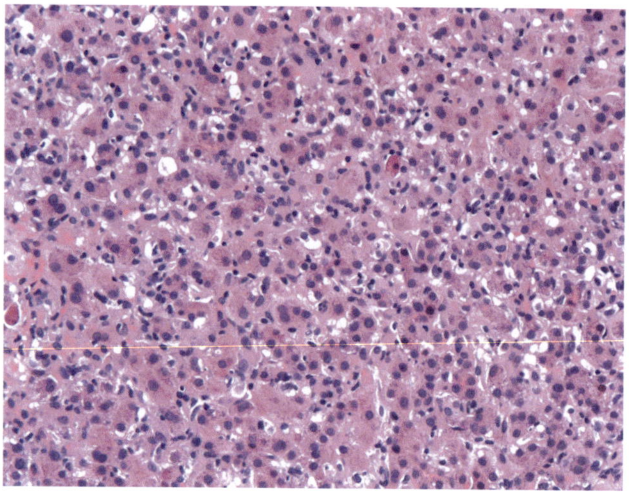

Fig. 8.5 Acute hepatitis induced by diclofenac. This image shows prominent lobular disarray with obvious hepatocytic regenerative changes, sinusoidal inflammatory infiltrate, and scattered apoptotic bodies. Drug/toxin-induced acute hepatitis accounts for 30% to 50% of all drug/toxin-induced liver injuries. It usually has an insidious onset, with latency between 2 and 24 weeks. Patients usually present with nausea and malaise, followed by abdominal pain and jaundice. Fever, skin rash, and hypereosinophilia may be found. Recovery after withdrawal of the agent for 2 to 4 weeks is common. Serum liver enzymes may rise for another week after withdrawal of the agent and then drop by 50% within a month.

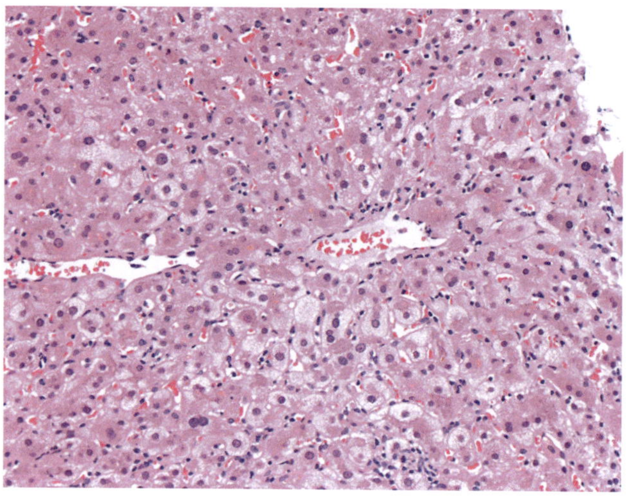

Fig. 8.6 Acute drug-induced hepatitis. Mild zone 3 hepatocytic hydropic swelling is seen together with a few foci of spotty necrosis and a moderate sinusoidal lymphocytic infiltrate. Differential histologic diagnoses include acute viral hepatitis (A, B, C, and E), reactivation of chronic hepatitis B, and acute Epstein-Barr viral hepatitis. Autoimmune hepatitis and Wilson disease uncommonly may present with an acute hepatitis–like histologic pattern.

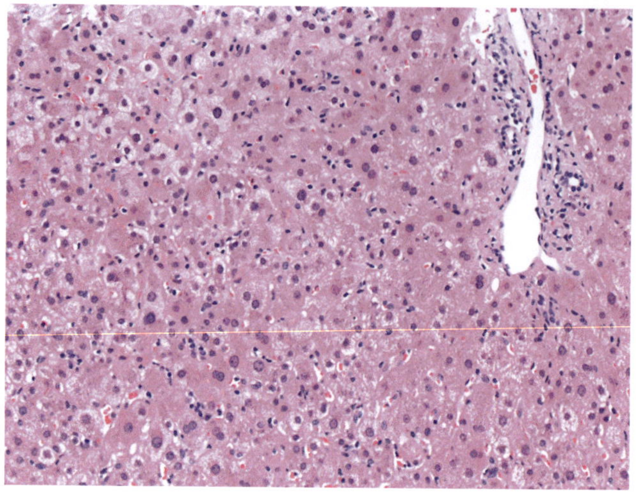

Fig. 8.7 Acute drug-induced hepatitis. Mild zone 3 hepatocytic hydropic swelling and rare foci of spotty necrosis are associated with moderate sinusoidal lymphocytic infiltrate. A normal portal tract is present.

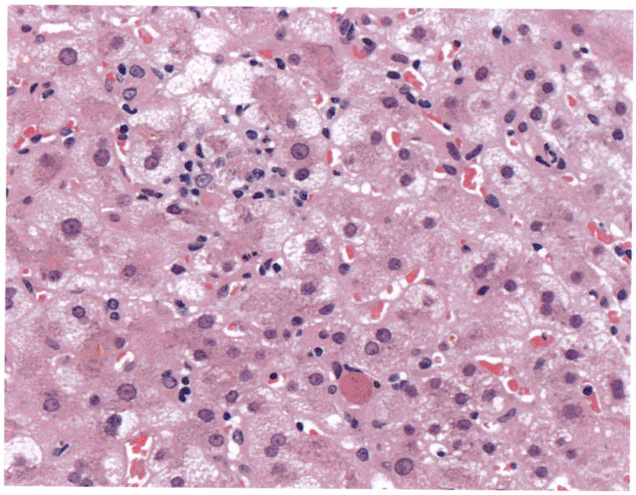

Fig. 8.8 Acute hepatitis. A focus of spotty necrosis (*upper*) and an apoptotic body (*lower*) are seen and are accompanied by mild hepatocytic hydropic swelling. There may be some overlapping clinical, biochemical, and histologic features between drug/toxin-induced acute hepatitis and drug/toxin-induced acute cholestatic hepatitis. The latter is characterised by a slower recovery, a low ratio of serum aminotransferase to serum alkaline phosphatase, and prominent bilirubinostasis on histology.

Table 8.2 Drugs and toxins associated with acute hepatitis

Acarbose	Cyclofenil	Halothane	Nevirapine	Sevoflurane
Acetylsalicylic acid	Danazol	Hydralazine	Nicotinic acid	Sibutramine
Acitretin	Dantrolene	Hydrazines	Nimesulide	Simvastatin
Adriamycin (doxorubicin)	Dapsone	Hydrochlorothiazide	Nitrofurantoin	Spironolactone
Amiodarone	Desflurane	Ibuprofen	Norfloxacin	Streptokinase
Amitriptyline	Desipramine	Imatinib mesylate	Oxacillin	Streptozotocin
Amlodipine	Diazepam	Indomethacin	Oxaprozin	Sulindac
Amodiaquine	Dichloromethotrexate	Infliximab	Oxyphenisatin	Suloctidil
Aprindine	Diclofenac	Interleukin-2	Papaverine	Sulphadiazine
Asparaginase	Diflunisal	Ipilimumab	Pemoline	Sulphadoxine-pyrimethamine
Atomoxetine	Dihydralazine	Isoniazid	Perhexiline maleate	Sulphamethizole
Benzarone	Disopyramide	Ketoconazole	Phenazopyridine	Sulphamethoxazole
Bromfenac	Disulfiram	Lamotrigine	Phenindione	Sulphasalazine
Captopril	Ecstasy	Lergotrile	Phenobarbital	Tacrine
Carbamazepine	Enflurane	Levofloxacin	Phenprocoumon	Telithromycin
Carbenicillin	Etodolac	Lisinopril	Phenylbutazone	Teniposide
Chlorpromazine	Etoposide	Losartan	Phenytoin	Thalidomide
Chlortetracycline	Etretinate	Mercaptopurine	Pirprofen	Thiotepa
Chlorzoxazone	Fenofibrate	Metformin	Probenecid	Ticrynafen (tienilic acid)
Cimetidine	Fluoxetine	Methimazole	Procainamide	Tolazamide
Cinchophen	Fluroxene	Methotrexate	Propylthiouracil	Trazodone
Ciprofloxacin	Gatifloxacin	Methoxyflurane	Pyrazinamide	Troglitazone
Cisplatin	Gemtuzumab	Methyldopa	Quetiapine	Trovafloxacin
Citalopram	Gliclazide	Minocycline	Rifampin	Verapamil
Clarithromycin	Glyburide (glibenclamide)	Mirtazapine	Riluzole	Ximelagatran
Clometacin	Gold	Mitomycin C	Rosuvastatin	
Cromolyn	Haloperidol	Naproxen	Sorafenib	

Adapted from Lewis JH, Kleiner DE. Hepatic injury due to drugs, herbal compounds, chemicals and toxins. In: Burt AD, Portmann BC, Ferrell LD, editors. MacSween's Pathology of the liver. 6th ed. London: Churchill-Livingstone; 2012 with permission.

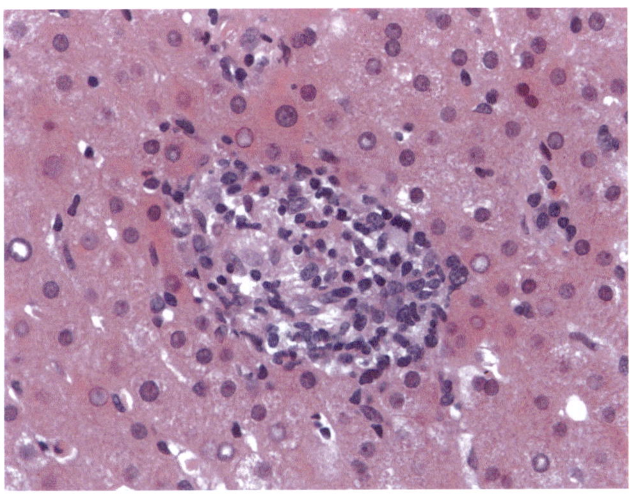

Fig. 8.9 Drug-induced hepatic granulomas. A small, discrete granuloma is present within the hepatic parenchyma. An eosinophil (*right middle*) is noted in the adjacent sinusoid. Drug/toxin-induced hepatic granulomas may be found alone or combined with other patterns of liver injury, including acute and chronic hepatitis, cholestatic hepatitis, and steatosis. They account for up to 29% of all hepatic granulomas. Microgranulomas, a collection of histiocytes (up to 10) often admixed with small lymphocytes and apoptotic hepatocytes, are nonspecific to all types of hepatic insults and drug/toxin-induced liver injuries and do not in themselves warrant a diagnosis of granulomatous hepatitis. The presence of epithelioid granulomas and, much less frequently, fibrin-ring granulomas signifies a genuine granulomatous hepatitis.

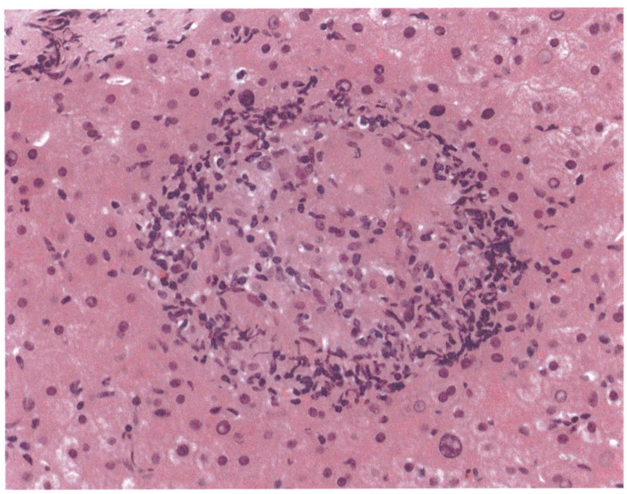

Fig. 8.10 Drug-induced hepatic granuloma. An epithelioid granuloma with a few scattered eosinophils is noted within the hepatic parenchyma. Differential diagnoses are other causes of hepatic granuloma, which may be grouped into infectious (e.g., mycobacterial infection, tertiary syphilis, parasitic infestation, fungal infection, and, rarely, viral infection) and noninfectious (e.g., primary biliary cirrhosis, drug-induced liver injury, foreign-body reaction, sarcoidosis, Hodgkin lymphoma, and chronic granulomatous disease).

Table 8.3 Drugs and toxins associated with granulomatous hepatitis or hepatic granuloma

Acetylsalicylic acid	Detajmium tartrate	Mestranol	Phenazone	Sulphadiazine
Acitretin	Diazepam	Methimazole	Phenprocoumon	Sulphadimethoxine
Allopurinol	Dicloxacillin	Methotrexate	Phenylbutazone	Sulphasalazine
Amiodarone	Didanosine	Methyldopa	Phenytoin	Sulphonylurea
Amoxicillin-clavulanate	Diltiazem	Metolazone	Prajmalium	Tacrine
Aprindine	Disopyramide	Nitrofurantoin	Probenecid	Tetrabamate
Azapropazone	Etanercept	Nomifensine	Procainamide	Thorotrast
Bacille Calmette-Guérin	Feprazone	Norethisterone	Procarbazine	Ticarcillin-clavulanate
Carbamazepine	Glyburide (glibenclamide)	Norethynodrel	Pronestyl	Tocainide
Carbutamide	Gold	Norfloxacin	Pyrazinamide	Tolbutamide
Cefalexin	Halothane	Norgestrel	Pyrimethamine- chloroquine	Trichlormethiazide
Chlorpromazine	Hydralazine	Oral contraceptives	Quinidine	Trimethoprim-sulphamethoxazole
Chlorpropamide	Imipramine	Oxacillin	Quinine	Troglitazone
Clavulanic acid	Interferon-α	Oxyphenbutazone	Ranitidine	Verapamil
Clometacin	Isoniazid	Oxyphenisatin	Rosiglitazone	
Cyclofenil	Mebendazole	Papaverine	Succinylsulphathiazole	
Dapsone	Mesalamine	Penicillin		

Adapted from Lewis JH, Kleiner DE. Hepatic injury due to drugs, herbal compounds, chemicals and toxins. In: Burt AD, Portmann BC, Ferrell LD, editors. MacSween's Pathology of the liver. 6th ed. London: Churchill-Livingstone; 2012 with permission.

8.2 Cholestatic Injury

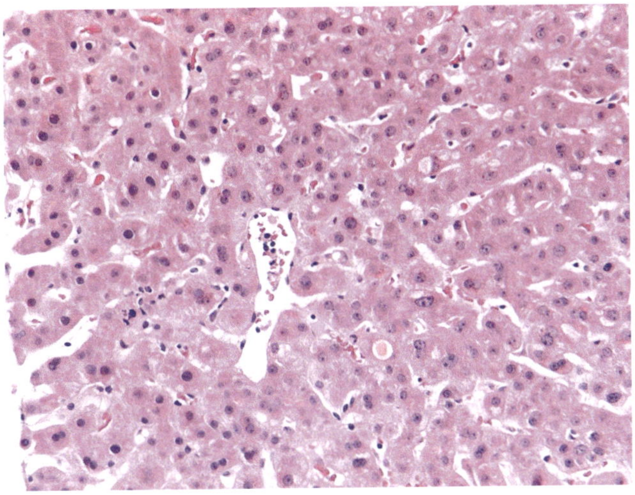

Fig. 8.11 Bland cholestasis induced by anabolic steroid use. Mild canalicular bilirubinostasis is present without any significant necroinflammatory activity, or portal features of large bile duct obstruction, underlying chronic cholangiopathy or ductopenia. Drug/toxin-induced bland cholestasis typically is insidious in onset, with a latency period of 4 to 24 weeks. Patients usually present with jaundice and pruritus. Hyperbilirubinaemia with normal or mildly elevated serum aminotransferase (<5× upper normal limit) and alkaline phosphatase (<2× upper normal limit) is the usual biochemical profile. Recovery is slow after withdrawal of the agent, and jaundice may persist for months.

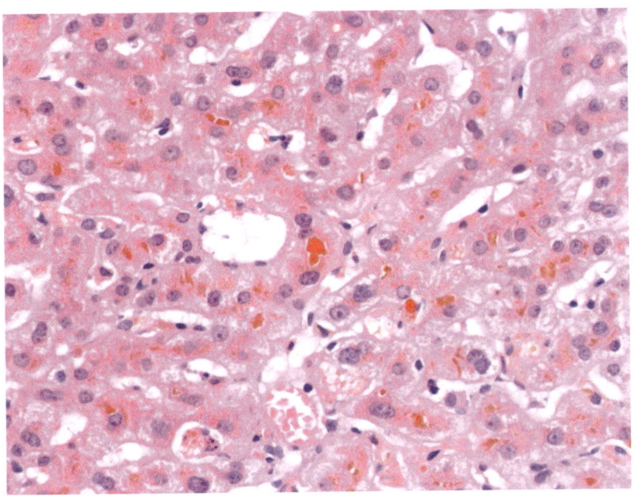

Fig. 8.12 Bland cholestasis. Marked hepatocellular and canalicular bilirubinostasis is present in the absence of significant inflammatory activity. Other causes of this pattern of bland cholestasis are sepsis, shock, early large duct obstruction, paraneoplastic syndrome, benign recurrent intrahepatic cholestasis, and cholestasis of pregnancy.

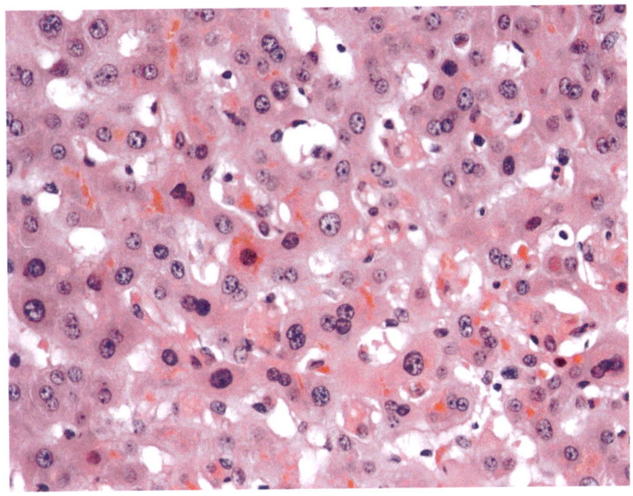

Fig. 8.13 Bland cholestasis induced by herbal medication. Marked hepatocellular and canalicular bilirubinostasis is present with minimal necroinflammatory activity. Some Kupffer cells also contain bilirubin pigment. There may be some overlapping clinical and biochemical features between drug/toxin-induced bland cholestasis and drug/toxin-induced acute cholestatic hepatitis. The latter is characterised by higher levels of serum alkaline phosphatase and the presence of necroinflammatory activity on histology.

Table 8.4 Drugs and toxins associated with bland cholestasis

Allopurinol	Chlorpropamide	Fluoxymesterone	Methyldopa	Phenytoin
Amsacrine	Chlortetracycline	Gatifloxacin	Methyltestosterone	Pioglitazone
Anastrozole	Cimetidine	Glyburide (glibenclamide)	Methylthiouracil	Piroxicam
Anabolic steroids	Cinnarizine	Gold	Nimesulide	Pravastatin
Aprindine	Ciprofloxacin	Haloperidol	Nitrofurantoin	Prochlorperazine
Azapropazone	Citalopram	Idoxuridine	Norethindrone (norethisterone)	Ritonavir
Azithromycin	Cloxacillin	Infliximab	Norethynodrel	Rosiglitazone
Benoxaprofen	Cyanamide	Interleukin-2	Norgestrel	Stavudine
Captopril	Cyclosporin	Interleukin-6	Oral contraceptives	Sulphadiazine
Carbamazepine	Danazol	Iprindole	Oxymetholone	Sulphamethoxazole
Celecoxib	Diazepam	Medroxyprogesterone	Paroxetine	Tamoxifen
Chloramphenicol	Disopyramide	Mercaptopurine	Penicillamine	Terfenadine
Chlordiazepoxide	Erythromycin	Mestranol	Perphenazine	Thioridazine
Chloropurine	Ethambutol	Metformin	Phenobarbital	Tolbutamide
Chlorozotocin	Ethchlorvynol	Methandrostenolone	Phenylbutazone	Trazodone
Chlorpromazine	Flucloxacillin	Methimazole		Warfarin

Adapted from Lewis JH, Kleiner DE. Hepatic injury due to drugs, herbal compounds, chemicals and toxins. In: Burt AD, Portmann BC, Ferrell LD, editors. MacSween's Pathology of the liver. 6th ed. London: Churchill-Livingstone; 2012 with permission.

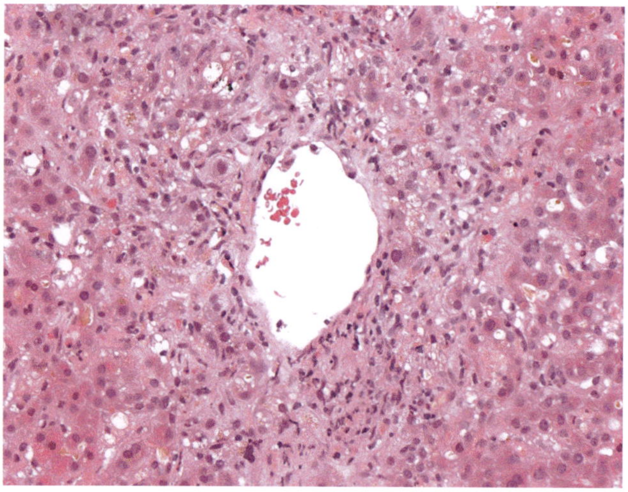

Fig. 8.14 Acute drug-induced cholestatic hepatitis. Perivenular necrosis is accompanied by marked hepatocellular and canalicular bilirubinostasis. Drug/toxin-induced acute cholestatic hepatitis accounts for one third of all drug/toxin-induced liver injuries. It typically has an insidious onset, with a latency period between 2 and 12 weeks. Patients usually present with nausea and malaise, followed by jaundice and pruritus. Fever, skin rash, and hypereosinophilia may be found. Recovery is slower than with drug/toxin-induced acute hepatitis. Serum liver enzymes may drop by 50% within 1 to 3 months. Some drug/toxin-induced cholestatic hepatitis may evolve into chronic cholestatic injury with varying degrees of bile duct injury, ductopaenia, and fibrosis.

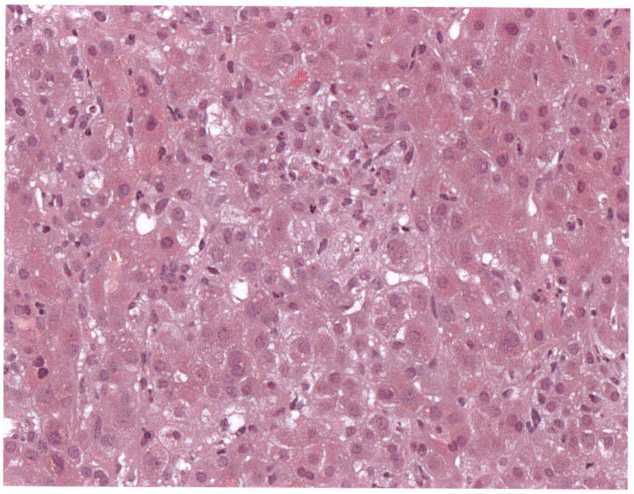

Fig. 8.15 Acute cholestatic hepatitis. Hepatocellular and canalicular bilirubinostasis is associated with focal necrosis and scattered eosinophils. Differential histologic diagnoses include extrahepatic or intrahepatic biliary obstruction, primary biliary cirrhosis, autoimmune cholangitis, primary sclerosing cholangitis, and progressive familial intrahepatic cholestasis. There may be some overlapping clinical, biochemical, and histologic features between drug/toxin-induced acute cholestatic hepatitis and drug/toxin-induced acute hepatitis. The latter is characterised by quicker recovery, a high ratio of serum aminotransferase to serum alkaline phosphatase, and minimal bilirubinostasis on histology.

Table 8.5 Drugs and toxins associated with acute cholestatic hepatitis

Acetohexamide	Clarithromycin	Haloperidol	Oral contraceptives	Rofecoxib
Allopurinol	Clavulanic acid	Halothane	Oestrogens, synthetic	Sulindac
Aminoglutethimide	Clometacin	Hycanthone	Oxacillin	Sulphadiazine
Amitriptyline	Clopidogrel	Hydralazine	Oxaprozin	Sulphamethoxazole
Amoxicillin-clavulanate	Clorazepate	Hydrochlorothiazide	Oxyphenisatin	Sulphasalazine
Ampicillin-sulbactam	Clozapine	Ibuprofen	Papaverine	Tamoxifen
Aprindine	Cyclosporin	Imatinib mesylate	Para-aminosalicylic acid	Telithromycin
Atenolol	Cyproterone	Imipramine	Penicillamine	Terbinafine
Atomoxetine	Dacarbazine	Indomethacin	Penicillin	Thiabendazole
Atorvastatin	Dantrolene	Iodipamide meglumine	Perphenazine	Thiopental sodium
Azathioprine	Dapsone	Iproclozide	Phenelzine	Thioridazine
Bromfenac	Dextropropoxyphene	Iproniazid	Phenindione	Ticarcillin-clavulanate
Bupropion	Diazepam	Irbesartan	Phenobarbital	Ticlopidine
Busulfan	Diclofenac	Isocarboxazid	Phenylbutazone	Tocainide
Captopril	Disopyramide	Isoniazid	Phenytoin	Tolazamide
Carbamazepine	Doxidan	Ketoconazole	Pioglitazone	Tolbutamide
Carbarsone	Duloxetine	Labetalol	Piroxicam	Total parenteral nutrition
Carbimazole	Enalapril	Loratadine	Pizotifen	Tranylcypromine
Cefadroxil	Erythromycin	Lovastatin	Polythiazide	Triazolam
Cefazolin	Ethchlorvynol	Meglumine antimoniate	Prajmalium	Trifluoperazine
Celecoxib	Ethionamide	Meprobamate	Procainamide	Trimethobenzamide
Chlorambucil	Floxuridine	Mercaptopurine	Prochlorperazine	Trimethoprim
Chloramphenicol	Flucloxacillin	Mesalamine (mesalazine)	Propafenone	Trimethoprim-sulphamethoxazole
Chlordiazepoxide	Fluoxymesterone	Metformin	Pyrazinamide	Tripelennamine
Chlorothiazide	Fluphenazine	Methyldopa	Quetiapine	Troglitazone
Chlorpromazine	Flurazepam	Naproxen	Quinethazone	Troleandomycin
Chlorpropamide	Flutamide	Nevirapine	Quinidine	Valproic acid
Chlorthalidone	Gatifloxacin	Nicotinic acid	Ramipril	Verapamil
Chlortetracycline	Gemcitabine	Nifedipine	Ranitidine	Zimelidine
Chlorzoxazone	Glyburide (glibenclamide)	Nimesulide	Repaglinide	
Cimetidine	Gold	Nitrofurantoin	Rifampin	
Cisplatin	Griseofulvin	Nomifensine	Risperidone	

Adapted from Lewis JH, Kleiner DE. Hepatic injury due to drugs, herbal compounds, chemicals and toxins. In: Burt AD, Portmann BC, Ferrell LD, editors. MacSween's Pathology of the liver. 6th ed. London: Churchill-Livingstone; 2012 with permission.

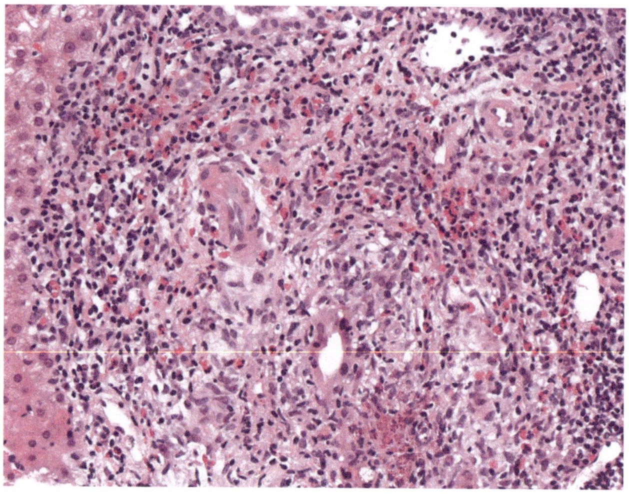

Fig. 8.16 Chronic cholestatic injury induced by trifluoperazine. A portal tract appears markedly expanded by an eosinophil-rich inflammatory infiltrate. An interlobular bile duct shows epithelial disarray and an intraepithelial inflammatory infiltrate. Poorly formed granulomas are seen. Drug/toxin-induced chronic cholestatic injury is characterised by various degrees of bile duct injury, ductopaenia, and fibrosis, mimicking primary biliary cirrhosis or primary sclerosing cholangitis. Some drug/toxin-induced chronic cholestatic injuries evolve from drug/toxin-induced acute cholestatic hepatitis. Patients present with prolonged jaundice and mildly elevated serum alkaline phosphatase levels for months to years after symptomatic recovery of drug/toxin-induced acute cholestatic hepatitis.

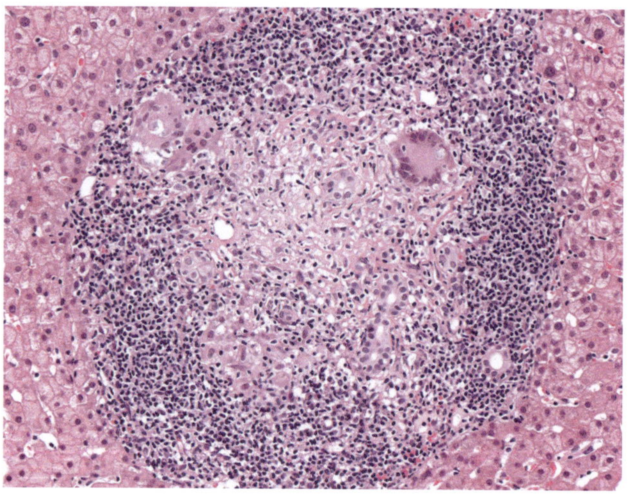

Fig. 8.17 Chronic cholestatic injury induced by trifluoperazine. A portal tract is markedly expanded by a lymphohistiocytic and granulomatous infiltrate. Multinucleated giant cells are present. Differential histologic diagnoses include primary biliary cirrhosis, autoimmune cholangitis, primary sclerosing cholangitis, chronic hepatitis C, HIV-associated cholangiopathy, Langerhans cell histiocytes, Hodgkin lymphoma, and progressive familial intrahepatic cholestasis.

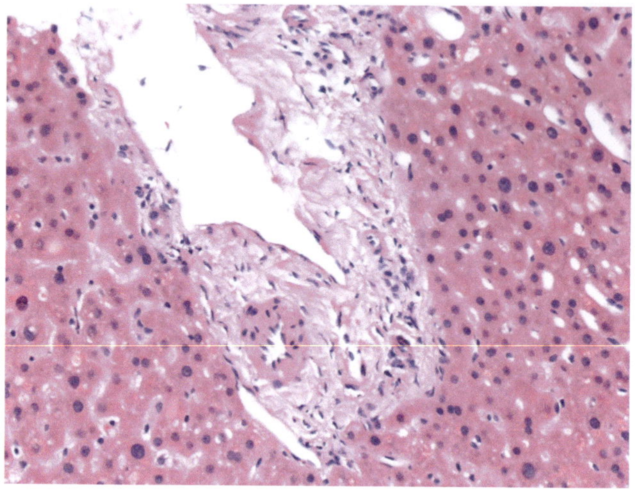

Fig. 8.18 Chronic cholestatic injury. This portal tract is devoid of an interlobular bile duct (ductopaenia). Other possible aetiologies of ductopaenia in an adult are primary biliary cirrhosis, primary sclerosing cholangitis, acquired sclerosing cholangitis, sarcoidosis, chronic rejection in liver allograft, chronic graft-versus-host disease, and idiopathic adult ductopaenia. The lack of a ductular reaction and deposits of copper-binding protein favour ductopaenia as part of a vanishing bile duct syndrome over conditions such as sclerosing cholangitis, sarcoidosis, and primary biliary cirrhosis.

Table 8.6 Drugs and toxins associated with chronic cholestatic injury

Ajmaline	Diazepam	Piroxicam
Amineptine	Dicloxacillin	Practolol
Amitriptyline	Enalapril	Prochlorperazine
Amoxicillin-clavulanate	Erythromycin	Ramipril
Ampicillin	Ezetimibe	Scolicides
Azathioprine	Floxuridine	Sulphonylurea
Candesartan	Flucloxacillin	Sulpiride
Carbamazepine	Gatifloxacin	Terbinafine
Carbutamide	Gold	Tetracycline
Chlorothiazide	Haloperidol	Thiabendazole
Chlorpromazine	Ibuprofen	Tiopronin
Chlorpropamide	Imipramine	Tolazamide
Cimetidine	Itraconazole	Tolbutamide
Cromolyn	Methyltestosterone	Total parenteral nutrition
Cyamemazine	Norandrostenolone	Trifluoperazine
Cyproheptadine	Phenylbutazone	Troleandomycin
Detajmium tartrate	Phenytoin	Xenalamine

Adapted from Lewis JH, Kleiner DE. Hepatic injury due to drugs, herbal compounds, chemicals and toxins. In: Burt AD, Portmann BC, Ferrell LD, editors. MacSween's Pathology of the liver. 6th ed. London: Churchill-Livingstone; 2012 with permission.

8.3 Steatosis and Steatohepatitis

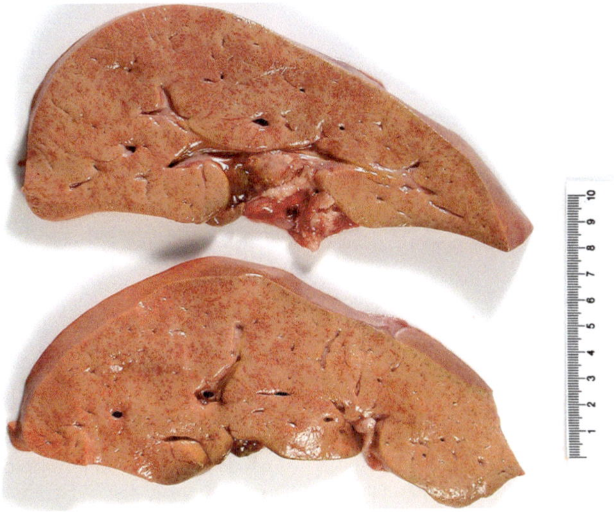

Fig. 8.19 Macrovesicular steatosis induced by prolonged corticosteroid treatment. This postmortem liver has a diffuse, yellowish, greasy appearance. Drug/toxin-induced steatosis usually is insidious. Patients either are asymptomatic or have mild, nonspecific symptoms. Mild elevated serum aminotransferase with normal serum bilirubin and alkaline phosphatase is the usual biochemical profile.

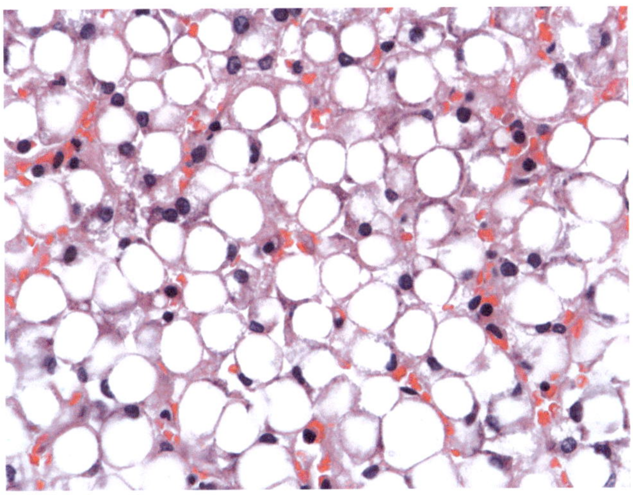

Fig. 8.20 Macrovesicular steatosis induced by corticosteroids. A diagnosis of drug-induced steatosis requires exclusion of other common causes. Correlation with alcoholic consumption and the presence of components of the metabolic syndrome (obesity, hypertension, hyperlipidaemia, impaired glucose tolerance, and diabetes mellitus) are essential to establish the proper diagnosis. However, coexisting nonalcoholic steatosis may, in fact, potentiate the prosteatotic effects of certain drugs.

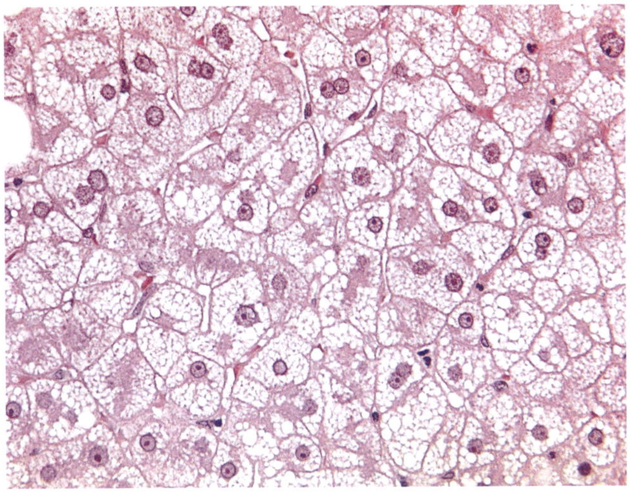

Fig. 8.21 Microvesicular steatosis induced by ethanol (acute alcoholic foamy degeneration). These hepatocytes contain multiple small fat droplets, which do not displace the nucleus. Drug/toxin-induced microvesicular steatosis has a variable onset depending on the agent. Latency is 1 to 4 weeks after exposure to agents directly inhibiting mitochondrial function or protein synthesis (e.g., acetylsalicylic acid) and 2 to 3 months after continuous use of agents inhibiting mitochondrial DNA synthesis (e.g., didanosine). Prodromal symptoms, including nausea, malaise, and abdominal discomfort, last for 1 to 4 weeks and are followed by rapid deteriorating and life-threatening liver failure, hepatic encephalopathy, lactic acidosis, and coagulopathy. Despite hypoalbuminaemia, prolonged prothrombin time, hyperammonaemia, and lactic acidosis, serum aminotransferase typically is elevated only minimally.

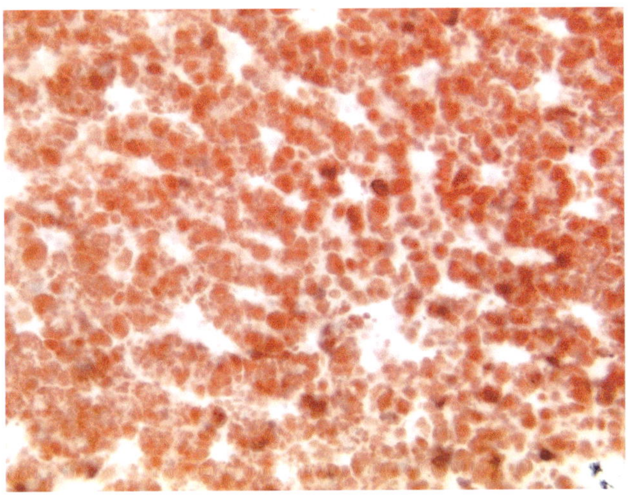

Fig. 8.22 Microvesicular steatosis induced by acetylsalicylic acid (Reye syndrome). Extensive steatosis is highlighted by oil red O staining, whereas no visible fat droplet was identified in the haematoxylin and eosin sections. Diffuse microvesicular steatosis is uncommon and associated with serious mitochondriopathies with fatty acid oxidation defects. Acute alcoholic foamy degeneration, and other drug/toxin-induced microvesicular steatosis, other causes of diffuse microvesicular steatosis are acute fatty liver of pregnancy, toxaemia of pregnancy, and various primary mitochondrial hepatopathies. Of note, cases originally attributed to acetylsalicylic acid were shown to be due to underlying metabolic disorders. Before concluding that microvescicular steatosis is drug induced, an underlying metabolic condition (e.g. mitochondriopathy) should always be considered.

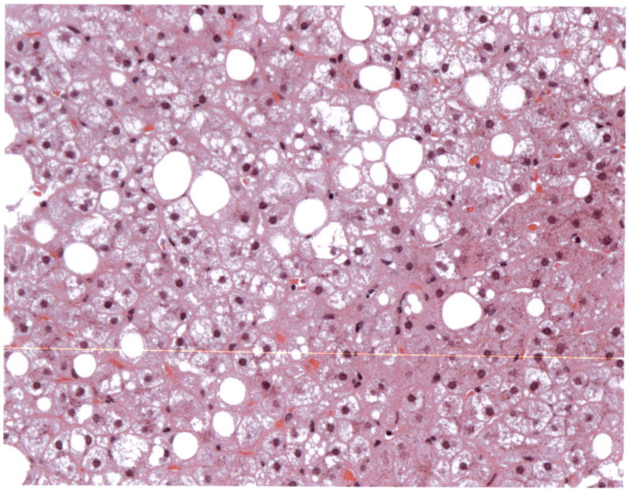

Fig. 8.23 Steatohepatitis induced by methotrexate. A ballooned hepatocyte (*centre*) is accompanied by many hepatocytes with macrovesicular steatosis. Drug/toxin-induced steatohepatitis usually has an insidious onset, with latency of 3 to 12 months. Patients either are asymptomatic or have mild, nonspecific symptoms.

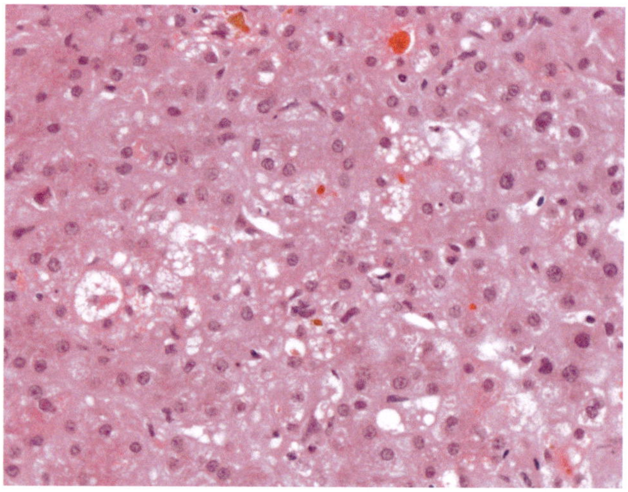

Fig. 8.24 Steatohepatitis induced by amiodarone. A ballooned hepatocyte containing a Mallory-Denk body (*left middle*) is accompanied by some hepatocytes showing macrovesicular and mediovesicular steatosis, as well as ballooning. Canalicular bilirubinostasis also is present.

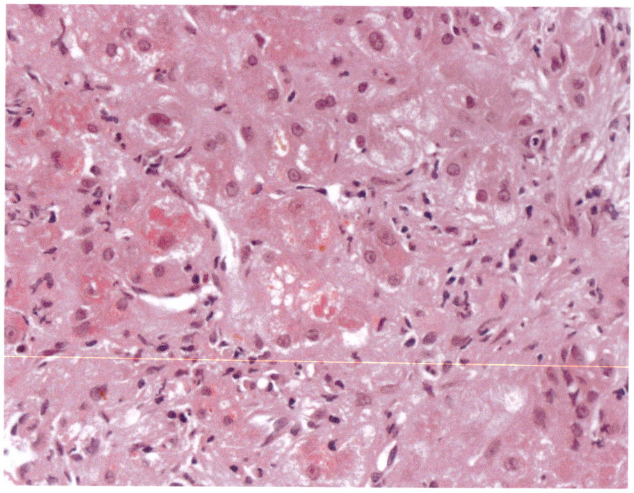

Fig. 8.25 Steatohepatitis induced by amiodarone. Two Mallory-Denk bodies (*middle* and *left middle*) are present. Ballooned hepatocytes and canalicular bilirubinostasis also are noted. Mallory-Denk bodies typically are associated with alcoholic, nonalcoholic, and drug-induced steatohepatitis, but also may be seen in chronic cholestatic disease, Wilson disease and other copper overload disorders, α_1-antitrypsin deficiency, focal nodular hyperplasia, and benign and malignant hepatocellular neoplasm.

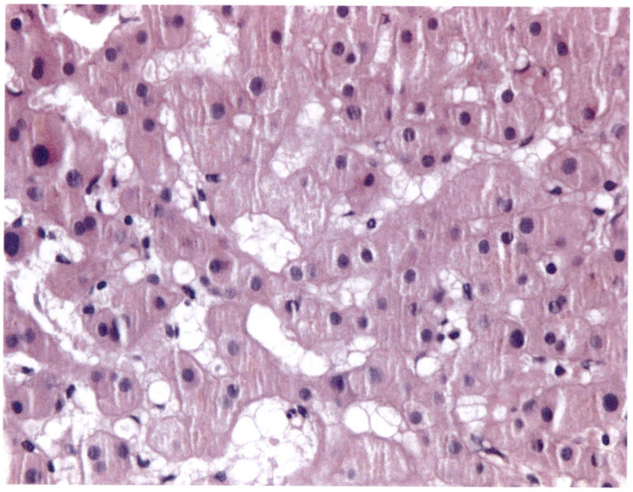

Fig. 8.26 Stellate cell lipidosis and hypertrophy induced by vitamin A. Stellate cells within the sinusoids contain multiple lipid droplets. Stellate cell lipidosis is estimated to occur in 1.1% of nontransplant liver biopsies. Patients usually are asymptomatic, with normal liver function tests or only mildly elevated serum alkaline phosphatase or aminotransferase levels. Many cases are associated with excessive vitamin A intake (e.g., through vitamin supplements, fish oil, or oral or tropical retinoid). However, patients with stellate cell lipidosis and excessive vitamin A intake typically do not show clinical and biochemical features of systemic hypervitaminosis A. Apart from excessive vitamin A intake, other causes associated with stellate cell lipidosis are cholestasis, alcoholic liver disease, primary biliary cirrhosis, chronic pancreatitis, diabetes mellitus, HIV infection, and certain drugs (methotrexate, corticosteroids, and valproic acid).

Table 8.7 Drugs and toxins associated with steatosis and steatohepatitis

MACROVESICULAR STEATOSIS			MICROVESICULAR STEATOSIS	STEATOHEPATITIS
2-Chloropropane	Dinitrobenzene	Mushrooms	Acetylsalicylic acid	Amiodarone
Acetylsalicylic acid	Dinitrotoluene	Naphthalene	Aflatoxins	Corticosteroids
Amanitin	Ethanol	Naproxen	Amineptine	Irinotecan
Amsacrine	Ethionine	Nifedipine	Amiodarone	Methotrexate
Antimony	Ethyl bromide	Nitrofurantoin	Camphor	Naproxen
Arsenic compounds	Ethyl chloride	Oestrogens, synthetic	Chlortetracycline	Oestrogens, synthetic
Asparaginase	Ethylene dibromide	Organic solvents	Demeclocycline	Perhexiline maleate
Azacytidine	Ethylene dichloride	Orotic acid	Desferoxamine	Raloxifene
Azaserine	Etretinate	Paracetamol	Didanosine	Risperidone
Azauridine	Fialuridine	Perhexiline maleate	Dimethylnitrosamine	Spironolactone
Bacillus cereus toxin	Flurazepam	Phosphorus	Ethanol	Sulphasalazine
Barium salts	Galactosamine	Puromycin	Ethyl chloride	Tamoxifen
Borates	Gold	Rifampin	Fialuridine	Vitamin A
Bromobenzene	Halogenated hydrocarbons	Risperidone	Hypoglycin A	
Cadmium	Hydralazine	Ritonavir	Ibuprofen	
Calcium hopantenate	Hydrazine	Safrole	Ketoprofen	
Carbon disulphide	Hydrazines	Spironolactone	Methyl salicylate	
Carbon tetrachloride	Ibuprofen	Stavudine	Mushrooms	
Chlorinated diphenyls	Indinavir	Streptozotocin	Oxytetracycline	
Chlorinated naphthalene	Indomethacin	Sulphasalazine	Phalloidin	
Chloroform	Interleukin-2	Sulindac	Phosphorus	
Chloroprene	Iodoform	Synthaline	Piroxicam	
Chromates	Irinotecan	Tamoxifen	Pirprofen	
Cisplatin	Isoniazid	Tetrachloroethane	Riluzole	
Clometacin	Luteoskyrin	Tetrachloroethylene	Rolitetracycline	
Cocaine	Mefloquine	Thiotepa	Stavudine	
Corticosteroids	Mercury	Total parenteral nutrition	Tetracycline	
Cortisone	Methimazole	Trichloroethylene	Tolmetin	
Cyanamide	Methotrexate	Trinitrotoluene	Warfarin	
Dantrolene	Methyl bromide	Uranium compounds		
DDT	Methyl chloride	Valproic acid		
Dichloroethylene	Methyl chlorobromide	Warfarin		
Dichloromethotrexate	Methyl dichloride	Zidovudine		
Dichloropropane	Methylchloroform			
Dimethylformamide	Methyldopa			
Dimethylhydrazine	Minocycline			
Dimethylnitrosamine	Mitomycin C			

Adapted from Lewis JH, Kleiner DE. Hepatic injury due to drugs, herbal compounds, chemicals and toxins. In: Burt AD, Portmann BC, Ferrell LD, editors. MacSween's Pathology of the liver. 6th ed. London: Churchill-Livingstone; 2012 with permission.

8.4 Vascular Lesions

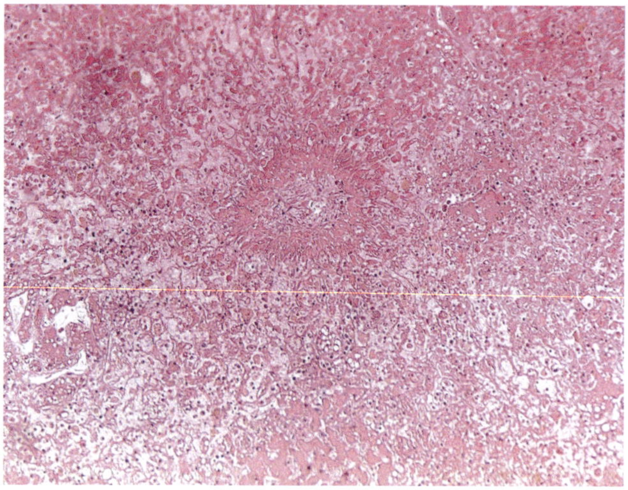

Fig. 8.27 Sinusoidal obstruction syndrome induced by chemotherapeutic agents. Hepatic vein obstruction with subintimal fibrin deposition is associated with extensive haemorrhagic necrosis. Sinusoidal obstruction syndrome, previously known as veno-occlusive disease, presents in acute, subacute, and chronic forms and is strongly associated with the use of chemotherapeutic agents and radiation. The acute form occurs within 1 to 3 weeks of exposure to the agent. Patients usually present with abdominal pain, weight gain, ascites, peripheral oedema, varices, and marked hepatitic liver function derangement. Mortality is up to 20% to 50%. The subacute and chronic forms have an insidious onset with a long latency, from weeks to years. Patients typically present with malaise, ascites, peripheral oedema, varices, hepatic encephalopathy, and mild hepatitic or mixed liver function derangement.

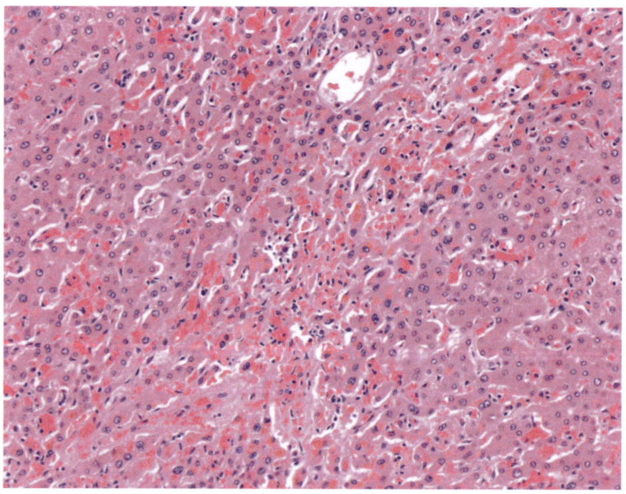

Fig. 8.28 Sinusoidal obstruction syndrome. Sinusoidal congestion and fibrin deposition are accompanied by hepatocyte drop-out and atrophy in the perivenular zone. Acute sinusoidal obstructive syndrome may be mimicked by acute Budd-Chiari syndrome with retrograde extension of thrombi into smaller venules. The differential histologic diagnoses of chronic sinusoidal obstruction essentially are the differential diagnoses of perivenular fibrosis, including alcoholic and nonalcoholic steatohepatitis, congestive heart failure, chronic Budd-Chiari syndrome, and sickle cell disease.

Table 8.8 Drugs and toxins associated with sinusoidal obstruction syndrome and Budd-Chiari syndrome

SINUSOIDAL OBSTRUCTION SYNDROME		BUDD-CHIARI SYNDROME
Actinomycin D (dactinomycin)	Daunorubicin	Cyclophosphamide
Adriamycin (doxorubicin)	Dimethylbusulfan	Dacarbazine
Azathioprine	Floxuridine	Oral contraceptive
Busulfan	Gemtuzumab	Vincristine
Carboplatin	Indicine	
Carmustine	Mercaptopurine	
Chlormethine (mechlorethamine)	Mitomycin C	
Cisplatin	Oxaliplatin	
Contraceptive steroids	Tamoxifen	
Cyclophosphamide	Thioguanine (thioguanine)	
Cysteamine	Urethane (ethyl carbamate)	
Cytarabine	Vinblastine	
Dacarbazine	Vincristine	
Danazol		

Adapted from Lewis JH, Kleiner DE. Hepatic injury due to drugs, herbal compounds, chemicals and toxins. In: Burt AD, Portmann BC, Ferrell LD, editors. MacSween's Pathology of the liver. 6th ed. London: Churchill-Livingstone; 2012 with permission.

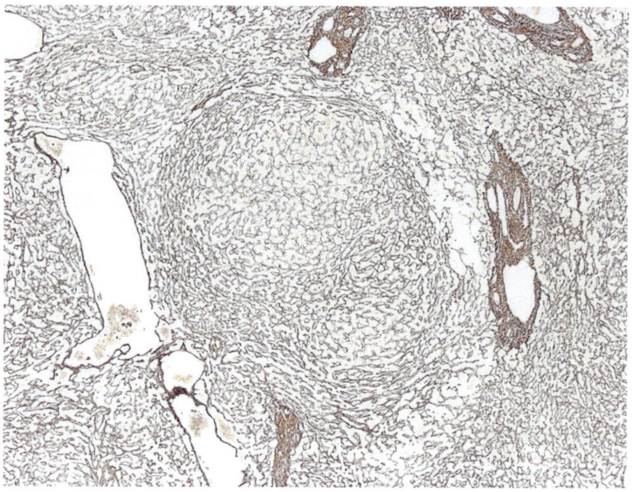

Fig. 8.29 Nodular regenerative hyperplasia. Parenchymal nodular change is present without any fibrosis (Gordon-Sweet reticulin stain). Drug/toxin-induced nodular regenerative hyperplasia usually has an insidious onset with a long latency, from 6 months to 6 years. Patients typically present with malaise, ascites, peripheral oedema, and varices. Normal or mildly elevated (<3× upper normal limit) serum aminotransferase and alkaline phosphatase levels are the typical biochemical profile.

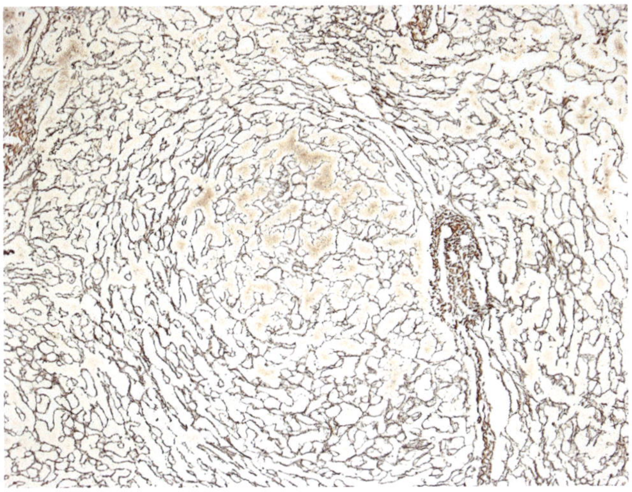

Fig. 8.30 Nodular regenerative hyperplasia. Parenchymal nodular change is present without any accompanying fibrosis (Gordon-Sweet reticulin stain). Other aetiologies of nodular regenerative hyperplasia include autoimmune diseases (e.g., rheumatoid arthritis, systemic lupus erythematosus, antiphospholipid syndrome, and polyarteritis nodosa), inflammatory diseases (e.g., inflammatory bowel disease, celiac disease, and sarcoidosis), haematologic diseases (e.g., myeloproliferative disease, lymphoma, macroglobulinaemia, mixed cryoglobulinaemia, and idiopathic thrombocytopaenic purpura), congenital or acquired immunodeficiency (e.g., chronic HIV infection, chronic granulomatous disease, and common variable immunodeficiency syndromes), extrahepatic neoplasms, primary biliary cirrhosis, cystinosis, and hereditary haemorrhagic telangiectasia. A possible pathogenetic mechanism is obstruction of small portal vein leading to atrophy of the downstream hepatic plates and regenerative hyperplasia of the properly perfused ones.

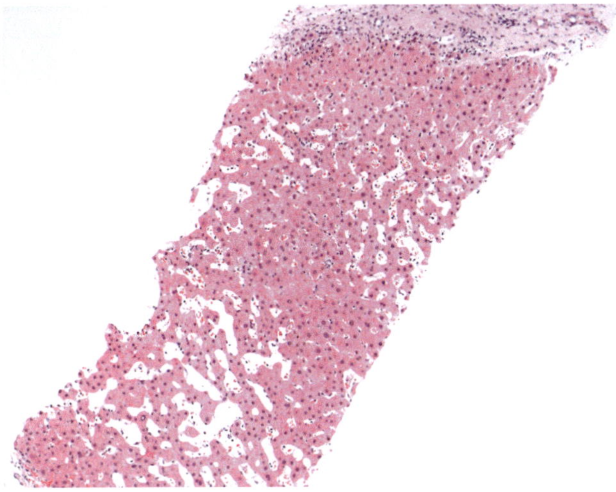

Fig. 8.31 Sinusoidal dilatation induced by azathioprine. There is marked midzonal sinusoidal dilatation. Drug/toxin-induced sinusoidal dilatation may be present in isolation or associated with peliosis and nodular regenerative hyperplasia.

Table 8.9 Drugs and toxins associated with nodular regenerative hyperplasia and hepatoportal sclerosis

NODULAR REGENERATIVE HYPERPLASIA	HEPATOPORTAL SCLEROSIS
Anabolic steroids	Azathioprine
Azathioprine	Arsenic compounds
Copper sulphate	Mercaptopurine
Corticosteroids	Methotrexate
Cytarabine	Oral contraceptives
Daunorubicin	Oxaliplatin
Didanosine	Vinyl chloride
Interleukin-2	
Mercaptopurine	
Oral contraceptives	
Oxaliplatin	
Thioguanine	
Thorotrast	
Toxic oil (rapeseed)	
Vinyl chloride	

Adapted from Lewis JH, Kleiner DE. Hepatic injury due to drugs, herbal compounds, chemicals and toxins. In: Burt AD, Portmann BC, Ferrell LD, editors. MacSween's Pathology of the liver. 6th ed. London: Churchill-Livingstone; 2012 with permission.

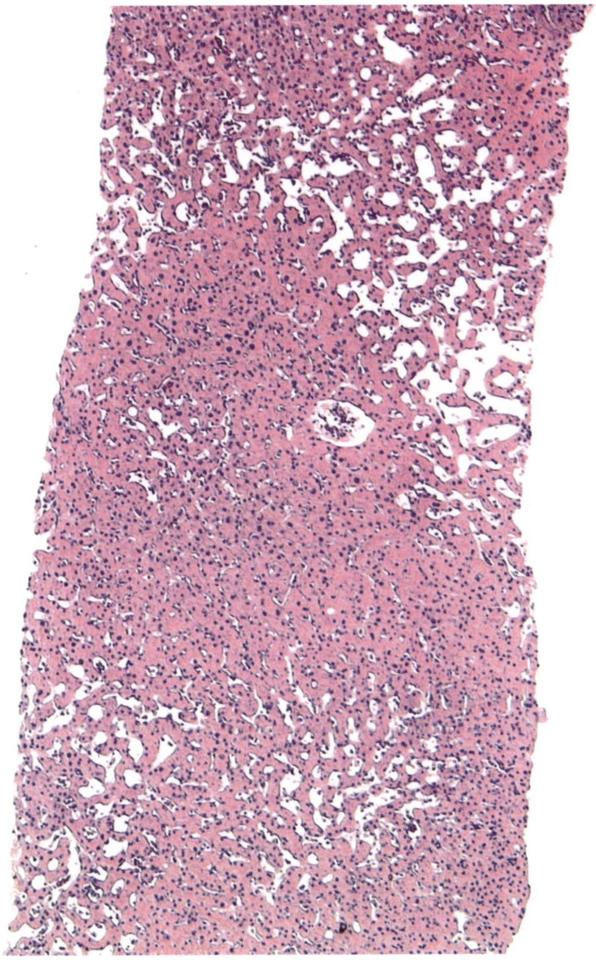

Fig. 8.32 Sinusoidal dilatation induced by oral contraceptive use. There is marked midzonal sinusoidal dilatation.

Table 8.10 Drugs and toxins associated with sinusoidal dilatation and peliosis

SINUSOIDAL DILATATION	PELIOSIS	
Anabolic steroids	Anabolic steroids	Methotrexate
Azathioprine	Azathioprine	Methyltestosterone
Carmustine	Busulfan	Oral contraceptives
Dacarbazine	Corticosteroids	Oestrogens, synthetic
Daunorubicin	Danazol	Oestrone sulphate
Metoclopramide	Diethylstilboestrol	Oxaliplatin
Mitomycin C	Fluoxymesterone	Tamoxifen
Oral contraceptives	Glucocorticoids	Testosterone
Oxaliplatin	Hydroxyprogesterone	Thioguanine
Thioguanine	Hydroxyurea	Thorotrast
Valproic acid	Medroxyprogesterone	Vinyl chloride
Vinblastine	Mercaptopurine	Vitamin A
Vitamin A	Methandrostenolone	

Adapted from Lewis JH, Kleiner DE. Hepatic injury due to drugs, herbal compounds, chemicals and toxins. In: Burt AD, Portmann BC, Ferrell LD, editors. MacSween's Pathology of the liver. 6th ed. London: Churchill-Livingstone; 2012 with permission.

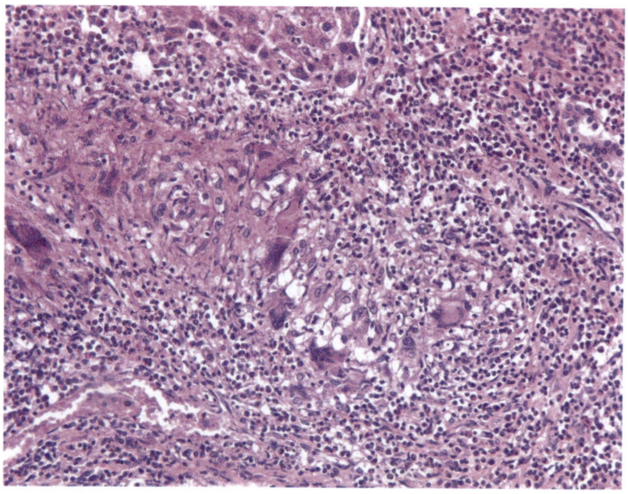

Fig. 8.33 Vasculitis induced by phenytoin. Granulomatous vasculitis is accompanied by a dense lymphoplasmacytic infiltrate in this portal tract. Agents associated with a drug/toxin-induced vasculitis include allopurinol, chlorothiazide, chlorpropamide, penicillin, phenylbutazone, phenytoin, and sulphonamide.

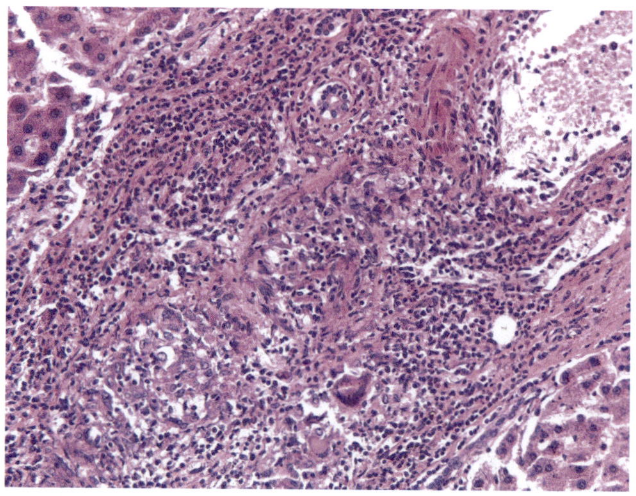

Fig. 8.34 Vasculitis induced by phenytoin. Granulomatous vasculitis is seen here accompanied by a dense lymphoplasmacytic infiltrate in the portal tract. Systemic vasculitis with hepatic involvement is another important differential diagnosis and includes polyarteritis nodosa, Takayasu arteritis, and giant cell arteritis.

8.5 Neoplasm and Tumour-like Lesions

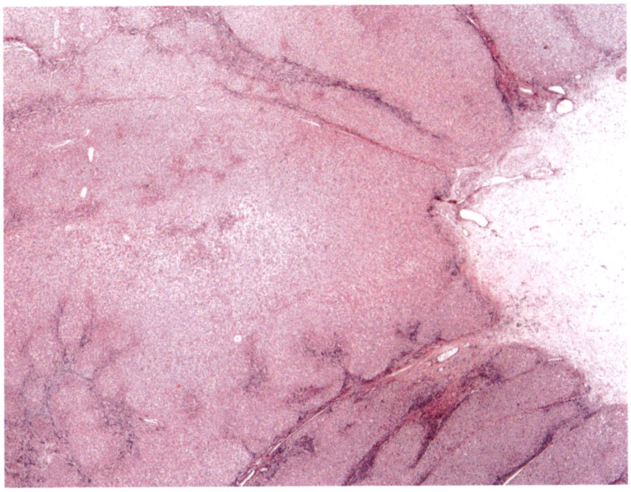

Fig. 8.35 Focal nodular hyperplasia. A central scar (*right*) with radiating fibrous septa separating regenerating hepatocytes is characteristic of focal nodular hyperplasia. Its definitive association with oral contraceptive use and synthetic oestrogens remains to be demonstrated.

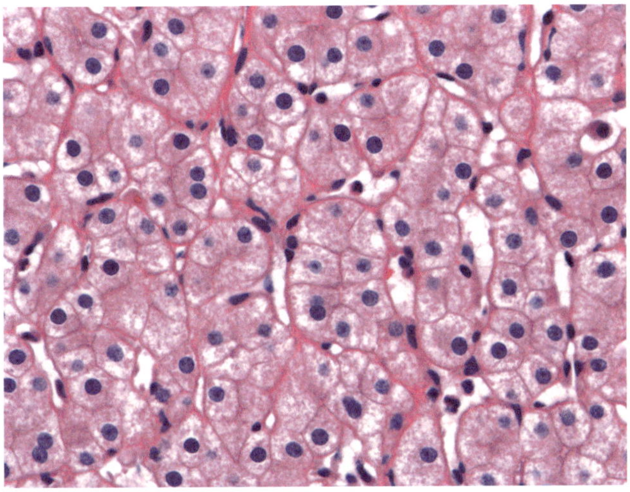

Fig. 8.36 Hepatocellular adenoma. Bland hepatocytes are arranged in trabeculae two cells thick. Hepatocellular adenoma may be associated with anabolic steroids, danazol, methyltestosterone, oral contraceptives, oxymetholone, rapeseed toxic oil, and synthetic oestrogens.

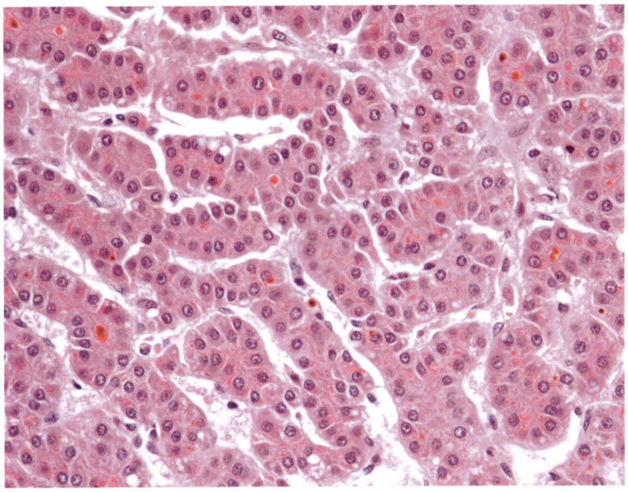

Fig. 8.37 Hepatocellular carcinoma. Neoplastic hepatocytes are arranged in trabeculae two to four cells thick with a marked sinusoidal vasculature. The tumour cells exhibit mild nuclear pleomorphism and hyperchromasia, prominent nucleoli, and bilirubinostasis. Aflatoxin and ethanol are two widely known agents associated with hepatocellular carcinoma. Other agents linked to hepatocellular carcinoma are anabolic steroids, arsenic compounds, methotrexate, methyltestosterone, oral contraceptives, oxymetholone, synthetic oestrogen, and thorotrast.

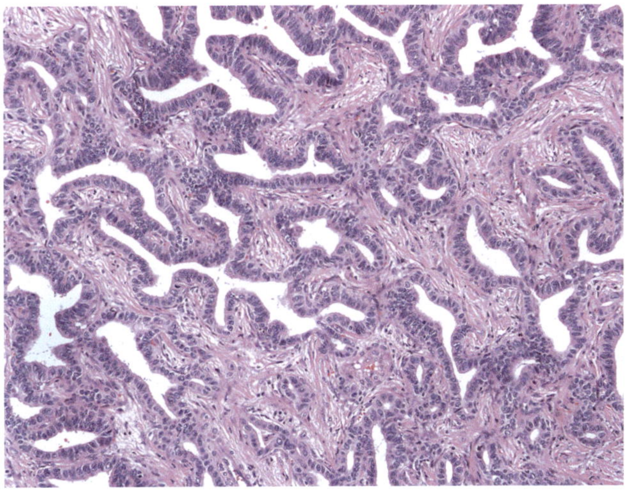

Fig. 8.38 Cholangiocarcinoma. Malignant glands with irregular, angulated contours are embedded in a fibroblastic stroma. Agents related to the development cholangiocarcinoma include anabolic steroids, isoniazid, methyldopa, oral contraceptives, synthetic oestrogen, and thorotrast.

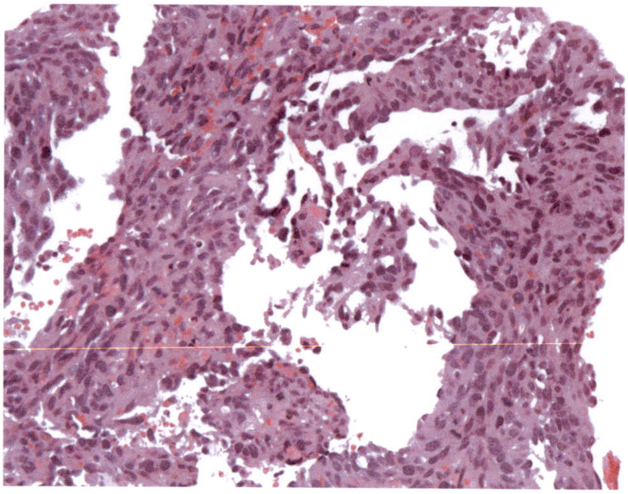

Fig. 8.39 Angiosarcoma. Sheets of malignant spindle cells possess slit-like vascular spaces containing red cells. Angiosarcoma is known to be associated with exposure to vinyl chloride, arsenic, and, historically, thorotrast (colloid thorium oxide used as a radiologic contrast medium in the 1930s to 1950s). Other agents related to angiosarcoma include anabolic steroids, copper sulphate, cyclophosphamide, diethylstilboestrol, oral contraceptives, and phenelzine.

8.6 Adaptive Change

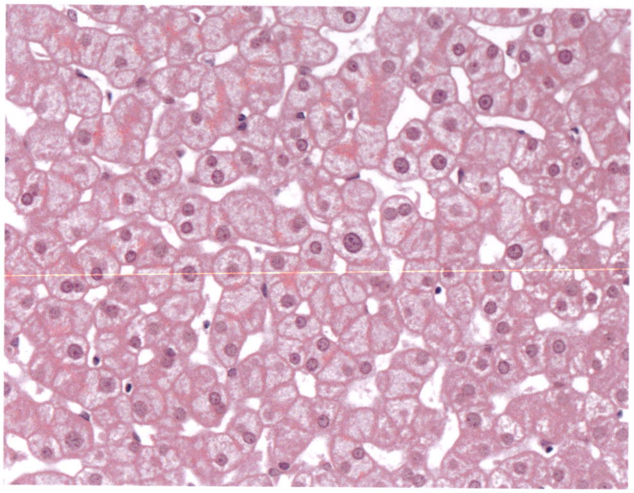

Fig. 8.40 Enzyme induction. Hepatocytes are enlarged and have pale, finely vesiculated cytoplasm. Enzyme induction is associated with long-term use of certain therapeutic agents leading to marked hypertrophy of the smooth endoplasmic reticulum and increased activity of microsomal enzymes. Examples of such agents include phenytoin, phenobarbital, rifampicin, ethanol, and warfarin. Patients usually are asymptomatic, with a mild elevation of serum alkaline phosphatase levels.

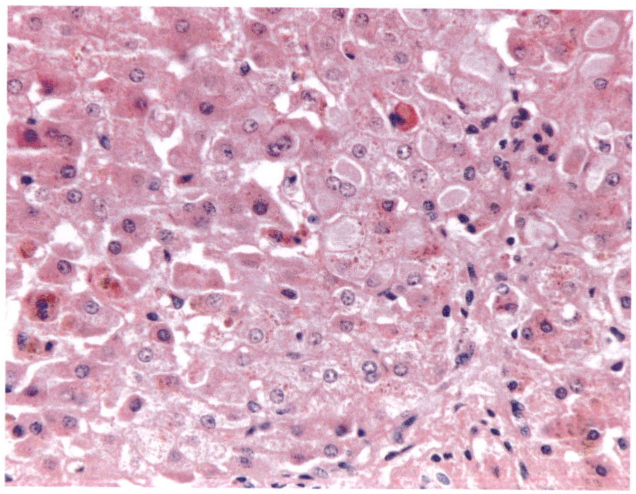

Fig. 8.41 Pseudo–ground-glass inclusion induced by thioguanine. Several hepatocytes contain a large palely eosinophilic, finely granular, and ground-glass–like intracytoplasmic inclusion with an occasional surrounding clear halo. The extreme form of enzyme induction is pseudo–ground-glass inclusion formation. Agents that may lead to this pattern include azathioprine, chlorpromazine, cyanamide, phenytoin, phenobarbital, and thioguanine. Pseudo–ground-glass inclusion also may be found in immunocompromised patients on multiple medications, glycogen storage disease type IV, and Lafora disease. It should be distinguished from genuine ground-glass inclusion associated with viral hepatitis B, which is positive on orcein or Victoria blue histochemical staining and on immunostaining for hepatitis B surface antigen.

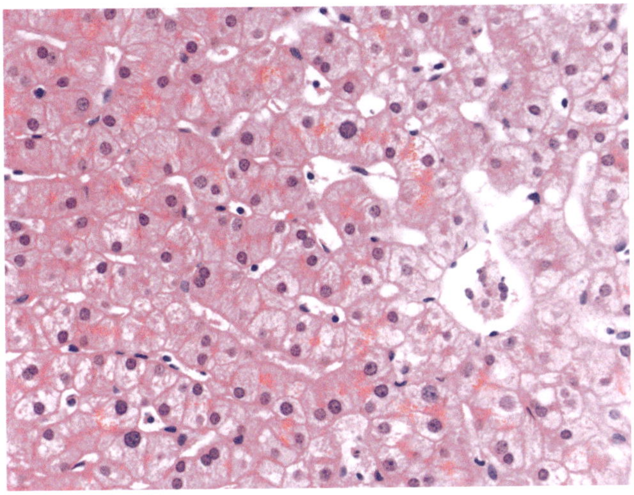

Fig. 8.42 Lipofuscin deposition. There are abundant golden-yellow, finely granular pigments in the pericanalicular cytoplasm of hepatocytes. Several distinct pigments may be deposited after exposure to certain drugs or toxins. Lipofuscin deposition is associated with aminopyrine, cascara sagrada, chlorpromazine, phenacetin, and phenothiazine. Accumulation of haemosiderin is associated with iron, cimetidine, ethanol, and hexachlorobenzene. Other pigments include gold, mercury, polyvinylpyrrolidone, silver, talc, thorotrast, and titanium.

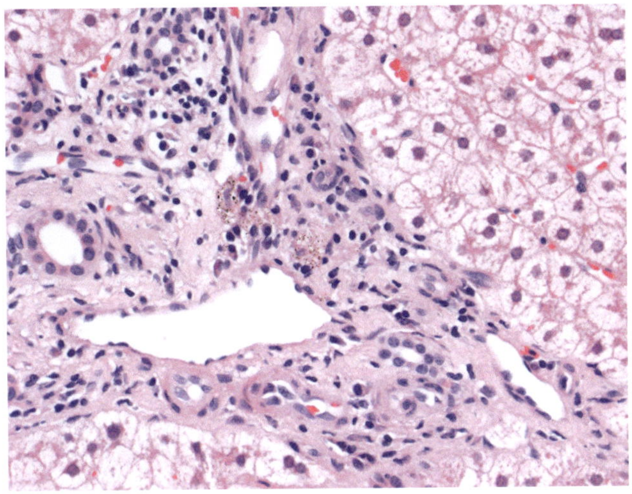

Fig. 8.43 Pigment deposition. Portal macrophages contain refractile brownish pigments in a liver biopsy sample from a patient with intravenous drug addiction.

9 Autoimmune Hepatitis

Autoimmune hepatitis (AIH) is considered the result of a loss of tolerance against one's own liver tissue, probably triggered by external factors in genetically predisposed patients. The diagnosis is based on a combination of clinical, laboratory, and histologic features, as well as the exclusion of other disorders, as illustrated in Fig. 9.16. The histologic manifestations of AIH vary depending on the presentation (e.g., acute hepatitis; asymptomatic, discovered during routine laboratory tests; fulminant hepatitis; chronic liver disease). AIH usually responds to immunosuppressive therapy, and liver biopsy may be used to monitor the response to treatment and decide when to stop treatment.

In some instances, AIH, primary biliary cirrhosis (PBC), and primary sclerosing cholangitis may be difficult to differentiate on clinical and laboratory grounds. The term *overlap syndrome* often is used in these cases. Other nonautoimmune conditions, such viral or drug-induced hepatitis or even steatohepatitis, may overlap serologically with AIH. In all these cases, liver histology may contribute to the final diagnosis.

A.W.H. Chan et al., *Atlas of Liver Pathology*, Atlas of Anatomic Pathology,
DOI 10.1007/978-1-4614-9114-9_9, © Springer Science+Business Media New York 2014

9.1 Autoimmune Hepatitis

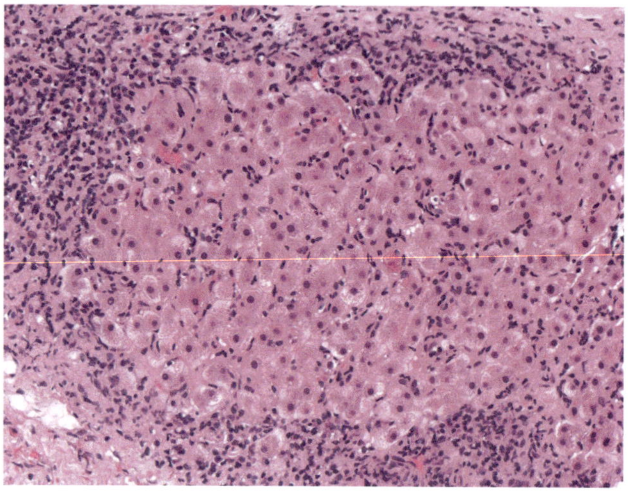

Fig. 9.1 Autoimmune hepatitis. A regenerative nodule in a cirrhotic liver is rimmed by dense septal lymphoplasmacytic infiltrate, with marked interface hepatitis; this is accompanied by prominent lobular necroinflammation. AIH commonly affects women, with a female-to-male ratio of 4:1. The usual age of presentation depends on the particular type of disease: bimodal (10–25 years and 45–70 years) for type 1, less than 15 years for type 2, and 37–43 years for type 3. Clinical manifestations vary widely and include asymptomatic deranged liver function (30%), acute hepatitic presentation (20%), fulminant liver failure, and cirrhosis. About half of patients suffer from concurrent autoimmune disorders, such as thyroiditis, or rheumatoid arthritis. Excellent clinical response to immunosuppression is characteristic in about 90% of patients. Different types of AIH depend on the autoantibody profile.

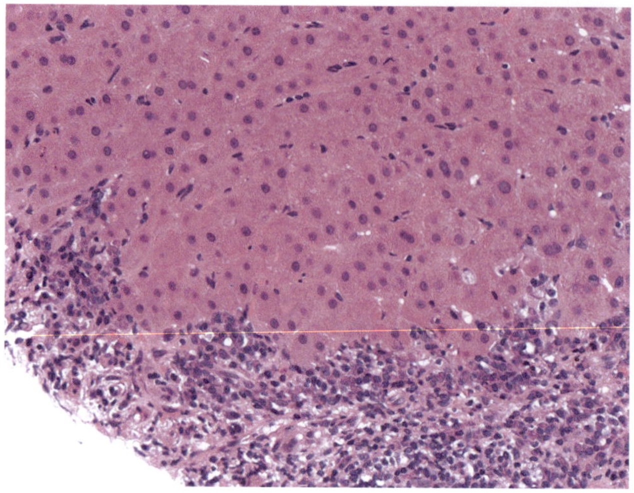

Fig. 9.3 Autoimmune hepatitis. A plasma cell–rich interface hepatitis is evident. Portal plasma cell–rich inflammation is not a consistent feature of AIH and may be absent in up to one third of cases, particularly in patients in remission on immunosuppressive therapy. The presence of a notable portal plasma cell infiltrate and interface hepatitis in patients who have been on immunosuppressive therapy usually is associated with disease relapse after stopping immunosuppressants.

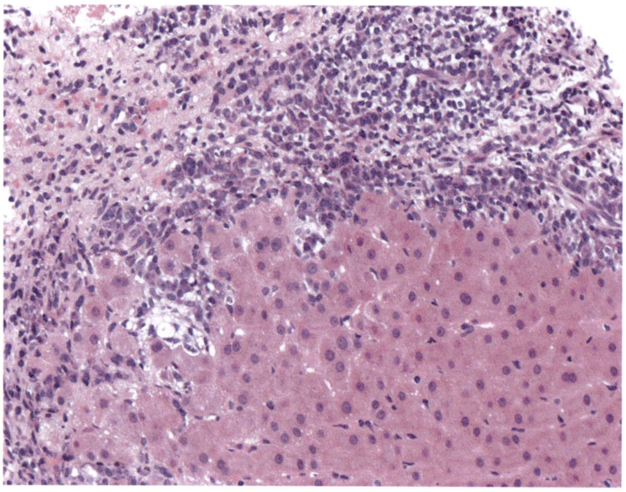

Fig. 9.2 Autoimmune hepatitis. A dense portal lymphoplasmacytic infiltrate and marked interface hepatitis are present. Portal plasma cell–rich inflammation typically is seen in AIH. Interface hepatitis, formerly referred to as piecemeal necrosis, is characterised by portal inflammatory cells eroding through the limiting plate between the portal tract and liver parenchyma, and surrounding individual and small groups of periportal hepatocytes. Significant interface hepatitis is a hallmark feature of AIH. Other characteristic features include emperipolesis and hepatocyte rosette formation.

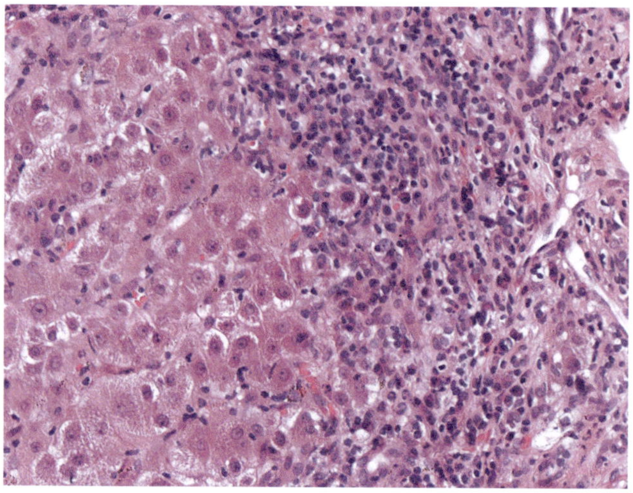

Fig. 9.4 Autoimmune hepatitis. Erosion of the limiting plate by a marked lymphoplasmacytic infiltrate. Although a portal plasma cell–rich inflammation typically is found in AIH, it also is associated with PBC and IgG4-related cholangiopathy. Acute hepatitis A, chronic hepatitis B, drug-induced liver injury, and plasma cell dyscrasia are other, less common causes of portal plasma cell–rich inflammation. Interface hepatitis should be differentiated from the simple spillover of portal inflammatory cells in acute hepatitis by the presence of periportal hepatocellular injury with apoptosis. Interface hepatitis also may be found in chronic viral hepatitis, PBC, Wilson disease, and drug-induced liver injury.

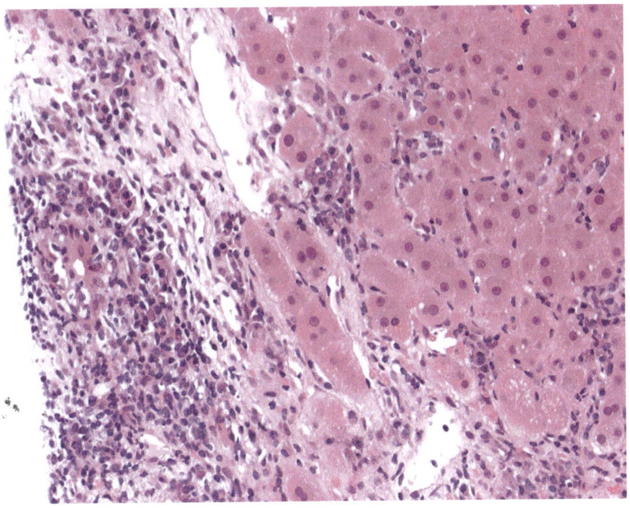

Fig. 9.5 Autoimmune hepatitis. An interlobular bile duct (*left*) shows epithelial disarray and lymphocytic infiltration. Focal bile duct injury does not exclude AIH because it is said to be present in up to 24% of classic AIH. However, chronic biliary disease or overlap syndrome must be considered in the presence of more extensive bile duct injury, florid duct lesion, ductular reaction, ductopaenia, chronic cholate stasis, portal granulomas, and/or periductal fibrosis.

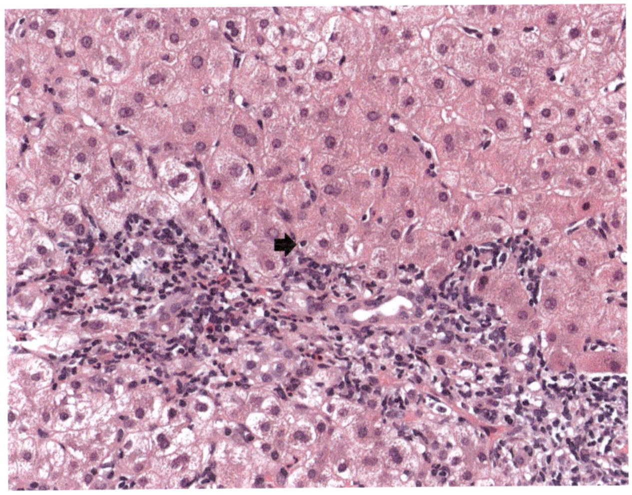

Fig. 9.7 Autoimmune hepatitis. Emperipolesis is characterised by the engulfment of lymphocytes by hepatocytes (*arrow*) in the periportal region, seen here with accompanying moderate interface hepatitis.

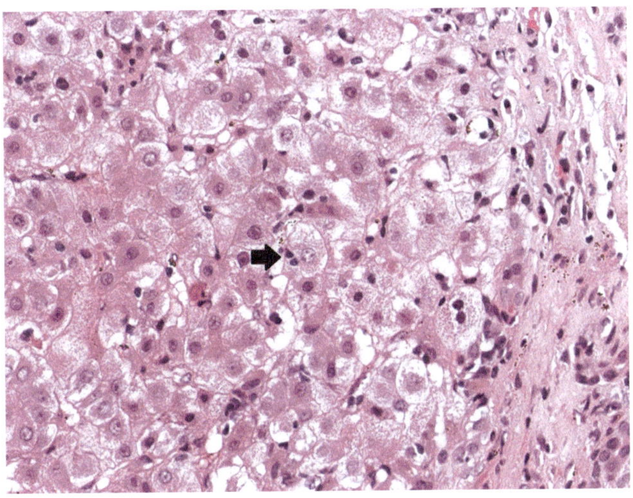

Fig. 9.6 Autoimmune hepatitis. Emperipolesis is featured by apparent engulfment of lymphocytes by hepatocytes (*arrow*) in background of ballooned hepatocytes and an apoptotic hepatocyte. Emperipolesis is regarded as one of the typical histologic features for the diagnosis of AIH; other features are interface hepatitis, portal lymphocytic/lymphoplasmacytic infiltrate, and hepatocyte rosette formation.

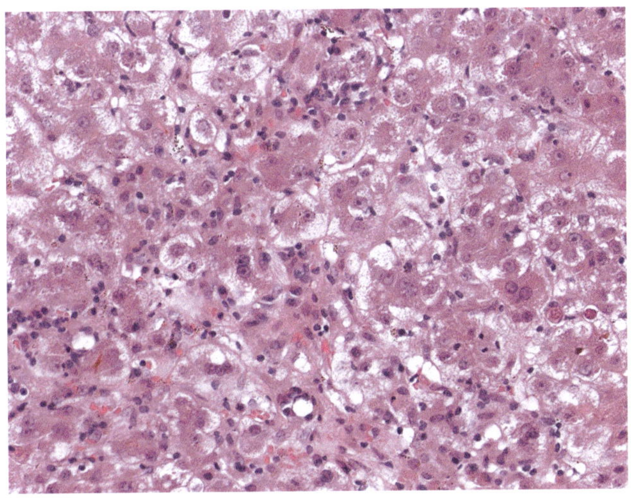

Fig. 9.8 Autoimmune hepatitis. Marked lobular disarray is noted, and this is associated with extensive ballooning degeneration, scattered apoptotic bodies, and a moderate lobular lymphocytic infiltrate. Variable degrees of lobular necroinflammation are observed in AIH and are composed of a combination of lobular lymphoplasmacytic infiltrates, ballooning degeneration, apoptotic bodies, spotty necrosis, confluent necrosis, and bridging necrosis.

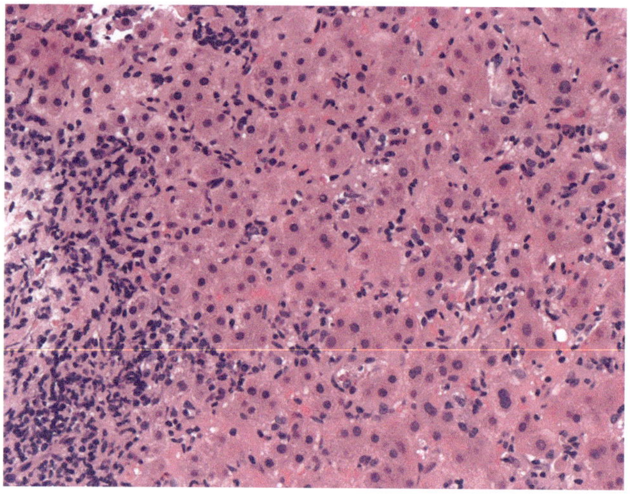

Fig. 9.9 Autoimmune hepatitis. Lobular disarray with a marked lobular lymphocytic infiltrate is seen here, with scattered foci of spotty necrosis and sinusoidal lymphocytosis. Prominent interface hepatitis also is noted. Lobular disarray usually is accompanied by typical portal and periportal changes in AIH. However, it occasionally presents as the predominant histologic pattern, often with a perivenular distribution (so-called central or terminal vein perivenulitis), and should be differentiated from acute viral hepatitis and drug-induced liver injuries by correlation with viral serology and the drug history.

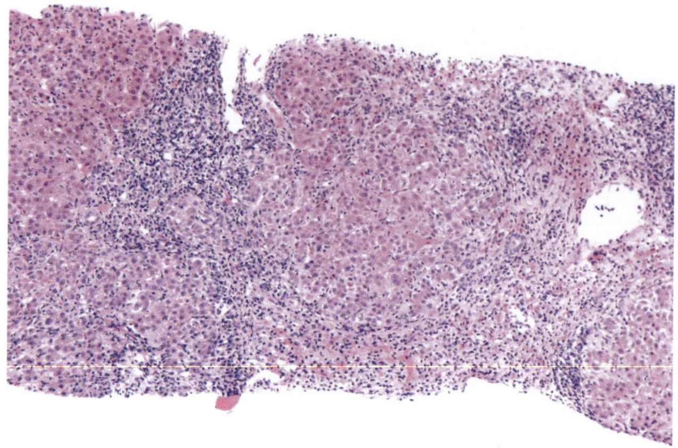

Fig. 9.11 Autoimmune hepatitis. Marked necroinflammatory activity is manifest here by the presence of bridging necrosis. Bridging necrosis signifies very marked damage to the liver parenchyma and may be seen in severe AIH. However, other causes of bridging necrosis, including acute viral hepatitis, drug-induced liver injury, rarely Wilson disease, seroconversion in chronic hepatitis B, superinfection of hepatitis D, and acute flare-up of chronic viral hepatitis, need to be considered in the absence of adequate clinical information.

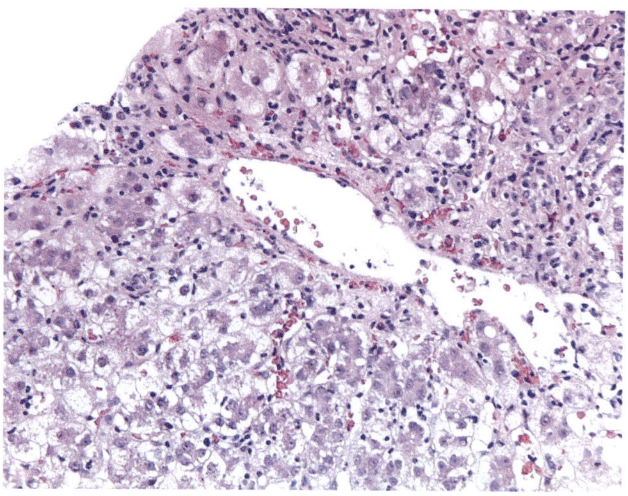

Fig. 9.10 Autoimmune hepatitis. Perivenular confluent necrosis is present in a background of extensive ballooning degeneration. Perivenular confluent necrosis is present in up to 17% of AIH with or without typical portal and periportal changes. Terminal hepatic venulitis sometimes may be found. AIH with perivenular confluent necrosis usually is associated with higher histologic grade, lower histologic stage, and more severe liver function derangement, including fulminant hepatic failure.

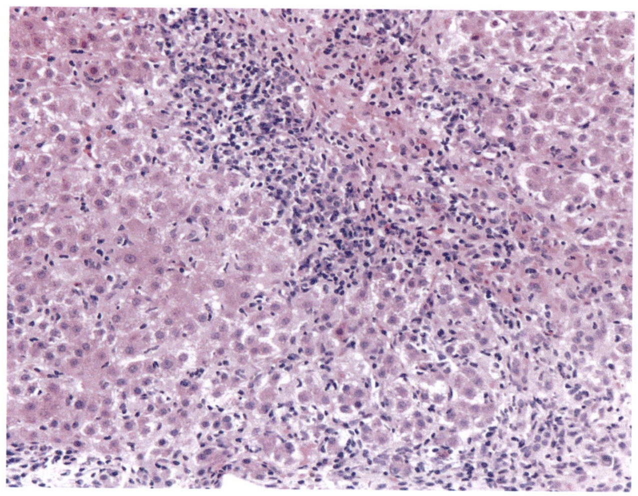

Fig. 9.12 Autoimmune hepatitis. Marked necroinflammatory activity is present with bridging necrosis. Distinction between bridging necrosis and bridging fibrosis may be challenging. Misdiagnosis of bridging necrosis as bridging fibrosis underestimates the activity and overestimates the chronicity. Histologic features in favour of bridging necrosis include the following: (1) the bridging region is more congested and haemorrhagic and contains more ceroid-laden macrophages; (2) the ductular reaction is present within the bridging region rather than at the parenchymal–stromal interface; (3) trichrome stain reveals a characteristic two-tone appearance, with darker staining in the residual portal tract and terminal hepatic venule wall and lighter staining in areas of recent collapse; (4) reticulin stain shows condensation of residual loosely aggregated reticulin fibres; and (5) orcein stain fails to highlight the presence of elastic fibres.

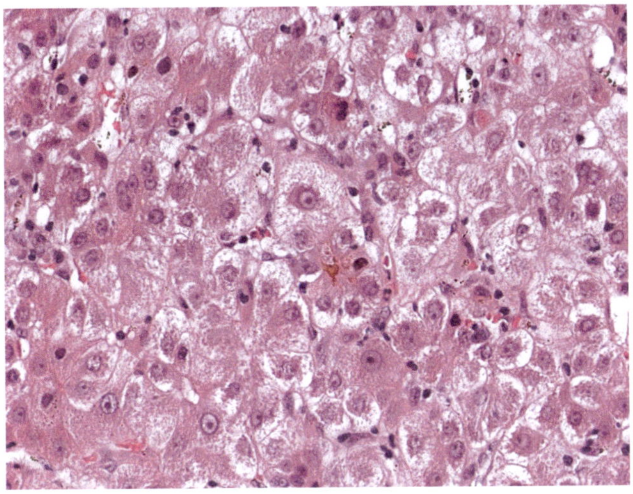

Fig. 9.13 Autoimmune hepatitis. Extensive ballooning degeneration is present with regenerating rosettes and canalicular bilirubinostasis. Hepatocyte rosette formation signifies active regeneration and is regarded as one of the typical histologic features for the diagnosis of AIH, in addition to interface hepatitis, a portal lymphocytic/lymphoplasmacytic infiltrate, and emperipolesis. Mild bilirubinostasis may be found in severe AIH with marked lobular necroinflammatory activity. However, prominent bilirubinostasis with lobular disarray (acute cholestatic hepatitis) is not typical for AIH, and drug-induced liver injury must be excluded with such a histologic pattern.

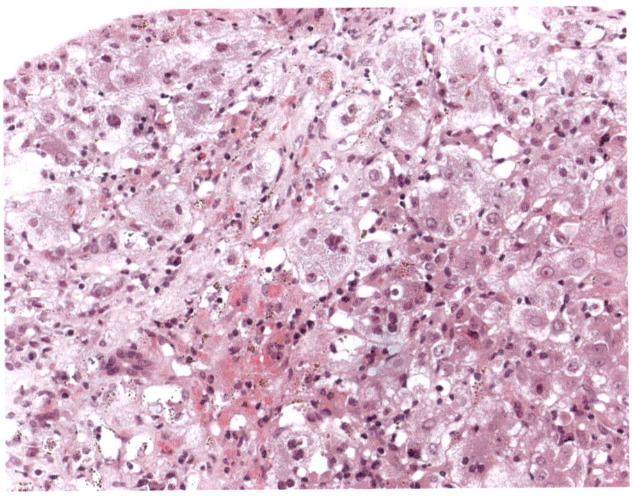

Fig. 9.14 Autoimmune hepatitis. Syncytial multinucleated hepatocyte giant cells are present in a background of marked ballooning degeneration and moderate lobular inflammatory infiltrate. Syncytial multinucleated hepatocytes are typical of neonatal giant cell hepatitis but may be found in autoimmune hepatitis and hepatitis of other aetiologies.

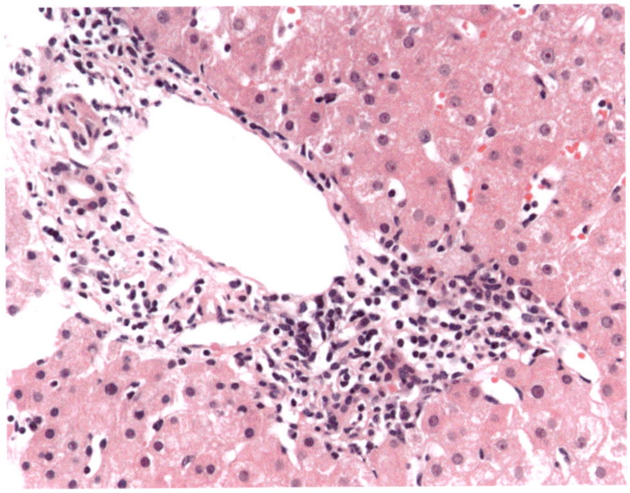

Fig. 9.15 Autoimmune hepatitis on immunosuppression. A mild portal lymphocytic infiltrate without interface hepatitis is present. The portal, periportal, and lobular necroinflammatory activities in AIH are reduced markedly after immunosuppression. Histologic remission is characterised by normal liver or mild nonspecific portal inflammation and typically lags behind clinical and biochemical remission. The presence of noticeable portal plasma cells and interface hepatitis in patients on immunosuppression usually is associated with disease relapse after stopping immunosuppressants.

PARAMETER	CUTOFF	POINTS
ANA/SMA+	≥ 1:40	1
or ANA/SMA+	≥ 1:80	2
or LKM	≥ 1:40	2
or SLA/LP	Positive	2
IgG	≥Upper limit of normal	1
	≥10% above upper limit of normal	2
Liver histology	Compatible with AIH	1
	Typical for AIH	2
Exclusion of viral hepatitis	Yes	2

Fig. 9.16 Simplified diagnostic criteria for autoimmune hepatitis. The diagnosis of AIH requires clinical, serologic, and histologic correlation. The International Autoimmune Hepatitis Group proposed a simplified scoring system in 2008 to replace the existing, more complex scoring system of 1999. The diagnostic cutoff values for probable AIH and definite AIH are six points (88% sensitivity and 97% specificity) and seven points (81% sensitivity and 99% specificity), respectively. Typical histology for AIH requires the presence of interface hepatitis, portal lymphocytic/lymphoplasmacytic infiltrate, emperipolesis, and hepatocyte rosette formation. Histology compatible with AIH is chronic hepatitis with lymphocytic infiltration without all the features considered typical.

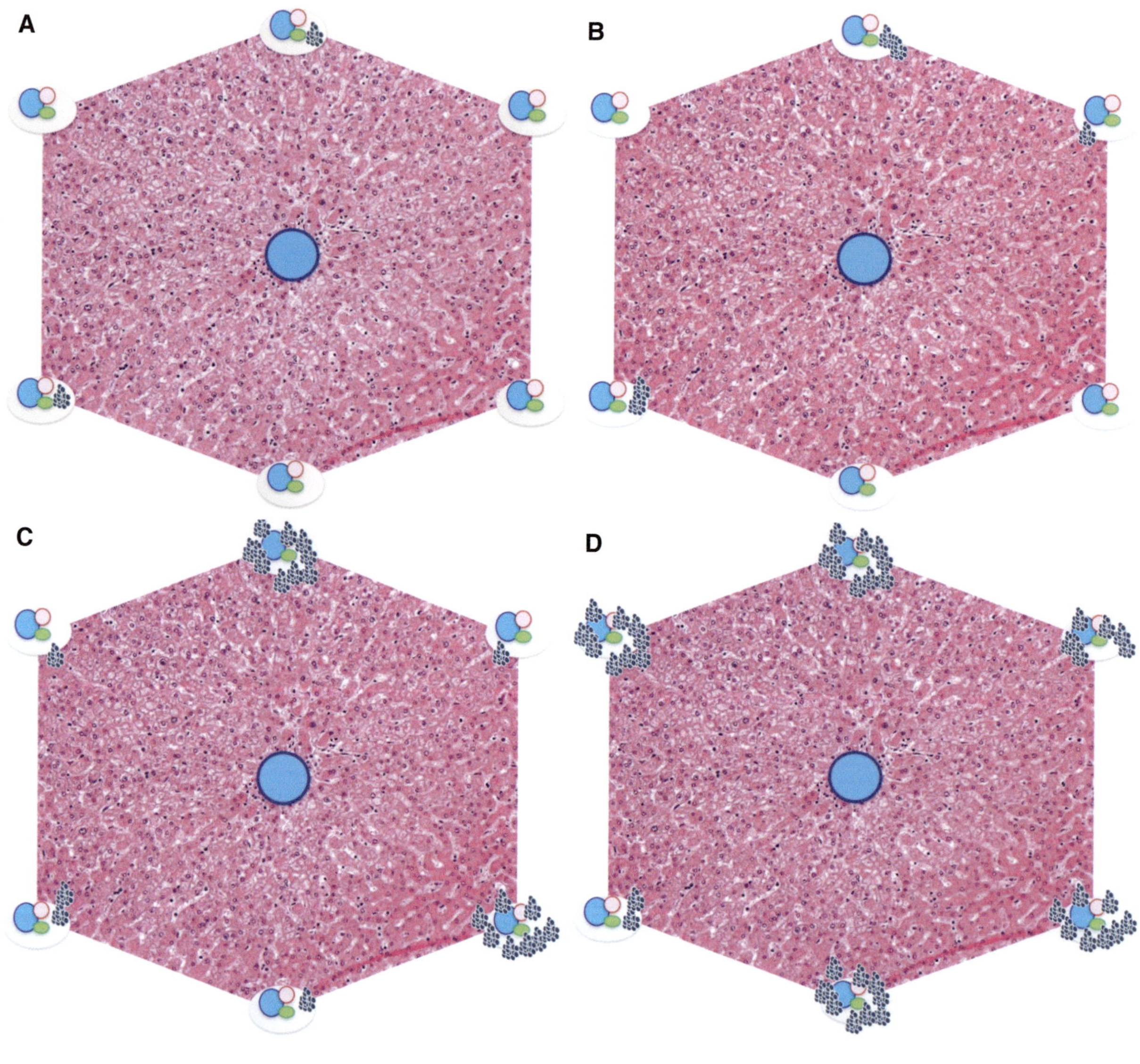

Fig. 9.17 Scheuer grading of portal–periportal activity (*blue dots* represent inflammatory cells). (**A**) Grade 1: portal inflammation only. (**B**) Grade 2: mild interface hepatitis. (**C**) Grade 3: moderate interface hepatitis. (**D**) Grade 4: severe interface hepatitis. The final Scheuer grade is determined by the higher grade of portal–periportal and lobular activities. No specific histologic scoring system has been developed for AIH, although Scheuer's system is entirely appropriate, as are other approaches, such as METAVIR.

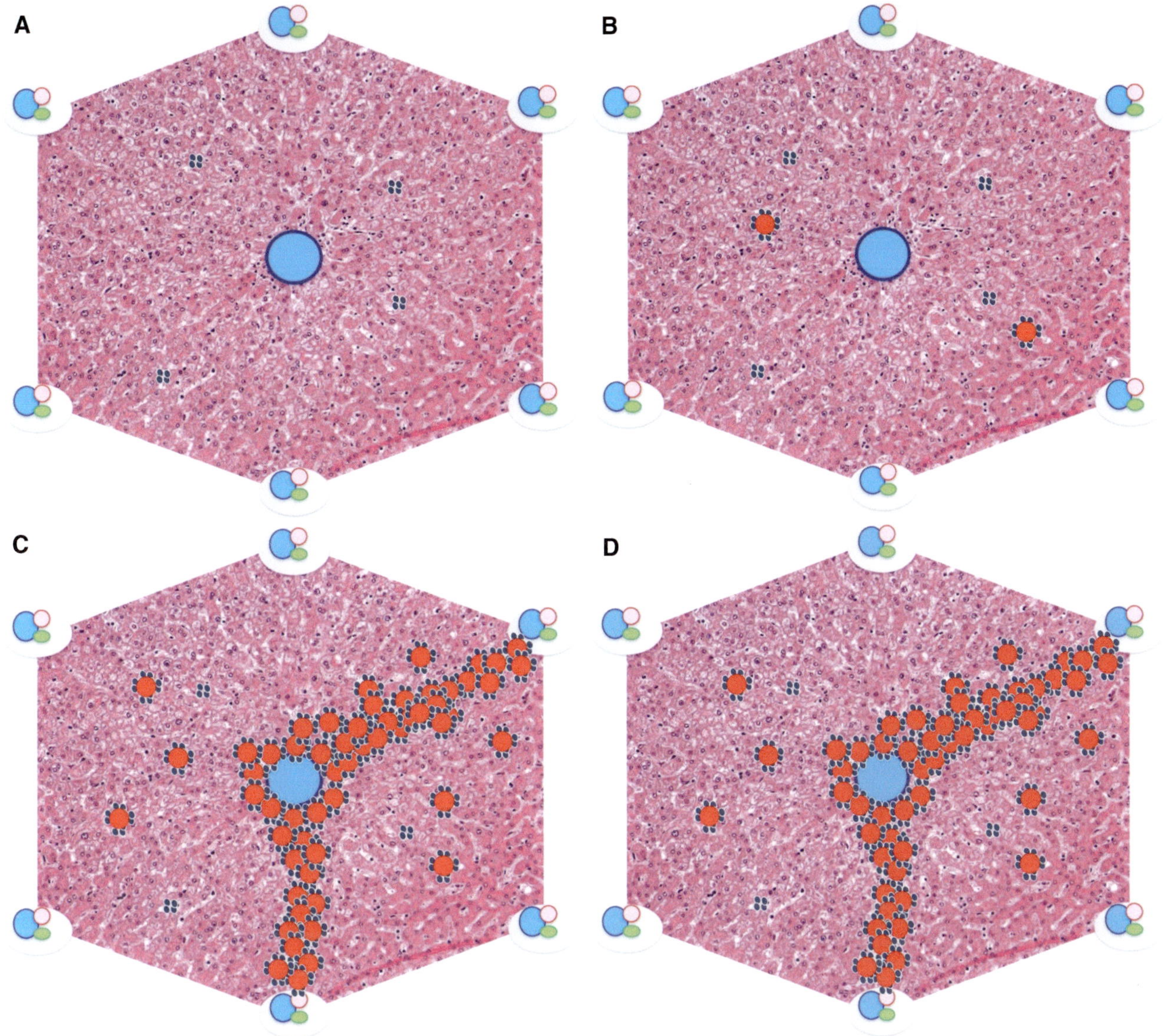

Fig. 9.18 Scheuer grading of lobular activity (*blue dots* and *red dots* represent inflammatory cells and hepatic necrosis, respectively). (**A**) Grade 1: inflammatory cells only, without any hepatocellular death. (**B**) Grade 2: focal necrosis or apoptotic bodies. (**C**) Grade 3: severe focal cell damage. (**D**) Grade 4: bridging necrosis. The final Scheuer grade is determined by the higher grade of portal–periportal and lobular activities.

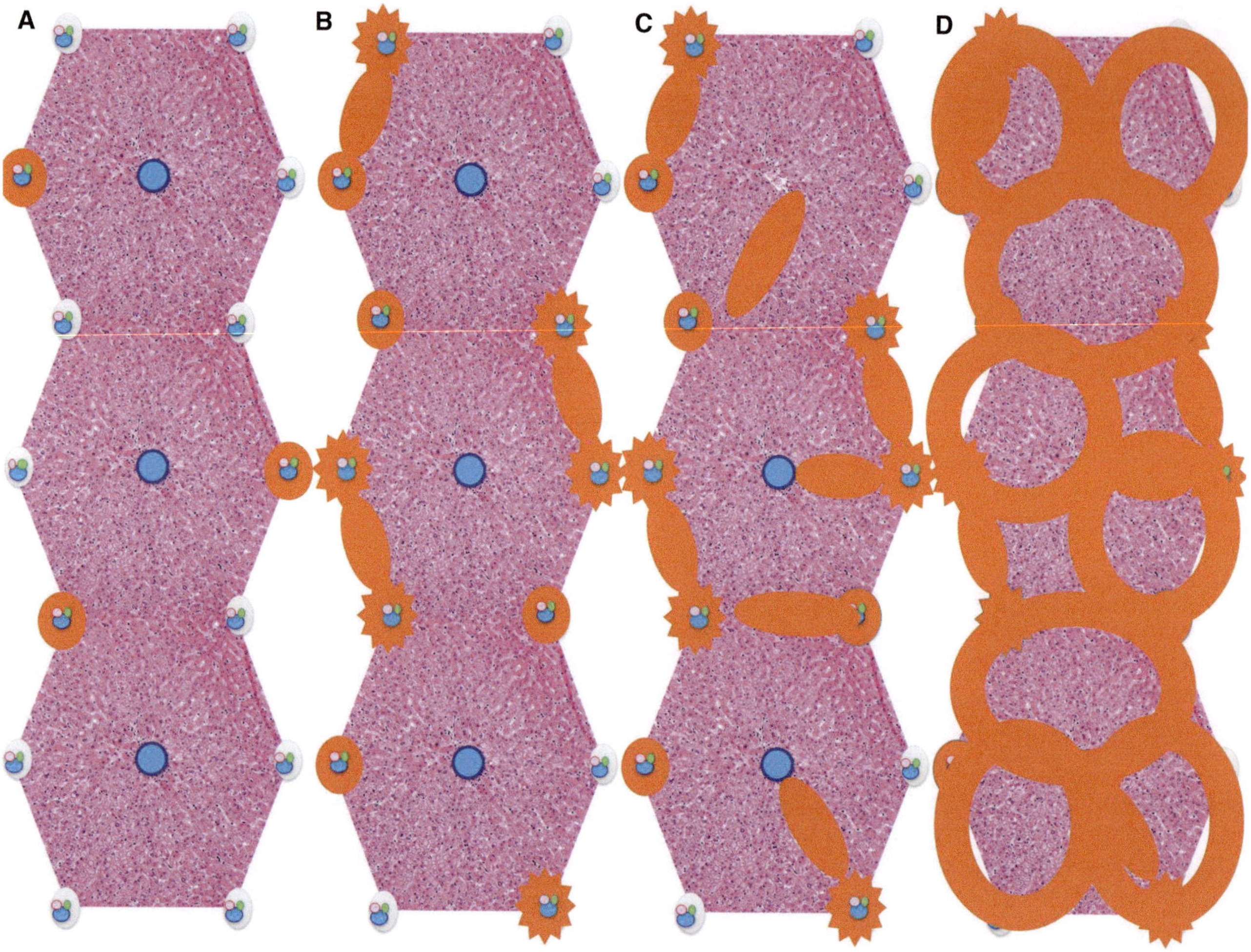

Fig. 9.19 Scheuer staging (orange region represents fibrosis). Stage 0: normal liver without any fibrosis. (**A**) Stage 1: enlarged fibrotic portal tracts. (**B**) Stage 2: periportal or portal–portal bridging septa but intact architecture. (**C**) Stage 3: fibrosis with architectural distortion but no obvious cirrhosis. (**D**) Stage 4: cirrhosis.

9.2 Overlap and Variant Syndromes

About 10% of autoimmune hepatitis shows coexisting features of immune-mediated biliary disease (overlap syndrome) or are associated with atypical features (variant syndrome). The overlap syndromes include autoimmune hepatitis-primary biliary cirrhosis (AIH-PBC) overlap syndrome and autoimmune hepatitis-primary sclerosing cholangitis (AIH-PSC; autoimmune sclerosing cholangitis) overlap syndrome, whereas the variant syndromes are seronegative autoimmune hepatitis and antimitochondrial antibody (AMA)-positive autoimmune hepatitis. A recent consensus document by an international study group indicates that these outlier conditions are probably best not considered to be separate specific conditions but rather reflect parts of a spectrum and that pragmatically they should be characterised on the predominant clinical and histological process present.

AUTOIMMUNE HEPATITIS FEATUES (2 OUT OF 3 REQUIRED	PRIMARY BILIARY CIRRHOSIS FEATURES (2 OUT OF 3 REQUIRED)
Serum ALT > 5x upper limit of normal	Serum ALP >2x upper limit of normal OR Serum GGT >5x upper limit of normal
Serum IgG >2x upper limit of normal OR Positive SMA	Positive AMA
Moderate to severe interface hepatitis or lobular necroinflammation in histology	Florid duct lesion in histolgy

Fig. 9.21 Diagnostic criteria for autoimmune hepatitis–primary biliary cirrhosis overlap syndrome by Chazouillères et al. Hepatology. 1998;28:296–301. The diagnostic criteria of AIH-PBC overlap syndrome have not been universally defined. One commonly used definition adopted in various studies was developed by Chazouillères et al. in 1998.

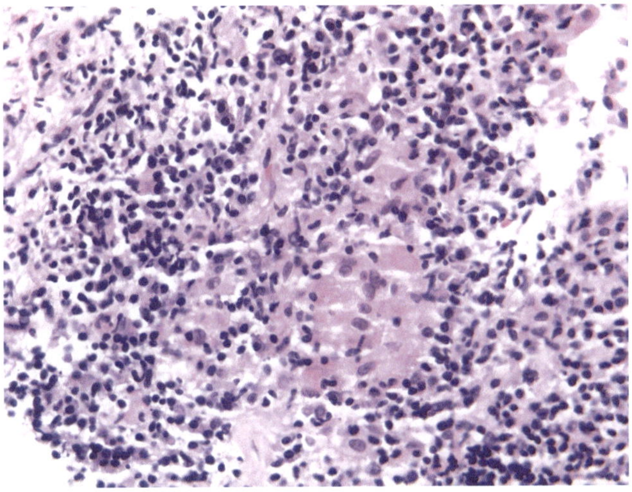

Fig. 9.20 Autoimmune hepatitis–primary biliary cirrhosis overlap syndrome. A poorly formed epithelioid granuloma is present in a portal tract with a surrounding dense lymphoplasmacytic infiltrate. Portal granulomas are not typical of AIH, and their presence in the background of otherwise typical AIH histologic changes should raise the possibility of AIH-PBC overlap syndrome or other aetiologies.

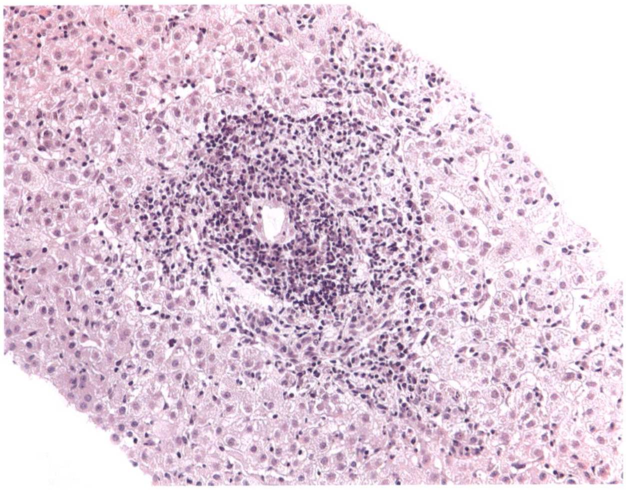

Fig. 9.22 Seronegative autoimmune hepatitis. A marked portal plasma-rich inflammatory infiltrate is accompanied by moderate interface hepatitis in a liver biopsy sample from a patient who was seronegative for autoantibodies. About 10% to 20% of AIH cases are seronegative for conventional autoantibodies but otherwise show no difference with respect to clinical presentation, biochemical profile, pathologic features, and treatment response compared with classic AIH. These patients subsequently may develop conventional autoantibodies after immunosuppression.

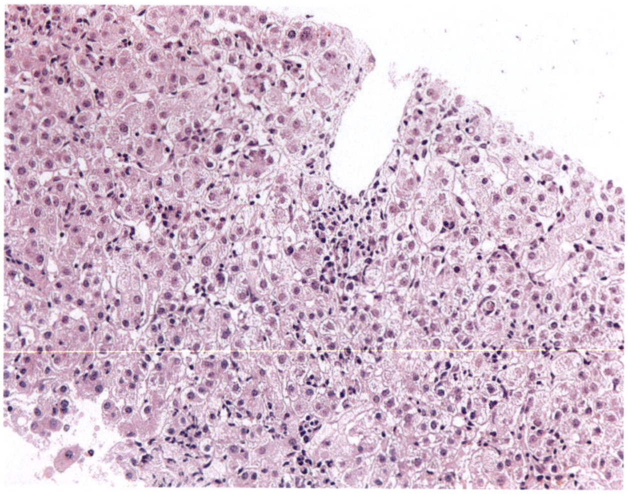

Fig. 9.23 Seronegative autoimmune hepatitis. A moderate to marked lobular lymphoplasmacytic infiltrate is accompanied by focal confluent necrosis, spotty necrosis, and hepatocyte rosette formation in a liver biopsy sample from a patient seronegative for autoantibodies.

10 Biliary Disease

Biliary disorders may affect the biliary tree at any site, from the smallest intrahepatic interlobular bile ducts to the ampulla of Vater. Disorders affecting the small intrahepatic bile ducts may be visualised directly on liver biopsy samples. If the pathology affects large intrahepatic or extrahepatic bile ducts, a liver biopsy sample may display only the indirect signs of the disease, the full histologic manifestation of which can be appreciated only on surgical specimens or at postmortem examination.

It is important for the histopathologist to be able to recognise the peripheral histologic signs of acute and chronic bile duct obstruction. This chapter also illustrates examples of the typical lesions of primary biliary cirrhosis (PBC) and primary sclerosing cholangitis (PSC), as well as examples of primary hepatolithiasis and recurrent pyogenic cholangitis. Langerhans cell histiocytosis and sarcoidosis may simulate PSC and PBC, respectively. IgG4-related disease is an increasingly recognised disorder often manifesting as a sclerosing cholangitis or simulating cholangiocarcinoma clinically and is included in this chapter.

A.W.H. Chan et al., *Atlas of Liver Pathology*, Atlas of Anatomic Pathology,
DOI 10.1007/978-1-4614-9114-9_10, © Springer Science+Business Media New York 2014

10.1 Primary Biliary Cirrhosis

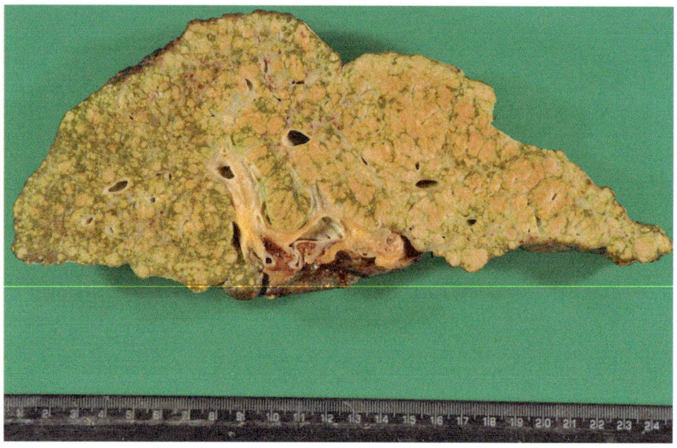

Fig. 10.1 Primary biliary cirrhosis. This explanted cirrhotic liver shows diffuse bile-stained discolouration, indicating prominent bilirubinostasis. PBC is a chronic cholestatic, destructive, and nonsuppurative disease of the intrahepatic bile ducts, progressively leading to cirrhosis. It commonly affects women, with female-to-male ratio of 9:1, and usually presents at age 40 to 60. Its onset typically is insidious, with fatigue and pruritus initially. It progresses slowly to cirrhosis and liver failure over 20 years. Elevation of serum IgM and antimitochondrial antibody (AMA; 90%–95% of patients), particularly the M2 fraction (pyruvate dehydrogenase E2 subunit), is typical. PBC is associated with other autoimmune processes, such as Sjögren syndrome, scleroderma, rheumatoid arthritis, and autoimmune thyroiditis. Bilirubinostasis occurs usually at a late stage, or earlier if other causes are superimposed (e.g., drug reaction).

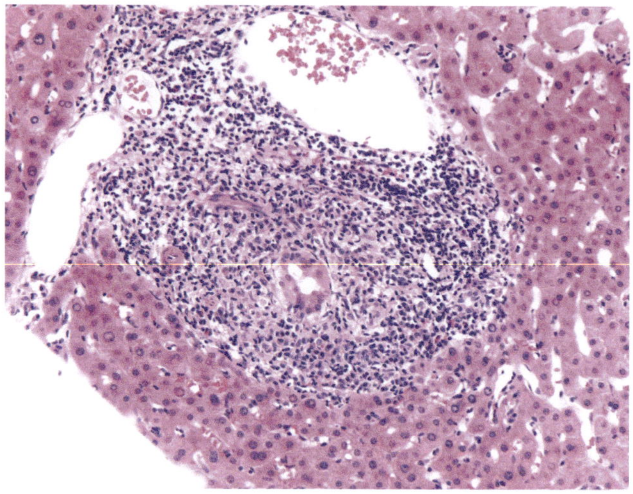

Fig. 10.3 Primary biliary cirrhosis. A damaged bile duct is present in a portal tract with a dense chronic inflammatory infiltrate of lymphocytes, plasma cells, histiocytes, and some eosinophils. Varying degrees of bile duct damage may be observed, in addition to the pathognomonic florid duct lesion. Lymphocytic cholangitis, characterised by an intraepithelial lymphocytic infiltrate associated with mild biliary epithelial damage, is found more commonly. However, this is not entirely specific for PBC and also may be found in chronic viral hepatitis C, drug-induced cholangiopathy, autoimmune hepatitis, PSC, HIV-associated cholangiopathy, lymphoproliferative disorders, acute cellular rejection in liver allograft, and graft-versus-host disease.

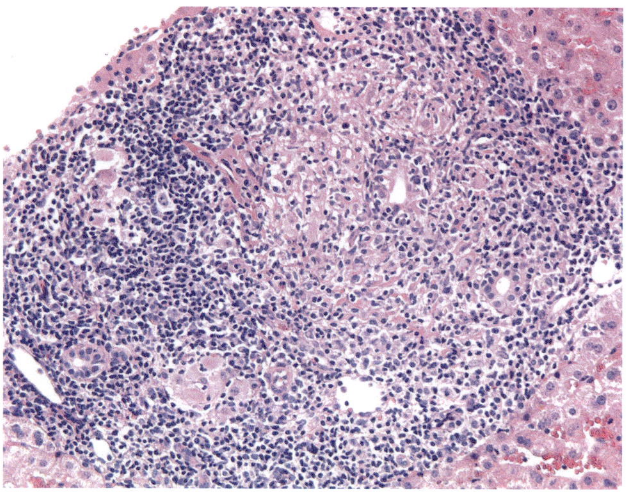

Fig. 10.2 Primary biliary cirrhosis. A florid duct lesion is seen here with a damaged duct surrounded by a dense lymphohistiocytic infiltrate. The florid duct lesion is the hallmark pathologic feature of PBC. It typically affects interlobular bile ducts of 40- to 80-μm calibre. The involved interlobular bile ducts show epithelial damage as evidenced by cytoplasmic vacuolation, apoptosis, and regenerative changes, with intraepithelial lymphocytic infiltration. Disruption of bile duct basement membrane may be highlighted by periodic acid-Schiff with diastase (PASD) stain. These bile ducts are surrounded by granulomatous inflammation comprising epithelioid histiocytes and small lymphocytes. Although the florid duct lesion is quite specific for PBC, certain drug/toxin-induced granulomatous chronic cholestatic injuries may produce a similar histologic appearance.

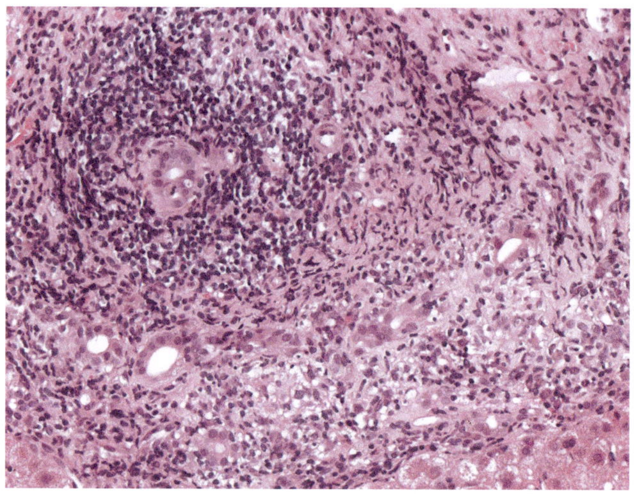

Fig. 10.4 Primary biliary cirrhosis. Damaged bile ducts are present in a portal tract with a dense chronic inflammatory infiltrate of lymphocytes, plasma cells, histiocytes, and a few eosinophils. A portal chronic inflammatory infiltrate commonly is associated with bile duct injuries and generally is composed mainly of lymphocytes, plasma cells, and a variable number of eosinophils. The presence of numerous plasma cells or scattered eosinophils is common in PBC and does not per se indicate autoimmune hepatitis or drug-induced cholangiopathy. Lymphoid aggregates and even follicles may also be seen. Portal inflammation with bile duct damage and/or florid duct lesion indicates stage I disease based on both Scheuer's and Ludwig's systems for assessing PBC.

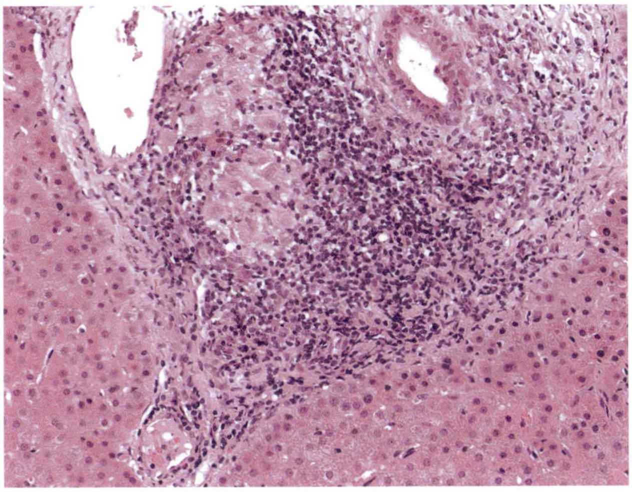

Fig. 10.5 Primary biliary cirrhosis. A noncaseating epithelioid granuloma is present within a portal tract with a mildly damaged bile duct and a dense chronic inflammatory infiltrate of lymphocytes, plasma cells, and histiocytes. Noncaseating epithelioid granulomas in portal tracts and, less commonly, lobules may be seen in a significant proportion of PBC cases. The presence of portal epithelioid granulomas with bile duct injury is typical for PBC, but also may be found in drug-induced liver injury and sarcoidosis. Granulomas in sarcoidosis usually are larger, more well-formed, and more numerous than those in PBC and are not associated with obvious bile duct injury in most cases.

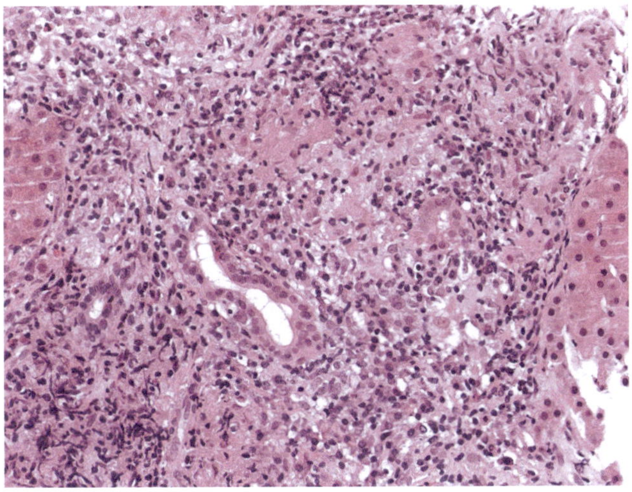

Fig. 10.6 Primary biliary cirrhosis. A poorly formed, noncaseating epithelioid granuloma is present within a portal tract with damaged bile ducts and a dense chronic inflammatory infiltrate of lymphocytes, plasma cells, histiocytes, and a few eosinophils.

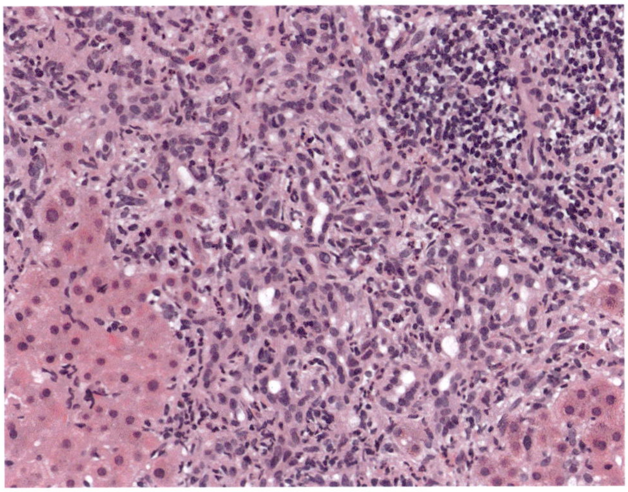

Fig. 10.7 Primary biliary cirrhosis. A prominent ductular reaction is accompanied by many neutrophils at the periphery of a portal tract. Ductular reaction occurs in PBC as the disease progresses and is driven by cholate stasis. Neutrophilic infiltrate commonly is seen in the vicinity, with proliferating bile ductules in ductular reactions. It is important to note that in this context, the presence of neutrophils does not indicate acute large duct obstruction or ascending cholangitis.

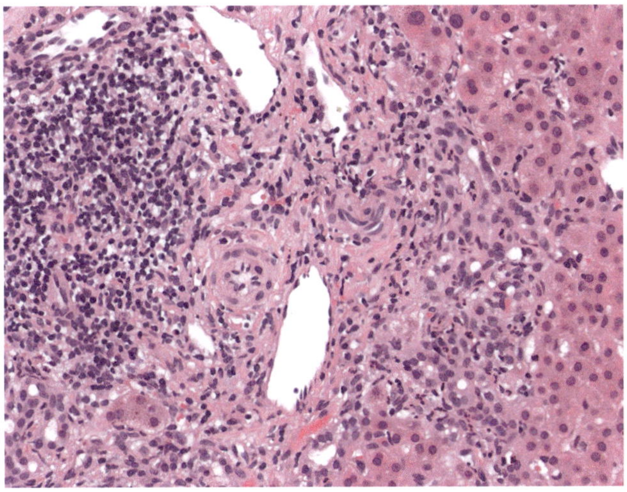

Fig. 10.8 Primary biliary cirrhosis. A moderate ductular reaction is seen with fibrotic expansion and is accompanied by many neutrophils at the periphery of this portal tract. The presence of a ductular reaction with some fibrosis indicates stage II disease in Scheuer's system for PBC.

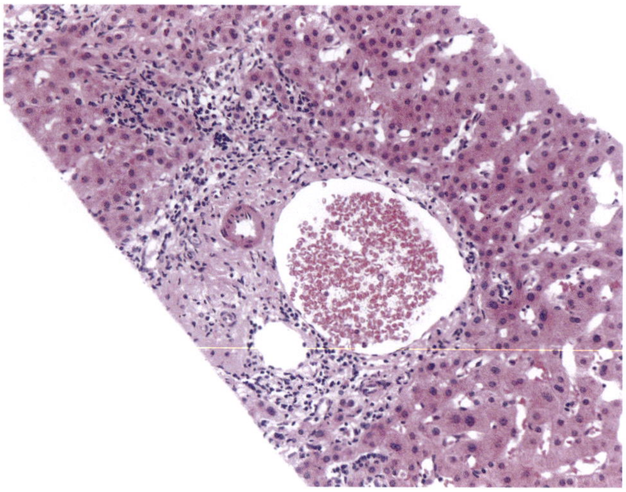

Fig. 10.9 Primary biliary cirrhosis. An unpaired hepatic artery without a bile duct is noted in a portal tract with a moderate lymphoplasmacytic infiltrate and focal interface hepatitis. Interface hepatitis may be found in PBC, particularly where there are florid duct lesions and prominent portal inflammation. Its presence should not in itself alter the diagnosis to autoimmune hepatitis or autoimmune hepatitis–PBC overlap syndrome, unless moderate to severe interface hepatitis or significant lobular necroinflammation with spotty necrosis and apoptotic bodies are observed, also in conjunction with the clinical picture.

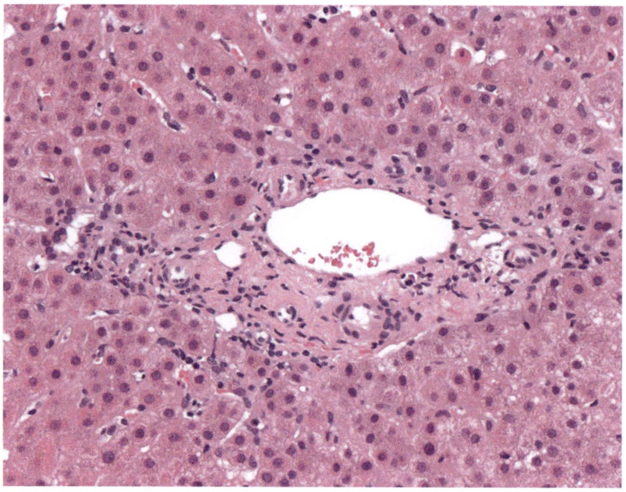

Fig. 10.10 Primary biliary cirrhosis. An unpaired hepatic artery without a bile duct is noted in this portal tract (ductopaenia). Ductopaenia traditionally is defined as the loss of interlobular ducts in more than 50% of portal tracts in an adequate sample containing at least 10 portal tracts or in 5 complete portal tracts. A recently proposed alternative diagnostic criterion is the presence of (1) an unpaired hepatic artery in at least 10% of portal tracts or (2) at least two unpaired hepatic arteries in different portal tracts regardless of the total number of portal tracts.

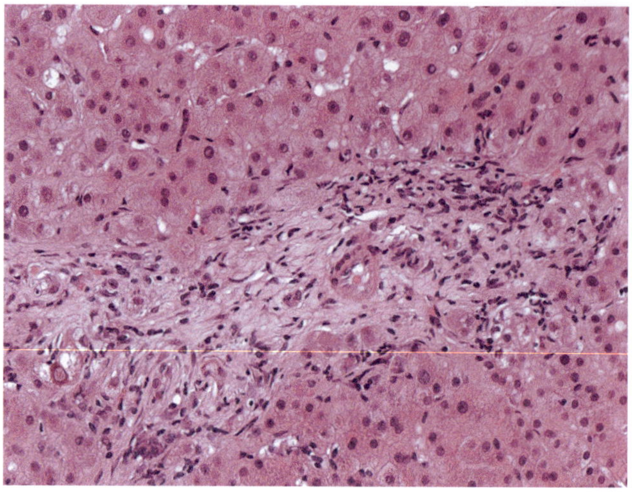

Fig. 10.11 Primary biliary cirrhosis. An unpaired hepatic artery without a bile duct is noted in a portal tract (ductopaenia). Ductopaenia is present in the later stages of PBC and not uncommonly is associated with portal, periportal, and/or bridging fibrosis. Other common causes of ductopaenia in adults include PSC, sarcoidosis, drug-induced cholangiopathy, chronic rejection in liver allograft, chronic graft-versus-host disease, and idiopathic adult ductopaenia.

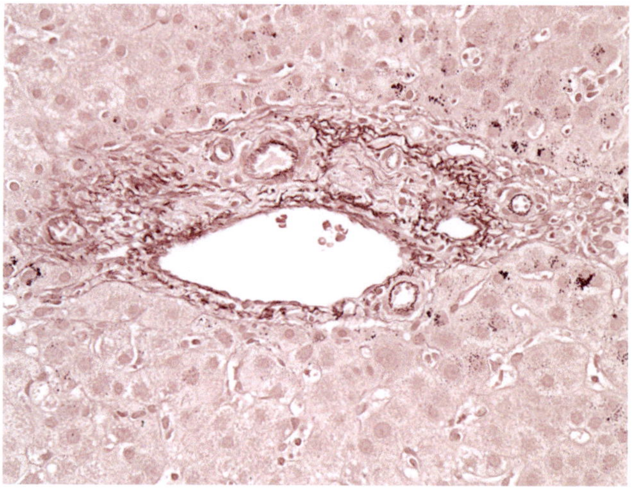

Fig. 10.12 Primary biliary cirrhosis (orcein stain). Chronic cholate stasis is evident by many of the periportal hepatocytes containing copper-associated protein. Deposition of copper or copper-associated proteins in periportal hepatocytes contributes to a constellation of histologic changes of chronic accumulation of bile acid (chronic cholate stasis), which also include feathery degeneration and Mallory-Denk bodies. The presence of chronic cholate stasis in periportal regions with minimal or mild fibrosis is indicative of PBC and other chronic cholestatic diseases.

STAGE	SCHEUER'S SYSTEM	LUDWIG'S SYSTEM
I	Florid duct lesion	Portal inflammation
II	Ductular reaction	Interface hepatitis
III	Bridging fibrosis	Bridging fibrosis
IV	Cirrhosis	Cirrhosis

Fig. 10.13 Staging systems for primary biliary cirrhosis. Pathologic staging systems developed by Scheuer and Ludwig have been adopted widely by pathologists and are applied to PBC and other chronic cholestatic diseases. Stage I disease is characterised by portal inflammation and bile duct damage including a florid duct lesion. Stage II disease is featured by progression of the portal inflammatory process to periportal interface activity (ductular reaction and interface hepatitis). Stage III disease is evidenced by fibrous scarring and usually accompanied by ductopaenia. Stage IV is the cirrhotic stage. The utility of these staging systems in biopsy specimens is controversial because of a heterogeneous distribution of histologic features and consequent sampling error. The stage is designated by the most advanced lesion.

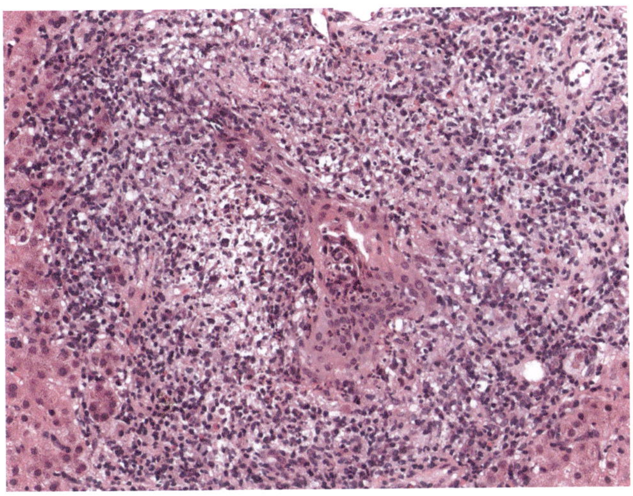

Fig. 10.14 Autoimmune cholangitis. A markedly damaged bile duct is noted in a portal tract in which there is a dense, chronic inflammatory infiltrate of lymphocytes, plasma cells, and eosinophils. This biopsy sample was taken from a patient who was seropositive for antinuclear antibody and seronegative for AMA. The term *autoimmune cholangitis*, also known as autoimmune cholangiopathy and AMA-negative primary biliary cirrhosis, is used for cases that demonstrate typical clinical, biochemical, and pathologic features, and treatment response to ursodeoxycholic acid but lacking serum AMA. It accounts for 5% to 10% of PBC. However, some investigators consider autoimmune cholangitis to be a broader heterogeneous group of diseases including AMA-negative PBC, variant forms of autoimmune hepatitis, and PSC.

10.2 Primary Sclerosing Cholangitis

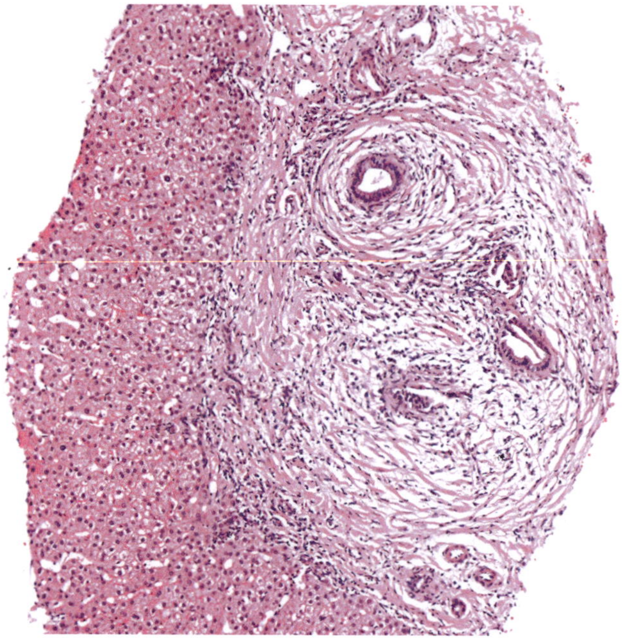

Fig. 10.15 Primary sclerosing cholangitis. Interlobular bile ducts are surrounded by periductal "onion-skin" concentric fibrosis and oedema, with a mild portal lymphocytic infiltrate. PSC is a chronic cholestatic, fibro-obliterative, inflammatory disease of the extrahepatic and intrahepatic bile ducts, progressively leading to cirrhosis. It commonly affects men, with a male-to-female ratio of 2:1, and presents at any age, including infancy and childhood. Its onset typically is one of intermittent episodes of jaundice, pruritus, and weight loss, progressing slowly to cirrhosis and liver failure. It is associated with inflammatory bowel disease (70% with ulcerative colitis), autoimmune pancreatitis (<25%), and retroperitoneal fibrosis. Cholangiography typically demonstrates multifocal irregularity, stricture, and dilatations ("beads-on-string" pattern).

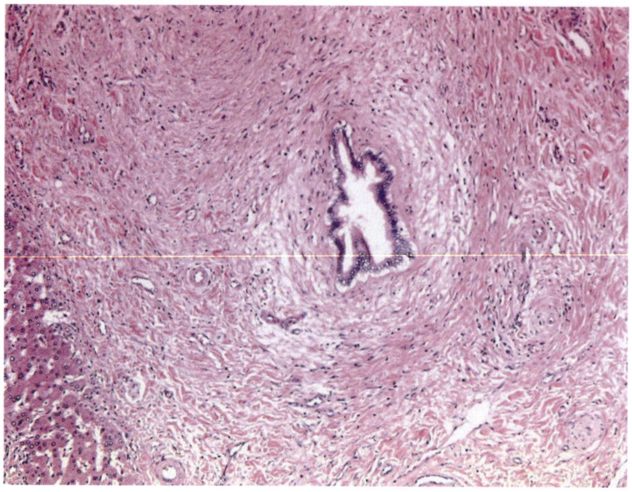

Fig. 10.16 Primary sclerosing cholangitis. A septal bile duct with an irregular contour is surrounded by periductal concentric fibrous tissue. The hallmark pathologic feature of PSC is a fibro-obliterative change in medium-sized to large bile ducts. The affected ducts are surrounded by periductal onion-skin concentric fibrosis and compressed to irregular contours and even complete fibrous obliteration. The biliary epithelial cells usually exhibit degenerative and atrophic changes. However, such characteristic lesions are present only in fewer than half of biopsy specimens, because such medium-sized to large ducts are sampled uncommonly in biopsy specimens.

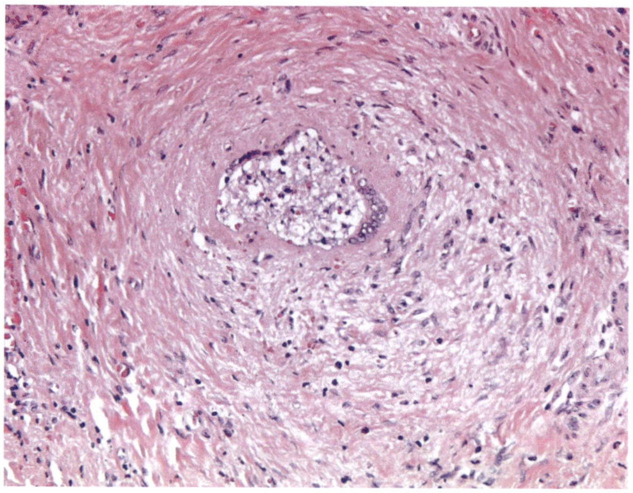

Fig. 10.17 Primary sclerosing cholangitis. The epithelial lining of a bile duct with periductal fibrosis is partially denuded. Some residual epithelial cells are attenuated with atrophic changes. Fibro-obliterative change of medium-sized to large bile ducts is not entirely specific for PSC and also may be found in secondary sclerosing cholangitis, such as IgG4-related sclerosing cholangitis, infectious cholangitis, recurrent pyogenic cholangitis, ischaemic cholangitis, Langerhans cell histiocytes, and portal biliopathy.

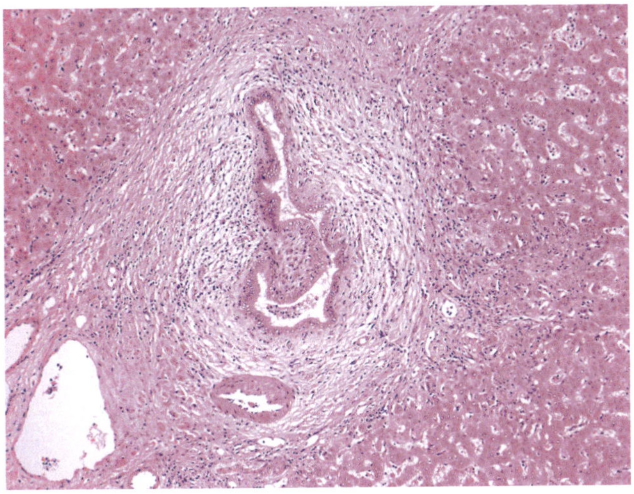

Fig. 10.18 Primary sclerosing cholangitis. A medium-sized bile duct with an irregular contour is surrounded by periductal onion-skin concentric fibrosis and oedema, with a mild portal lymphocytic infiltrate. In addition to diagnostic fibro-obliterative bile duct lesions, other typical changes in portal tracts include a mixed inflammatory infiltrate, xanthogranulomatous inflammation, and portal vein phlebitis. Prominent fibrosis and inflammation in the hilar region may lead to the development of an inflammatory pseudotumour. Xanthogranulomatous inflammation may result from duct ulceration and bile extravasation. Portal vein phlebitis also may be present but occurs less frequently than in IgG4-related sclerosing cholangitis.

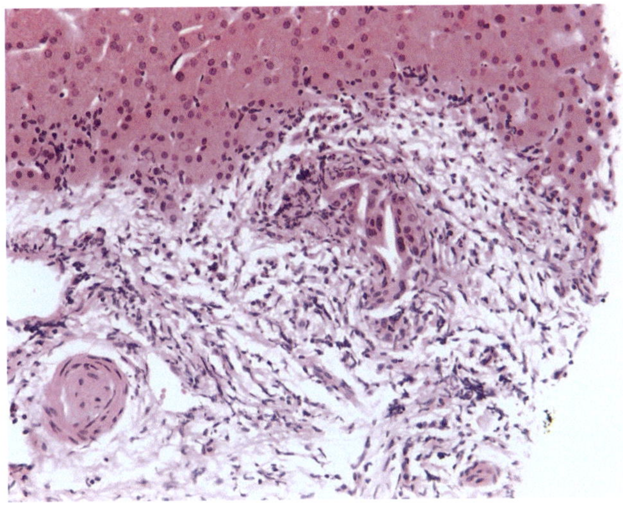

Fig. 10.20 Primary sclerosing cholangitis. This interlobular bile duct has an irregular contour and is embedded in an oedematous stroma with a mixed inflammatory infiltrate. Some interface hepatitis also is present. Small duct PSC is a variant of PSC affecting small septal or interlobular ducts only. The characteristic beads-on-string cholangiographic feature is absent. Interface hepatitis may be found in PSC. Its presence should not per se signify a diagnosis of autoimmune hepatitis or autoimmune hepatitis–PSC overlap syndrome, unless moderate to severe interface hepatitis or significant lobular necroinflammation with spotty necrosis and apoptotic bodies also is observed.

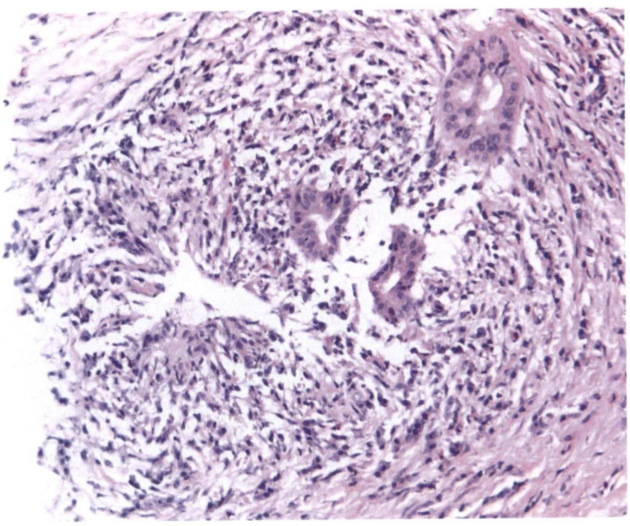

Fig. 10.19 Primary sclerosing cholangitis. These interlobular bile ducts show irregular contours with regenerative and degenerative epithelial changes. They are surrounded by a moderate chronic inflammatory infiltrate mainly of small lymphocytes, a few plasma cells, and eosinophils. No periductal onion-skin concentric fibrosis is identified. Small septal ducts and interlobular bile ducts may be primarily involved in some cases of PSC (small duct variant) or may be affected secondarily as the result of fibro-obliteration of larger bile ducts. Direct involvement is characterised by irregular bile duct contours, degenerative and atrophic epithelial changes, and periductal fibrosis. Characteristic onion-skin concentric fibrosis may be absent because of the heterogeneous distribution of the disease process. Indirect involvement is evidenced by portal oedema and fibrosis, mild portal mixed inflammation, and a ductular reaction.

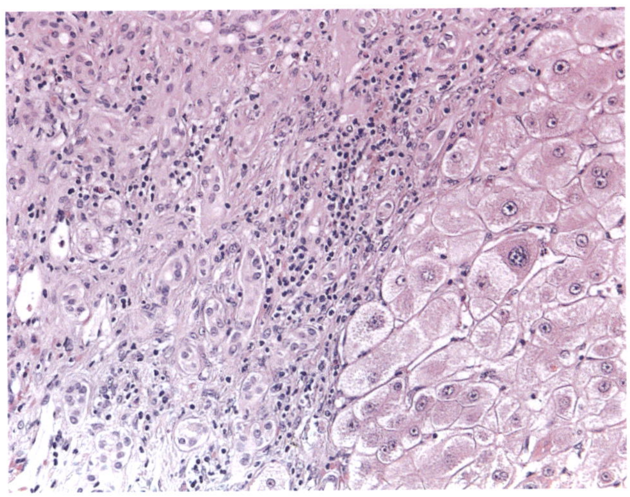

Fig. 10.21 Primary sclerosing cholangitis. Ductular reaction is associated with feathery degeneration of periportal hepatocytes. Ductular reaction is common in PSC and other chronic cholestatic diseases in later stages, corresponding to chronic bile duct injury. However, as noted elsewhere, it also occurs in acute hepatitis with bridging/panacinar necrosis, chronic hepatitis with bridging fibrosis/cirrhosis, acute ascending cholangitis, focal nodular hyperplasia, and inflammatory hepatocellular adenoma.

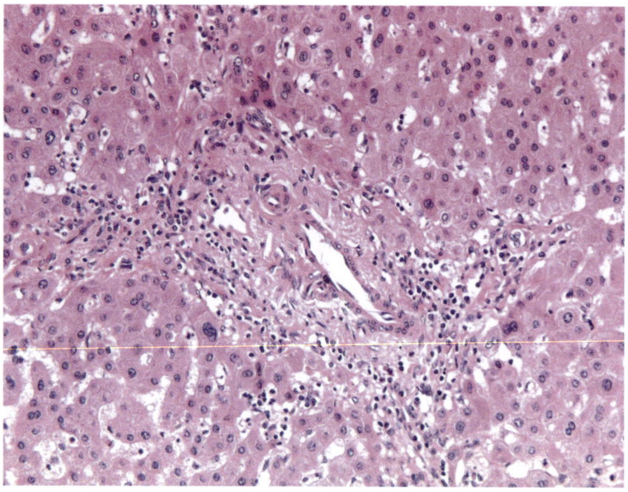

Fig. 10.22 Primary sclerosing cholangitis. An unpaired hepatic artery without a bile duct is noted within this portal tract (ductopaenia). Ductopaenia is present in the later stages of PSC and is not uncommonly associated with portal, periportal, or bridging fibrosis. Other common causes of ductopaenia in adults include PBC, sarcoidosis, drug-induced cholangiopathy, chronic rejection in liver allograft, chronic graft-versus-host disease, and idiopathic adulthood ductopaenia.

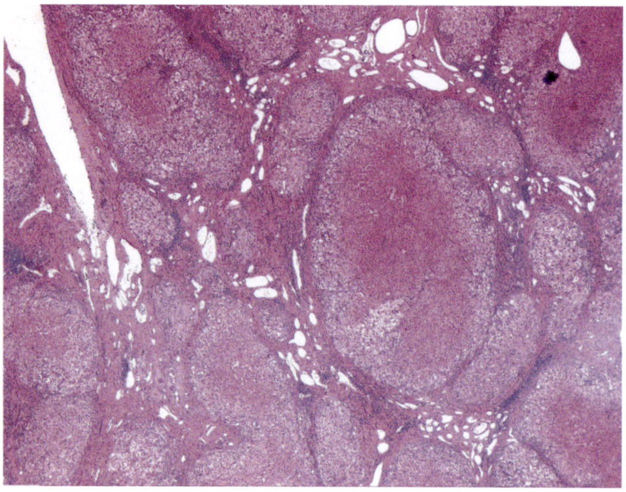

Fig. 10.23 Primary sclerosing cholangitis. Regenerative nodules of variable size and shape are noted. These contain a characteristic peripheral, pale biliary halo. The biliary halo is a characteristic feature of biliary cirrhosis and results from periseptal oedema, loosely packed fibrous tissue at the interface, ductular reaction, and feathery degeneration in periseptal hepatocytes.

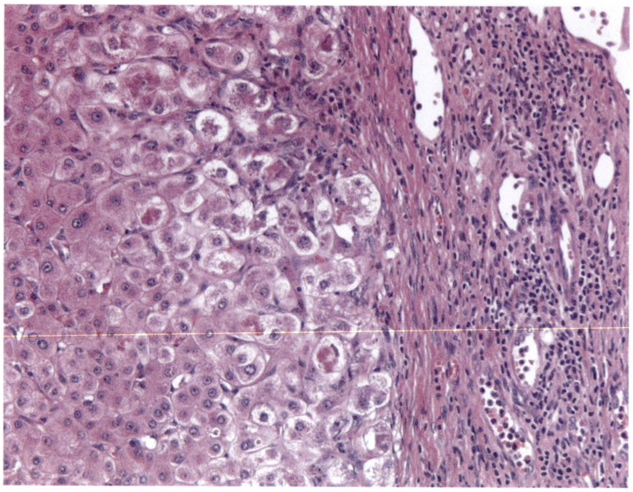

Fig. 10.24 Primary sclerosing cholangitis. Periseptal hepatocytes show feathery degeneration and contain many Mallory-Denk bodies. Feathery degeneration and Mallory-Denk bodies in periportal hepatocytes contribute to a constellation of histologic changes of chronic accumulation of bile acid (chronic cholate stasis), which also includes deposition of copper or copper-associated proteins. Full-blown features of chronic cholate stasis are typical in primary biliary cirrhosis and other chronic cholestatic diseases. Accumulation of copper is observed in Wilson disease, Indian childhood cirrhosis, and idiopathic copper toxicosis.

10.3 Other Biliary Diseases

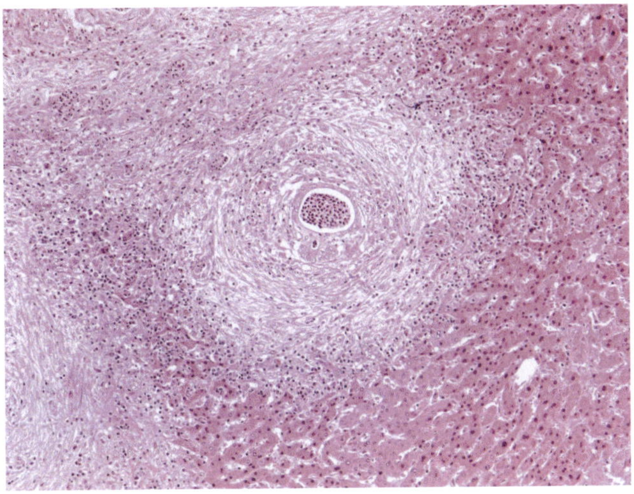

Fig. 10.25 Acute large duct obstruction. A bile duct is infiltrated and distended by neutrophils (acute cholangitis). The portal tract is oedematous and contains a mixed inflammatory infiltrate of neutrophils and lymphocytes. Obstruction of hilar or extrahepatic large bile ducts may lead to different pathologic features, depending on the duration of the problem. In the early stages of obstruction (within the first 2 weeks), one typically sees zone 3 canalicular and cytoplasmic bilirubinostasis, portal oedema, portal mixed inflammation, and ductular reaction. Acute cholangitis and abscess may result from superimposed ascending infection. Intermediate stages of obstruction (after weeks to months) are characterised by more prominent bilirubinostasis, cholestatic hepatocyte rosettes, feathery degeneration, bile infarct, chronic cholate stasis, ductular reaction, and portal and periductal fibrosis.

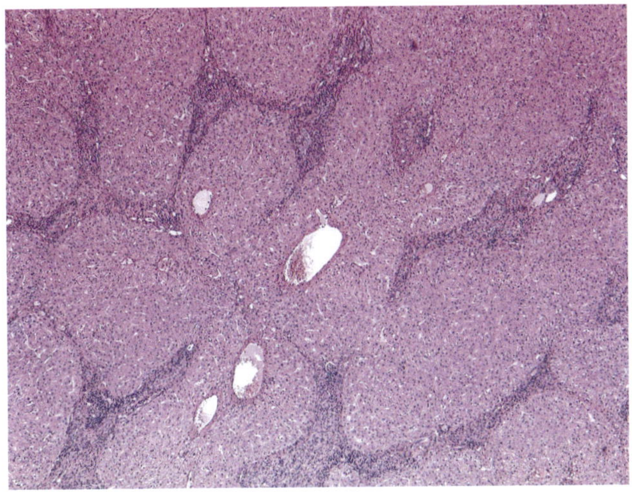

Fig. 10.27 Chronic large duct obstruction with biliary cirrhosis. In the later stages of large duct obstruction (i.e., after months to years), there generally is bridging fibrosis. The bridging is porto-portal with preservation of the porto-central relationships.

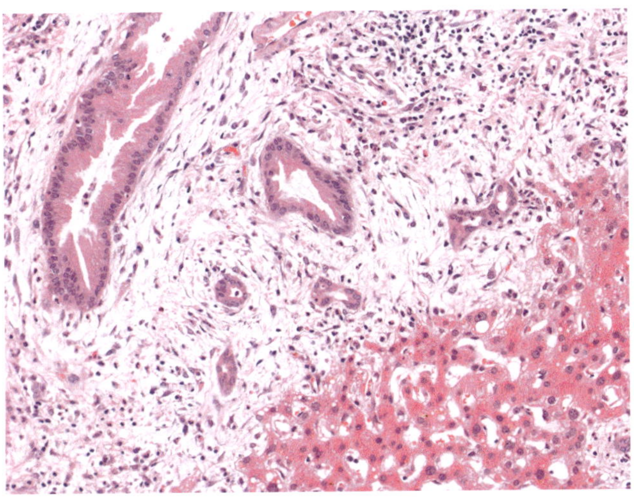

Fig. 10.26 Acute large duct obstruction. A moderate ductular reaction and mixed inflammatory infiltrate are seen in a portal tract. Common causes of large duct obstruction in adults include choledocholithiasis, recurrent pyogenic cholangitis, PSC, secondary sclerosing cholangitis, iatrogenic biliary stricture, and neoplasms of the hilar and extrahepatic bile ducts, pancreatic head, ampulla of Vater, and duodenum. The principal aetiologies of large duct obstruction in children are biliary atresia, choledochal cysts, PSC, and secondary sclerosing cholangitis. The diagnosis of large duct obstruction usually is established by radiologic investigations with clinical correlation. Liver biopsy now is seldom required.

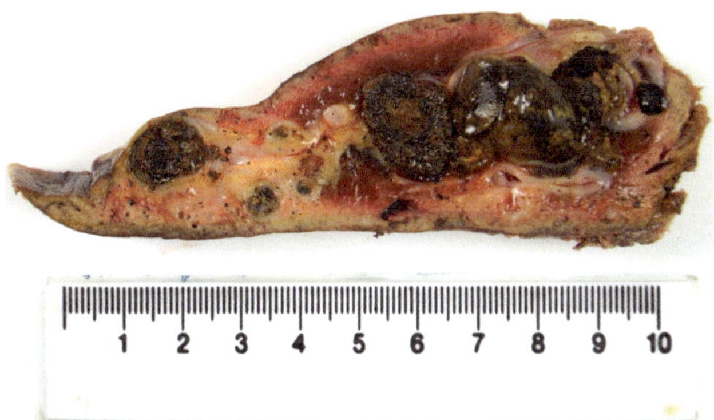

Fig. 10.28 Primary hepatolithiasis/recurrent pyogenic cholangitis. This atrophic liver segment shows dilated bile ducts with multiple dark brown/black calculi. Primary hepatolithiasis and recurrent pyogenic cholangitis are two closely related entities that probably represent pathologic and clinical aspects of the same disease. Primary hepatolithiasis is defined by de novo formation of calculi within the intrahepatic bile ducts, whereas recurrent pyogenic cholangitis, also known as oriental cholangiohepatitis, is characterised by repeated attacks of acute suppurative cholangitis due to primary hepatolithiasis. It is endemic in East Asia, with a prevalence of 4.1% to 52.0% compared with <1% in Western countries.

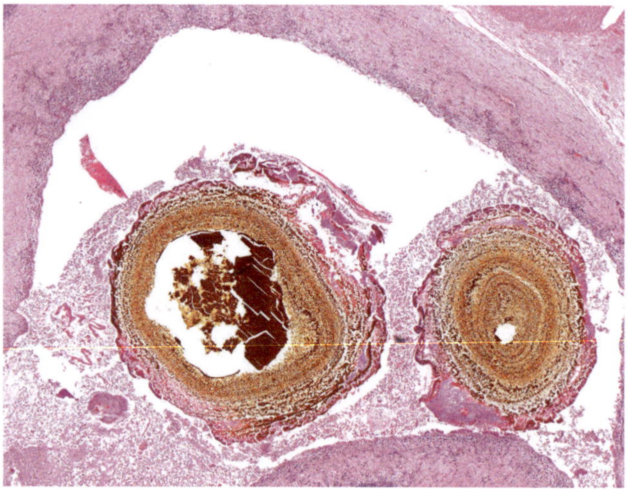

Fig. 10.29 Primary hepatolithiasis/recurrent pyogenic cholangitis. Calculi with concentric lamellar brown-pigmented layers are present within a markedly dilated bile duct. Primary hepatolithiasis is characterised by the presence of multiple small calculi within the intrahepatic bile ducts. These calculi are composed primarily of calcium bilirubinate with variable amounts of fatty acid and cholesterol. Calcium bilirubinate stones appear brownish to black, soft and friable grossly, and as concentric lamellar brown-pigmented layers microscopically.

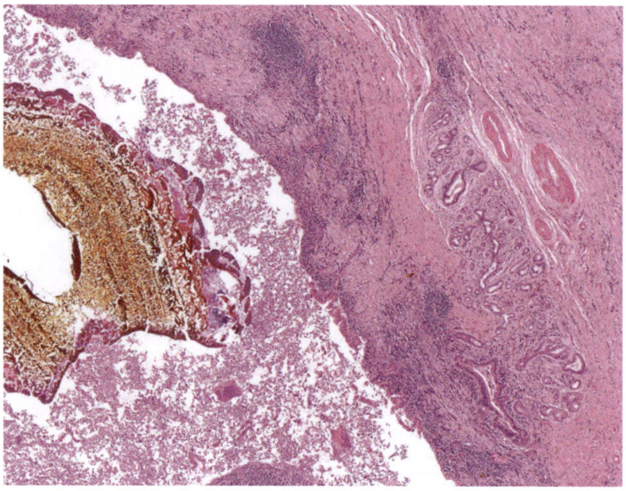

Fig. 10.30 Primary hepatolithiasis/recurrent pyogenic cholangitis. Calculi with concentric lamellar brownish-pigmented layers are present within a markedly dilated bile duct. The bile duct contains a moderate chronic inflammatory infiltrate, peribiliary gland hyperplasia, and fibrous thickening of the wall. The stone-containing bile ducts in primary hepatolithiasis show varying degrees of chronic inflammation, lymphoid follicle, and peribiliary gland hyperplasia, with mural and periductal fibrosis.

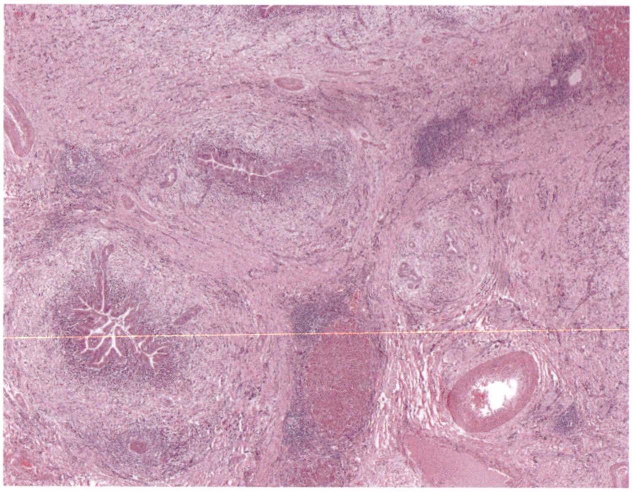

Fig. 10.31 Primary hepatolithiasis/recurrent pyogenic cholangitis. Segmental and septal bile ducts show irregular contours with periductal onion-skin concentric fibrosis, oedema, and chronic inflammatory infiltrate. Bile ducts proximal to the stone-containing ducts exhibit fibro-obliterative change with periductal onion-skin concentric fibrosis and often are compressed, leading to an irregular contour and even complete fibrous obliteration (secondary sclerosing cholangitis). Reactive hyperplastic (and, less commonly, atrophic) changes of biliary epithelial cells may be found. Parasitic infestations, such as clonorchiasis, opisthorchiasis, and ascariasis, may be present in some cases.

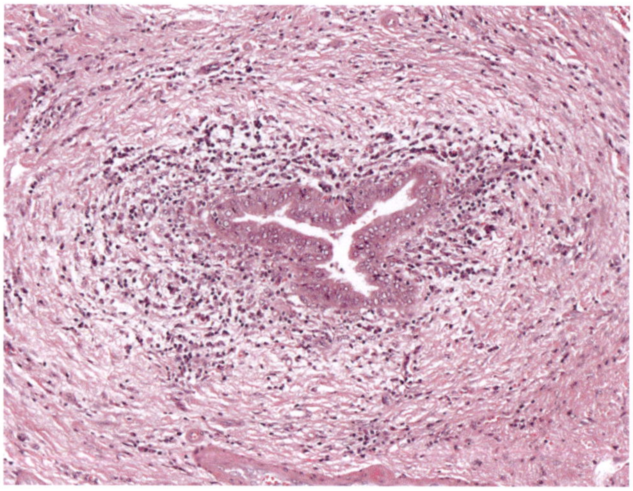

Fig. 10.32 Primary hepatolithiasis/recurrent pyogenic cholangitis. This segmental bile duct shows an irregular contour with periductal onion-skin concentric fibrosis, oedema, and chronic inflammatory infiltrate. In contrast to PSC, primary hepatolithiasis less commonly leads to ductopaenia (20%). Ductular reaction rarely is present. Interface hepatitis, chronic cholate stasis, and biliary cirrhosis also are not typical in primary hepatolithiasis. In Asian patients, a left lobe predilection, disproportionate dilatation of the intrahepatic bile ducts on cholangiography, and the presence of liver flukes and peribiliary gland hyperplasia favour a diagnosis of primary hepatolithiasis over PSC.

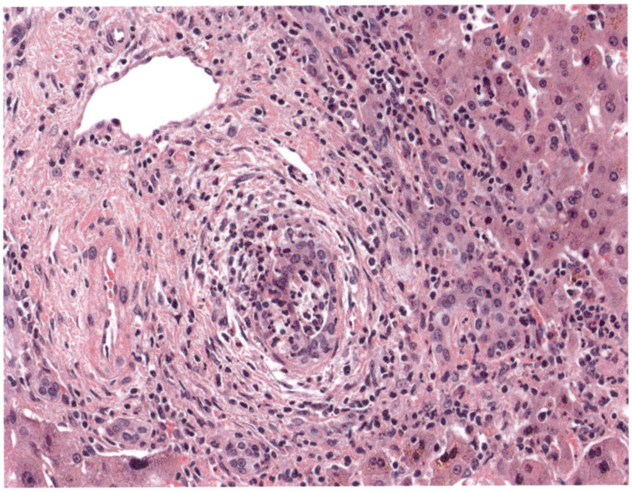

Fig. 10.33 Primary hepatolithiasis/recurrent pyogenic cholangitis. This bile duct is infiltrated and distended by neutrophils (acute cholangitis) and accompanied by a portal mixed inflammatory infiltrate and ductular reaction. Primary hepatolithiasis may be complicated by secondary bacterial infection and results in acute ascending cholangitis, pyogenic abscess, inflammatory pseudotumour, thrombophlebitis of the hepatic or portal vein, and septicaemia. Repeated episodes of acute suppurative cholangitis are characteristic. *Escherichia coli* may be isolated from the bile in 95% of patients with acute attacks.

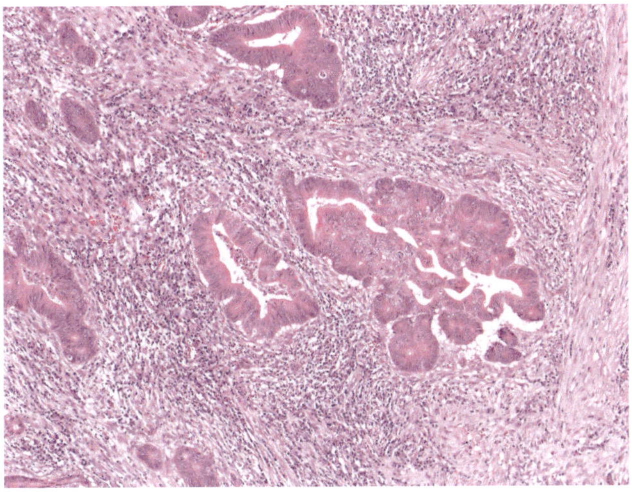

Fig. 10.34 Cholangiocarcinoma arising in primary hepatolithiasis/recurrent pyogenic cholangitis. Irregular complex and angulated malignant glands are embedded in an inflamed fibroblastic stroma. Premalignant precursors, namely biliary intraepithelial neoplasia and, less commonly, intraductal papillary neoplasm of bile ducts, and frank invasive cholangiocarcinoma, are long-term complications of primary hepatolithiasis.

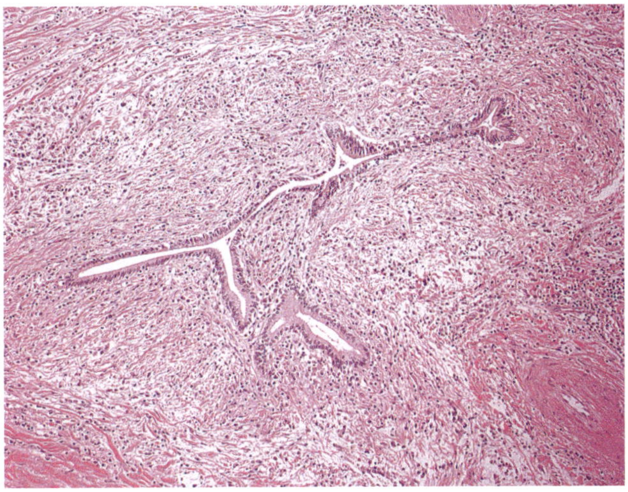

Fig. 10.35 Immunoglobulin G4 (IgG4)-related sclerosing cholangitis (courtesy of Dr. Yoh Zen). Septal bile ducts show irregular contour with periductal fibrosis, oedema and chronic inflammatory infiltrate. IgG4-related sclerosing cholangitis commonly affects men with a male-to-female ratio of 5:1. It usually presents in adulthood and the majority of patients are older than 50 years old. It is associated with other IgG4-related diseases including chronic sclerosing sialadenitis, autoimmune pancreatitis and retroperitoneal fibrosis. Cholangiography typically demonstrates multifocal irregularity, stricture and dilatations ("beads on string" pattern) similar to the findings of primary sclerosing cholangitis. Serum IgG4 level is typically elevated.

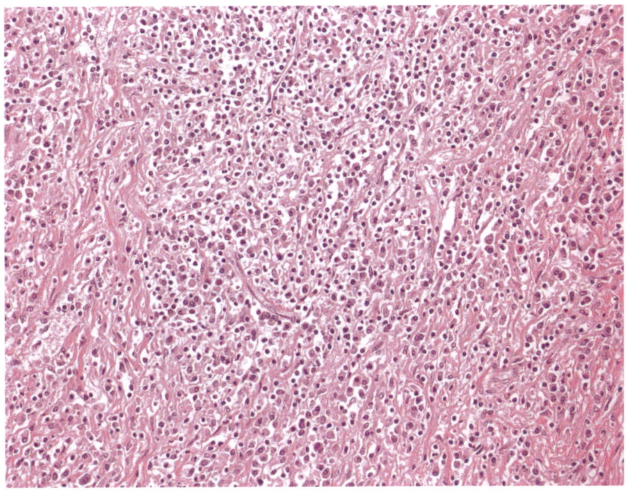

Fig. 10.36 Immunoglobulin G4 (IgG4)-related sclerosing cholangitis (courtesy of Dr. Yoh Zen). The portal tract is markedly infiltrated by a plasma cell-rich inflammatory infiltrate. The pathological hallmark of IgG4-related sclerosing cholangitis is the presence of dense lymphoplasmacytic infiltrate with predominantly IgG4-containing plasma cells. In contrast to primary sclerosing cholangitis, periductal "onion-skin" concentric fibrosis and ductopaenia are rare, while portal vein phlebitis is more commonly found. In some cases, mass-forming inflammatory pseudotumours are present in the hilar region and may mimic cholangiocarcinoma.

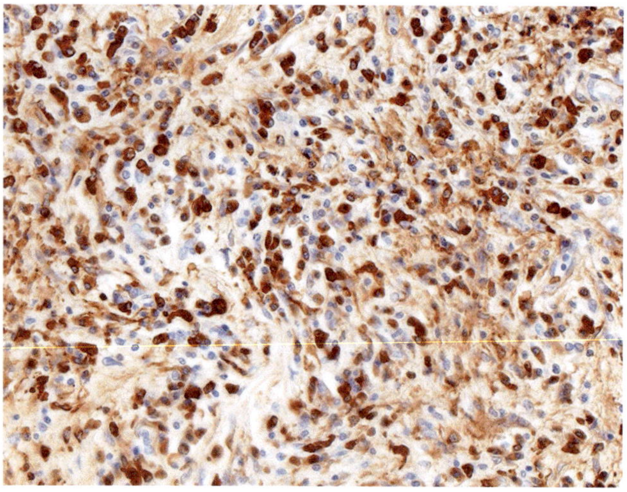

Fig. 10.37 Immunoglobulin G4 (IgG4)-related sclerosing cholangitis (IgG4 stain; courtesy of Dr. Yoh Zen). This portal tract is infiltrated by numerous IgG4-containing plasma cells. Demonstration of elevated IgG4-containing plasma cells is diagnostic for IgG4-related cholangitis. There is no consensus on the cut-off value. Commonly used criteria include more than 10 IgG4-positive plasma cells in a high power field, and a ratio of IgG4-positive plasma cells to IgG-positive plasma cells of greater than 40%.

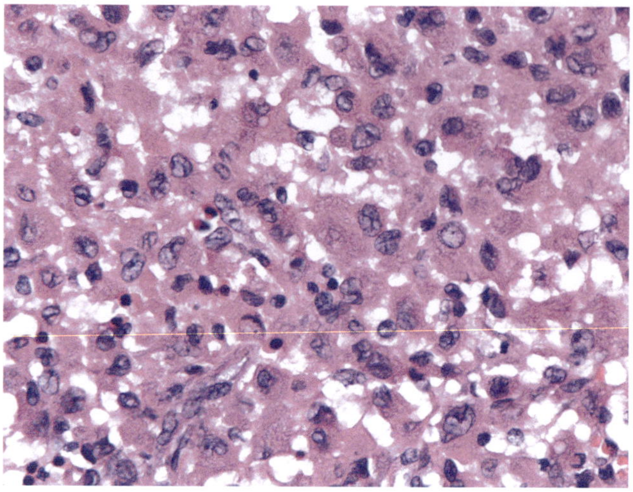

Fig. 10.39 Langerhans cell histiocytosis. There are aggregates of plump epithelioid Langerhans cells with a reniform nucleus and abundant eosinophilic cytoplasm. A few scattered eosinophils are present. The hallmark feature of Langerhans cell histiocytosis is the presence of Langerhans cells, which exhibit a reniform nucleus, nuclear groove, inconspicuous nucleoli, and abundant eosinophilic cytoplasm. Immunoreactivity for CD1a, langerin/CD207, and S100 and the presence of the pathognomonic ultrastructural structure of Birbeck granules are essential diagnostic features. Langerhans cells usually are accompanied by an eosinophil-rich inflammatory infiltrate.

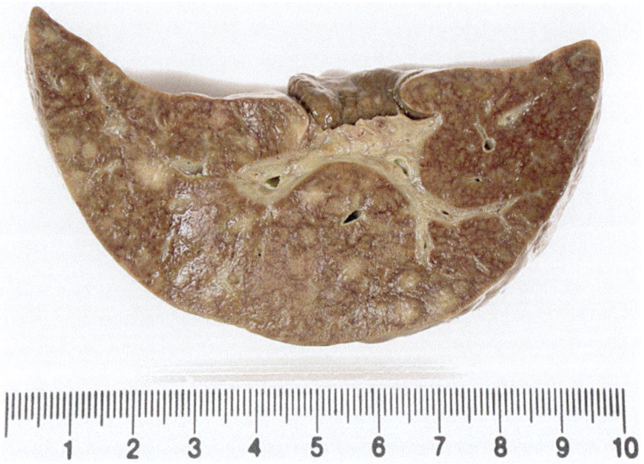

Fig. 10.38 Langerhans cell histiocytosis. An enlarged infant liver contains multiple white nodules. Langerhans cell histiocytosis, previously referred to as histiocytosis X and Langerhans cell granulomatosis, has a wide spectrum of clinical presentations. Hepatic involvement is common in disseminated multisystem Langerhans cell histiocytosis (Letterer-Siwe disease), which is rapidly progressive and potentially fatal and mainly affects children under 2 years old. Fever, pancytopaenia, skin and bone lesions, and hepatosplenomegaly are typical clinical manifestations. About 10% to 15% of these patients develop secondary sclerosing cholangitis. The prognosis is poor, with 66% mortality for those who fail to respond to treatment.

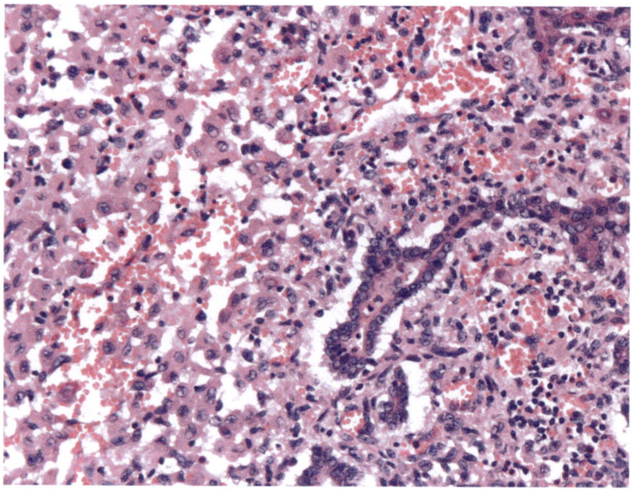

Fig. 10.40 Langerhans cell histiocytosis. An interlobular bile duct is surrounded by sheets of plump epithelioid Langerhans cells with a reniform nucleus and abundant eosinophilic cytoplasm. Bile duct injury is typical in Langerhans cell histiocytosis. Bile ducts are surrounded and infiltrated by Langerhans cells and exhibit varying degrees of epithelial disarray. The affected ducts may be surrounded by periductal onion-skin concentric fibrosis and, in some, complete fibrous obliteration (secondary sclerosing cholangitis). Disease progression with ductular reaction, ductopaenia, chronic cholate stasis, bridging fibrosis, and even biliary cirrhosis also may be present.

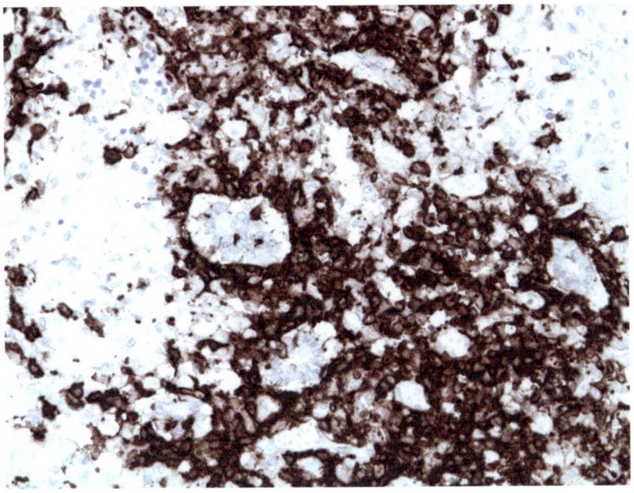

Fig. 10.41 Langerhans cell histiocytosis (CD1a stain). Two bile ducts are surrounded and infiltrated by CD1a-positive Langerhans cells. Differential diagnoses of Langerhans cell histiocytosis include neonatal sclerosing cholangitis, PSC, and secondary sclerosing cholangitis related to X-linked immunodeficiency with hyperimmunoglobulin M. Demonstration of Langerhans cells is essential to distinguish Langerhans cell histiocytosis from other possible causes of sclerosing cholangitis.

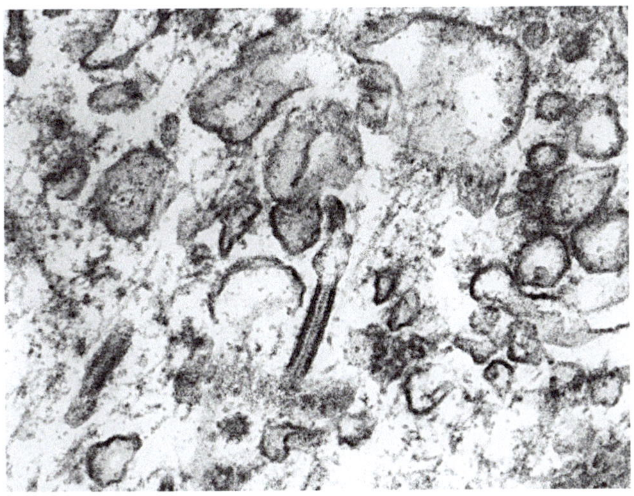

Fig. 10.42 Langerhans cell histiocytosis (electron microscopy). A typical "tennis-racquet"–like Birbeck granule is present. Birbeck granules are the ultrastructural hallmark of Langerhans cell histiocytes. They have a distinctive tennis-racquet–like configuration. The "racquet handle" is 200 to 400 nm long and 33 nm wide with a characteristic trilaminar profile. The presence of Birbeck granules may be confirmed by immunostaining for langerin/CD207.

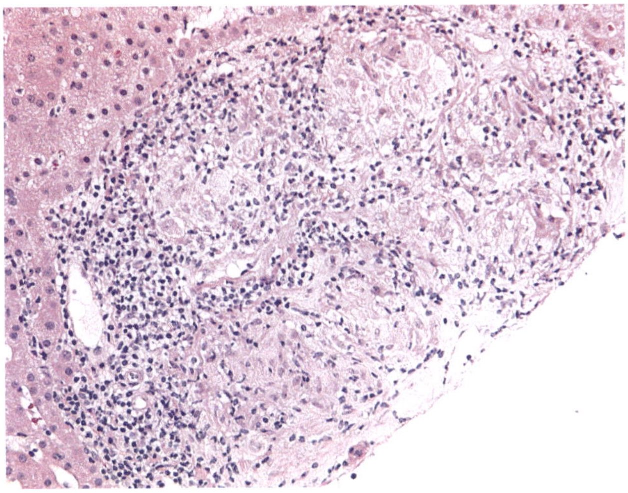

Fig. 10.43 Sarcoidosis. Multiple noncaseating epithelioid granulomas are present in a portal tract. The interlobular bile duct is absent. Sarcoidosis is a systemic granulomatous disease of unknown aetiology. It occurs worldwide, with the highest prevalence in northern European countries. It usually affects young patients, with a peak in the age group of 20 to 29 years. A slight female predominance is observed. The liver is involved in 55% to 90% of cases of sarcoidosis and follows lungs and lymph nodes in the frequency of involvement. Most patients are asymptomatic, but a small proportion may present with chronic cholestatic disease resembling PBC or PSC, or portal hypertension with or without cirrhosis.

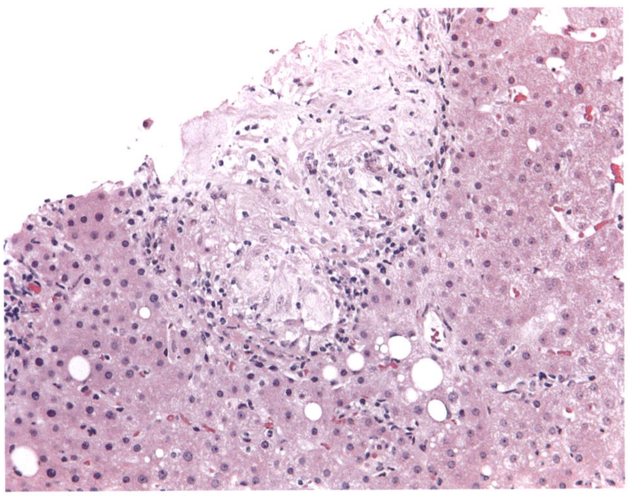

Fig. 10.44 Sarcoidosis. There is a noncaseating epithelioid granuloma with a rim of small lymphocytes. Hepatic sarcoidosis is characterised by multiple noncaseating epithelioid granulomas located predominantly in the portal and periportal regions. Sarcoid granulomas generally are well-demarcated aggregates of epithelioid histiocytes with a rim mainly of lymphocytes, occasionally plasma cells, and eosinophils. Asteroid and Schaumann bodies are uncommon, in contrast to pulmonary sarcoidosis. Central fibrinoid necrosis may occur, but caseation typically is absent. Older granulomas may undergo fibrosis with lamellar collagen fibres, or coalesce to elicit an extensive, irregular fibrous scar. Nonspecific portal and lobular necroinflammation also may be found.

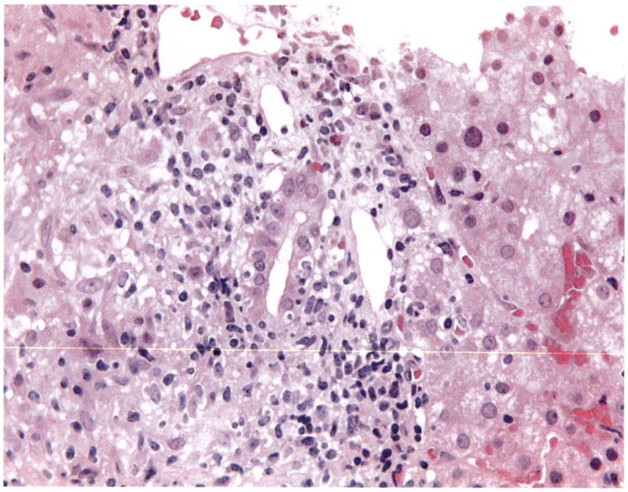

Fig. 10.45 Sarcoidosis. This damaged interlobular duct is infiltrated by small lymphocytes, and there is an adjacent noncaseating epithelioid granuloma (*left*). Up to half of hepatic sarcoidosis cases exhibit bile duct injury. Lymphocytic cholangitis, portal granuloma, and ductopaenia may mimic primary biliary cirrhosis, whereas fibro-obliteration of small bile ducts secondary to compression of hilar large bile ducts by sarcoid granulomas may resemble PSC. A small proportion of hepatic sarcoidosis cases exhibit vascular disorders including sinusoidal dilatation, nodular regenerative hyperplasia, and Budd-Chiari syndrome due to obliteration of hepatic vessels or sinusoids by sarcoid granulomas.

11 Vascular Disorders

Vascular disorders usually are divided into disorders affecting the portal veins, the sinusoids, the hepatic veins, and the hepatic arteries, although these components rarely are affected in isolation. Portal and hepatic vein thrombosis usually is the result of elements of the Virchow triad, including hypercoagulative states, endothelial injury, and stasis. Signs of portal vein obliteration may be too patchy and subtle to be recognised, particularly on a liver biopsy. In more advanced cases, parenchymal signs of vein obliteration include atrophy, extinction, or hyperplasia. Vascular obliterative changes now are considered an essential step in the progression of fibrosis in chronic liver disease, and their resolution may have a role in the regression of fibrosis.

Injury to the sinusoids may be induced by several causes, with chemotherapeutic agents representing the commonest risk factor. The term *sinusoidal obstruction syndrome* is now preferred over *veno-occlusive disease*.

The liver parenchyma is relatively resistant to ischaemia, as it is protected by its dual portal and arterial blood supply. The biliary tree, however, is only arterialised and therefore more sensitive to alterations of the arterial blood flow.

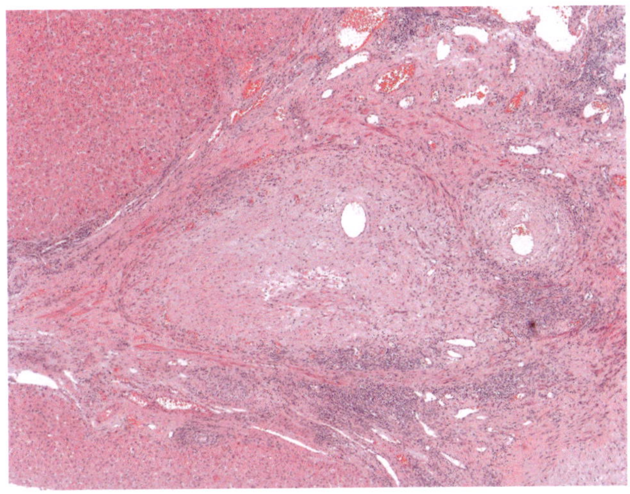

Fig. 11.1 Portal vein thrombosis. A thrombosed portal vein shows partial recanalisation with a small lumen. Thrombosis is the commonest disease of the large portal veins; its predisposing factors are those of classic Virchow's triad: hypercoagulative status, endothelial injury, and stasis. Thrombophilic conditions may be found in about 60% of cases, whereas local predisposing conditions may be identified in about 30% of cases. Cirrhosis and malignancy are the most frequent local predisposing factors in adults. Portal vein thrombosis may present acutely with a sudden onset of severe abdominal pain, or chronically with clinical features of portal hypertension (varices, ascites, and splenomegaly) and/or portal biliopathy (jaundice, biliary colic, cholangitis, and pancreatitis).

A.W.H. Chan et al., *Atlas of Liver Pathology*, Atlas of Anatomic Pathology,
DOI 10.1007/978-1-4614-9114-9_11, © Springer Science+Business Media New York 2014

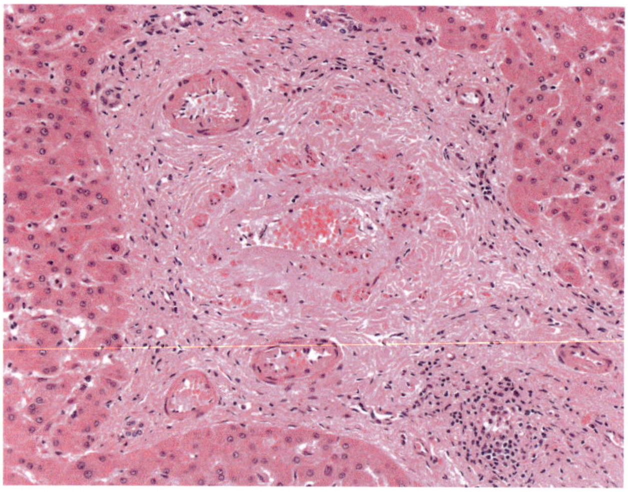

Fig. 11.2 Portal vein thrombosis. A small portal vein radicle is involved by extension of thrombosis from a larger vein. An organizing thrombus is present, with incorporation of a fibrous scar into the muscular wall of the involved vein. Portal vein thrombosis typically is found in portal veins larger than 200 μm, which rarely are found in liver biopsy specimens. Complete fibrous obliteration, organisation with subtle intimal fibrosis or mural calcification, or recanalisation with complex fibrous webs may be found. Recurrent thrombosis is evidenced by multiple layers of mural fibrosis. Portal vein thrombi may extend into smaller portal veins, which may be obstructed by thrombi or replaced by a fibrous scar. Uninvolved small portal veins may be dilated and even herniate into the periportal hepatic parenchyma.

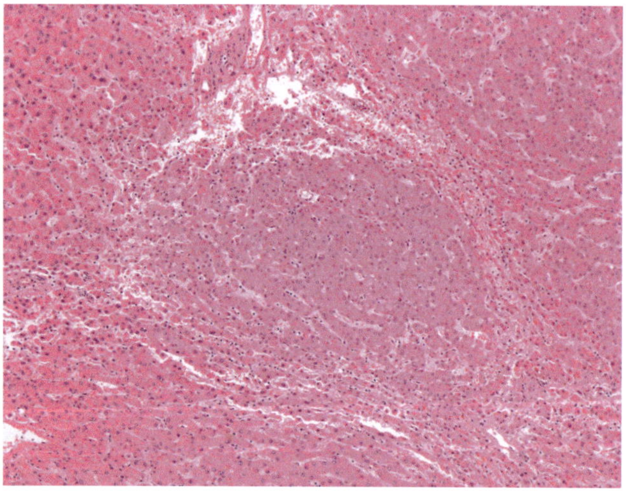

Fig. 11.3 Nodular regenerative hyperplasia in portal vein thrombosis. Parenchymal nodular change is present without any fibrosis. Nodular regenerative hyperplasia is characterised by diffuse benign transformation of the hepatic parenchyma into small regenerative nodules with minimal or no fibrosis. It sometimes is associated with thrombotic or nonthrombotic obliteration of small portal veins and, occasionally, small hepatic veins. Gordon-Sweets reticulin stain highlights the characteristic peripheral condensation of reticulin fibres in nodular regenerative hyperplasia. Drugs and toxins are major causes of nodular regenerative hyperplasia; others include autoimmune diseases, inflammatory diseases, haematologic diseases, congenital or acquired immunodeficiency, primary biliary cirrhosis, and cystinosis.

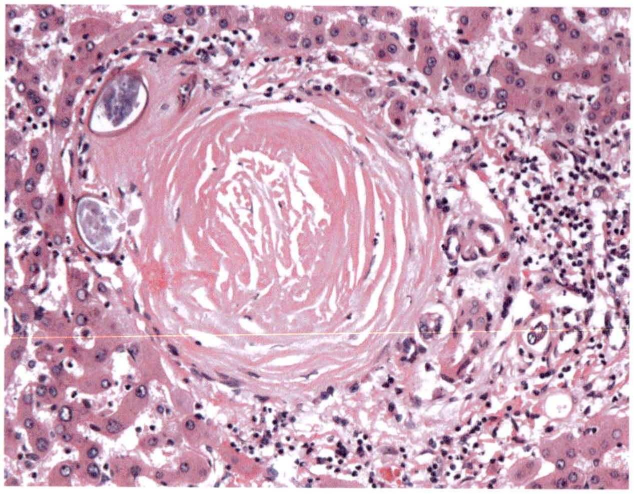

Fig. 11.4 Obliterative portal venopathy in schistosomiasis. This portal tract contains a fibrous obliterated portal vein and *Schistosoma* ova. Obliterative portal venopathy is a rare cause of portal hypertension secondary to the obstruction of small portal veins. It is associated with portal-based inflammation (e.g., primary biliary cirrhosis, primary sclerosing cholangitis, sarcoidosis, schistosomiasis, and congenital hepatic fibrosis), vasculitis (e.g., polyarteritis nodosa, rheumatic arthritis, and systemic lupus erythematosus), thrombosis (e.g., extension from large portal vein thrombosis, local stasis in cirrhosis), congestive portal venopathy (e.g., Budd-Chiari syndrome, cirrhosis), and drug-induced vascular injury (e.g., from azathioprine, arsenic compounds, mercaptopurine, methotrexate, oral contraceptives, oxaliplatin, and vinyl chloride).

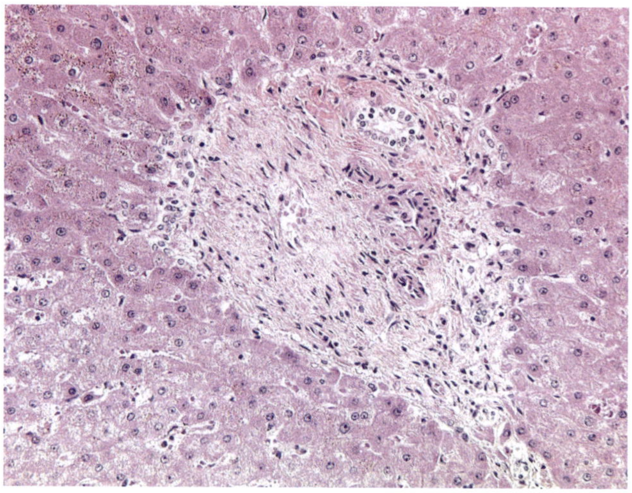

Fig. 11.5 Hepatoportal sclerosis. This portal tract contains a largely obliterated portal vein and is accompanied by mild portal fibrosis. Hepatoportal sclerosis may be regarded as an idiopathic form of obliterative portal venopathy. Many synonyms exist in the literature, including noncirrhotic portal hypertension, idiopathic portal hypertension, (benign) intrahepatic portal hypertension, noncirrhotic portal fibrosis, and Banti disease. Clinically, patients present with features of portal hypertension in the absence of chronic liver disease, cirrhosis, or obstructed extrahepatic portal vein obstruction.

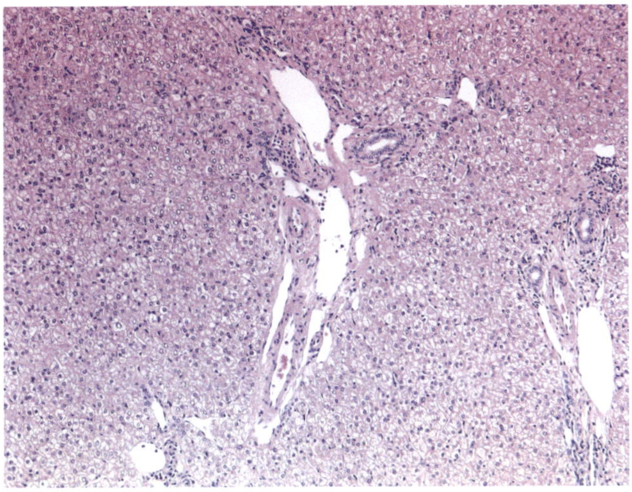

Fig. 11.6 Hepatoportal sclerosis. Multiple dilated portal venous channels are present. In obliterative portal venopathy and hepatoportal sclerosis, occluded small portal veins largely are replaced by fibrous tissues and may disappear. The involved portal tracts usually are expanded by fibrosis. Uninvolved small portal veins may be dilated and may increase in number, with herniation into the periportal hepatic parenchyma. Sinusoidal dilatation, a variable degree of parenchymal atrophy, and occasional bridging fibrosis may be found.

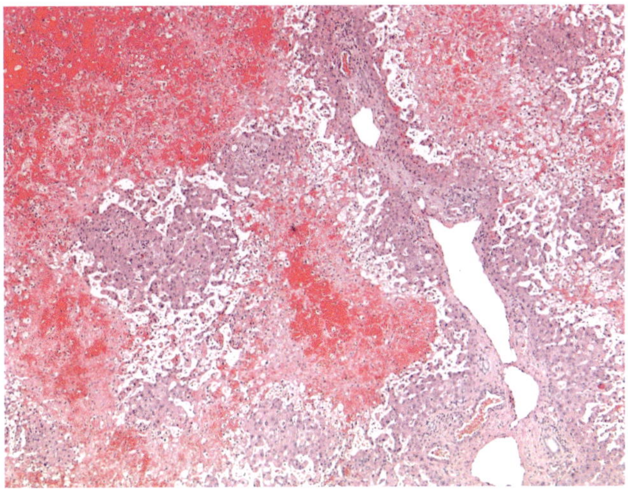

Fig. 11.8 Liver in Budd-Chiari syndrome. This thrombosed hepatic vein is associated with perivenular haemorrhagic necrosis and sinusoidal dilatation. Budd-Chiari syndrome currently is defined as a broad spectrum of diseases associated with hepatic venous outflow tract obstruction, irrespective of the level or aetiology of obstruction. Cardiac and pericardial diseases and sinusoidal obstruction syndrome are excluded from this definition. Budd-Chiari syndrome is classified as primary (intramural obstruction by thrombosis or phlebitis) or secondary (extramural obstruction by space-occupying lesion). Thrombosis is the commonest cause of large hepatic vein obstruction and is associated with hypercoagulative status, endothelial injury, and stasis. The classical clinical triad of acute Budd-Chiari syndrome is painful hepatomegaly, ascites, and liver dysfunction. However, up to 20% of patients are asymptomatic.

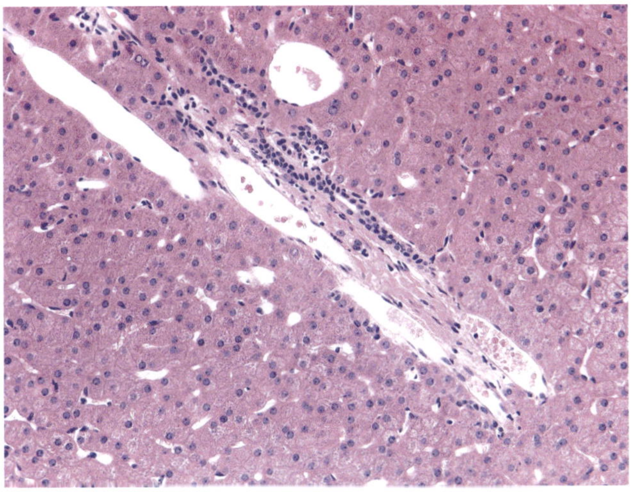

Fig. 11.7 Hepatoportal sclerosis. Dilated portal venous channels herniate into the periportal hepatic parenchyma. Hepatoportal sclerosis essentially is a diagnosis of exclusion. Clinical, serologic, radiologic, and histologic correlations are required to eliminate other aetiologies of small portal vein obliteration. Careful histologic examination should be performed to rule out primary biliary cirrhosis (florid duct lesions, portal granulomas), primary sclerosing cholangitis (fibro-obliterative bile duct lesions), sarcoidosis (noncaseating granulomas), schistosomiasis (ova and haemozoin pigments), congenital hepatic fibrosis (ductal plate malformation), and polyarteritis nodosa (active or healed vasculitis). Exclusion of cirrhosis also is crucial to establish the diagnosis of hepatoportal sclerosis.

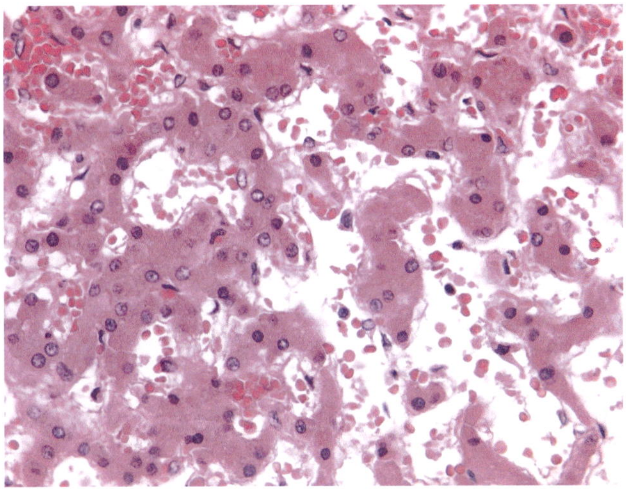

Fig. 11.9 Liver in Budd-Chiari syndrome. Dilated sinusoids and extravasation of red cells into the space of Disse may be seen. Acute hepatic vein thrombosis is associated with perivenular congestion, necrosis, sinusoidal dilatation, and extravasation of red cells into the space of Disse. Thrombosed hepatic veins later may become completely obliterated, organised with subtle intimal fibrosis, or recanalised with multiple venous lumina. Recurrent thrombosis is characterised by multiple layers of mural fibrosis. Pericellular/perisinusoidal fibrosis and atrophy of hepatocytes may be found. Fibrous septa bridging occluded hepatic veins may produce a venocentric cirrhosis or so-called reversed lobulation cirrhosis. Secondary portal vein thrombosis frequently is found. Nodular regenerative hyperplasia and focal nodular hyperplasia-like large regenerative nodules also may be observed.

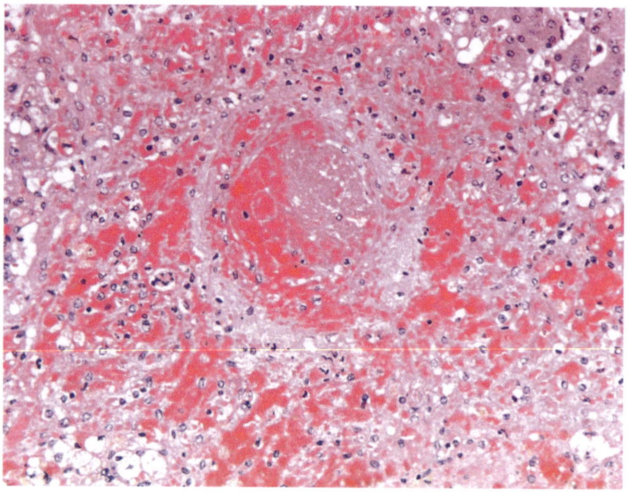

Fig. 11.10 Liver in Budd-Chiari syndrome. A thrombosed hepatic vein may be seen, associated with prominent perivenular haemorrhagic necrosis. Pathologically, Budd-Chiari syndrome may be indistinguishable from sinusoidal obstruction syndrome, obliterative hepatic venopathy, and congestive hepatopathy secondary to heart failure or constrictive pericarditis. Demonstration of thrombosis in large hepatic veins is difficult on liver biopsy, as sampling of large hepatic veins is uncommon in needle biopsy specimens.

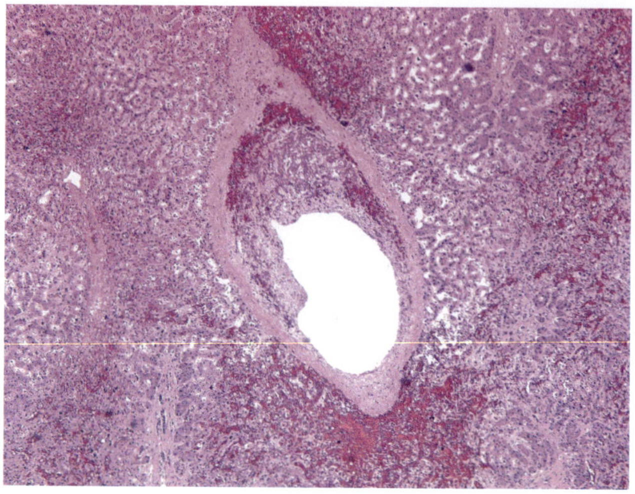

Fig. 11.12 Liver in Budd-Chiari syndrome. A large hepatic vein is partially occluded by a fibrin clot containing basophilic immune complex material in a patient with antiphospholipid syndrome. Clinical, serologic, radiologic, and histologic correlations are required to establish the underlying aetiology of Budd-Chiari syndrome. Liver biopsy is useful in confirming the diagnosis, excluding other aetiologies of liver dysfunction, assessing disease severity in terms of necrosis and fibrosis, and determining the underlying cause (e.g., vasculitis, sarcoid noncaseating granuloma, pyogenic abscess, mycetoma, or neoplasm). To minimize the problems associated with sampling, biopsy cores from two or more sites are recommended.

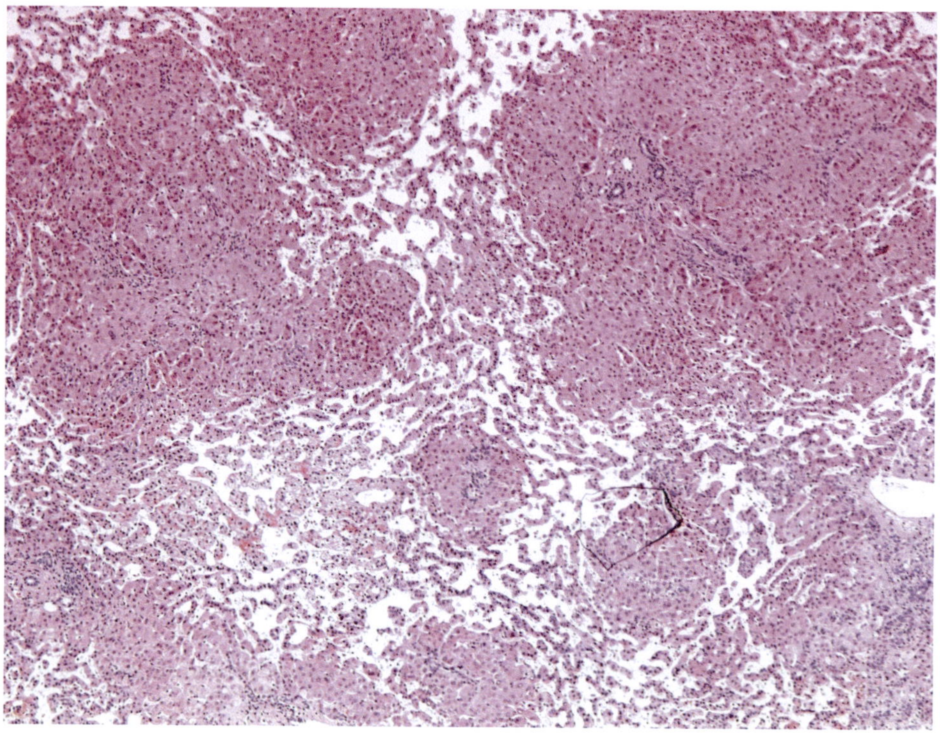

Fig. 11.11 Liver in Budd-Chiari syndrome. Prominent sinusoidal dilatation of zones 3 and 2 is associated with atrophied hepatocytes. Sinusoidal dilatation usually is accompanied by atrophy of hepatocytes and may be caused by hepatic venous outflow tract obstruction, portal vein obstruction, or increased arterial flow. Oral contraception, pregnancy, sickle cell anaemia, and various chronic wasting illnesses (e.g., tuberculosis, HIV, Hodgkin lymphoma, renal cell carcinoma) also may be associated with sinusoidal dilatation.

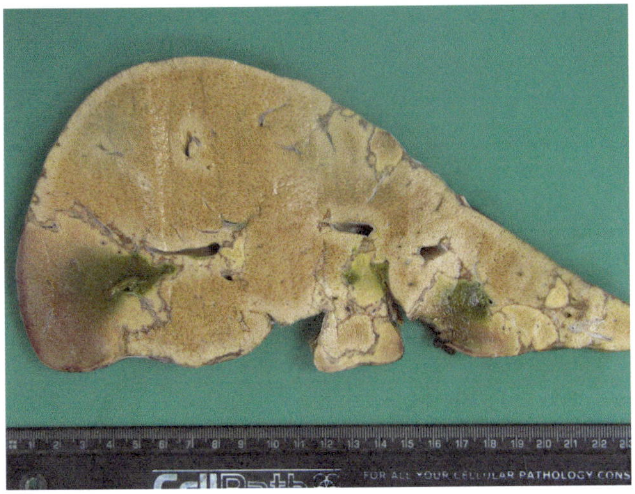

Fig. 11.13 Acute hepatic artery thrombosis. There are wedge-shaped infarcts in the subcapsular region, associated with extravasation of bile. Hepatic artery thrombosis is uncommon but important in two situations, namely liver transplantation and transarterial chemoembolization for hepatic tumour. Hepatic artery thrombosis is the commonest vascular complication in liver allograft and affects 2.5% to 11% of patients post transplantation, particularly children and patients receiving reduced-size grafts. Transarterial chemoembolisation is a regional treatment for primary hepatocellular carcinoma and, occasionally, metastases. Pathologically, hepatic artery thrombosis is characterised by ischaemic hepatic necrosis of varying sizes and ischaemic cholangitis.

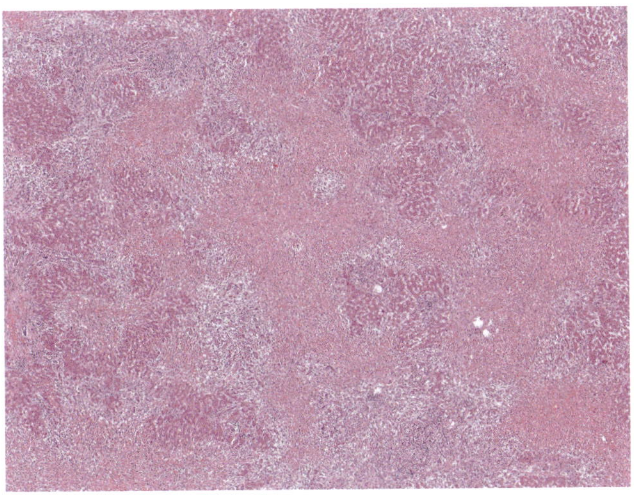

Fig. 11.14 Acute hepatic ischaemia in a patient with shock secondary to ruptured hepatocellular carcinoma. Ischaemic necrosis is present in zones 3 and 2 and is accompanied by marked congestion. Hepatic infarction is defined as ischaemic necrosis of at least two contiguous acini. The dual blood supply from the hepatic artery and portal vein generally protects the liver from ischaemic injury. However, generalised hepatic infarction may occur in shock, disseminated intravascular coagulation, toxaemia of pregnancy, and combined thrombosis of the hepatic artery/portal vein, hepatic artery/hepatic vein, and hepatic vein/portal vein.

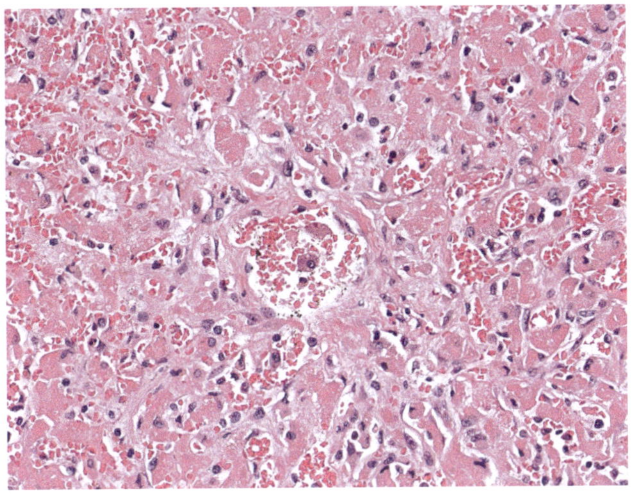

Fig. 11.15 Acute hepatic ischaemia in a patient with shock secondary to ruptured hepatocellular carcinoma. Coagulative necrosis may be seen in the perivenular region and accompanied by sinusoidal congestion. The differential diagnosis of the histologic picture of acute hepatic ischaemia includes other vascular disorders (e.g., Budd-Chiari syndrome, sinusoidal obstructive syndrome), drug/toxin-induced acute hepatic necrosis (e.g., acetaminophen), and necrosis associated with nonhepatotropic viral infections (e.g., herpes simplex virus and adenovirus).

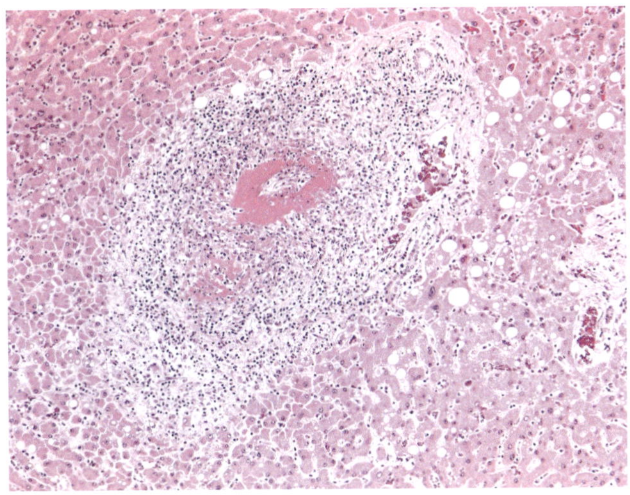

Fig. 11.16 Arteritis in polyarteritis nodosa. Fibrinoid necrosis of the hepatic arterial wall is seen, associated with a dense inflammatory infiltrate. The hepatic arteries may be involved by a vasculitic process in polyarteritis nodosa, Churg-Strauss syndrome, Wegener granulomatosis, systemic lupus erythematosus and rheumatoid arthritis. Certain drugs, including allopurinol, chlorothiazide, chlorpropamide, penicillin, phenylbutazone, phenytoin, and sulphonamide, also may cause arteritis in the liver. Most cases are asymptomatic, but a few cases may be complicated by hepatic artery aneurysm, hepatic rupture, and infarction. Obliteration of small portal veins secondary to small hepatic artery vasculitis may lead to nodular regenerative hyperplasia and portal hypertension.

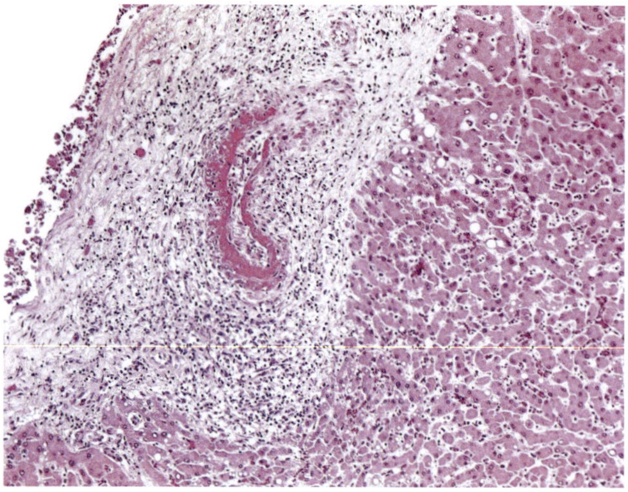

Fig. 11.17 Arteritis in polyarteritis nodosa. Fibrinoid necrosis of the hepatic arterial wall. The features of arteritis in the liver are the same as those in other organs.

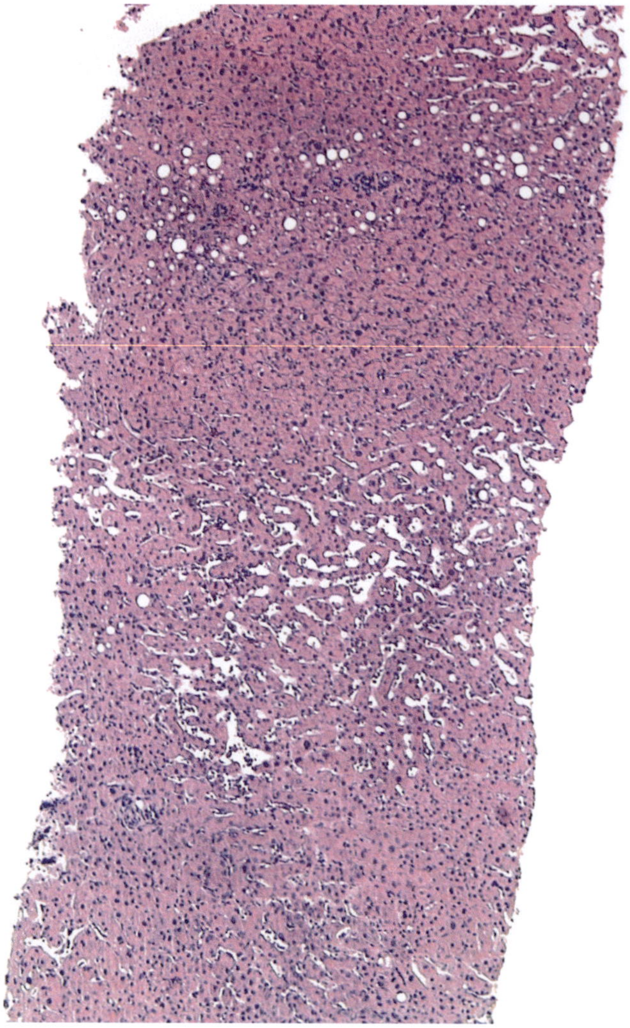

Fig. 11.18 Sinusoidal dilatation induced by oral contraceptive use. There is marked midzonal sinusoidal dilatation. Sinusoidal dilatation may be caused by hepatic venous outflow tract obstruction, portal vein obstruction, or increased arterial flow. Oral contraceptive treatment, pregnancy, sickle cell anaemia, and various chronic wasting illnesses (e.g., tuberculosis, HIV, Hodgkin lymphoma, renal cell carcinoma) also may be associated with sinusoidal dilatation. Sinusoidal dilatation may be accompanied by atrophy of the hepatocytes, focal apoptosis, and pericellular/perisinusoidal fibrosis. *Infarct of Zahn* is the term often used for localized sinusoidal dilatation and hepatocytic atrophy associated with regional portal vein obstruction. Sinusoidal dilatation is also seen in the inflammatory type of hepatocellular adenoma commonly associated with oral contraceptive use.

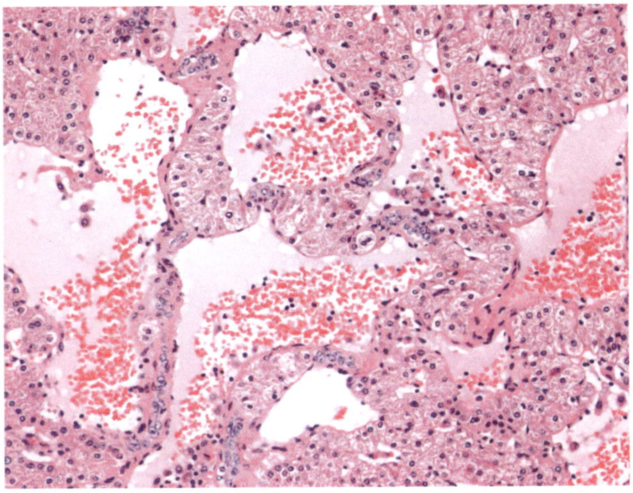

Fig. 11.19 Peliosis hepatis. Dilated sinusoidal spaces are separated by benign hepatocyte plates and partially lined by bland endothelial cells. Peliosis hepatis is the presence of cystic blood-filled spaces due to loss of integrity of the sinusoidal wall. Most cases represent incidental findings, but rarely, it may present with haemoperitoneum secondary to rupture. It is associated with certain drugs (e.g., anabolic steroids, oestrogenic steroids, corticosteroids, azathioprine, methotrexate, and 6-mercaptopurine), infection (e.g., bartonellosis, tuberculosis, and leprosy), and hairy cell leukaemia. Peliosis hepatis associated with *Bartonella* species also is referred to as bacillary peliosis and is restricted to patients with AIDS and other immunocompromised states. Bacillary peliosis is manifest by peliosis of the spleen and lymph nodes, in addition to the liver, and commonly is associated with bacillary angiomatosis of the skin and other organs.

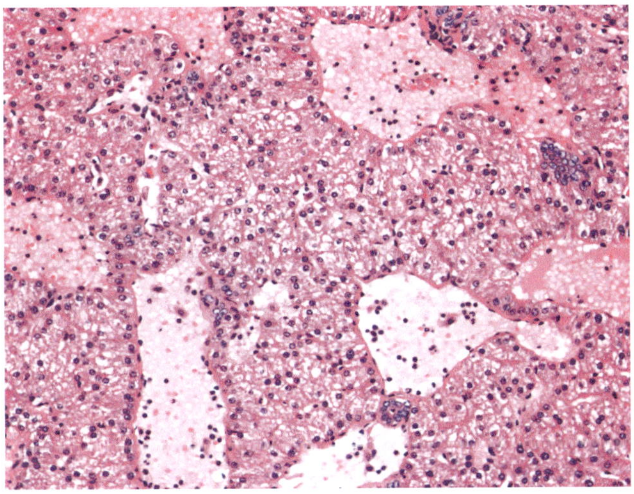

Fig. 11.20 Peliosis hepatis. Peliosis hepatis is composed of cystic blood-filled spaces from millimetres to a few centimetres. The endothelial lining may be absent initially but reappears after reendothelialisation. Rupture of the sinusoidal wall is evident by disruption of reticulin fibres, demonstrated by Gordon-Sweets reticulin stain. Warthin-Starry stain and immunostains for *Bartonella* may be helpful in ruling out bacillary peliosis.

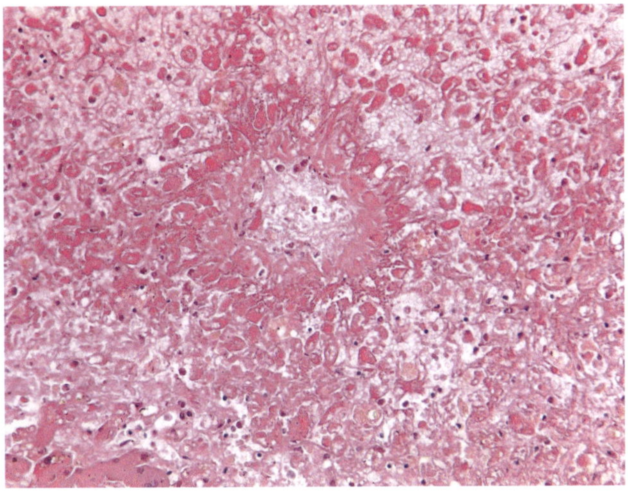

Fig. 11.21 Acute sinusoidal obstruction syndrome. Hepatic vein obstruction with subintimal fibrin deposition is associated with extensive zone 3 haemorrhagic necrosis. Sinusoidal obstruction syndrome, previously referred to as veno-occlusive disease or toxic sinusoidal injury, is strongly associated with the use of chemotherapeutic agents and radiation. A similar and somewhat confusing term, *veno-occlusive lesion*, sometimes is used to describe obliteration of small hepatic veins by injuries other than those associated with drugs or radiation; *obliterative hepatic venopathy* perhaps is a better term. Sinusoidal obstruction syndrome may present clinically in acute, subacute, or chronic form. Mortality is up to 20% to 50% with acute sinusoidal obstruction syndrome.

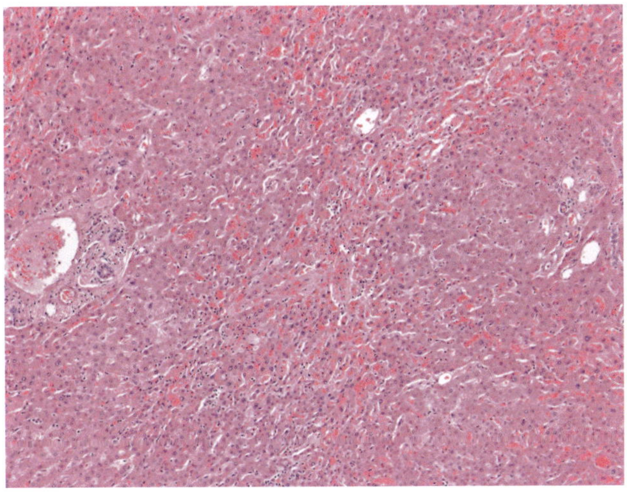

Fig. 11.22 Acute sinusoidal obstruction syndrome. Sinusoidal congestion and fibrin deposition are accompanied by hepatocyte drop-out. Sinusoidal obstruction syndrome is characterised pathologically by subintimal oedema, haemorrhage, and fibrin deposition in sinusoids and small hepatic veins less than 300 μm. Sinusoidal congestion and haemorrhagic necrosis usually are found. As the disease advances, involved hepatic veins may become completely obliterated, organised with subtle intimal fibrosis, or recanalised with multiple venous lumina. Pericellular/perisinusoidal fibrosis and atrophy of hepatocytes may be found.

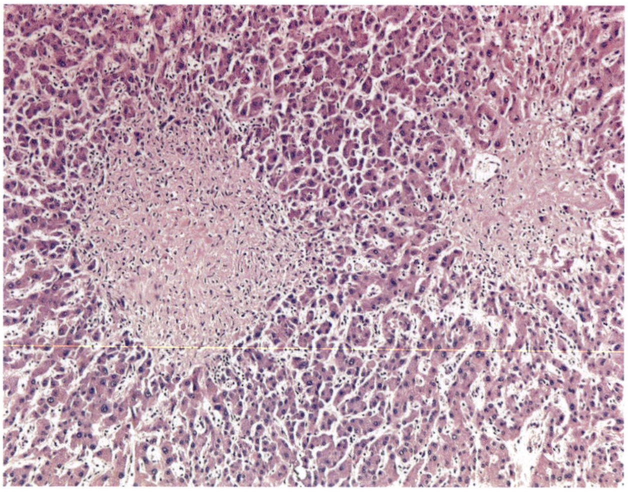

Fig. 11.23 Chronic sinusoidal obstruction syndrome. Fibrous obliteration of small hepatic veins is associated with perivenular fibrosis and hepatocellular atrophy. Acute sinusoidal obstructive syndrome may be mimicked by acute Budd-Chiari syndrome with retrograde extension of thrombi into smaller venules. Absence of thrombi in large hepatic veins on imaging excludes acute Budd-Chiari syndrome. The histologic differential diagnoses of chronic sinusoidal obstruction are the conditions associated with perivenular fibrosis, including alcoholic and nonalcoholic steatohepatitis, congestive heart failure, chronic Budd-Chiari syndrome, and sickle cell disease.

12 Premalignant Lesions

Like other epithelial neoplasms, both hepatocellular carcinoma (HCC) and cholangiocarcinoma arising in the background of cirrhosis and chronic inflammatory biliary disorders are thought to originate from a premalignant stage.

The histologic appearance of the precursor lesions of HCC has been the subject of extensive investigations and debate for many years. This probably results from the complex tridimensional structure of the hepatic plates and the architectural changes characteristic of cirrhosis, which result in a complex array of premalignant hepatocellular changes, clonal expansions, and nodular proliferations, with a blurred transition to overt malignancy. During the process of hepatocarcinogenesis, several phenotypic changes arise, often designated as premalignant lesions, including hepatocellular cytologic changes, microscopic expansile foci (dysplastic foci, up to 1 mm), and macroscopic nodular lesions (dysplastic nodules).

In contrast, biliary dysplasia is conceptually and morphologically similar to dysplasia of other "luminal" epithelium, and follows similar rules and criteria. Infiltration through the basal membrane marks the transition from in situ disease to invasive malignancy. Biliary premalignant lesions bear considerable similarities to their pancreatic counterparts, probably the result of their common embryologic origin.

A.W.H. Chan et al., *Atlas of Liver Pathology*, Atlas of Anatomic Pathology,
DOI 10.1007/978-1-4614-9114-9_12,

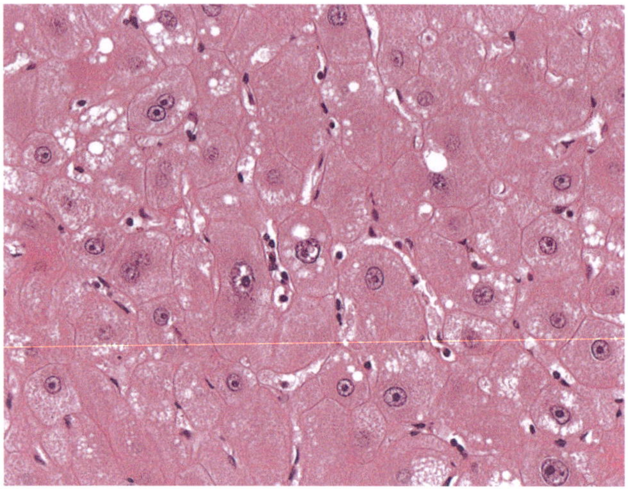

Fig. 12.1 Large cell change. These hepatocytes exhibit cellular and nuclear enlargement, nuclear pleomorphism and binucleation, prominent nucleoli, and a preserved nucleocytoplasmic ratio. Large cell change, formerly known as large cell dysplasia, now is believed to represent a pathophysiologic nuclear polyploidy, a degenerative senescent change occurring as a consequence of chronic liver injury, and in particular cholestasis. Large cell change is best regarded as a predictive marker associated with the risk of HCC rather than a genuine premalignant lesion. However, recent data suggest that large cell change, in some situations, may be a genuine premalignant lesion.

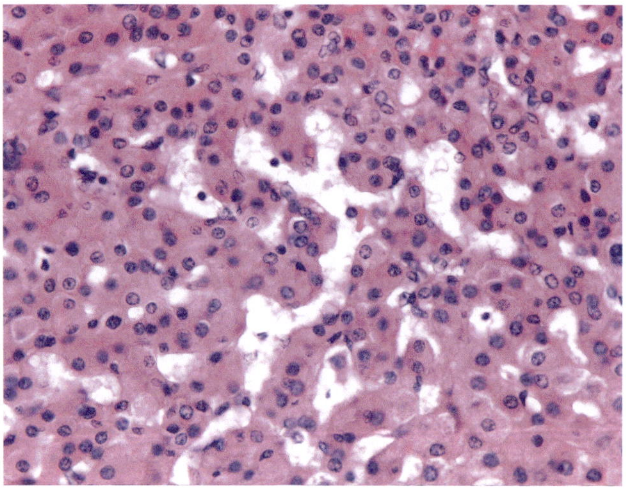

Fig. 12.2 Small cell change. Hepatocytes exhibit decreased cell volume, minimal nuclear pleomorphism, increased nucleocytoplasmic ratio, and increased nuclear density. Small cell change generally is believed to be an early premalignant lesion because of its higher prevalence in cirrhotic livers with HCC than in those without, high proliferative activity, a morphologic continuum between small cell change and HCC, an immunophenotype similar to that of hepatic progenitor cells, and similar chromosomal alterations in small cell change and adjacent HCC. Markedly reduced expression of p16 and p21 and an accumulation of DNA damage occur in small cell change and HCC compared with large cell change, suggesting that small cell change represents a more "advanced" lesion than large cell change.

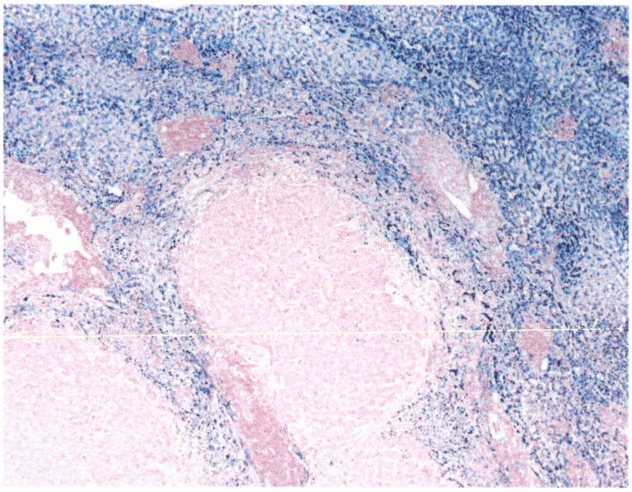

Fig. 12.3 Iron-free foci. Several hepatic nodules are free of haemosiderin deposition in a liver explant of hereditary haemochromatosis. Iron-free foci in hereditary haemochromatosis are shown to be more frequent in livers with HCC (50.0%) than in those without (8.3%) and to have a higher proliferative index and coexisting large cell change/small cell change (71.4%). HCCs in hereditary haemochromatosis not uncommonly are iron-free, and the sequential development from iron-free nodules to iron-free HCC in a recent rat model supports these foci as premalignant lesions. However, the underlying mechanisms of iron resistance in these foci and subsequent malignant transformation remain unknown.

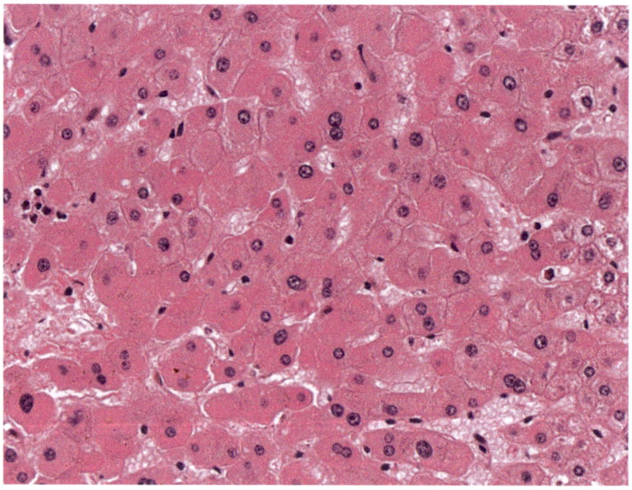

Fig. 12.4 Oncocytic focus. A group of hepatocytes exhibit deeply eosinophilic granular cytoplasm. Apart from these well-documented atypias, there are other hepatocellular cytologic changes, collectively termed *foci of altered hepatocytes*, described in several animal models in early hepatocarcinogenesis caused by chemicals, radiation, and chronic infection with hepadnaviruses. Although some foci of altered hepatocytes, including glycogen-storing clear cell foci, clear cell–predominated mixed cell foci, and oncocytic foci, also have been observed in chronic liver disease with or without HCC in humans, there is insufficient evidence to establish their definite role in human hepatocarcinogenesis.

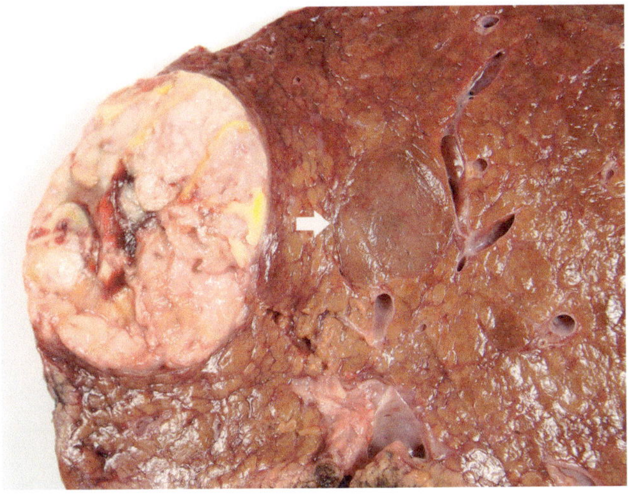

Fig. 12.5 Dysplastic nodule. A 1.7-cm vague tan nodule (*arrow*) is seen arising in a cirrhotic background and is adjacent to an HCC. Dysplastic nodules are macroscopically distinct from surrounding cirrhotic regenerative nodules by their size (varying from a few millimetres to a few centimetres), colour, texture, and degree of bulging. They are classified as low or high grade according to the degree of architectural and cytologic atypia. Histologically, both low-grade and high-grade dysplastic nodules are hypercellular; increased cell density in high-grade lesions may be up to twice that of the surrounding liver. Both also often exhibit features suggesting clonal-like cell population, such as iron or copper accumulation, or steatosis in a background liver without significant fatty change.

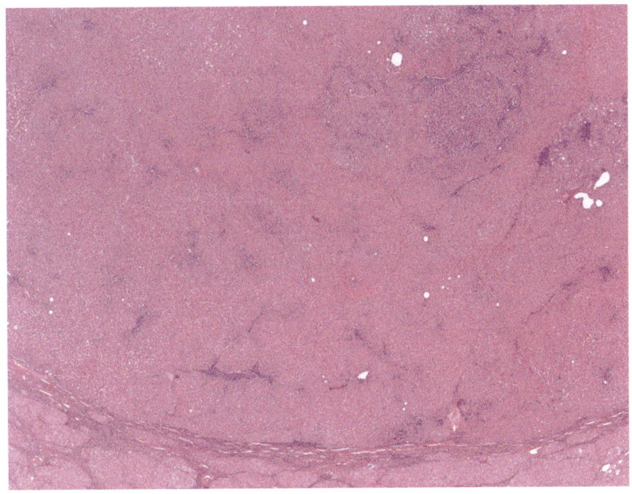

Fig. 12.7 High-grade dysplastic nodule. A 2-cm hepatic nodule demonstrate a nodule-in-nodule pattern with a few subnodules (*upper right*). High-grade dysplastic nodules usually are vaguely nodular and contain significant architectural and/or cytologic atypia. Atypical architectural features include a nodule-in-nodule pattern, pseudo-acinar formation, and thickened trabeculae up to three cells thick. Cytologic changes comprise focal or diffuse small cell change, iron-free foci, focal steatosis with Mallory-Denk bodies or intracellular hyaline inclusions, and clear cell change.

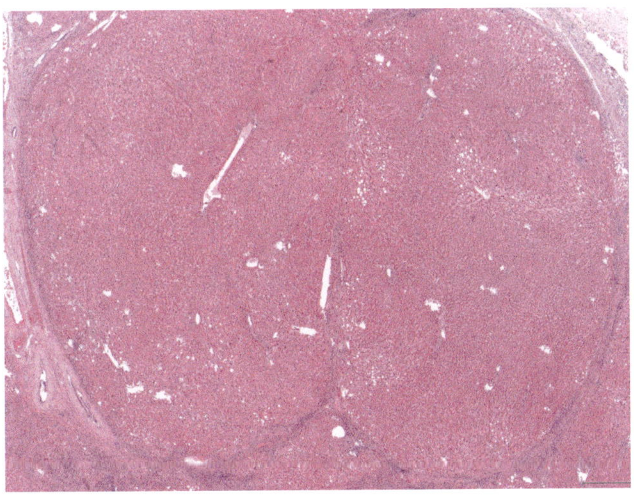

Fig. 12.6 Low-grade dysplastic nodule. An 8-mm hepatic nodule is surrounded by a fibrous pseudo-capsule and contains some intranodular portal tracts. Apart from scattered foci of large cell change, there is no other noticeable architectural or cytologic atypia. Low-grade dysplastic nodules usually are distinct rather than vaguely nodular because of the presence of a condensed fibrous scar at its periphery. Architectural atypia is absent, whereas cytologic atypia is minimal, with occasional large cell changes and absent mitoses. It often contains intranodular portal tracts, with only very rare aberrant unpaired or nontriad arterioles. It is impossible to distinguish between low-grade dysplastic and large regenerative nodules confidently by morphology alone in the current consensus, and it has been argued that the latter term should no longer be used.

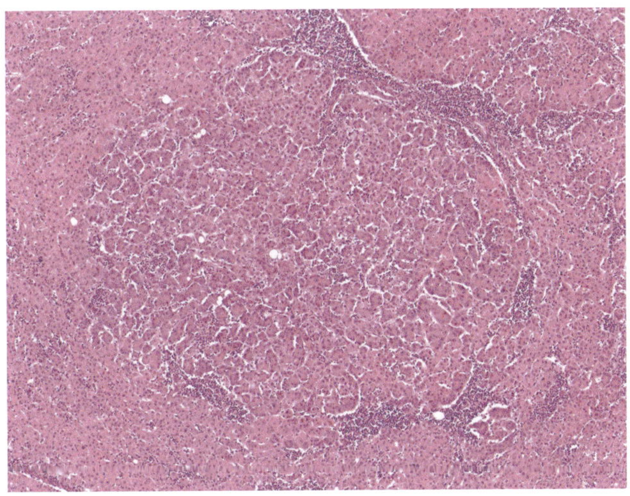

Fig. 12.8 High-grade dysplastic nodule. Shown is a small distinct subnodule within a dysplastic nodule (nodule-in-nodule pattern). Subnodules represent foci of clonal expansion. Among all the atypical changes found in high-grade dysplastic nodules, the nodule-in-nodule pattern is the most worrisome feature, because HCC not uncommonly emerges from such subnodules.

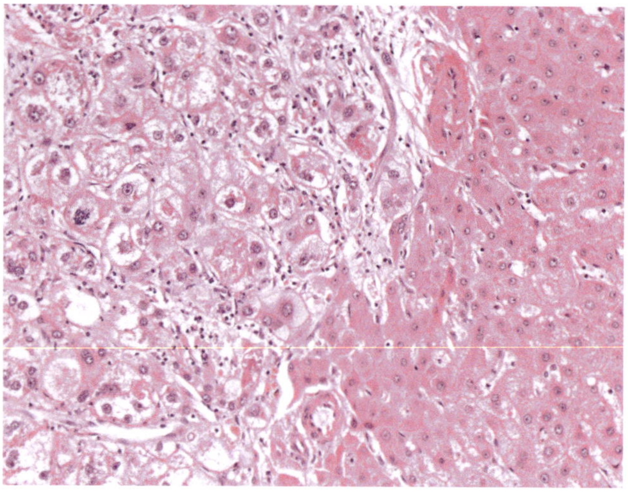

Fig. 12.9 High-grade dysplastic nodule. A subnodule of swollen hepatocytes with clear cytoplasm and some Mallory-Denk bodies is present within a dysplastic nodule (nodule-in-nodule pattern). Two unpaired arterioles also are noted.

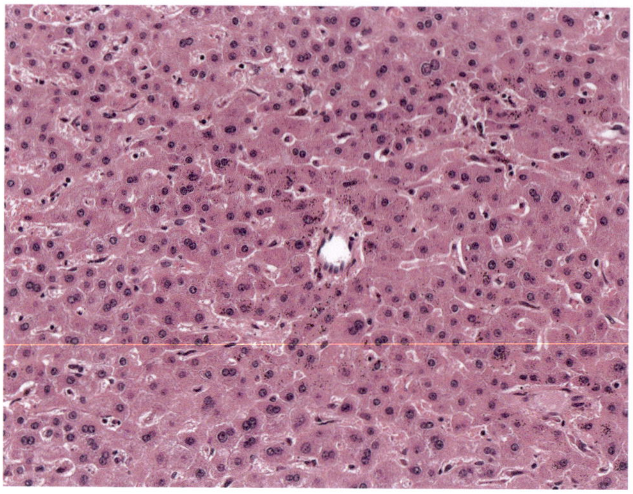

Fig. 12.11 High-grade dysplastic nodule. An unpaired or nontriad arteriole is present. Unpaired or nontriad arterioles are common findings in hepatocellular adenoma and HCC. High-grade dysplastic nodules occasionally contain unpaired arterioles, but low-grade dysplastic nodules usually do not. Unpaired arterioles indicate neovascularisation in tumourigenesis. Complete sinusoidal capillarisation, characterised by diffuse immunoreactivity to CD34 in the sinusoids, is a frequent phenomenon in HCC (82.5%–100%) associated with neovascularisation. This pattern is observed in only 20% and 2% of hepatocellular adenomas and high-grade dysplastic nodules, respectively. Patchy capillarisation may be observed in cirrhosis and low-grade dysplastic nodules. Immunostaining for CD34 serves as a useful diagnostic tool to differentiate HCC, dysplastic and large regeneration nodules.

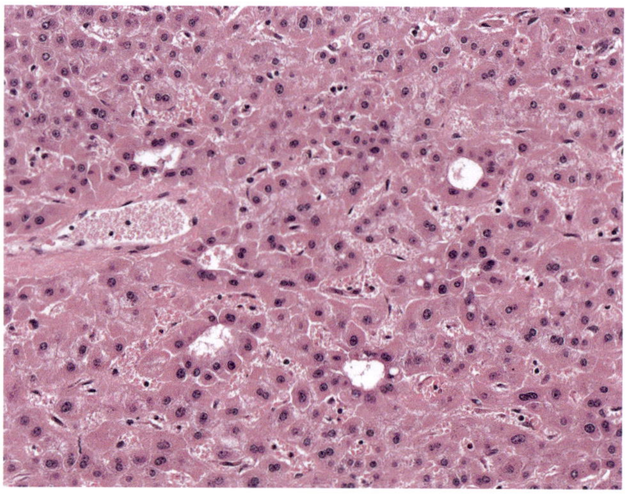

Fig. 12.10 High-grade dysplastic nodule. Several groups of hepatocytes are arranged in a pseudo-acinar pattern. Hepatocytes in the normal adult liver are arranged in single-cell plates. In rapidly proliferating foci, the hepatocyte plate is distorted to form a rosette, a pseudo-acinus, or a pseudo-gland. Such an abnormal architectural change may be observed in neoplastic (high-grade dysplastic nodule and well-differentiated carcinoma) and sometimes in very active nonneoplastic regenerating processes.

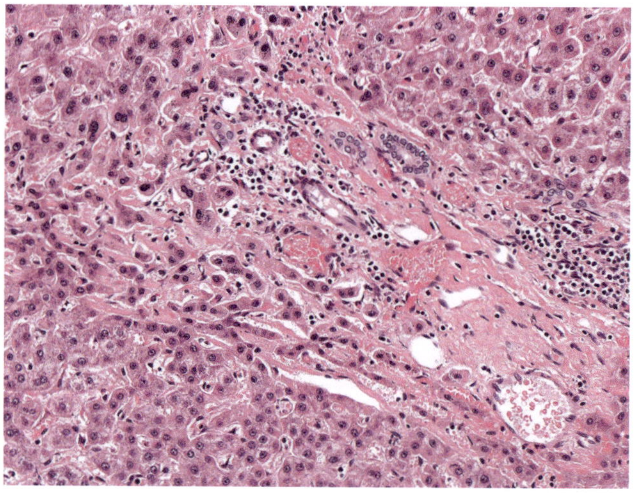

Fig. 12.12 Early hepatocellular carcinoma. An intratumoural portal tract is infiltrated by atypical hepatocytes without any ductular reaction. This phenomenon is designated as stromal invasion. Early HCC is also known as "small hepatocellular carcinoma of vaguely nodular type" and "small hepatocellular carcinoma with indistinct margin." There is a marked overlap in pathologic features between early HCCs and high-grade dysplastic nodules. Stromal invasion is considered to be helpful in differentiating early HCC from a high-grade dysplastic nodule. The absence of significant ductular reaction (with the aid of immunostains for cytokeratin 7/19) favours genuine stromal invasion rather than pseudo-invasion, but the distinction is often not straightforward.

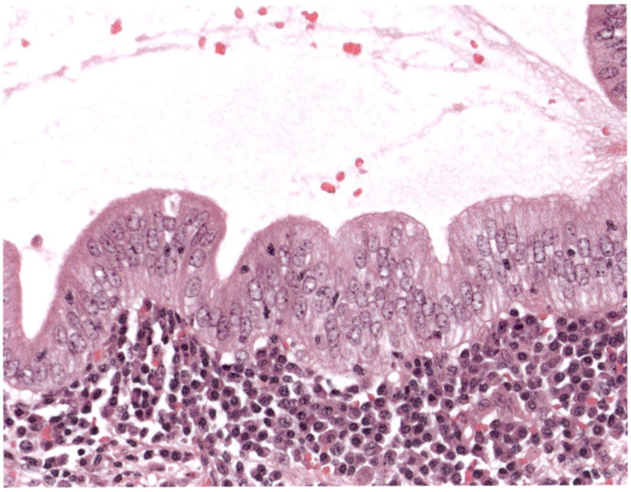

Fig. 12.13 Hyperplastic biliary epithelial cells. Benign biliary epithelial cells of a large intrahepatic duct exhibit uniform, round to oval-shaped and vesicular nuclei, mild nuclear pseudo-stratification, small distinct nucleoli, and preserved normal polarity. Reactive or hyperplastic change of biliary epithelial cells not uncommonly is encountered in chronic biliary diseases, and may be differentiated from biliary intraepithelial neoplasia (BilIN) by the bland cytologic appearance of the former.

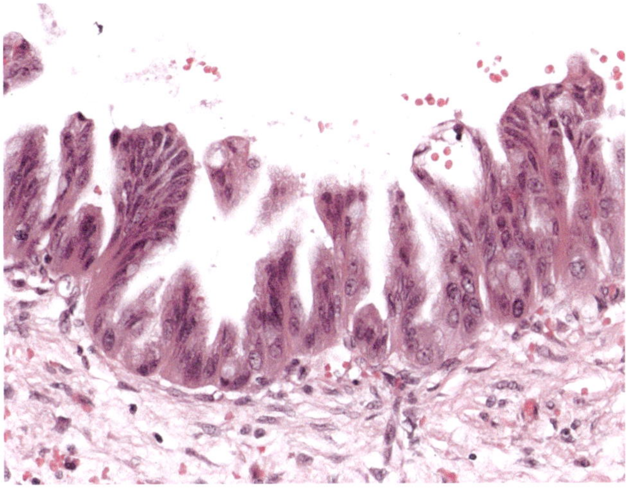

Fig. 12.15 Biliary intraepithelial neoplasia, grade 2 (BilIN-2). Moderately dysplastic biliary epithelial cells demonstrate round to oval-shaped vesicular nuclei, focal loss of polarity, mild nuclear pleomorphism, distinct nucleoli, and micropapillary growth. BilIN is thought to be a precursor to cholangiocarcinoma. It may be found in both extrahepatic and intrahepatic bile ducts. BilINs arising in intrahepatic bile ducts are associated mainly with chronic biliary disease such as primary sclerosing cholangitis, recurrent pyogenic cholangitis, congenital biliary diseases, and liver fluke infection, but also may be found in chronic hepatitis C, alcoholic cirrhosis, and thorotrast deposition to a lesser extent.

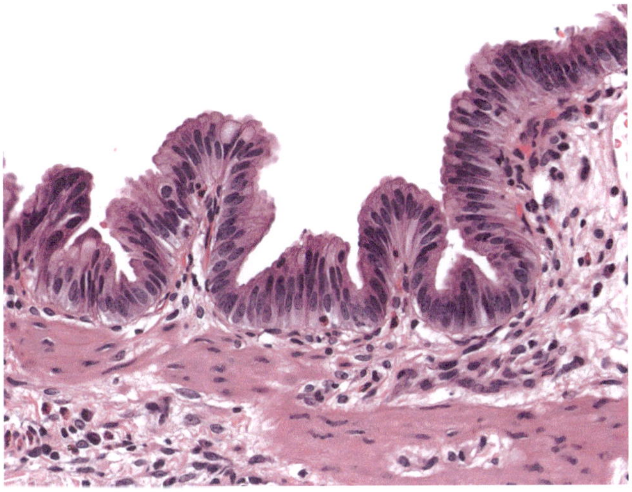

Fig. 12.14 Biliary intraepithelial neoplasia, grade 1 (BilIN-1). Mildly dysplastic biliary epithelial cells exhibit elongated hyperchromatic nuclei, largely preserved polarity, mild nuclear pseudo-stratification, and focal micropapillary growth. In the latest World Health Organization (WHO) classification, the terminology of BilIN is similar to that used in the exocrine pancreas (pancreatic intraepithelial neoplasia [PanIN]; note, however, that BilIN-1 is not equivalent to its pancreatic counterpart, PanIN-1, mucinous metaplasia). The three-tiered grading system (BilIN-1 to BilIN-3) depends mainly on the degree of cytologic atypia and corresponds to mild, moderate, and severe dysplasia, respectively. Such terms are applied to microscopic atypical biliary lesions with a flat or micropapillary growth pattern.

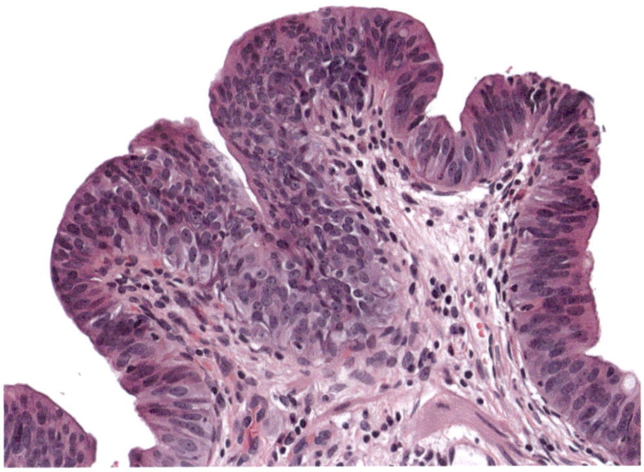

Fig. 12.16 Biliary intraepithelial neoplasia, grade 3 (BilIN-3). Severely dysplastic biliary epithelial cells are characterised by round to oval-shaped hyperchromatic nuclei, a marked loss of polarity, moderate nuclear pleomorphism, and distinct nucleoli. Although BilIN and intraductal papillary neoplasm of bile ducts (IPNB) both are considered precursor lesions of cholangiocarcinoma and share some similar pathologic characteristics, they are different in that (1) BilIN is a microscopic lesion with a flat or micropapillary configuration, whereas IPNB is a grossly or radiologically identifiable lesion with a papillary structure; (2) BilIN is associated with tubular cholangiocarcinoma, whereas IPNB is related to mucinous cholangiocarcinoma in addition to tubular neoplasms; and (3) BilIN typically is negative for MUC2 and CK20, but IPNB commonly is immunoreactive for MUC2 and CK20.

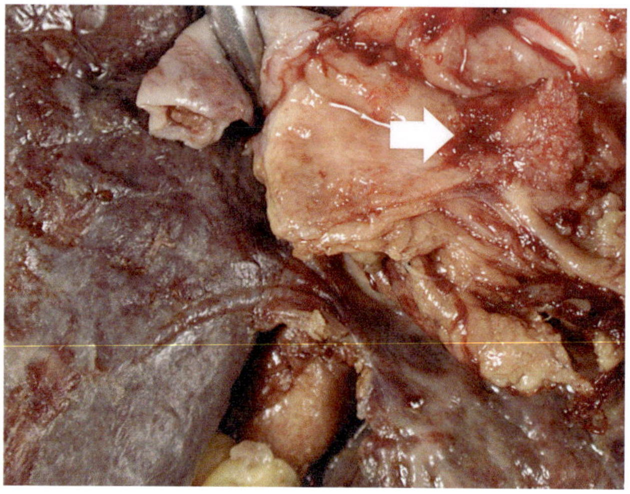

Fig. 12.17 Intraductal papillary neoplasm of bile ducts. A 0.6-cm friable, tan, polypoid, papillary mass is present in the common hepatic duct. IPNB, previously referred to as biliary papilloma or papillomatosis, was a term adopted in the latest WHO classification (4th edition, 2010), paralleling its pancreatic counterpart (intraductal papillary mucinous neoplasm). It is a grossly identifiable neoplasm characterised histologically by prominent papillary growth of atypical biliary epithelium with delicate fibrovascular cores, arising within the bile duct lumen. It commonly affects patients in the sixth to seventh decades. It usually is found in extrahepatic hilar or intrahepatic large bile ducts. It may arise from apparently normal bile ducts but more frequently is associated with primary sclerosing cholangitis, recurrent pyogenic cholangitis, congenital biliary diseases, and liver fluke infection.

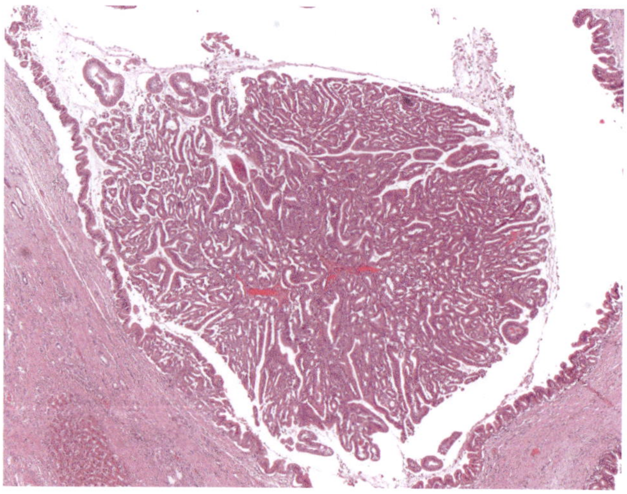

Fig. 12.18 Intraductal papillary neoplasm of bile ducts. A cystically dilated bile duct contains a papillary growth. IPNB is classified as low-, intermediate-, or high-grade IPNB according to the degree of cytologic atypia. IPNB may be categorized into invasive and noninvasive types, depending on whether invasive cholangiocarcinoma is present. Invasive IPNB also is referred to as IPNB with an associated invasive carcinoma. IPNB has a better clinical outcome than conventional cholangiocarcinoma. The 5-year survival of patients with noninvasive IPNB, invasive IPNB, and conventional cholangiocarcinoma is 100%, 53%, and 0%, respectively. Favourable prognostic factors for invasive IPNB include grossly visible mucin production, mucinous cholangiocarcinoma as the invasive component, and nonexpression of MUC1.

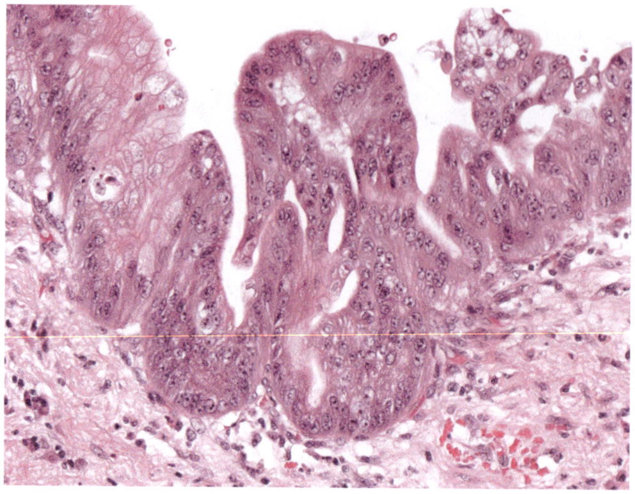

Fig. 12.19 Intraductal papillary neoplasm of bile ducts, pancreatobiliary type. A high-grade component (*centre* and *right*) is composed of atypical epithelial cells with roundish vesicular nuclei, prominent nucleoli, and a complete loss of polarity, whereas the low-/intermediate-grade component (*left*) is composed of atypical epithelial cells with roundish vesicular nuclei, prominent nucleoli, preserved polarity, and abundant apical mucin. IPNB has four distinct phenotypes: pancreatobiliary (50%), intestinal (40%), gastric (5%), and oncocytic (5%). Their associated invasive carcinomas usually show similar phenotypes. The oncocytic type is thought to be a variant of the pancreatobiliary type. About 70% to 80% of IPNB is associated with invasive tumour. The pancreatobiliary type commonly is associated with tubular cholangiocarcinoma, whereas the intestinal type typically is related to mucinous (colloid) carcinoma.

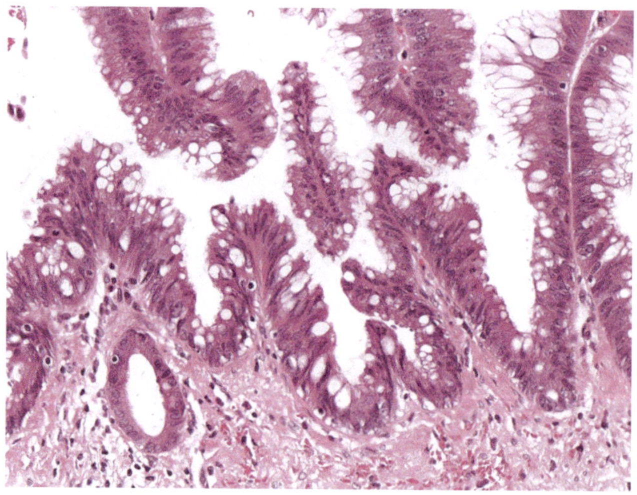

Fig. 12.20 Intraductal papillary neoplasm of bile ducts, intestinal type. The lining epithelial cells exhibit mild cytologic atypia. Some goblet cells also are present. More than 80% of IPNB cases show a MUC1⁻/MUC2⁺ immunophenotype. MUC2 is expressed more commonly in the intestinal type than in the pancreatobiliary and gastric types, whereas MUC1 expression usually is observed in the pancreatobiliary type. IPNB-associated tubular and mucinous invasive tumours are MUC1⁺/MUC2⁺ (70%) and MUC1⁻/MUC2⁺ (90%), respectively.

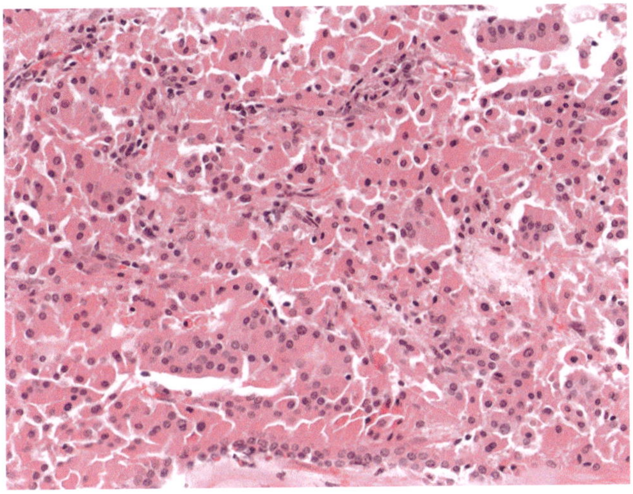

Fig. 12.21 Intraductal papillary neoplasm of bile ducts, oncocytic type. The lining epithelial cells exhibit mild cytologic atypia with abundant eosinophilic granular cytoplasm. IPNB is distinguished from BilIN by the presence of macroscopically visible intraductal lesions. The cystic type of IPNB, which is characterized by cystic ductal dilatation with prominent intraductal mucin accumulation, is differentiated from mucinous cystic neoplasm by the presence of direct luminal connection to the bile ducts and absence of an ovarian-type mesenchymal stroma.

13 Neoplasm-like Liver Lesions

Neoplasm-like liver lesions are mass-forming lesions that may develop in normal as well as diseased liver. They generally are considered to carry a low risk for neoplastic progression. They may be solid or cystic, solitary or multifocal. Hepatocellular lesions include focal nodular hyperplasia (FNH), a localised hyperplastic mass probably secondary to a vascular insult. Nodular regenerative hyperplasia has a similar pathogenesis but affects the liver more diffusely. In some cases, areas of nodular regenerative hyperplasia become dominant and form nodular lesions, which may be evident on imaging and cause diagnostic difficulties. Large regenerative nodules usually are observed in cirrhosis. They are similar to the background regenerative nodules, although larger, and are visible macroscopically in surgical specimens or on imaging. Inflammatory pseudotumour is a localised mass-forming inflammatory reaction. It usually is associated with other conditions, although in rare cases it has been shown to be neoplastic.

Mass-forming nonneoplastic tumour-like lesions in the liver may be solid or cystic, and solitary or multiple. Solid tumour-like lesions include FNH, nodular regenerative hyperplasia, large regenerative nodule, and inflammatory pseudotumour. Cystic neoplasm-like lesions include solitary bile duct cyst, obstructive dilatation of bile duct, ciliated foregut cyst, haemorrhagic cyst, and infective cyst (see Chapter 7).

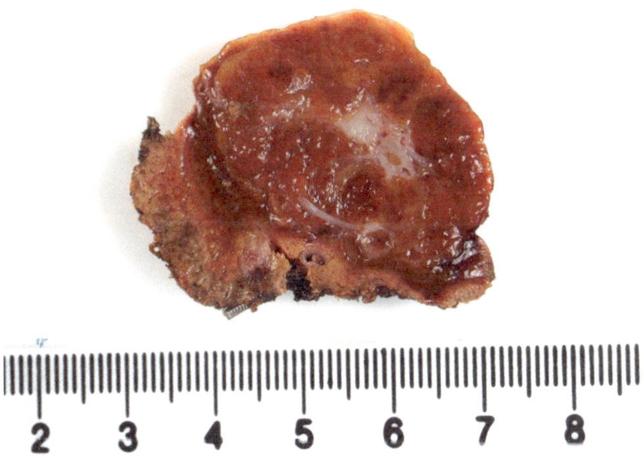

Fig. 13.1 Focal nodular hyperplasia. A tan, well-demarcated, nonencapsulated, and multilobulated subcapsular mass appears to contain a central whitish fibrous scar. FNH is the second commonest benign liver "tumour" following haemangioma and accounts for 8% of all primary liver masses. It affects 0.4% to 3% of the general population. The typical age of presentation is between 20 and 40 years. A marked female predominance (4:1 to 9:1) is observed. FNH may be solitary (67%) or multiple. It varies in size from a few millimetres to >10 cm. It usually is a well-demarcated, nonencapsulated, and multilobulated lesion. Central scar with radiating fibrous septa is characteristic but may be absent in some cases, particularly in variant FNH.

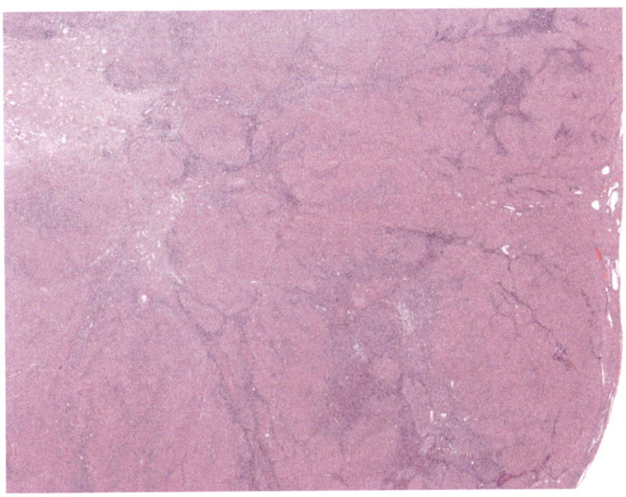

Fig. 13.2 Focal nodular hyperplasia. A multilobulated lesion contains a central scar with radiating fibrous septa that divide the surrounding hepatocytes into multiple lobules. In classical FNH, the central scar contains abnormal tortuous thick-walled arteries, whereas the radiating fibrous septa contain abnormal arterioles and a prominent ductular reaction. Interlobular bile ducts and portal veins typically are absent. The hepatic lobules are composed of hepatocytes arranged in plates one to two cells thick with an intact reticulin framework. Focal steatosis, mild inflammatory infiltrate, and chronic cholate stasis also may be found. The background liver usually is normal. A "map-like" staining pattern of glutamine synthetase is characteristic.

A.W.H. Chan et al., *Atlas of Liver Pathology*, Atlas of Anatomic Pathology,
DOI 10.1007/978-1-4614-9114-9_13, © Springer Science+Business Media New York 2014

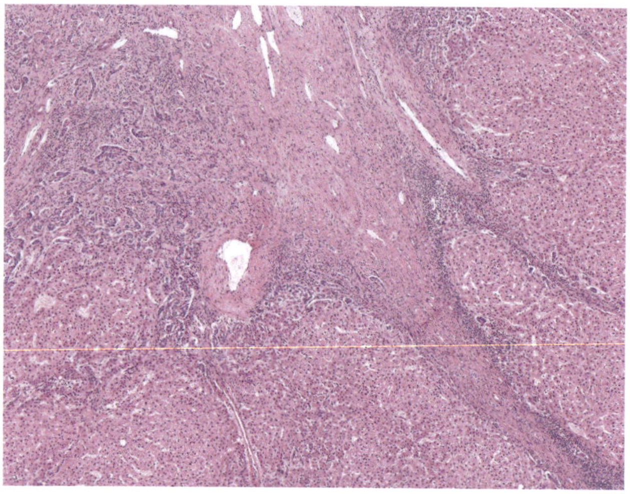

Fig. 13.3 Focal nodular hyperplasia. Radiating fibrous septa with thick-walled arteries divide the surrounding hepatocytes into multiple lobules and contain abnormal arterioles and a prominent ductular reaction. Variant forms of FNH exist, but there is no universal consensus regarding diagnostic criteria. Several different terms have been used: *early FNH*, *pre-FNH*, *subtle FNH*, and *FNH-like nodule*. These are characterised by the presence of diffuse steatosis, Mallory-Denk bodies, large cell change, and/or sinusoidal dilatation. A central scar usually is absent, whereas the ductular reaction in fibrous septa is minimal. The background liver is normal or contains coexisting vascular disorders (e.g., portal vein thrombosis or agenesis, hepatic vein thrombosis, hereditary haemorrhagic telangiectasia).

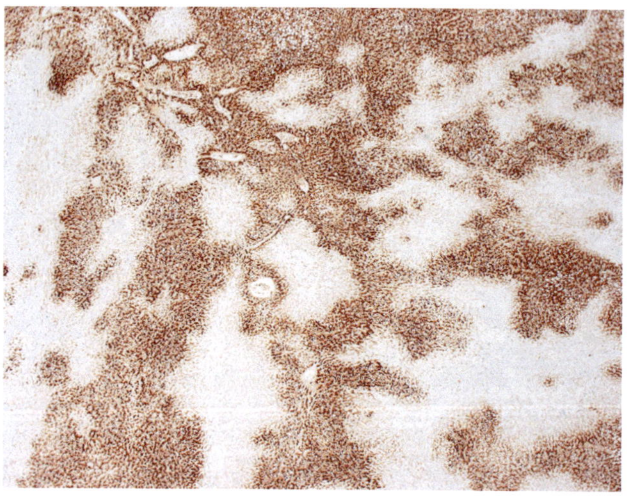

Fig. 13.4 Focal nodular hyperplasia exhibits a characteristic map-like staining pattern of glutamine synthetase. The key differential diagnosis is inflammatory hepatocellular adenoma, which previously considered a morphological (telangiectatic) variant of FNH. These are characterised by a focal or diffuse inflammatory infiltrate, sinusoidal dilatation, peliosis, and thick-walled arteries with a ductular reaction. FNH and inflammatory adenoma therefore share some morphologic features, which may present diagnostic difficulties. The characteristic map-like staining pattern of glutamine synthetase in FNH and immunoreactivity for serum amyloid A and C-reactive protein in inflammatory hepatocellular adenoma are useful for differentiating between these two entities.

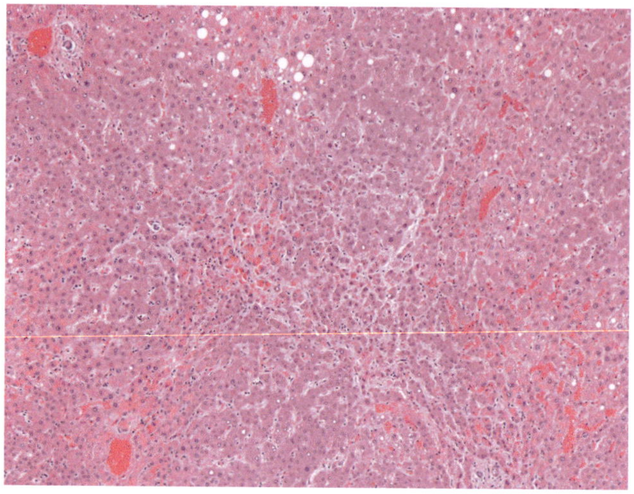

Fig. 13.5 Nodular regenerative hyperplasia. Parenchymal nodular change is present without any fibrosis. The periphery of these nodules is composed of atrophic hepatocytes. Nodular regenerative hyperplasia is an uncommon liver disease, with a prevalence of 0.72% to 2.6% in autopsy series and 0.52% in biopsy series. It is observed in 14% to 27% of cases of noncirrhotic portal hypertension. It mainly affects patients older than 60, although rare cases have been reported in children and even fetuses. Nodular regenerative hyperplasia is characterised pathologically by a diffuse benign transformation of the hepatic parenchyma into small regenerative nodules with minimal or no fibrosis. Obliteration of small portal veins and occasionally small hepatic veins may be found. Gordon-Sweets reticulin stain highlights the characteristic peripheral condensation of reticulin fibres in nodular regenerative hyperplasia.

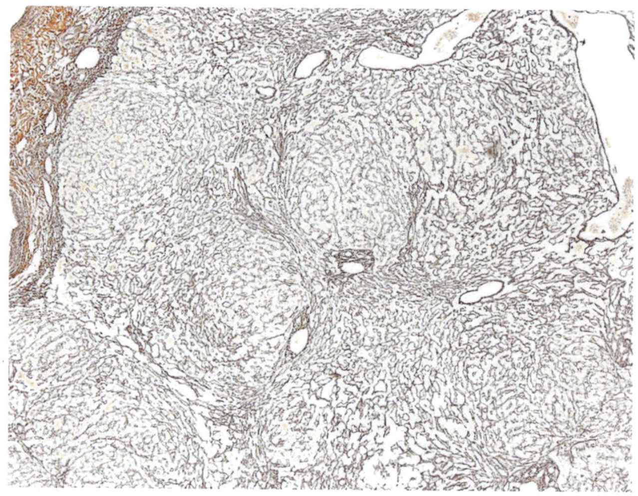

Fig. 13.6 Nodular regenerative hyperplasia (Gordon-Sweets reticulin stain). Parenchymal nodular change is present without any fibrosis. Drugs and toxins are the major aetiologies of nodular regenerative hyperplasia; other causes include autoimmune diseases (e.g., rheumatoid arthritis, systemic lupus erythematosus, antiphospholipid syndrome, and polyarteritis nodosa), inflammatory diseases (e.g., inflammatory bowel disease, celiac disease, and sarcoidosis), haematologic diseases (e.g., myeloproliferative disease, lymphoma, macroglobulinaemia, mixed cryoglobulinaemia, and idiopathic thrombocytopaenic purpura), congenital or acquired immunodeficiency (e.g., chronic HIV infection, chronic granulomatous disease, and common variable immunodeficiency syndromes), primary biliary cirrhosis, and cystinosis.

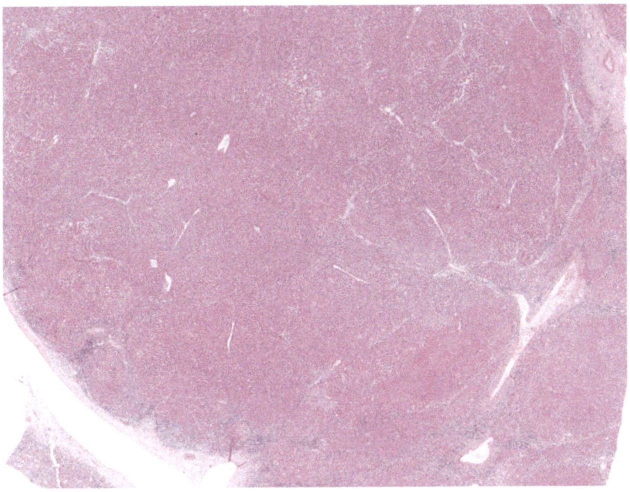

Fig. 13.7 Large regenerative nodule. A 1.3-cm distinctive regenerative nodule is present against a background of cirrhosis. No significant cytologic or architectural atypia is present. Large regenerative nodule, or macroregenerative nodule in older terminology, is a lesion with a minimum diameter of 5 mm. It is more distinctive and larger than surrounding cirrhotic regenerative nodules. Large regenerative nodules are cytologically bland, with no architectural or cytologic atypia.

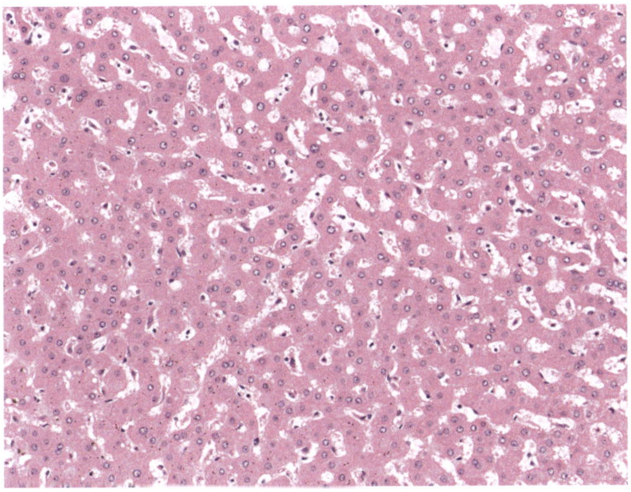

Fig. 13.8 Large regenerative nodule. The lesional hepatocytes are bland, and there is no architectural or cytologic atypia. Differential diagnoses include low-grade dysplastic nodule and hepatocellular adenoma. It may be impossible to confidently distinguish between low-grade dysplastic and large regenerative nodules by morphology alone in the current consensus, and it has been argued that the latter term should be dropped. The presence of intranodular portal tracts/fibrous septa favours large regenerative nodule, whereas the presence of intranodular unpaired arterioles is more suggestive of a dysplastic nodule.

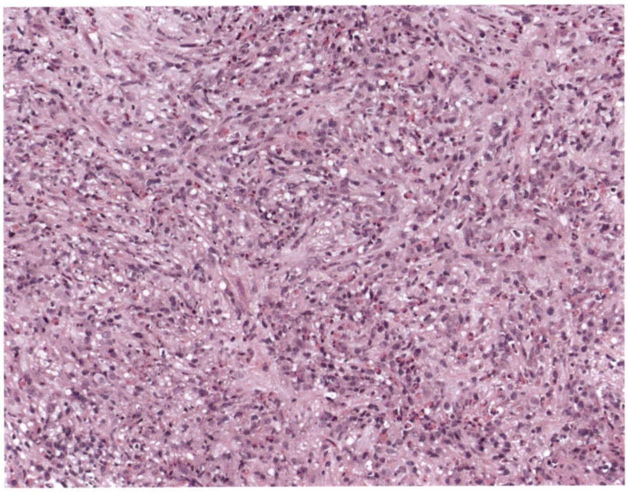

Fig. 13.9 Inflammatory pseudotumour. Fascicles of fibroblasts and myofibroblasts are admixed with many small lymphocytes, eosinophils, and a scattering of neutrophils. So-called inflammatory pseudotumours represent a heterogeneous group of reactive or neoplastic hepatic lesions. The true neoplastic form is better designated as inflammatory myofibroblastic tumour. Inflammatory pseudotumours occur at all ages, with a mean age of presentation of 37 years. The male-to-female ratio is about 3:1. Inflammatory pseudotumours are mainly solitary (80%) and have a variable size. They are composed of a proliferation of fibroblasts and myofibroblasts admixed with a mixed inflammatory infiltrate. Granulomatous or xanthogranulomatous inflammation also may be present.

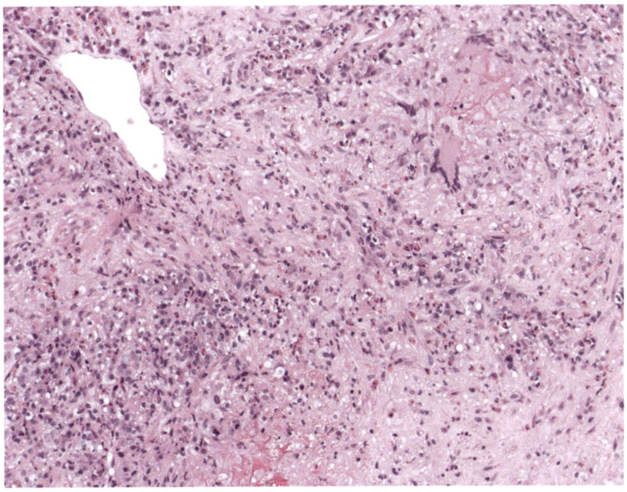

Fig. 13.10 Inflammatory pseudotumour. Small lymphocytes, eosinophils, and multinucleated giant cells are present between fibroblasts and myofibroblasts. The exact pathogenesis remains uncertain. Some suggest that inflammatory pseudotumours represent a reactive process to infective organisms and/or adjacent abscess. In most patients, however, no specific organism can be cultured or identified in tissue sections. Several cases are associated with primary sclerosing cholangitis or IgG4 sclerosing cholangiopathy and in the latter are characterised by the presence of abundant IgG4-positive plasma cells. One fifth of cases are found to have underlying malignancy in the hepatobiliary tract, gastrointestinal tract, and other sites. However, a proportion of cases are neoplastic in nature by demonstrating monoclonality and aberrant expression and translocation of ALK1.

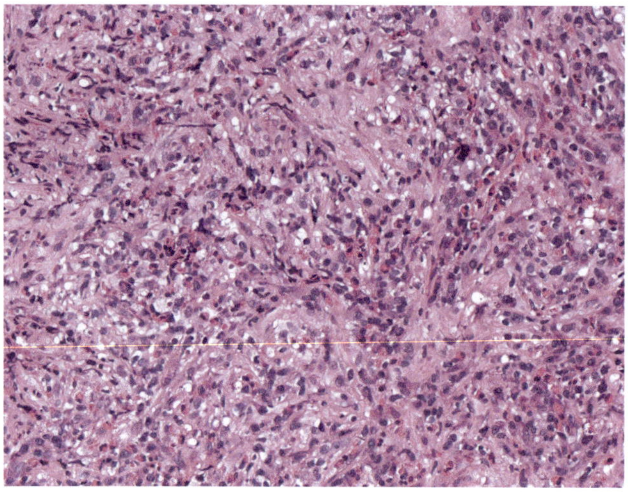

Fig. 13.11 Inflammatory pseudotumour. Fascicles of fibroblasts and myofibroblasts are admixed with a polymorphous inflammatory infiltrate. Inflammatory pseudotumour-like follicular dendritic cell tumour is the main differential diagnosis. This rare hepatic tumour is characterised by a marked female predominance (4:1 to 9:1), proliferation of spindle cells (which are immunoreactive to CD21 and CD35) in fascicles, whorls or a storiform pattern, and a strong association with Epstein-Barr virus.

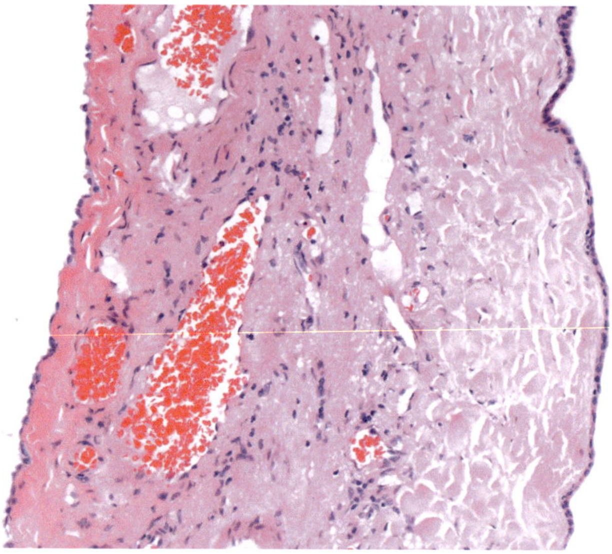

Fig. 13.13 Solitary bile duct cyst. A unilocular cystic lesion is lined by a single layer of bland nonciliated cuboidal cells. Differential diagnoses include other epithelial-lined benign cystic lesions: ciliated foregut cyst, mucinous cystic neoplasm, and cystic-type intraductal papillary neoplasm of the bile duct (IPNB). Ciliated foregut cysts are lined by pseudostratified ciliated columnar cells. Mucinous cystic neoplasms are lined by mucinous epithelial cells with variable cytologic and architectural atypia and a characteristic underlying ovarian-type stroma. The cystic type of IPNB is characterised by ductal dilatation by mucinous epithelial cells with a variable cytologic and architectural atypia with prominent intraductal mucin accumulation, direct luminal connection to the bile ducts, and an absence of ovarian-type stroma.

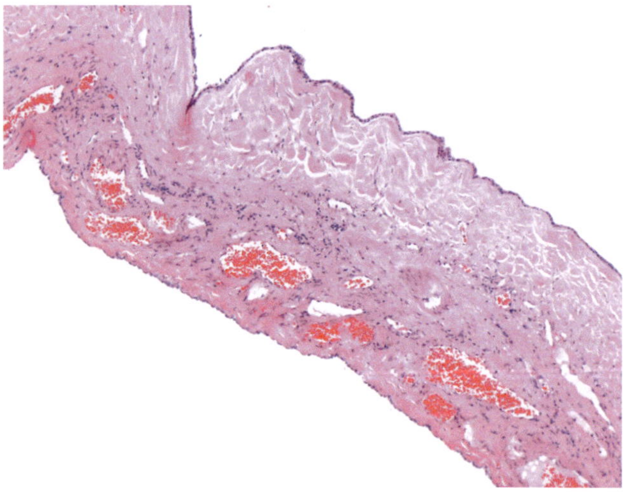

Fig. 13.12 Solitary bile duct cyst. A unilocular cystic lesion is lined by a single layer of bland nonciliated cuboidal cells. Solitary bile duct cyst, also known as solitary hepatic cyst and solitary nonparasitic cyst, usually is an incidental finding. It may represent a limited form at one end of the spectrum of fibropolycystic liver disease (ductal plate malformation). The usual age of presentation is 30 to 50 years. A female predominance (4:1) is observed. Most solitary bile duct cysts (95%) are unilocular. They are lined by a single layer of nonciliated cuboidal, columnar, or attenuated cells, which are immunoreactive to cytokeratin 7 and 19. Malignant transformation is extremely rare.

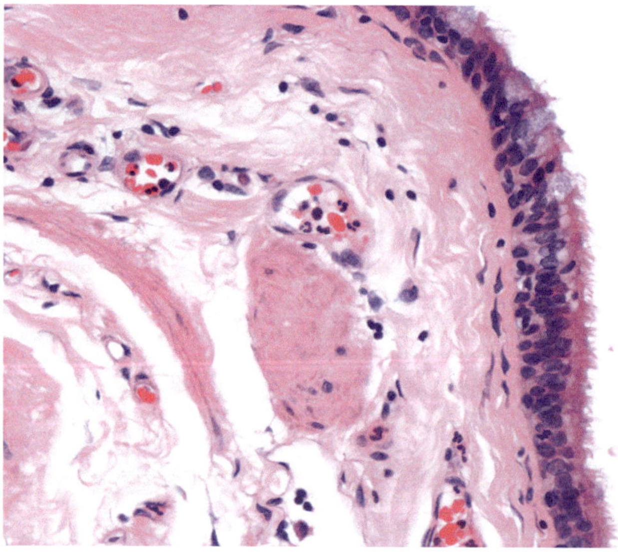

Fig. 13.14 Ciliated foregut cyst. A unilocular cystic lesion is lined by benign pseudostratified ciliated columnar cells. This is an uncommon entity, with about 100 reported cases. It is a developmental malformation and resembles bronchogenic cyst or other ciliated cysts from other embryonal foregut derivatives (e.g., sublingual region, oesophagus, and stomach). Although it is a developmental malformation, the mean age of presentation is about 48 years and it usually presents as an incidental finding in imaging studies or at surgery. Ciliated foregut cysts are unilocular in most cases (93%). They are lined by pseudostratified ciliated columnar cells. Squamous metaplasia and a smooth muscle layer may be found. Rare cases of malignant transformation to squamous cell carcinoma have been reported.

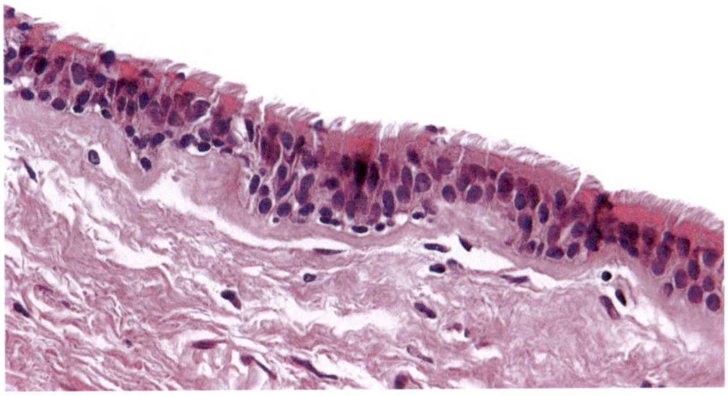

Fig. 13.15 Ciliated foregut cyst. A unilocular cystic lesion is lined by benign pseudostratified ciliated columnar cells. Differential diagnoses are other epithelial-lining benign cystic lesions: solitary bile duct cyst, mucinous cystic neoplasm, and cystic-type IPNB.

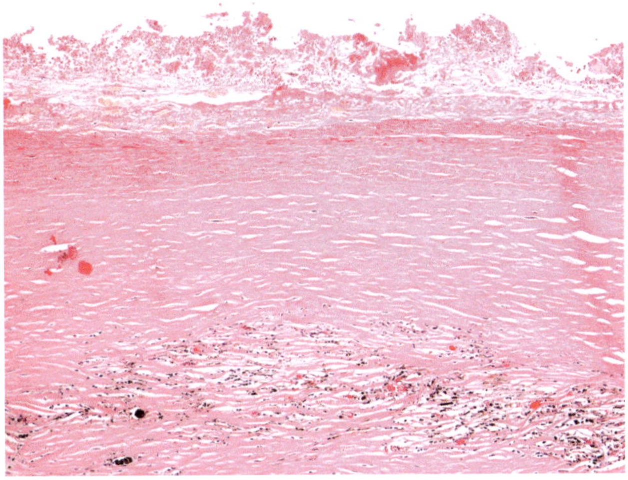

Fig. 13.16 Haemorrhagic cyst. A unilocular cyst containing a fibrous wall and scattered haemosiderin-laden macrophages. The cyst is lined by haemorrhage and fibrin only, without any epithelial lining. Haemorrhagic cysts without any epithelial lining may represent cystic degeneration of organising haematoma, haemorrhagic cystic degeneration of any tumour, and hepatic endometriosis. The latter two require proper sampling to reveal more diagnostic pathologic features of the corresponding lesions.

14 Epithelial Liver Neoplasms

Primary liver epithelial neoplasms are defined according to their similarity to the ambient epithelial cells, that is, hepatocytes and biliary epithelial cells. Neoplasms with mixed hepatocellular and biliary phenotypes do exist and probably derive from progenitor cells capable of dual differentiation.

The hepatocellular tumours include hepatocellular adenoma (HCA) and hepatocellular carcinoma (HCC). The association between HCA and the oral contraceptive pill has long been known, although recent studies have shown that HCA may be divided into four main subtypes according to their clinical, histologic and molecular characteristics. HCC usually originates in cirrhotic livers and, more rarely, in mildly diseased noncirrhotic or sometimes entirely normal livers. Fibrolamellar carcinoma is an unusual variant of HCC, usually observed in young adults without underlying liver disease.

Cholangiocarcinomas usually are separated into hilar and intrahepatic subtypes depending on their anatomic location. Chronic biliary inflammatory conditions are the main risk factors. Cholangiocarcinoma also may arise in cirrhosis of the nonbiliary type.

A.W.H. Chan et al., *Atlas of Liver Pathology*, Atlas of Anatomic Pathology,
DOI 10.1007/978-1-4614-9114-9_14, © Springer Science+Business Media New York 2014

14.1 Hepatocellular Epithelial Neoplasms

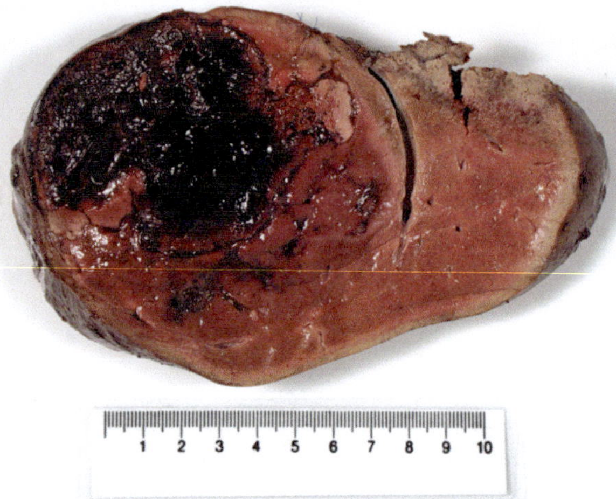

Fig. 14.1 Hepatocellular adenoma. A haemorrhagic tumour is present in a noncirrhotic liver. HCAs are primary benign hepatocellular neoplasms. Their annual incidence in long-term contraceptive users is 3 to 4 in 100,000, as opposed to only 0.1 in 100,000 in nonusers or women with less than 2 years of exposure. About 85% of cases in Western countries occur in females. The usual age of presentation is 30 to 40 years. The major risk factor is use of oestrogenic or androgenic steroids. Other risk factors include glycogen storage types Ia and III, galactosaemia, tyrosinaemia, familial polyposis coli, iron overload related to beta thalassemia, maturity onset diabetes of the young type 3 (MODY3), and obesity.

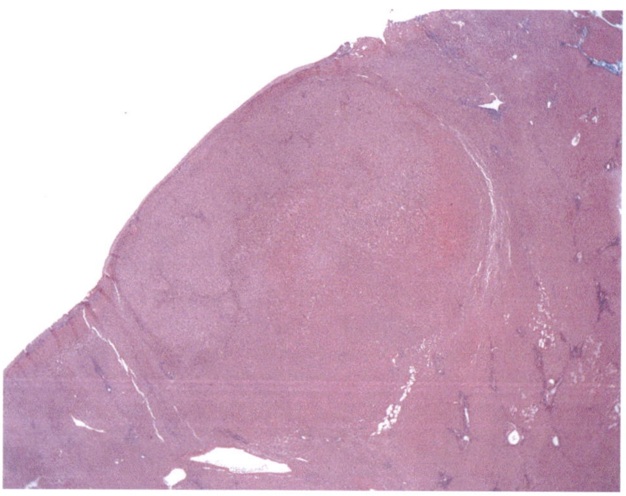

Fig. 14.2 Hepatocellular adenoma. A solitary well-circumscribed nonencapsulated hepatocellular neoplasm is present in a noncirrhotic liver. HCAs usually are solitary. Multiple adenomas and adenomatosis (10 or more adenomas) are found predominantly in females and most commonly associated with glycogen storage disease type I. However, the complication rates of haemorrhage (27%), rupture (18%), and reported malignant transformation (up to 7%) of solitary HCA are similar to those of multiple adenomas. HCAs are highly variable in size, with a mean diameter of 8.5 cm. The cut surface is ill defined, soft, and white to brownish, with little or no fibrous capsule. Congestion, haemorrhage, necrosis, and fibrosis are not infrequent.

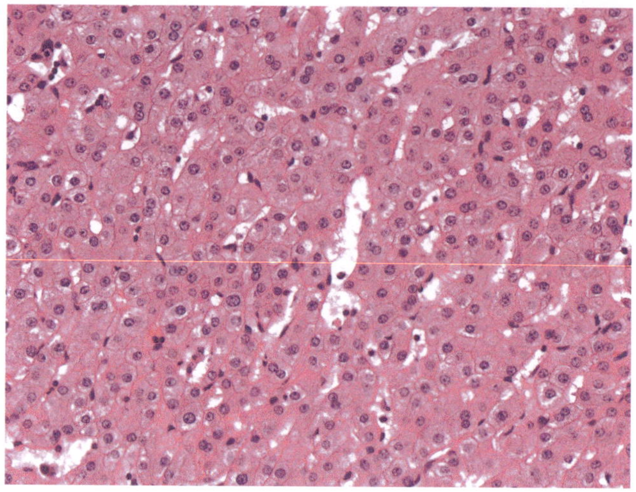

Fig. 14.3 Hepatocellular adenoma. Bland hepatocytes are arranged in trabeculae one to two cells thick with a sinusoidal vasculature. HCAs are composed of trabeculae of benign hepatocytes in one- to two-cell–thick plates, very occasionally with pseudoacini. The hepatocytes may be normal or loaded by steatosis, glycogen (clear cytoplasm), or haemosiderosis. Cytoplasmic or canalicular bilirubinostasis, lipofuscin, Dubin-Johnson pigment, and, rarely, Mallory-Denk bodies also may be found. Cytologic atypia or mitotic activity is uncommon. Unpaired or nontriad arterioles typically are found.

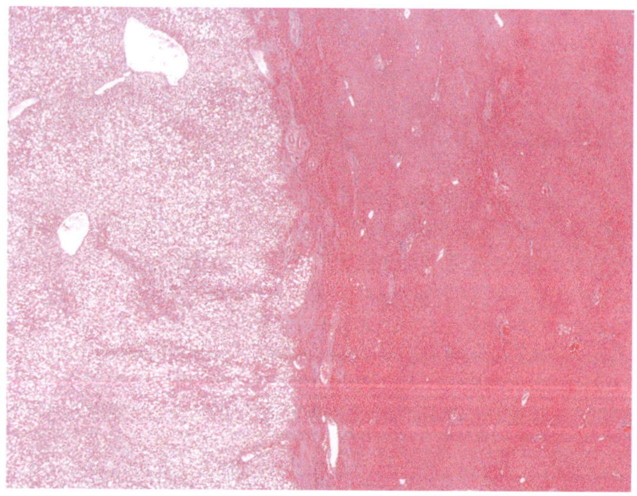

Fig. 14.4 Hepatocellular adenoma, hepatocyte nuclear factor 1α (HNF1α)-inactivated subtype. An HCA with marked steatosis appears well-demarcated from the background of a nonsteatotic liver. HCA is subclassified into four major subtypes according to phenotype and genotype: HNF1α-inactivated, β-catenin–activated, inflammatory, and unclassified. Unclassified HCA accounts for only <10% of all adenomas and does not exhibit specific genetic or phenotypic changes.

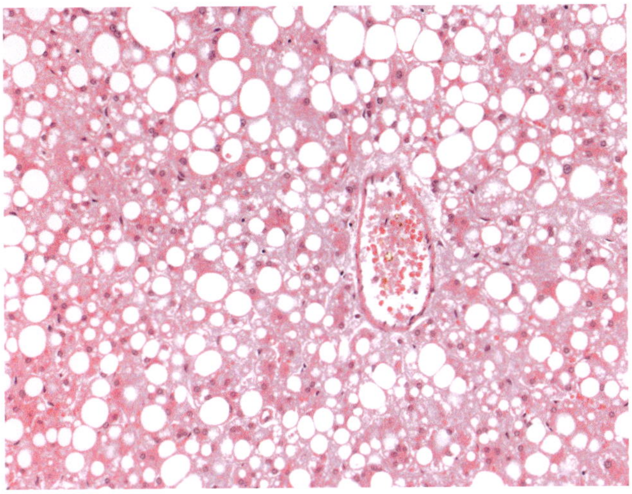

Fig. 14.5 Hepatocellular adenoma, HNF1α-inactivated subtype. The lesional hepatocytes exhibit marked steatosis. An unpaired arteriole is noted. HNF1α-inactivated HCAs account for 35% to 40% of all adenomas. They usually are found in women and are associated with marked steatosis and adenomatosis. Negativity of immunostaining for liver fatty acid–binding protein (L-FABP) is characteristic. A heterozygous germline mutation of HNF1α accounts for 10% of HNF1α-inactivated HCAs and is associated with autosomal dominant MODY3. Heterozygous germline mutations of *CYP1B1* also account for 14% of HNF1α-inactivated HCAs.

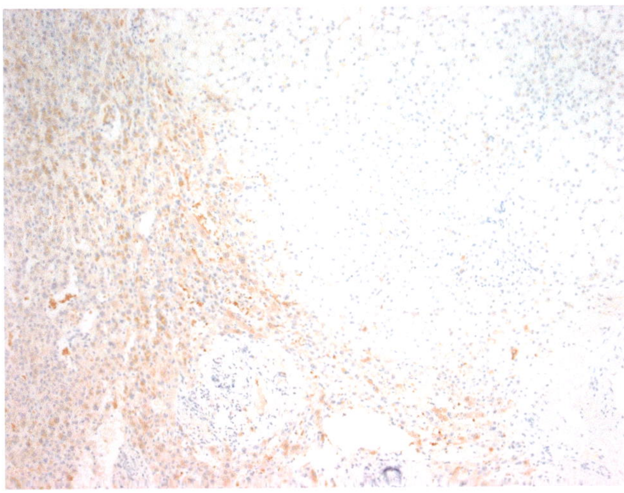

Fig. 14.6 Hepatocellular adenoma, HNF1α-inactivated subtype (L-FABP). The lesional hepatocytes exhibit a characteristically negative pattern, in contrast to nontumorous hepatocytes in the background.

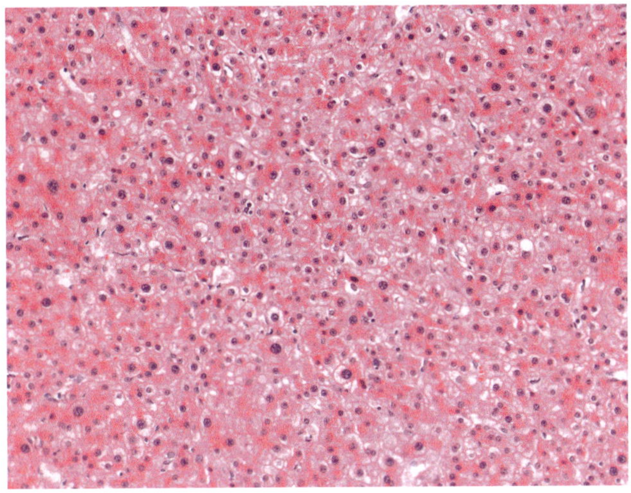

Fig. 14.7 Hepatocellular adenoma, β-catenin–activated subtype. Mild cytologic atypia with mild nuclear pleomorphism and enlargement is noted. β-Catenin–activated HCA accounts for 10% to 15% of all adenomas. It typically is found in men and may be associated with glycogen storage disease and use of androgenic steroids. Significant cytologic atypia and pseudoacinar formation are common pathologic features, whereas steatosis and inflammation usually are lacking. Aberrant cytoplasmic and nuclear staining of β-catenin and diffuse staining of glutamine synthetase are typical findings. β-Catenin–activated HCA is considered to be at higher risk for malignant transformation than other subtypes.

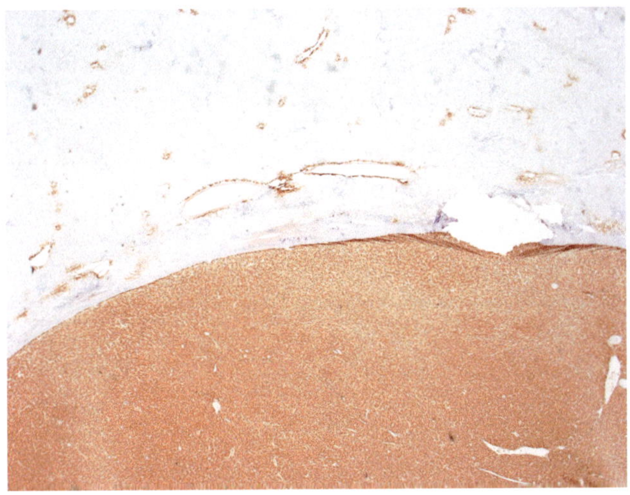

Fig. 14.8 Hepatocellular adenoma, β-catenin–activated subtype (glutamine synthetase). The lesional hepatocytes show diffuse immunoreactivity. Distinction between HCA and well-differentiated HCC may be difficult and sometimes impossible, particularly in small biopsy samples. Although immunoreactivities towards glypican-3 and CD34 (with a complete sinusoidal capillarisation pattern) favour HCC, a small portion of HCAs share similar immunostaining patterns. Cytologic atypia, diffuse cytoplasmic staining of glutamine synthetase, and nuclear staining of β-catenin overlap between β-catenin–activated HCA and well-differentiated HCC.

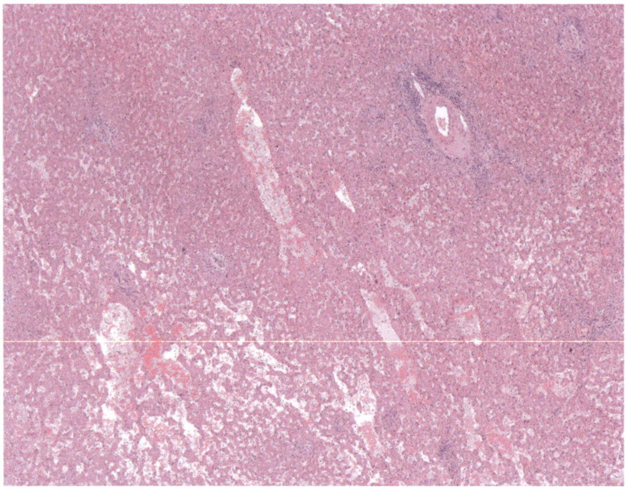

Fig. 14.9 Hepatocellular adenoma, inflammatory subtype. This HCA contains areas of sinusoidal dilatation, congestion, and peliosis. Inflammatory HCA, previously referred to as telangiectatic focal nodular hyperplasia, accounts for 45% to 60% of all adenomas. It is associated with elevation of serum C-reactive protein and the erythrocyte sedimentation rate in half the cases. Focal or diffuse inflammatory infiltrates, sinusoidal dilatation, peliosis, and thick-walled arteries with ductular reaction are typical pathologic findings. Immunoreactivity towards inflammation-associated protein, such as serum amyloid A and C-reactive protein, is the hallmark feature. About 60% of inflammatory HCAs are associated with a gp130 gene mutation, and 15% of this subgroup show coexisting β-catenin mutations.

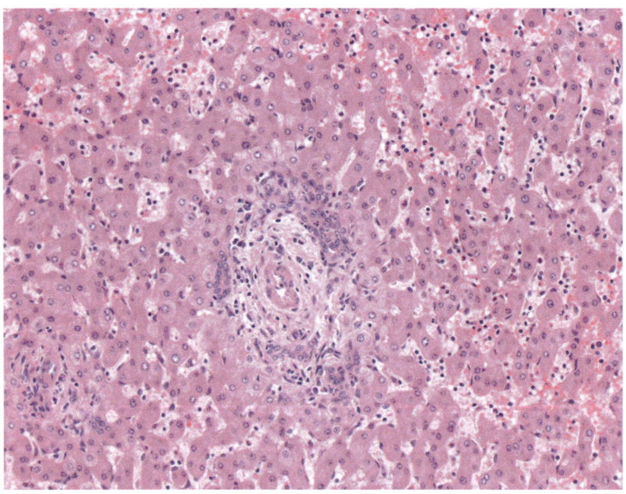

Fig. 14.10 Hepatocellular adenoma, inflammatory subtype. An abnormal thick-walled artery is accompanied by a mild ductular reaction. Such a histologic feature together with sinusoidal dilatation and peliosis led to the misnomer of *telangiectatic focal nodular hyperplasia* in the past. Focal nodular hyperplasia and inflammatory HCA sometimes are difficult to distinguish from each other. The presence of a fibrous scar with large arteries suggests focal nodular hyperplasia. The characteristic "map-like" staining pattern of glutamine synthetase in focal nodular hyperplasia and immunoreactivity for serum amyloid A and C-reactive protein in inflammatory HCA are useful in difficult cases.

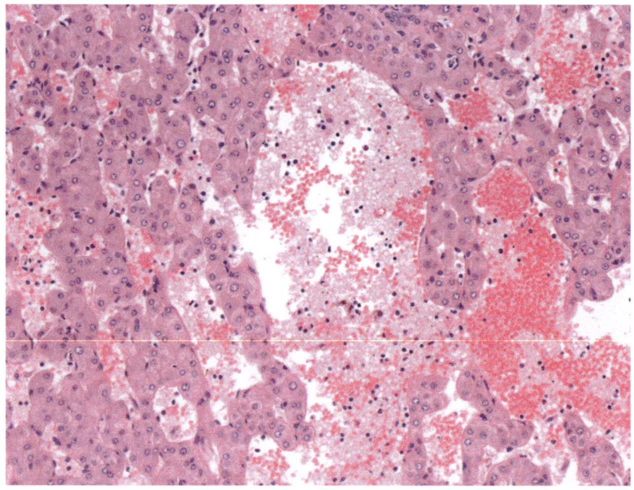

Fig. 14.11 Hepatocellular adenoma, inflammatory subtype. An area of sinusoidal dilatation, congestion, and peliosis is highlighted. Another differential diagnosis of HCA is hepatic angiomyolipoma. Differentiation of hepatic angiomyolipoma from HCA may be straightforward if all three histologic components of hepatic angiomyolipoma are present. However, the myomatous type of angiomyolipoma with unusual growth patterns, namely trabecular, pelioid, and inflammatory, can mimic an HCA, particularly the inflammatory subtype. Immunoreactivity for HMB45 or Melan-A in angiomyolipoma is helpful in difficult cases.

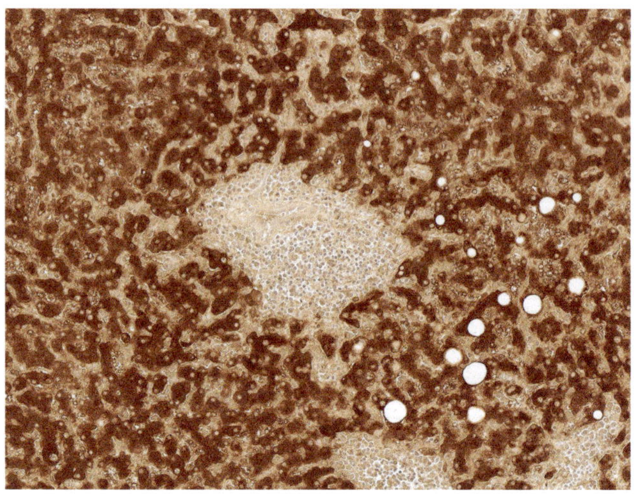

Fig. 14.12 Hepatocellular adenoma, inflammatory subtype (serum amyloid A). The lesional hepatocytes are diffusely immunoreactive towards serum amyloid A. An unpaired thick-walled artery surrounded by moderate inflammatory infiltrate also is noted.

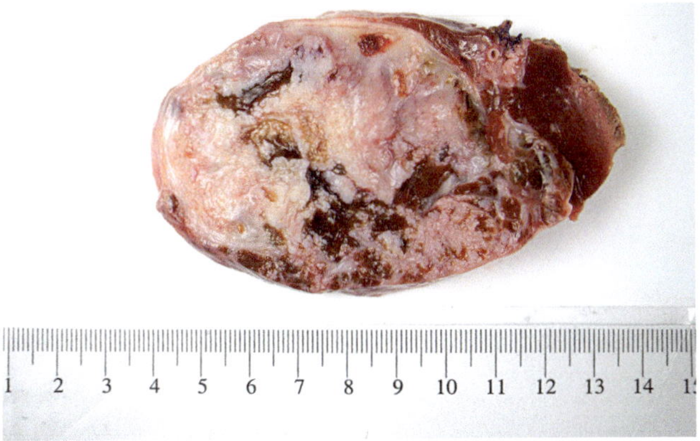

Fig. 14.13 Hepatoblastoma. A mixed epithelial and mesenchymal hepatoblastoma shows a variegated cut surface. Hepatoblastoma is a rare primary malignant hepatic neoplasm with an annual incidence of 0.1 in 100,000. It is the commonest paediatric primary liver tumour. About 90% of cases present before the age of 5 years. Neonatal presentation accounts for only 4% of cases, whereas rare cases of prenatal presentation have been reported. Hepatoblastoma is strongly associated with prematurity and low birth weight. About 5% of cases are associated with congenital renal or gastrointestinal anomalies, as well as inherited syndromes, including Beckwith-Wiedemann syndrome, familial adenomatous polyposis coli, trisomy 18, trisomy 21, Prader-Willi syndrome, and glycogen storage disease type Ia.

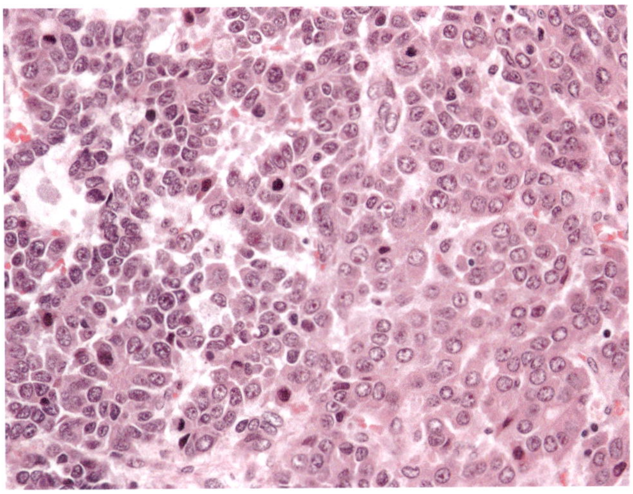

Fig. 14.14 Hepatoblastoma. Mixed foetal (*lower right*) and embryonal epithelial components (*upper left*) are present. Hepatoblastoma usually is solitary and varies in size from a few centimetres to >20 cm. Histologically, it may be grouped into a wholly epithelial type (55%), a mixed epithelial and mesenchymal (MEM) type (45%), and a not-otherwise specified type. The wholly epithelial type is subclassified into fetal (30%), mixed fetal and embryonal (20%), macrotrabecular (3%), and small cell undifferentiated (<2%) subtypes. The MEM type also is divided into MEM with and without teratoid features.

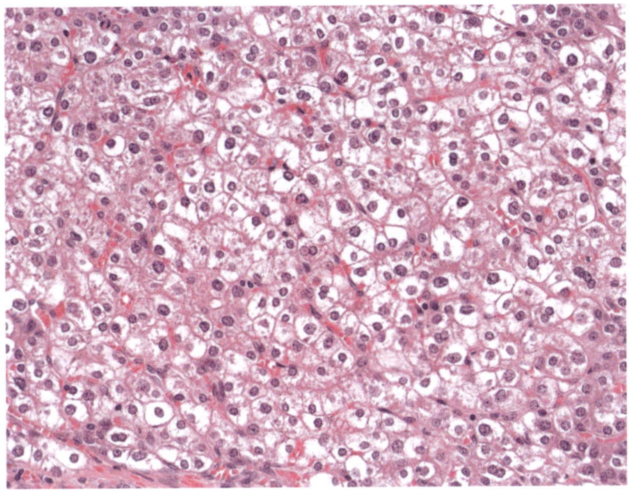

Fig. 14.15 Hepatoblastoma. A fetal epithelial component is composed of trabeculae of fetal hepatocytes with clear or eosinophilic cytoplasm. Pure fetal hepatoblastoma is composed of trabeculae and nests of hepatoblasts with round nuclei, fine chromatin, inconspicuous to small distinct nucleoli, and moderate amounts of clear or eosinophilic granular cytoplasm. The presence of a clear cytoplasm is associated with varying degrees of cytoplasmic glycogen. Alternating tumour cells with clear and eosinophilic cytoplasm give a "light-and-dark" pattern at low powers. A subset of fetal hepatoblastomas with mitotic rates greater than two per 10 high-power fields is noted and usually is associated with larger, more pleomorphic nuclei, less cytoplasmic glycogen, and more cellular crowding. This type sometimes is designated a *mitotically active* or *crowded* fetal hepatoblastoma.

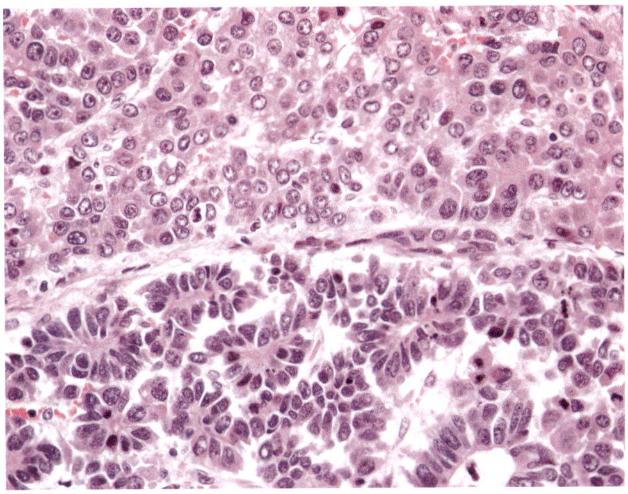

Fig. 14.16 Hepatoblastoma. Mixed fetal (*upper*) and embryonal components (*lower*) are present. Mixed fetal and embryonal hepatoblastomas are composed of both fetal and embryonal epithelial components. The embryonal component is featured by solid nests, rosettes, and pseudoacini of embryonal hepatoblasts with irregular nuclei, coarse chromatin, and a small amount of eosinophilic granular cytoplasm. Mitosis usually is more frequent in the embryonal component.

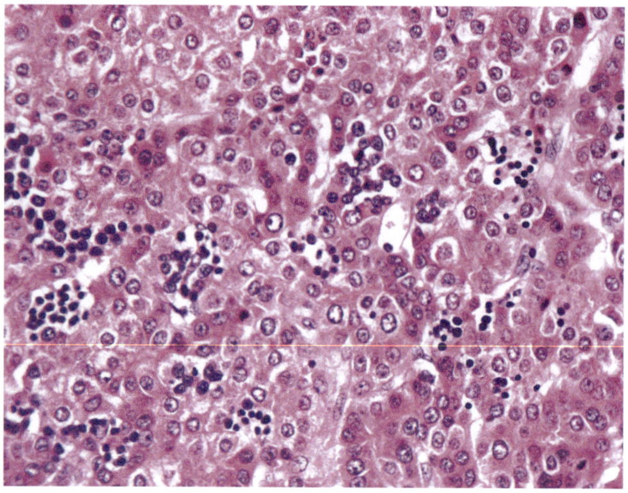

Fig. 14.17 Hepatoblastoma. Many foci of extramedullary haematopoiesis are scattered among the tumour cells. Clusters of extramedullary haematopoietic cells are found more commonly in the fetal epithelial than the embryonal epithelial component, and more often in pretreatment biopsies than posttreatment excisional specimens.

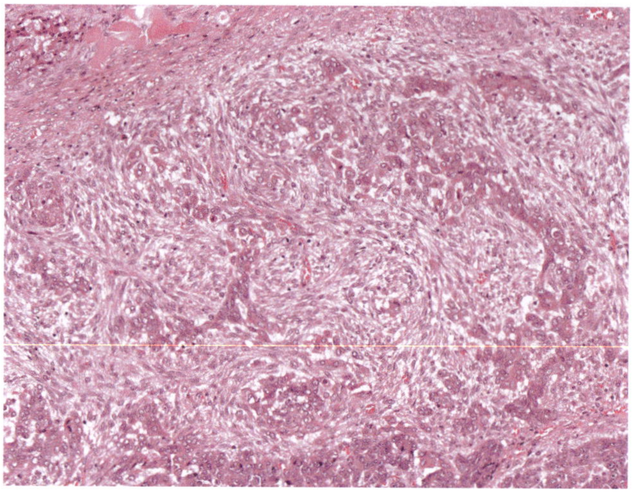

Fig. 14.19 Hepatoblastoma. The epithelial component is intimately mixed with the fibroblastic mesenchymal component. MEM hepatoblastomas consist of both epithelial and mesenchymal components. The epithelial component usually is fetal- or mixed fetal/embryonal-type neoplastic tissue. The mesenchymal component most commonly is composed of mature/immature fibrous tissue, osteoid-like tissue, and hyaline cartilage. The remainder include heterologous tissues of all germ cell layers, such as melanin-containing epithelium, mucinous epithelium, neuroglial tissue, and skeletal muscle. Hepatoblastoma with the latter mesenchymal component is referred to as MEM hepatoblastoma with teratoid features, although the prognostic significance of this component is uncertain.

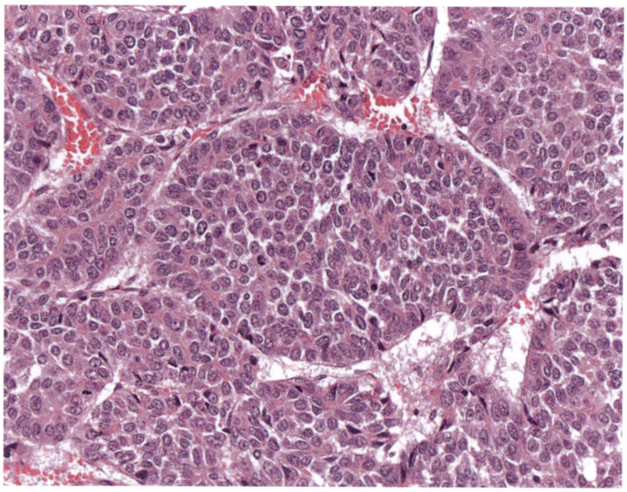

Fig. 14.18 Hepatoblastoma. Macrotrabeculae are seen here with broad trabeculae of embryonal hepatoblasts more than 10 cells thick. Macrotrabecular hepatoblastoma is composed predominantly of trabeculae of tumour cells 10 or more cells thick. A focal macrotrabecular growth pattern may be found in other types of hepatoblastoma. Macrotrabecular hepatoblastoma may be subclassified further as MT-1 (composed predominantly of hepatocytes with vesicular nuclei and prominent nucleoli; poorer prognosis) and MT-2 (composed of fetal/embryonal hepatoblasts). The MT-1 subtype may be difficult to differentiate from HCC in older children.

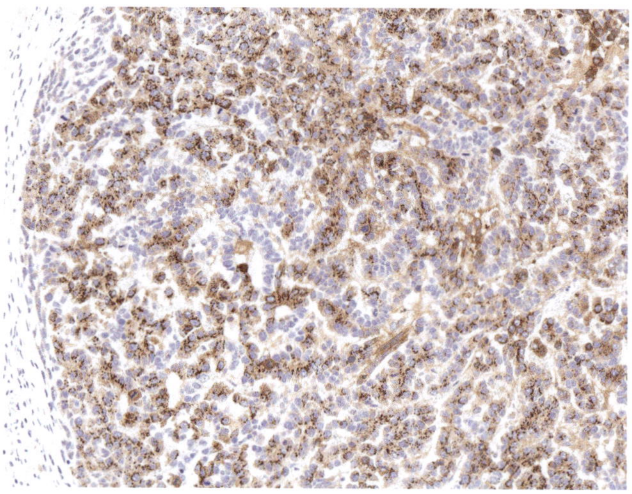

Fig. 14.20 Hepatoblastoma (α-fetoprotein). The tumour cells show patchy positivity. AFP is a major plasma glycoprotein produced by the yolk sac and liver during normal fetal development. About half of hepatoblastomas show patchy immunoreactivity for AFP. Hepatoblastoma also shows variable expression of markers of hepatocellular differentiation, including HepPar-1 and α_1-antitrypsin.

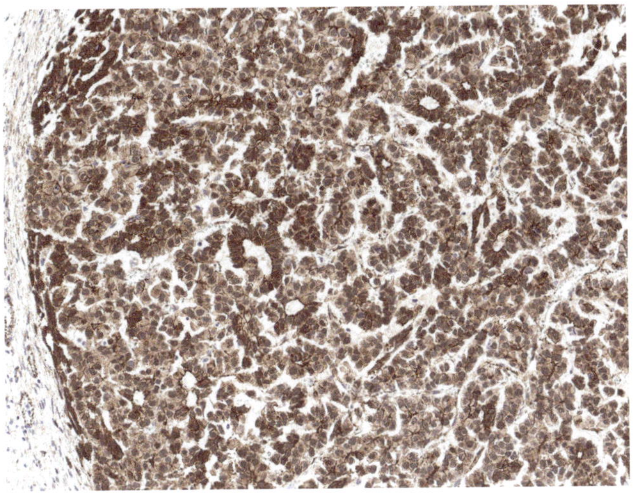

Fig. 14.21 Hepatoblastoma (β-catenin). The tumour cells show nuclear, cytoplasmic, and membranous positivity. The Wnt/β-catenin pathway is one of the key signalling pathways in the tumourigenesis of hepatoblastoma. Translocation of β-catenin to the nucleus, a marker of activation of the canonical Wnt/β-catenin pathway, is present in 70% to 90% of hepatoblastomas, particularly in areas with a fetal epithelial component.

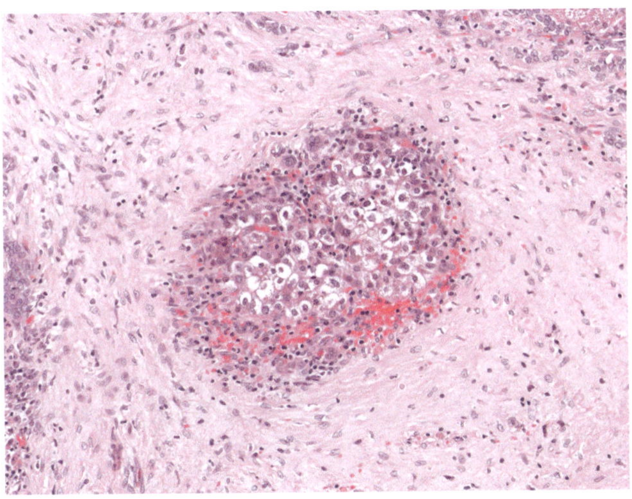

Fig. 14.22 Hepatoblastoma, post chemotherapy. A small cluster of fetal hepatoblasts with a clear cytoplasm is present in fibrous stroma. Neoadjuvant chemotherapy before surgery or transplantation is commonly is used in the treatment of hepatoblastoma. Microscopically, the treated tumour may be completely absent of viable tumour cells and replaced by necrosis, old and recent haemorrhage, and fibrous spheres. However, most cases contain varying amounts of residual tumour. Residual fetal hepatoblastoma typically is composed of small nests of clear or eosinophilic hepatoblasts in fibrous stroma, which sometimes are difficult to distinguish from entrapped normal liver. Residual embryonal, macrotrabecular, and small cell undifferentiated components are more easily identified.

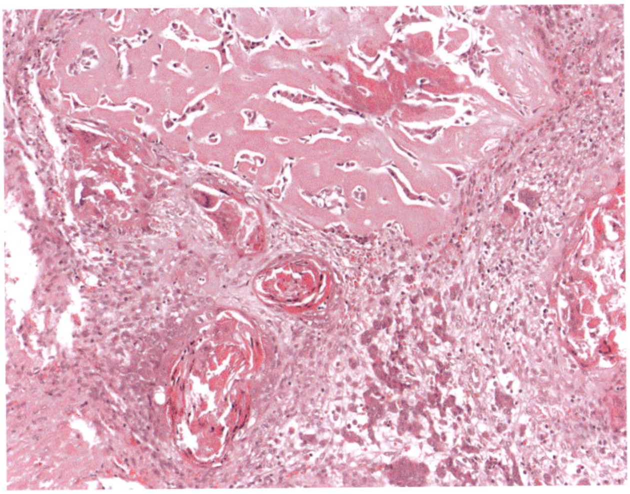

Fig. 14.23 Hepatoblastoma, post chemotherapy. Osteoid tissue, keratinised squamous epithelial tissue, foreign-body reaction, and residual cords of fetal hepatoblasts are present. Osteoid commonly is seen in hepatoblastoma after chemotherapy. Some treated lesions may be composed of foci of osteoid tissue only with no residual epithelial component. Keratinised squamous epithelium also is a typical post-chemotherapy change and usually is associated with foreign-body reaction. Its presence does not signify the diagnosis of MEM hepatoblastoma with teratoid features.

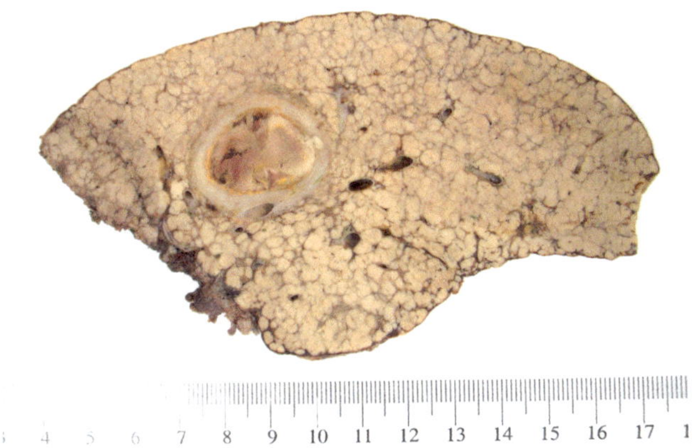

Fig. 14.24 Hepatocellular carcinoma, nodular type. A necrotic tumour with a fibrous pseudo-capsule is present within a cirrhotic liver. HCC is the commonest primary hepatic malignancy. It is the fifth commonest cancer in men and the seventh in women worldwide, and the third commonest cause of cancer death. Most cases (85%) occur in developing countries in East and Southeast Asia and middle and western Africa. The age-specific incidence varies significantly among countries. Male-to-female ratios range from 2:1 to 5:1. Cirrhosis of any cause, chronic viral hepatitis, alcohol, nonalcoholic fatty liver disease, various metabolic diseases (e.g., hereditary haemochromatosis, α_1-antitrypsin deficiency, and tyrosinaemia), and aflatoxin B1 are known risk factors for HCC.

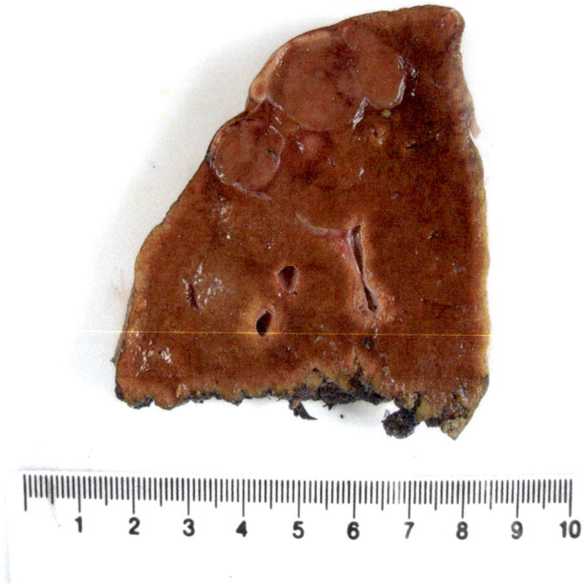

Fig. 14.25 Hepatocellular carcinoma, nodular type. Unencapsulated multilobulated tumour nodules are present in a noncirrhotic liver. HCCs vary in size from a few millimetres to >30 cm. Small HCCs are defined as lesions less than 2 cm and are subdivided further into early HCC and progressed HCC. The former is a well-differentiated HCC with vague nodulation, an indistinct border, and a better prognosis, whereas the latter is a moderately differentiated HCC with distinct nodularity, often a fibrous pseudo-capsule, and a poorer outcome. HCCs may be solitary or multiple. Multiple nodules may represent multicentric HCC (multiple independent HCCs) or a single primary HCC with intrahepatic metastases. A fibrous pseudo-capsule may be seen in HCC, particularly in those arising from cirrhotic liver.

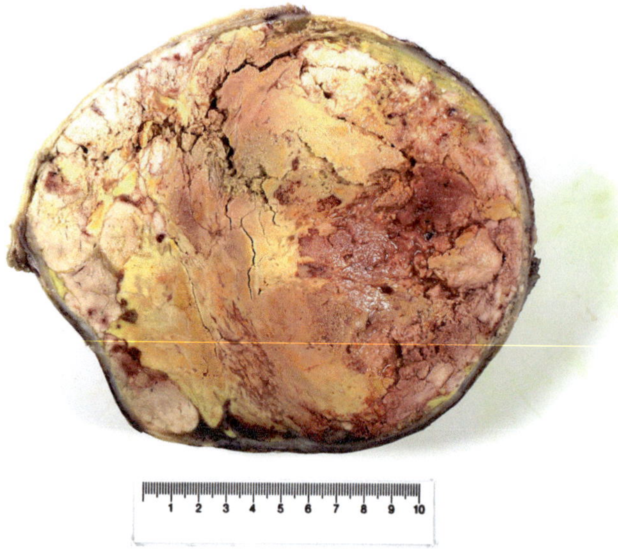

Fig. 14.26 Hepatocellular carcinoma, massive type. A huge necrotic tumour almost replaces the entire right hepatic lobe in this specimen. HCC may be classified macroscopically according to the growth pattern. The nodular type is the commonest pattern. It is characterised by solitary or multiple tumour nodules and usually associated with cirrhosis. The so-called massive type is characterised by a poorly circumscribed, large dominant mass with or without satellite nodules occupying a significant portion of the liver, and is seen frequently in noncirrhotic livers. The diffuse type is rare and characterised by numerous small tumour masses infiltrating throughout the liver. They may simulate regenerative nodules in cirrhotic livers (cirrhotomimetic), and may not be identifiable on imaging even if widespread. The pedunculated type also is rare and represents a tumour mass protruding from the liver surface with or without a pedicle.

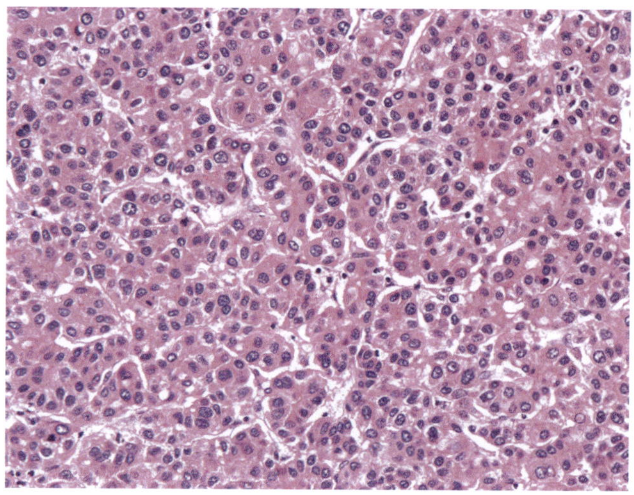

Fig. 14.27 Hepatocellular carcinoma, trabecular pattern. A moderately differentiated HCC is present here and is composed of thickened trabeculae of minimally pleomorphic tumour cells. Histologically, HCC exhibits various architectural patterns, including trabecular, pseudoacinar, and compact patterns. Trabecular growth is the commonest pattern in well- and moderately differentiated HCCs. Tumour cells are arranged in trabeculae at least three cells thick with a sinusoidal vasculature. The thickness of trabeculae correlates with tumour dedifferentiation. The reticulin framework may be focally or completely depleted.

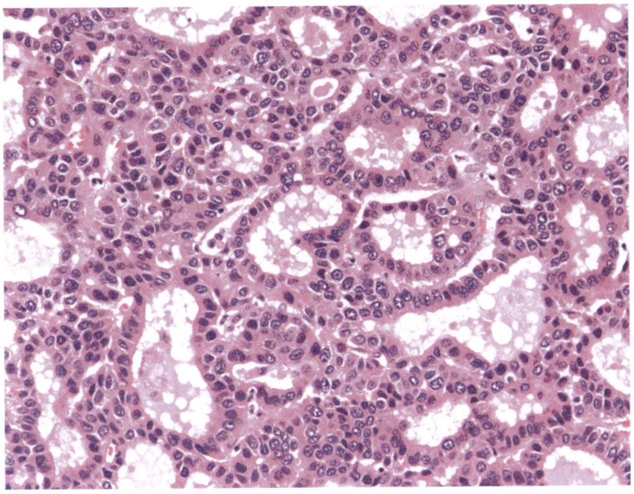

Fig. 14.28 Hepatocellular carcinoma, pseudoacinar pattern. This moderately differentiated HCC is focally composed of gland-like structures filled with pale eosinophilic proteinaceous fluid. Pseudoacinar/pseudoglandular areas commonly coexist with trabecular areas in well- and moderately differentiated HCCs. It is characterised by gland-like structures that arise through abnormal dilatation of bile canaliculi or degeneration of thick trabeculae. Proteinaceous fluid, often positive for periodic acid-Schiff and negative for mucicarmine, and bile may be found within the lumina of gland-like structures. Sometimes, markedly dilated sinusoids or peliotic changes in HCC may mimic pseudoacinar growth. Pseudoacinar growth of HCCs must be distinguished from genuine glandular formation in cholangiocarcinoma or metastatic adenocarcinoma.

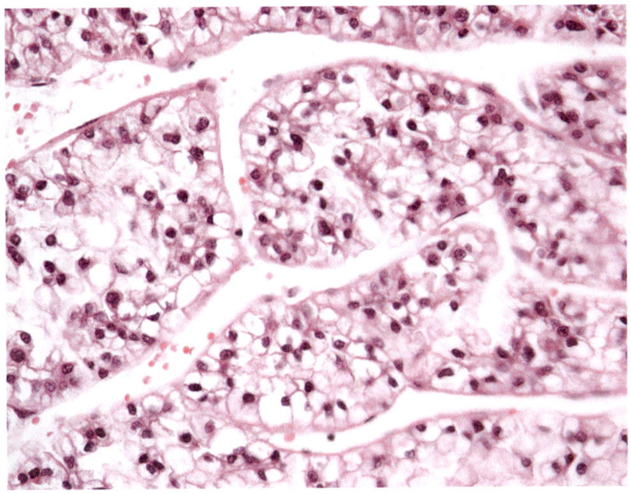

Fig. 14.30 Hepatocellular carcinoma, clear cell type. There are thick trabeculae of tumour cells with a clear cytoplasm. Cytologically, malignant tumour cells of HCC usually are polygonal cells with enlarged nuclei, prominent nucleoli, and abundant eosinophilic granular cytoplasm. There are several variants depending on their cytologic appearance, including the presence of cytoplasmic deposits and inclusions. Clear HCC cells are tumour cells with abundant glycogen. Differentiation between HCC with predominant clear cells and clear cell renal cell carcinoma may be difficult by routine light microscopy alone. Immunohistochemistry may be necessary to make the distinction.

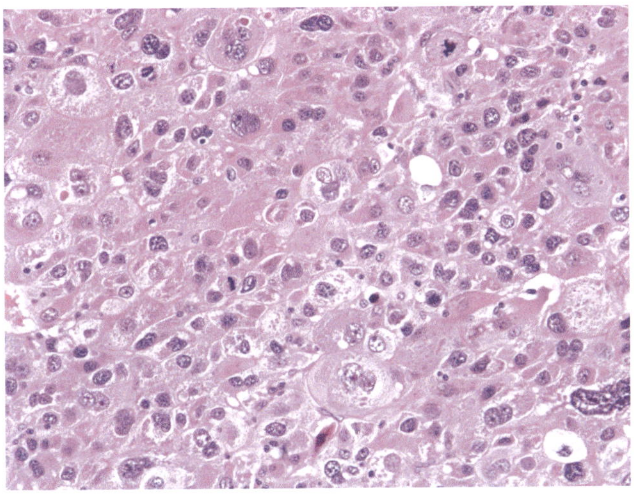

Fig. 14.29 Hepatocellular carcinoma, compact pattern. This poorly differentiated HCC is composed of solid sheets of markedly pleomorphic tumour cells with giant nuclei and multinucleation. A sinusoidal vasculature is inconspicuous. A compact growth is common in poorly differentiated HCCs and is characterised by solid sheets of tumour cells with an inconspicuous sinusoidal vasculature. Histologic grading of HCC is based on the degree of tumour differentiation. The Edmondson and Steiner system classifies HCCs as grade I to grade IV, whereas the World Health Organisation (WHO) system divides HCCs into well-differentiated, moderately differentiated, poorly differentiated, and undifferentiated types. However, tumour grade is not in itself a good independent prognostic marker and is not highly reproducible. Moreover, heterogeneity of tumour grades in a single tumour is a common phenomenon and increases with tumour size.

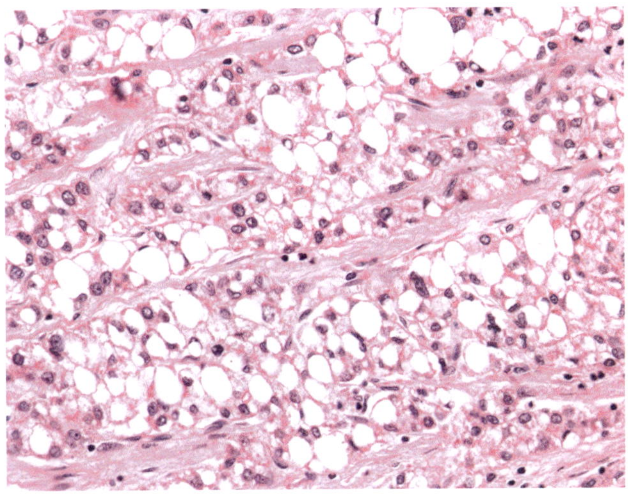

Fig. 14.31 Hepatocellular carcinoma, steatotic or steatohepatitic type. There are thick trabeculae of tumour cells with macrovesicular steatosis. Diffuse steatosis commonly is found in small HCCs. The extent of steatosis usually decreases with the tumour size. HCCs with diffuse steatosis must be differentiated from steatotic HCAs (HNF1α-inactivated subtype) and angiomyolipomas. Focal fatty change, rarely lipoma, myelolipoma, and coelomic fat ectopia are other possible differential diagnoses.

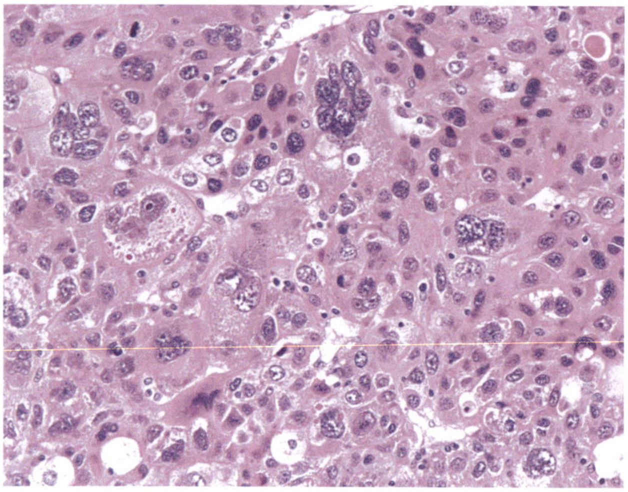

Fig. 14.32 Hepatocellular carcinoma, pleomorphic type. This image shows a solid sheet of markedly pleomorphic tumour cells with giant nuclei or multinucleation. Pleomorphic cells show marked variation in nuclear and cellular size and shape. Bizarre mononuclear and multinucleated giant tumour cells and, rarely, osteoclast-like tumour cells may be found. Pleomorphic cells commonly are present in poorly differentiated HCCs.

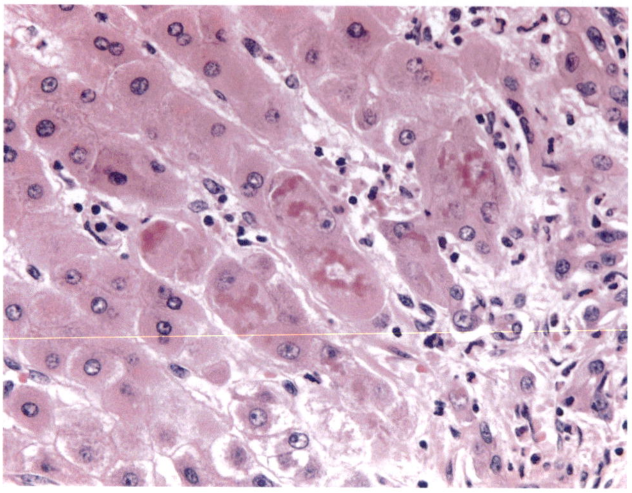

Fig. 14.34 Hepatocellular carcinoma with Mallory-Denk bodies. There are deeply eosinophilic, ropey, intracytoplasmic inclusions within malignant hepatocytes. Mallory-Denk bodies are misfolded and aggregated intermediate filaments (mainly cytokeratin [CK] 8/18) combined with other different classes of proteins, including p62 and ubiquitin. Apart from HCCs, they may be found in focal nodular hyperplasia and HCAs. Intracellular hyaline bodies, also known as globular hyaline bodies, are deeply eosinophilic globular intracytoplasmic inclusions usually surrounded by a clear halo, and they also are immunoreactive for CK8/18, p62, and ubiquitin. They occasionally may be seen in cholangiocarcinoma.

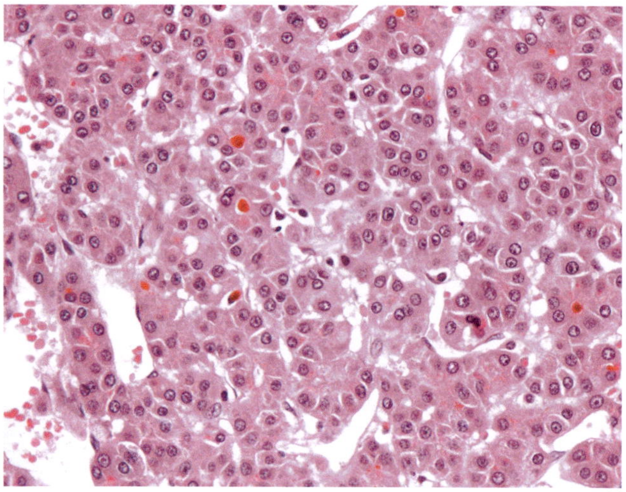

Fig. 14.33 Hepatocellular carcinoma with bile production. Bile plugs are present in the dilated canaliculi among tumour cells. Bile production is a diagnostic feature of hepatocellular differentiation. It usually is found in well-differentiated HCCs. Bile plugs are present in either canaliculi or pseudoacini.

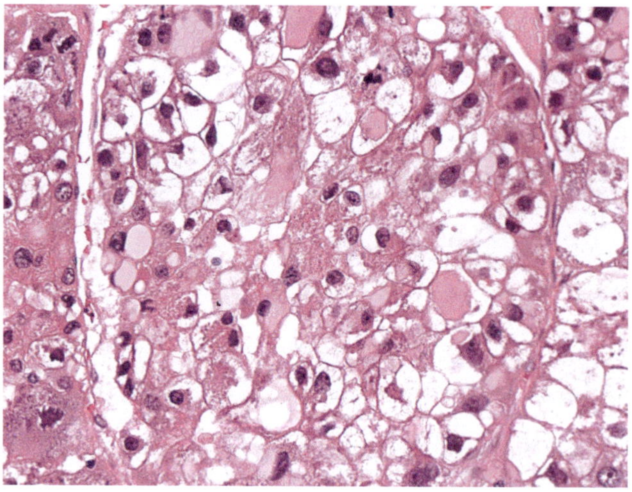

Fig. 14.35 Hepatocellular carcinoma with pale bodies. There are lightly eosinophilic globular homogenous intracytoplasmic inclusions within malignant hepatocytes in this tumour. Pale bodies may vary from light to deeply eosinophilic inclusions and resemble α_1-antitrypsin globules, intracellular hyaline bodies, and ground-glass change. Immunoreactivity to fibrinogen is the key discriminating feature. It may be found in HCC, especially the fibrolamellar variant.

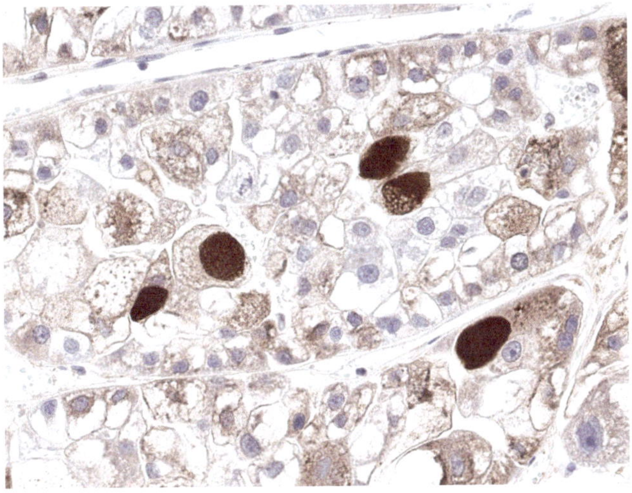

Fig. 14.36 Hepatocellular carcinoma with pale bodies (fibrinogen). Pale bodies in malignant hepatocytes are immunoreactive to fibrinogen. In addition to Mallory-Denk bodies, intracellular hyaline bodies, and pale bodies, HCCs also may contain ground-glass inclusions (hepatitis B surface antigen), α_1-antitrypsin globules, and α_1-antichymotrypsin globules.

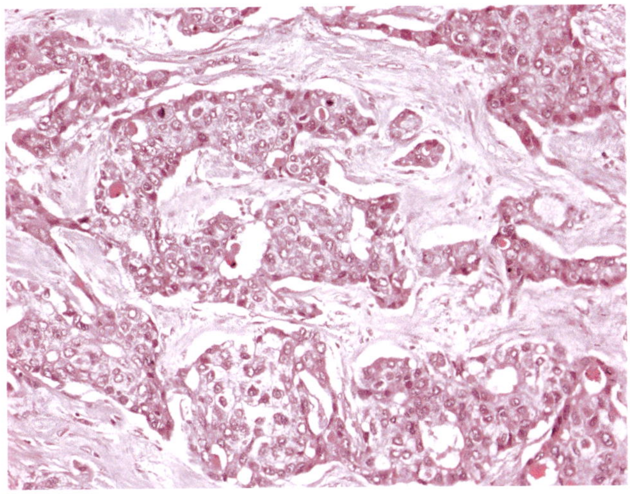

Fig. 14.38 Hepatocellular carcinoma, scirrhous type. Nests and sheets of malignant hepatocytes are embedded in sclerotic fibrous stroma. Scirrhous HCC is another variant and accounts for 5% of all HCCs. It clinically and cytologically resembles classic HCC. It differs from fibrolamellar HCC by the absence of typical large polygonal eosinophilic tumour cells with voluminous cytoplasm and pale bodies.

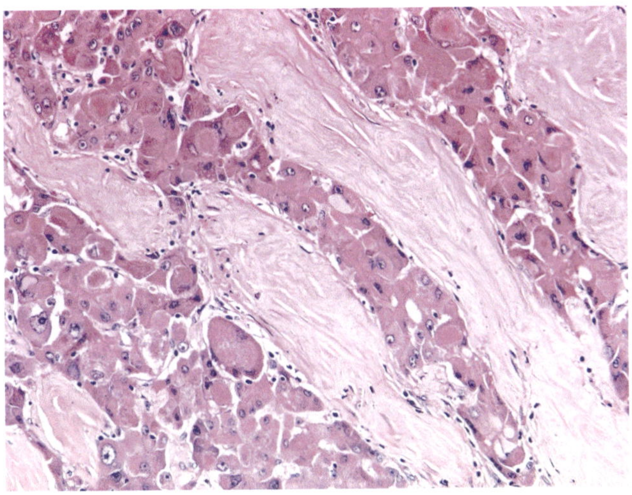

Fig. 14.37 Hepatocellular carcinoma, fibrolamellar type. Trabeculae of large polygonal eosinophilic tumour cells with voluminous cytoplasm and pale bodies are separated by lamellar fibrous bands. Fibrolamellar HCC is a variant accounting for 0.5% to 9.0% of all primary hepatic malignancies. It is less frequent in Asia and Africa than in Western countries. It affects both sexes equally and presents at a younger age (median age of 25 years) than classical HCC. It is not associated with cirrhosis, and its underlying causes and risk factors remain uncertain.

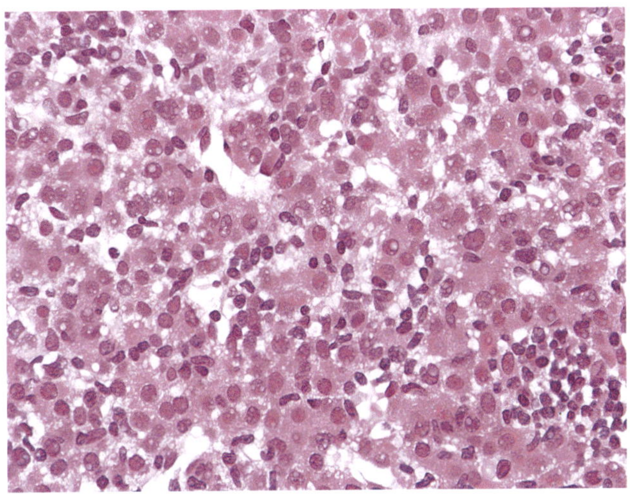

Fig. 14.39 Hepatocellular carcinoma, lymphoepithelioma-like. Trabeculae of malignant hepatocytes are infiltrated by abundant lymphocytes. Lymphoepithelioma-like HCC, also known as lymphocyte-rich HCC, is a rare variant, with fewer than 20 cases reported in the literature. The median age of presentation is 58 years. It commonly arises within a cirrhotic liver. It frequently is associated with hepatitis C (68.4%) and, rarely, Epstein-Barr virus (EBV; 5.3%).

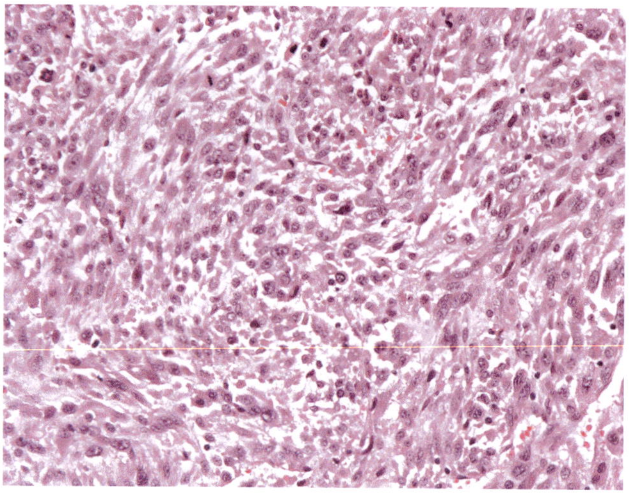

Fig. 14.40 Hepatocellular carcinoma, sarcomatoid type. The tumour is composed of markedly pleomorphic malignant spindle cells. Mitotic figures are seen readily. Sarcomatoid HCC is an uncommon variant that is either focally or entirely composed of malignant spindle cells. Most sarcomatoid HCCs exhibit areas of classic HCC and therefore require adequate sampling to be recognised. Sarcomatoid transformation commonly has been described in association with neoadjuvant systemic chemotherapy or transarterial chemoembolisation (TACE).

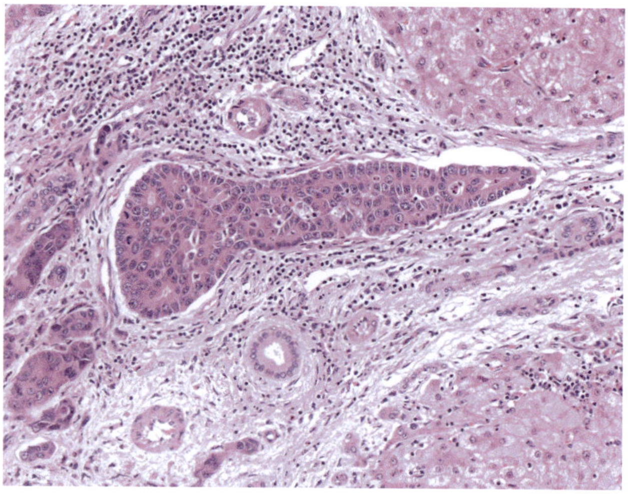

Fig. 14.41 Hepatocellular carcinoma. Microscopic vascular invasion is evident. Vascular invasion, both macroscopic and microscopic, is an important independent prognostic factor for overall and disease-free survival, and its presence or absence should be stated routinely in the pathology report. Macroscopic or microscopic tumour thrombosis in the portal venous system is the crucial route for intrahepatic metastases and recurrences. Vascular invasion correlates with tumour size and tumour grade. Microscopic vascular invasion is present in >50% and 25% of tumours more than 5 cm and less than 3 cm, respectively.

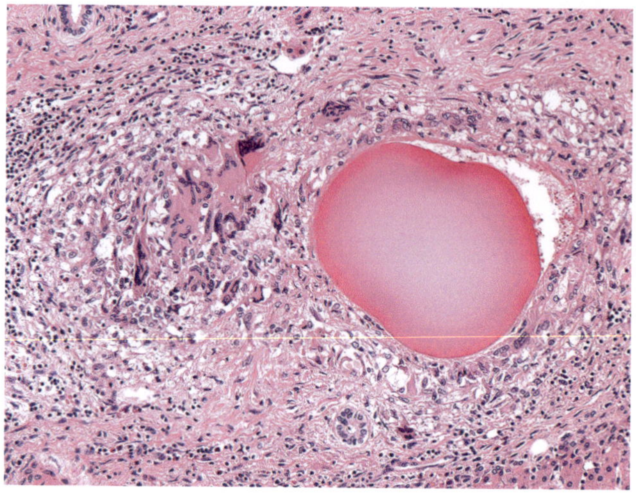

Fig. 14.42 Transarterial chemoembolisation. An extravasated therapeutic embolus is associated with foreign-body reaction. TACE is a regional treatment used mainly for HCC and occasionally metastatic neoplasms. It may be used as curative therapy to eradicate the entire tumour or as neoadjuvant therapy to shrink the tumour before surgical excision. HCC after TACE undergoes necrosis, but any residual tumour tends to exhibit a combined hepatocholangiocellular phenotype with ductular, glandular, or spindle cell (sarcomatoid) growth and expression of stemness markers (CD56/NCAM, EpCAM, and CD133).

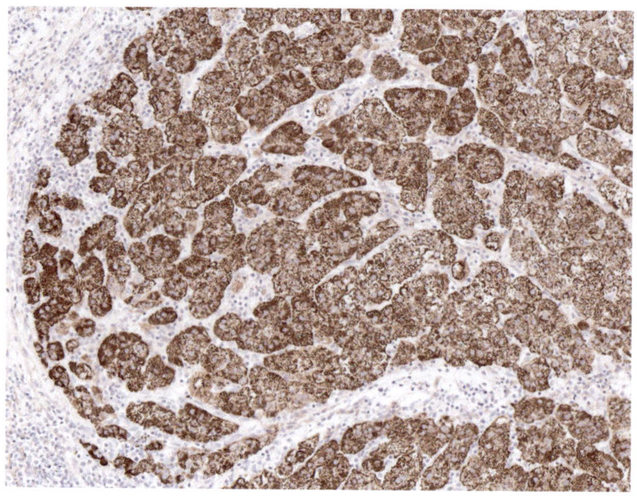

Fig. 14.43 Hepatocellular carcinoma (HepPar-1 stain). Hepatocellular differentiation is confirmed by immunoreactivity towards HepPar-1. Immunostaining for HepPar-1 is helpful in demonstrating hepatocellular differentiation. About 85% of well- and moderately differentiated HCCs are immunoreactive to HepPar-1, whereas less than 40% of poorly differentiated tumours are positive. However, this immunostain is not entirely specific because it is positive in hepatoid adenocarcinoma from other primary sites, and a small portion (<5%) of cholangiocarcinomas. Canalicular immunoreactivity for polyclonal carcinoembryonic antigen (pCEA) and CD10 also indicates hepatocellular differentiation, with overall sensitivity and specificity of 70% and nearly 100%.

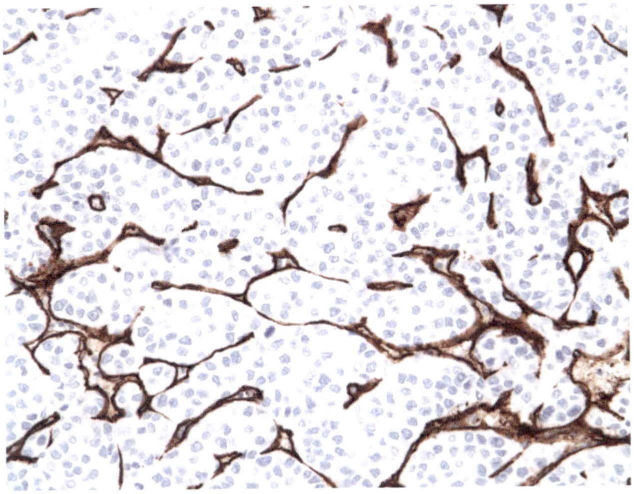

Fig. 14.44 Hepatocellular carcinoma (CD34 stain). Complete capillarisation is featured by diffuse sinusoidal expression of CD34. Sinusoidal endothelium in normal liver is devoid of CD34 immunoreactivity. However, many nonneoplastic and neoplastic liver diseases lead to distortion of the normal hepatic microcirculation and the formation of aberrant new vessels, resulting in sinusoidal capillarisation. Two distinct patterns of capillarisation may be demonstrated by immunostaining for CD34: complete and incomplete patterns. The former is characterised by a diffuse sinusoidal expression of CD34 within the entire lesion and is helpful in differentiating HCCs from benign hepatocellular lesions, with an overall sensitivity of 93.2% and specificity of 96.2%.

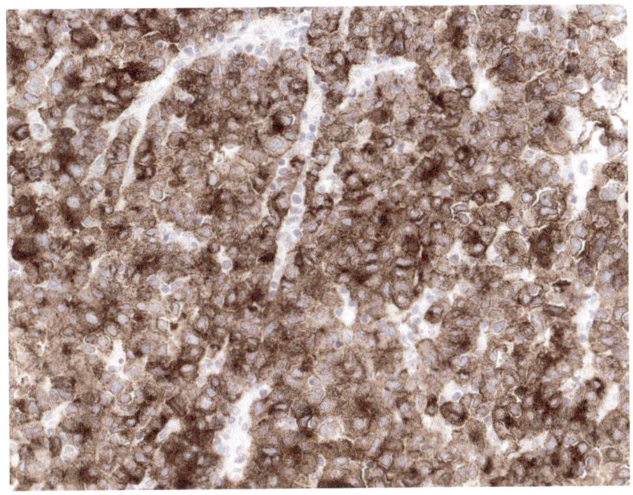

Fig. 14.45 Hepatocellular carcinoma (glypican-3 stain). The malignant tumour cells in this moderately differentiated HCC are highlighted with both membranous and cytoplasmic patterns. Glypican-3, a member of the glycosylphosphatidylinositol-anchored heparin sulphate proteoglycans, is normally expressed in fetal but not adult liver. It promotes the growth of HCC by activating the Wnt/β-catenin and insulin-like growth factor signalling pathways. It differentiates HCC from benign hepatocellular lesions, with an overall sensitivity of 78.6% and specificity of 92.9%. Other markers (glutamine synthetase, heat shock protein 70, and clathrin heavy chain) have been studied to use independently or in combination with the others to help the distinction between benign and malignant hepatocellular lesions.

PRIMARY TUMOUR (T)	
T1	Solitary tumour without vascular invasion
T2	Solitary tumour without vascular invasion; or multiple tumours none more than 5 cm in greatest dimension
T3a	Multiple tumours more than 5 cm in greatest dimension
T3b	Tumour involving a major branch of the portal or hepatic veins (right or left portal vein or right, middle or left hepatic vein)
T4	Tumour with direct invasion of adjacent organs other than the gallbladder or with perforation of visceral peritoneum
REGIONAL LYMPH NODE (N)	
N0	No regional lymph node metastasis
N1	Regional lymph node(s) metastasis
DISTANT METASTASIS (M)	
M0	No distant metastasis
M1	Distant metastasis

Fig. 14.46 American Joint Committee on Cancer (AJCC) tumour-node-metastasis (TNM) system of hepatocellular carcinoma, seventh edition. Treatment selection for HCC patients considers ablative as well as surgical management and requires a staging system based not only on tumour extent but also on underlying liver disease, cirrhotic status, and functional liver reserve. Several clinical staging systems, such as the Okuda classification, the Cancer of the Liver Italian Program (CLIP) system, the Barcelona Clinic Liver Cancer (BCLC) system, and the Chinese University Prognostic Index (CUPI), have been developed to attempt better stratification of HCC patients.

14.2 Biliary Epithelial Neoplasms

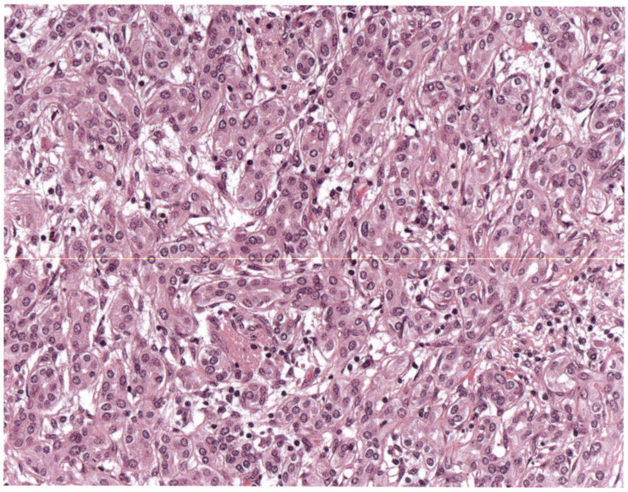

Fig. 14.47 Bile duct adenoma. There is proliferation of small tubular glands lined by a single layer of cuboidal epithelial cells with uniform bland nuclei. A mild lymphocytic infiltrate is noted. Bile duct adenoma, also known as peribiliary gland hamartoma, typically is an incidental finding. It usually is solitary (80%) and varies in size from 1 to 20 mm. It is a well-circumscribed unencapsulated nodule, located mainly in the subcapsular region and not uncommonly in the target of frozen section during abdominal surgery to exclude metastatic malignancy. Microscopically, it is composed of a proliferation of small tubular glands lined by a single layer of cuboidal to columnar epithelial cells with uniform bland nuclei. Varying degrees of fibrosis and inflammatory infiltrate usually are present. The lumina of tubular glands typically are small, without irregular dilatation or inspissated bile. Intraluminal mucin may be found.

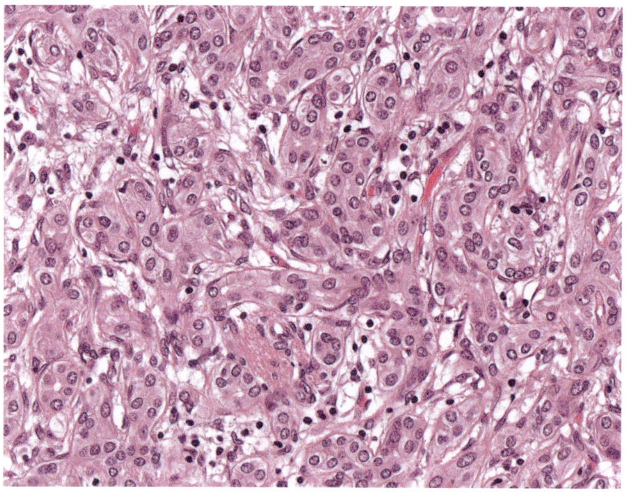

Fig. 14.48 Bile duct adenoma. There is a proliferation of small tubular glands lined by bland cuboidal epithelial cells with uniform nuclei. The main differential diagnoses of bile duct adenoma are von Meyenburg complexes, cholangiocarcinoma, and metastatic adenocarcinoma. Although von Meyenburg complexes usually are small and often are also situated in the subcapsular region, their ductal structures are irregularly dilated and occasionally inspissated bile or eosinophilic material. Cholangiocarcinoma and metastatic adenocarcinoma differ from bile duct adenoma by the presence of abnormal glandular architecture and malignant cytology.

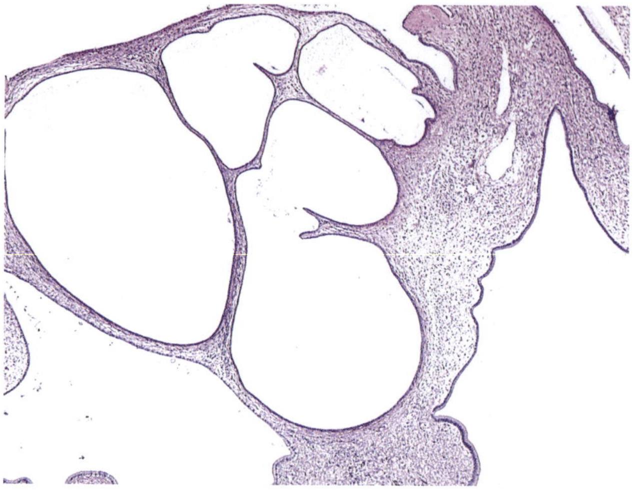

Fig. 14.49 Mucinous cystic neoplasm (MCN), low-grade intraepithelial neoplasia. A multilobular cyst is lined by a single layer of bland mucinous epithelial cells. *Mucinous cystic neoplasm*, previously referred to as bile duct cystadenoma and cystadenocarcinoma, is a term adopted in the latest WHO classification (fourth edition, 2010) paralleling its pancreatic counterpart. As with intraductal papillary neoplasm of the bile duct (IPNB), MCN may be categorized into invasive and noninvasive subtypes. Noninvasive MCN is classified further into MCN with low/intermediate-grade and high-grade intraepithelial neoplasia according to the degree of architectural cytologic atypia. Invasive MCN also is referred to as MCN with an associated invasive carcinoma (formerly mucinous cystadenocarcinoma).

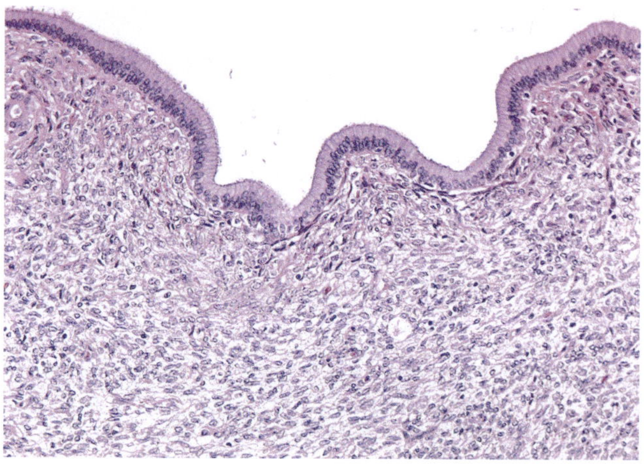

Fig. 14.50 Mucinous cystic neoplasm, low-grade intraepithelial neoplasia. A single layer of bland mucinous epithelial cells lies on an ovarian-type mesenchymal stroma. MCN is an uncommon cyst-forming epithelial neoplasm accounting for less than 5% of all hepatic cystic lesions. Noninvasive MCN is seen almost exclusively in females, with a mean age of 45 years. It is a benign neoplasm with an excellent prognosis after complete excision. Invasive MCN occurs in older patients with a mean age of 59 years. Invasive MCN with ovarian type mesenchymal stroma or residual noninvasive MCN components seems to have a much better prognosis than classic cholangiocarcinoma.

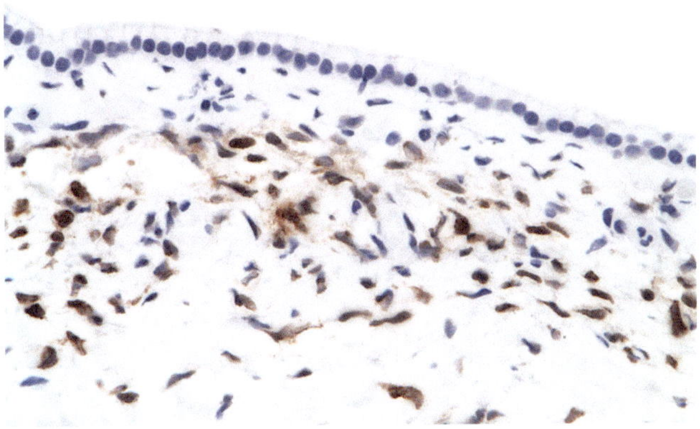

Fig. 14.51 Mucinous cystic neoplasm, low-grade intraepithelial neoplasia (progestrogen receptor [PR] stain). Spindle cells in the ovarian-type mesenchymal stroma are highlighted. MCN typically is multilocular and varies in size from 2.5 to 28 cm. It does not have any direct communication with large bile ducts. Papillary and solid growths may be present in MCN with high-grade intraepithelial neoplasia and MCN with an associated invasive carcinoma. Microscopically, MCN is lined by mucinous epithelial cells with varying degrees of architectural and cytologic atypia. The ovarian-type mesenchymal stroma is characteristic, and the stromal cells typically are immunoreactive to oestrogen receptor and progestrogen receptor. The invasive component of most invasive MCNs usually is adenocarcinoma with tubulopapillary or tubular growth patterns.

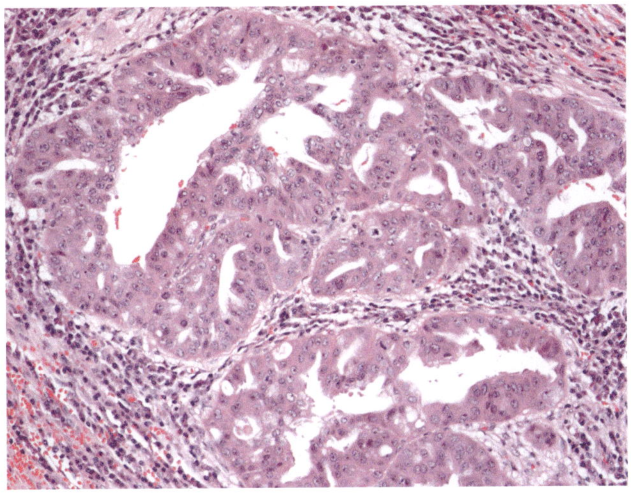

Fig. 14.53 Mucinous cystic neoplasm with an associated invasive carcinoma. There are neoplastic cystic lesions that may be considered as differential diagnoses of MCN. The cystic type of IPNB is characterised by cystic ductal dilatation with prominent intraductal mucin accumulation. Varying degrees of architectural and cytologic atypia and areas of invasive carcinoma may be found. The cystic type of IPNB differs from MCN by the presence of a direct luminal connection to the bile ducts and the absence of the ovarian-type stroma. Serous microcystic adenoma is a multilobular cyst lined by a single layer of bland cuboidal epithelial cells with clear cytoplasm and lacking the ovarian-type stroma.

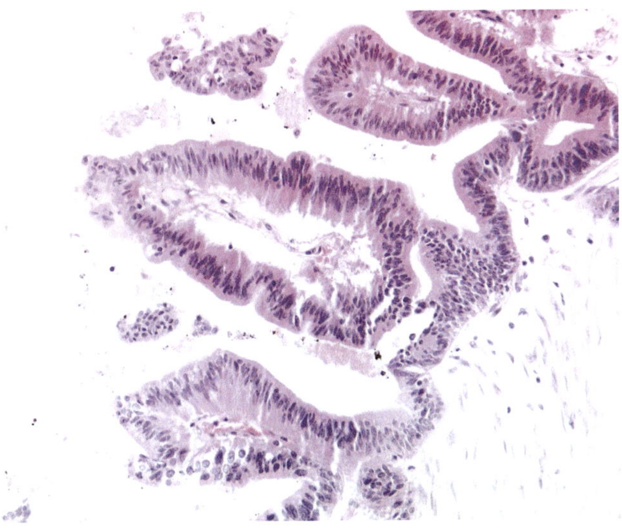

Fig. 14.52 Mucinous cystic neoplasm, high-grade intraepithelial neoplasia. Papillary fronds are lined by atypical mucinous epithelial cells with nuclear stratification, enlargement, and pleomorphism. Some non-neoplastic cysts may be considered as differential diagnoses. Solitary bile duct cyst is a unilocular cyst lined by a single layer of nonmucinous cuboidal or columnar cells without the ovarian-type stroma. Polycystic liver disease is characterised by multiple cysts lined by attenuated or cuboidal cells and usually accompanied by von Meyenburg complexes and/or corpora albicantes–like collapsed cysts. Endometriosis is composed of endometrium-type nonmucinous epithelium and stroma with varying degrees of haemorrhage and haemosiderin-laden macrophages. Peribiliary cyst is a multilocular cyst at the perihilar region and is lined by mucinous epithelial cells with an absence of the ovarian-type stroma.

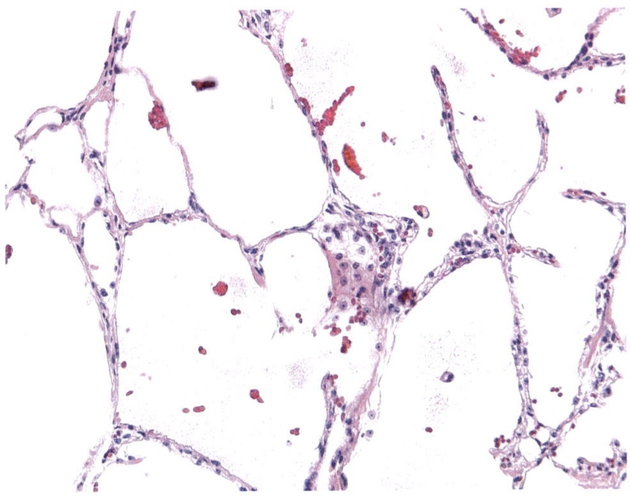

Fig. 14.54 Serous microcystic adenoma. Multiple small cystic spaces are separated by thin septa, which are lined by bland cuboidal epithelial cells with clear cytoplasm. Serous microcystic adenoma is an exceedingly uncommon benign hepatic neoplasm, much rarer than its pancreatic counterpart. Grossly, it is a well-circumscribed sponge-like tumour with multiple microcysts filled with clear serous fluid. Microscopically, it is composed of multiple small cystic spaces separated by thin septa, which are lined by bland cuboidal epithelial cells with glycogen-rich clear cytoplasm.

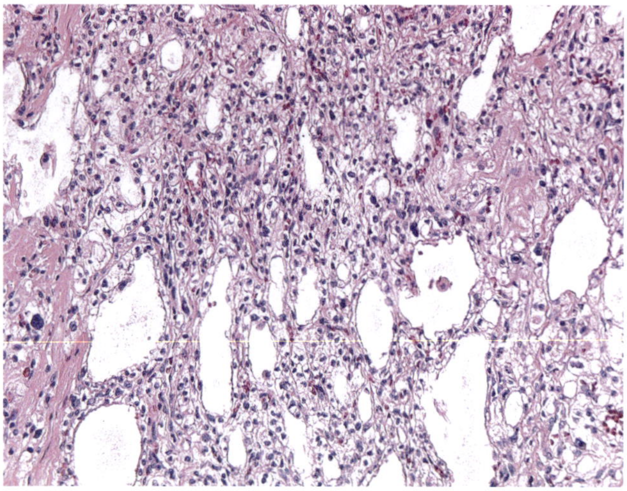

Fig. 14.55 Serous microcystic adenoma. Multiple small cystic spaces are separated by thin septa, which are lined by bland cuboidal epithelial cells with clear cytoplasm. Serous microcystic adenoma exhibits quite characteristic microscopic features and seldom is confused with other entities. Metastatic clear cell renal cell carcinoma is the only important differential diagnosis. Clinicoradiologic correlation and immunohistochemical stains for renal cell markers (CD10, PAX2, and PAX8) are helpful in difficult cases.

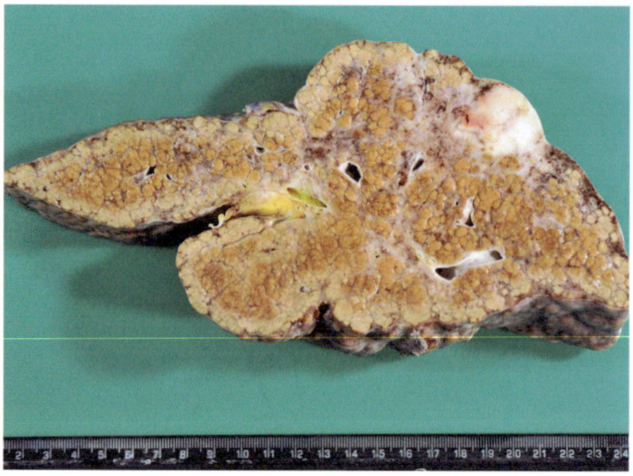

Fig. 14.57 Intrahepatic cholangiocarcinoma, mass-forming type. A firm white tumour is present within a cirrhotic liver. Intrahepatic cholangiocarcinoma may be solitary or multiple. It may be classified macroscopically according to the growth pattern. The mass-forming type is featured by solitary or multiple tumour nodules. The periductal-infiltrating type is characterised by diffuse longitudinal tumour infiltration along the biliary tree. The intraductal growth type is featured by a polypoid or papillary lesion within a dilated bile duct. The mixed type is a combination of any three growth patterns. Intrahepatic cholangiocarcinomas arising from small to medium-sized bile ducts in the liver parenchyma (peripheral cholangiocarcinoma) usually are the mass-forming type (60%), mixed mass-forming and periductal-infiltrating type (20%), or periductal infiltrating type (20%).

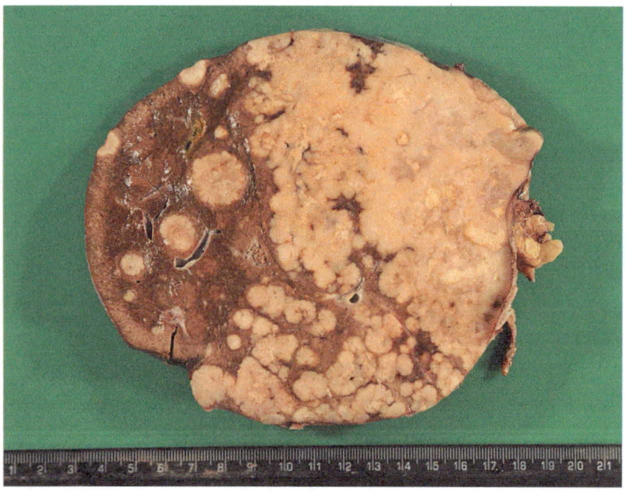

Fig. 14.56 Intrahepatic cholangiocarcinoma, mass-forming type. Multiple tan-coloured tumour masses of varied sizes are present in a noncirrhotic liver. Intrahepatic cholangiocarcinoma is the second commonest primary hepatic malignancy (5%–15%). A wide geographic variation in incidence is observed, with the highest incidence in Thailand, Laos, southern China, and Korea. Intrahepatic cholangiocarcinoma usually affects the elderly population, with a slight male predilection. Chronic biliary diseases (primary sclerosing cholangitis, hepatolithiasis, and parasitic biliary infestation), congenital biliary abnormalities (fibrocystic liver disease and choledochal cyst), nonbiliary cirrhosis, hereditary haemochromatosis, and thorotrast are known risk factors for cholangiocarcinoma. Biliary intraepithelial neoplasia and IPNB are considered precursors of cholangiocarcinoma.

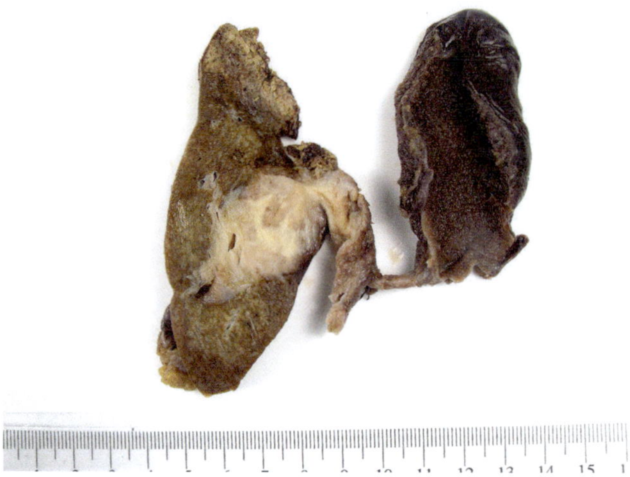

Fig. 14.58 Intrahepatic cholangiocarcinoma, mass-forming and periductal-infiltrating type. In the perihilar region of a noncirrhotic liver, a whitish mass with periductal infiltration of the common hepatic duct is present. The presence of periductal-infiltrating growth, whether pure or mixed with other growth patterns, currently is classified as T4 tumour in the seventh edition of the AJCC TNM system. The mixed type with a periductal-infiltrating component has a high rate of macroscopic vascular invasion (61%), perineural invasion (80%), and lymph node metastasis (50%). This type has a 0% 5-year survival rate, whereas the mass-forming and intraductal growth types have 39% and 69% survival rates, respectively.

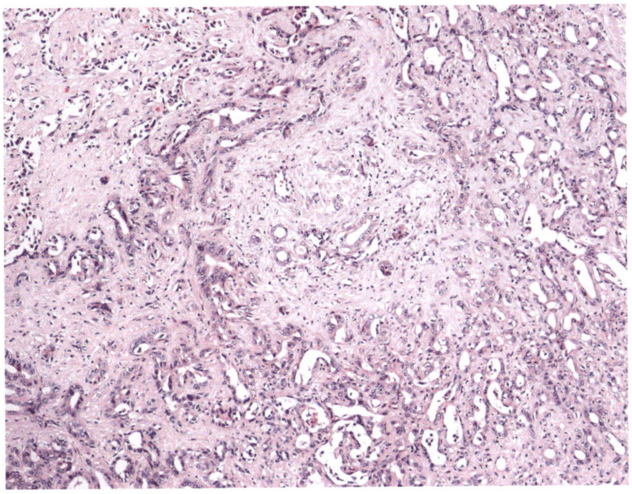

Fig. 14.59 Intrahepatic cholangiocarcinoma. Irregular and angulated glands are embedded in fibrous stroma. Most intrahepatic cholangiocarcinomas are adenocarcinomas with variable differentiation and fibroplasia. Most are well differentiated and predominantly composed of tubules and glands. Complex cribriform glands, micropapillae, solid nests, and infiltrative cords also may be present. The tumour cells usually are cuboidal or columnar cells with small nuclei and nucleoli. Mucin seldom is abundant, except in the mucinous variant, in which there may be prominent luminal and extravasated mucin. Fibroplasia is typical for intrahepatic cholangiocarcinoma, in contrast to HCC. Fibroplasia usually is more prominent in the central portion of the tumour. Lymphovascular permeation and perineural invasion are frequent.

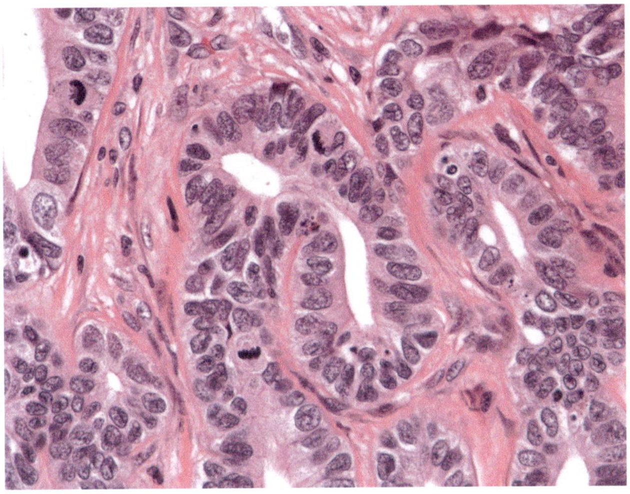

Fig. 14.61 Intrahepatic cholangiocarcinoma. These tumour cells exhibit moderate nuclear pleomorphism, inconspicuous nucleoli, and frequent mitosis. Several differential diagnoses for intrahepatic cholangiocarcinoma exist, including von Meyenburg complexes and bile duct adenomas. HCC with a prominent pseudoacinar growth may mimic intrahepatic cholangiocarcinoma, but recognition of a more typical trabecular growth and immunoreactivity to HepPar-1, pCEA, and CD10 make the distinction. Metastatic adenocarcinoma is indistinguishable in haematoxylin and eosin sections only; hence, immunohistochemistry and clinicoradiologic correlation are essential.

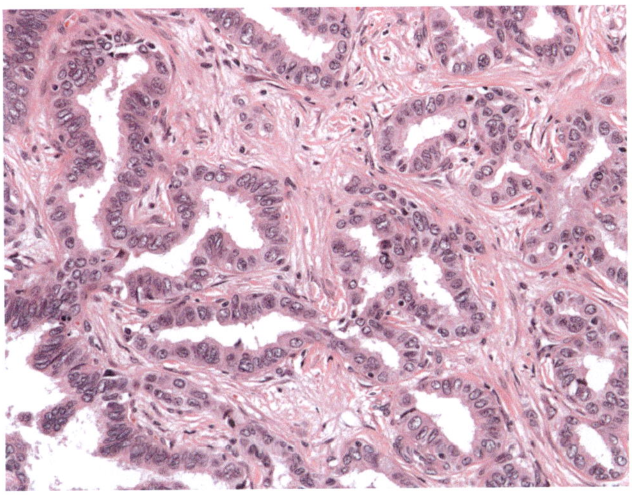

Fig. 14.60 Intrahepatic cholangiocarcinoma. Irregular and angulated glands are embedded in a fibrous stroma. Intrahepatic cholangiocarcinomas are classified as well-differentiated, moderately differentiated, or poorly differentiated tumours according to their glandular differentiation in the WHO system. Well-differentiated tumours typically are composed of tubules with or without micropapillary growth. Moderately differentiated tumours usually consist of irregular and dilated tubules with cribriform glands and infiltrative cords. Poorly differentiated tumours tend to be composed of complex glands, infiltrative cords, and solid sheets of markedly pleomorphic tumour cells.

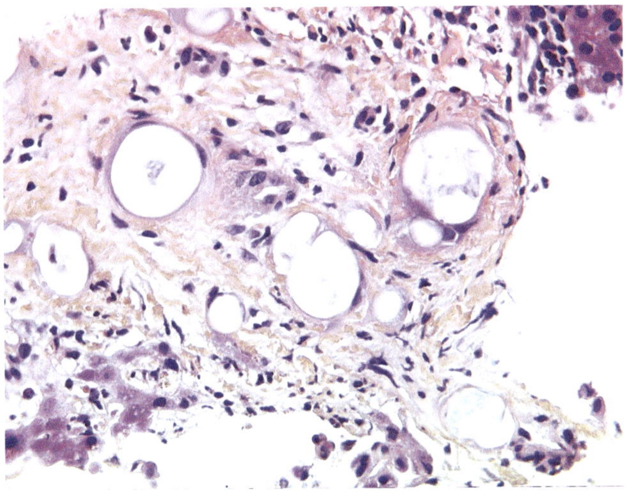

Fig. 14.62 Intrahepatic cholangiocarcinoma, signet ring cell type. Signet ring tumour cells are scattered in fibrous stroma. There are several histologic variants of intrahepatic cholangiocarcinoma, including adenosquamous carcinoma, squamous carcinoma, mucinous carcinoma, signet ring cell carcinoma, clear cell carcinoma, mucoepidermoid carcinoma, lymphoepithelioma-like carcinoma, and sarcomatoid carcinoma.

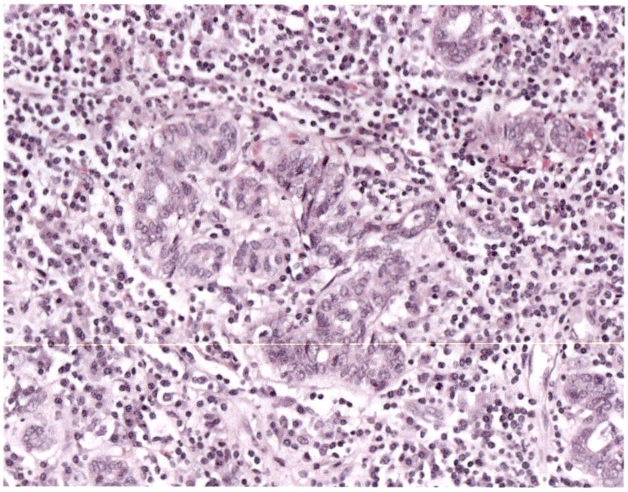

Fig. 14.63 Intrahepatic cholangiocarcinoma, lymphoepithelioma-like. Irregular and complex glands and tubules are admixed with a dense lymphoplasmacytic infiltrate. Lymphoepithelioma-like cholangiocarcinoma is a rare variant of intrahepatic cholangiocarcinoma, with fewer than 25 cases reported in the literature. Most (81%) of these cases have been associated with EBV. The EBV-associated tumours predominantly affect women, with a male-to-female ratio of 1:7.5. The median age of presentation is 56 years. It seems to have a much more favourable prognosis than conventional intrahepatic cholangiocarcinoma.

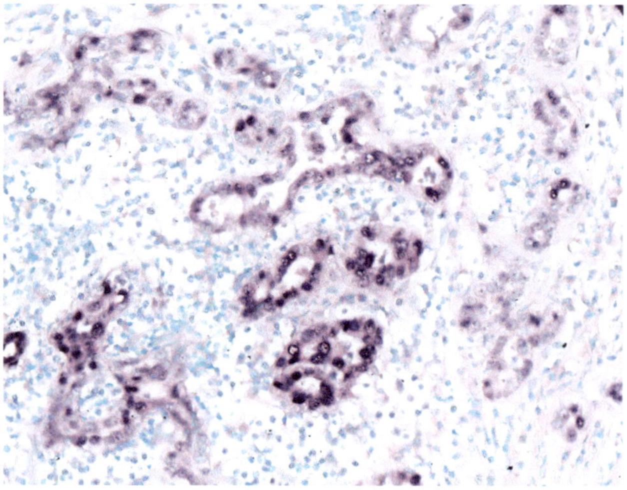

Fig. 14.64 Intrahepatic cholangiocarcinoma, lymphoepithelioma-like (in situ hybridization of EBV-encoded RNA [EBER]). The malignant tumour cells in this lymphoepithelioma-like cholangiocarcinoma are highlighted. Lymphoepithelioma-like cholangiocarcinoma consists of a malignant glandular component with a variable amount of undifferentiated tumour. Half of purely glandular lymphoepithelioma-like cholangiocarcinomas are well differentiated, with relatively bland architectural and cytologic features.

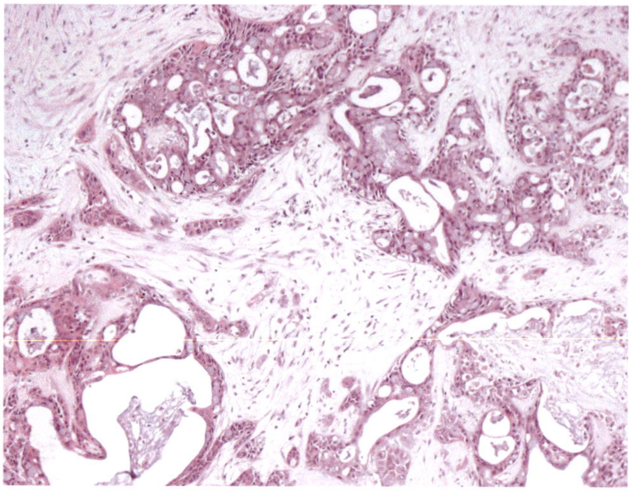

Fig. 14.65 Intrahepatic cholangiocarcinoma, mucoepidermoid. There are irregular solid and cystic nests of squamoid (epidermoid), intermediate, and mucinous tumour cells in fibrous stroma. Mucoepidermoid cholangiocarcinoma is a rare variant of intrahepatic cholangiocarcinoma, with 17 cases reported in the literature. A slight male predominance is observed, with a male-to-female ratio of 1.4:1. The median age at presentation is 63 years. It seems to have an extremely poor prognosis, and more than 60% of patients die within 6 months of the initial diagnosis.

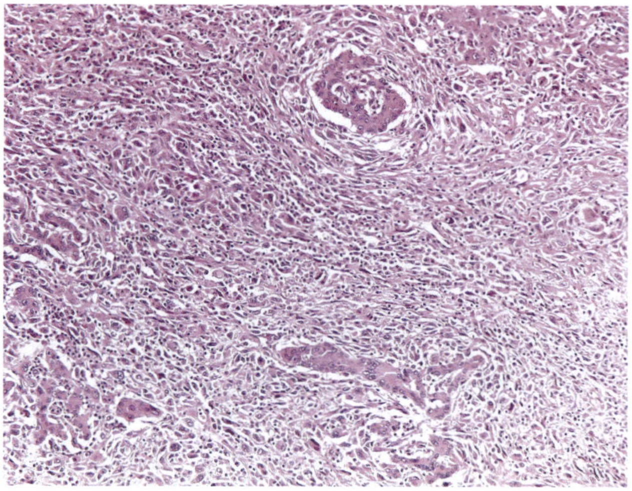

Fig. 14.66 Intrahepatic cholangiocarcinoma, sarcomatoid type. Malignant glands are seen, surrounded by a malignant spindle cell proliferation. Sarcomatoid cholangiocarcinoma is an uncommon variant of intrahepatic cholangiocarcinoma that is either focally or entirely composed of sarcomatoid components; it accounts for 4.5% of intrahepatic cholangiocarcinomas. The sarcomatoid component mainly is a malignant spindle cell proliferation, resembling fibrosarcoma or malignant fibrous histiocytoma. Heterologous elements, such as osteoid or chondroid tissue, may be seen, however, albeit rarely.

PRIMARY TUMOUR (T)	
Tis	Carcinoma in situ (intraductal tumour)
T1	Solitary tumour without vascular invasion
T2a	Solitary tumour without vascular invasion
T2b	Multiple tumours with or without vascular invasion
T3	Tumour perforating the visceral peritoneum or involving the local extrahepatic structures by direct invasion
T4	Tumour with periductal invasion
REGIONAL LYMPH NODE (N)	
N0	No regional lymph node metastasis
N1	Regional lymph node(s) metastasis
DISTANT METASTASIS (M)	
M0	No distant metastasis
M1	Distant metastasis

Fig. 14.67 The AJCC TNM system of intrahepatic cholangiocarcinoma, seventh edition. This staging system is new for the seventh edition and is independent of the staging system for HCC and extrahepatic biliary malignancy. This system also applies to combined hepatocellular-cholangiocarcinoma (HCC-CC).

PRIMARY TUMOUR (T)	
Tis	Carcinoma in situ (intraductal tumour)
T1	Tumour confined to the bile duct, with extension up to the muscle layer or fibrous tissue
T2a	Tumour invades beyond the wall of the bile duct to surrounding adipose tissue
T2b	Tumour invades adjacent hepatic parenchyma
T3	Tumour invades unilateral branches of portalvein or hepatic artery
T4	Tumour invades main portal vein or its branches bilaterally; or the common hepatic artery; or the second-order biliary radicals bilaterally; or unilateral second-order biliary radicals with contralateral portal vein or hepatic artery involvement
REGIONAL LYMPH NODE (N)	
N0	No regional lymph node metastasis
N1	Regional lymph node(s) metastasis
DISTANT METASTASIS (M)	
M0	No distant metastasis
M1	Distant metastasis

Fig. 14.68 The AJCC TNM system for perihilar cholangiocarcinoma, seventh edition.

14.3 Combined Hepatocellular–Cholangiocarcinoma

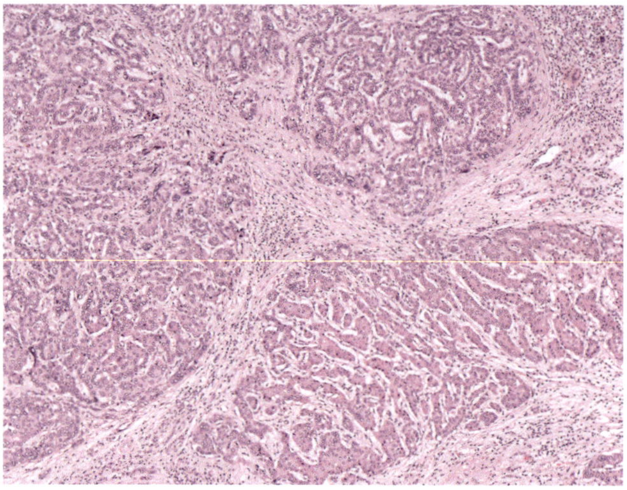

Fig. 14.69 Classic-type combined hepatocellular-cholangiocarcinoma. This tumour exhibits dual differentiation with both hepatocellular (*lower*) and cholangiocellular (*upper*) components. Combined HCC-CC, also known as mixed HCC-CC, is defined as a tumour with unequivocal, intimately mixed hepatocellular and biliary components. It differs from "collision tumours," which are separate HCCs and cholangiocarcinomas arising in the same liver. A true combined HCC-CC is rare and accounts for <1% of all primary hepatic malignancies. Geographic variation, age of presentation, and sex predilection are the same as those of conventional HCC. In the latest WHO classification (fourth edition, 2010), it is classified further into classic-type combined HCC-CC and combined HCC-CC with stem cell features.

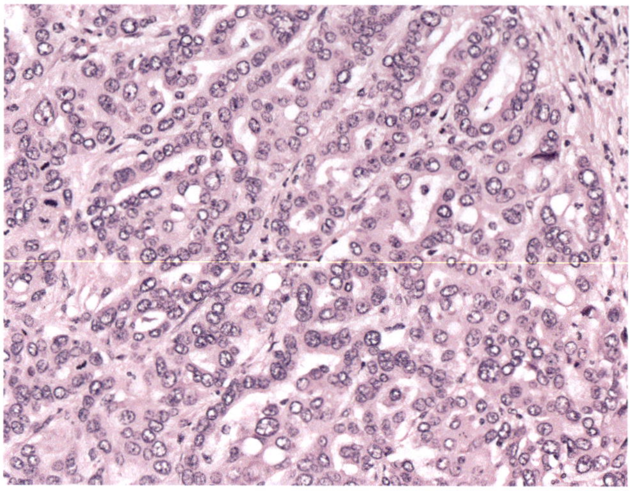

Fig. 14.71 Classic-type combined hepatocellular-cholangiocarcinoma (CK19 stain). In contrast to HepPar-1, the hepatocellular component shows focal positivity, whereas the cholangiocellular component shows diffuse positivity. When considered in parallel with Fig. 14.69, there clearly are some tumour cells coexpressing HepPar-1 and CK19. They may represent an intermediate component between HCC and cholangiocarcinoma.

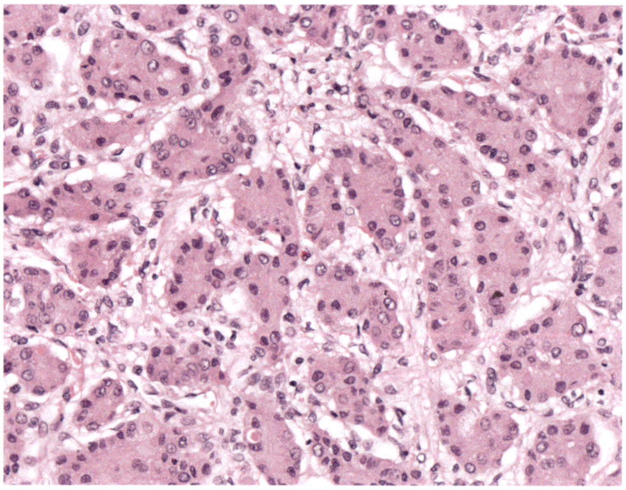

Fig. 14.70 Classic-type combined hepatocellular-cholangiocarcinoma (HepPar-1 stain). The hepatocellular component shows diffuse positivity, whereas the cholangiocellular component shows only focal positivity. Classic-type combined HCC-CC is believed to have less favourable prognosis than classic HCC. HCC expressing biliary keratins (CK7 and CK19) without a genuine glandular component also carries a poorer outcome than classic HCC.

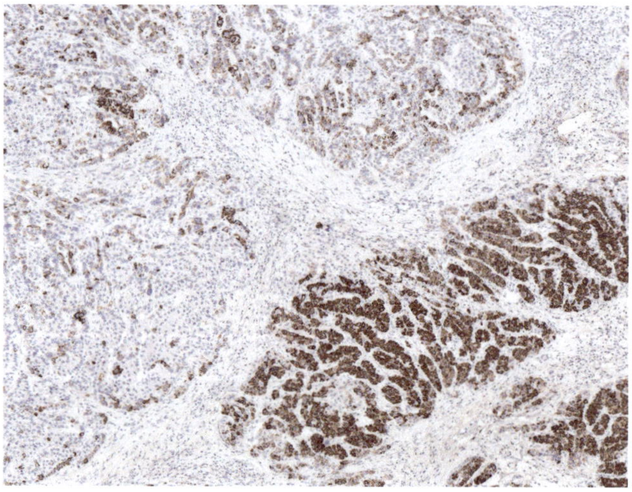

Fig. 14.72 Classic-type combined hepatocellular-cholangiocarcinoma. The hepatocellular component is composed of trabeculae of malignant hepatocytes. Classic-type combined HCC-CC is composed of regions of typical HCC and regions of typical cholangiocarcinoma. The hepatocellular component may be well to poorly differentiated. Definite hepatocellular differentiation may be demonstrated by the presence of bile, immunoreactivity to HepPar-1 and α-fetoprotein, and canalicular positivity to pCEA and CD10.

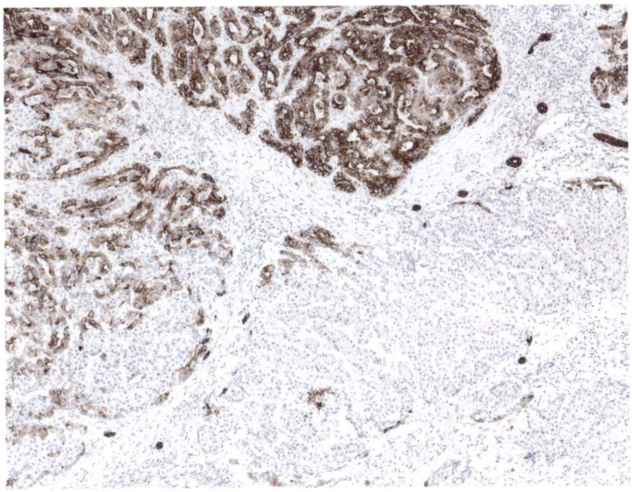

Fig. 14.73 Classic-type combined hepatocellular-cholangiocarcinoma. The cholangiocellular component is composed of closely packed, irregular glands. Some tumour cells (*left*) are small oval-shaped cells with a high nucleocytoplasmic ratio and may represent an intermediate component between HCC and cholangiocarcinoma. Classic-type combined HCC-CC is composed of regions of typical HCC and regions of typical cholangiocarcinoma. The cholangiocarcinoma component can be well to poorly differentiated. Definite cholangiocarcinoma differentiation may be demonstrated by the presence of genuine glandular formation with mucin production. Immunoreactivity to "biliary" keratins (CK7 and CK19) may be helpful but are not entirely specific, because the hepatocellular component may demonstrate focal immunoreactivity.

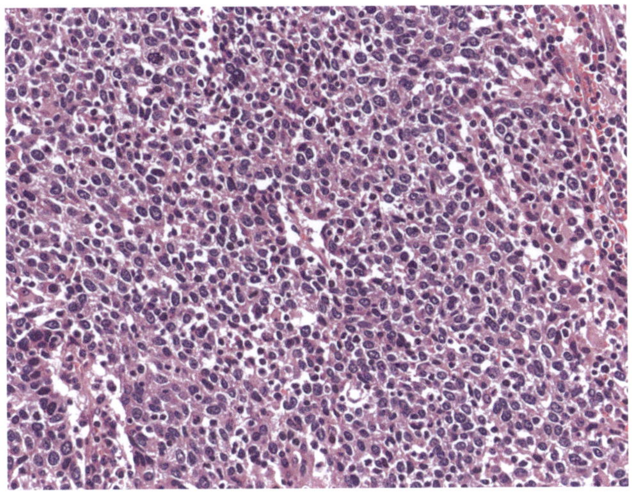

Fig. 14.75 Intermediate cell–subtype combined hepatocellular-cholangiocarcinoma with stem cell features. There is a sheet of small oval-shaped tumour cells with hyperchromatic nuclei and a high nucleocytoplasmic ratio. *Combined HCC-CC with stem cell features* is a new entity in the latest WHO classification (fourth edition, 2010). It is a term applied to tumours with a significant component with features suggesting a stem/progenitor phenotype. It is classified further into three subtypes by morphology: typical, intermediate cell, and cholangiolocellular subtypes. However, the biological differences among these subtypes are uncertain.

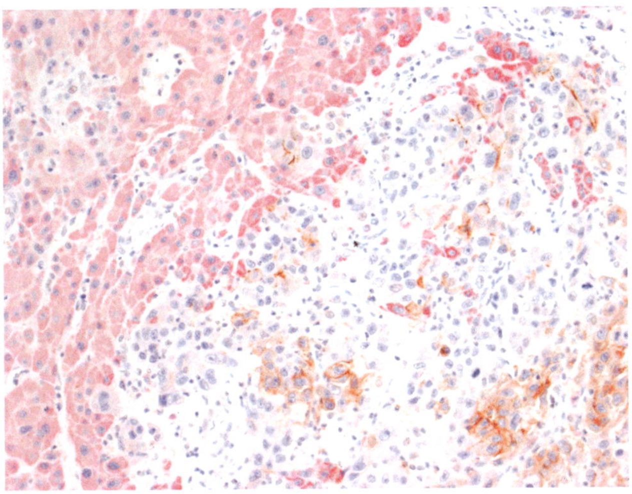

Fig. 14.74 Classic-type combined hepatocellular-cholangiocarcinoma (CD133 stain: brown; HepPar-1 stain: red). In the vicinity of the hepatocellular component (*left*), small oval-shaped tumour cells with hyperchromatic nuclei and a high nucleocytoplasmic ratio are seen to express CD133 (a stemness marker). The intermediate component between HCC and cholangiocarcinoma may express stemness markers (CD56/NCAM, EpCAM, and CD133). If this intermediate component with stem/progenitor cell phenotype predominates, a diagnosis of combined HCC-CC with stem cell features should be considered. Expression of stemness markers also may be found in one third of residual HCCs after TACE.

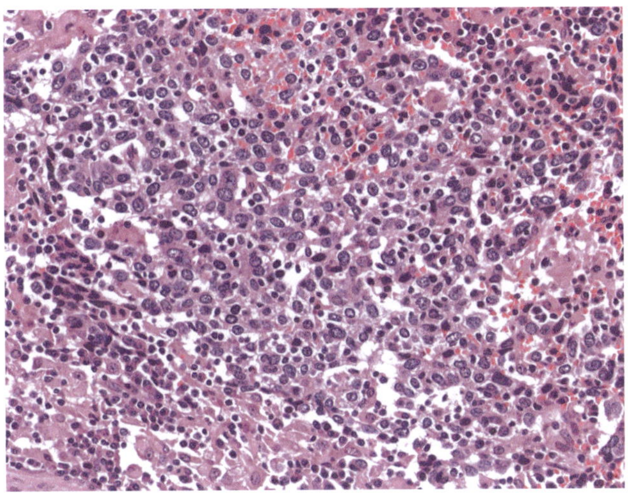

Fig. 14.76 Intermediate cell subtype of combined hepatocellular-cholangiocarcinoma with stem cell features. There is a sheet of small oval-shaped tumour cells with hyperchromatic nuclei and a high nucleocytoplasmic ratio. The intermediate subtype of combined HCC-CC with stem cell features is composed of sheets, trabeculae, or strands of small oval-shaped cells with hyperchromatic nuclei and a high nucleocytoplasmic ratio. Coexpression of hepatocellular markers (HepPar-1) and cholangiocellular markers (CK7/19) usually are found. Stemness markers (CD56/NCAM, EpCAM, and CD133) are variably expressed.

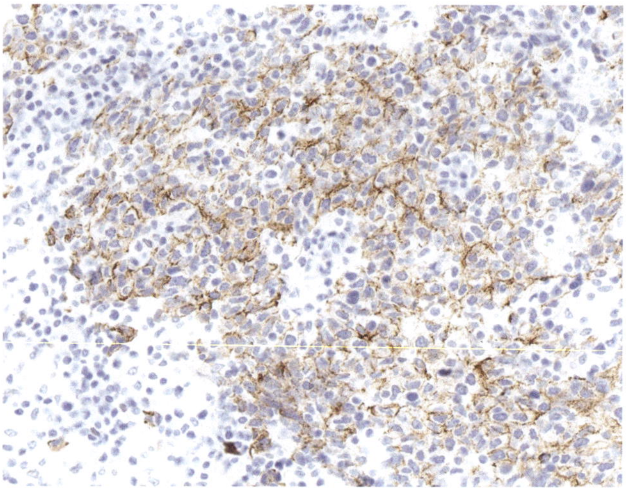

Fig. 14.77 Intermediate cell subtype of combined hepatocellular-cholangiocarcinoma with stem cell features (immunohistochemistry for EpCAM). Focal expression of this stemness marker is demonstrated. In contrast to the microscopic growth pattern of the immediate cell subtype, the typical subtype of combined HCC-CC with stem cell features is composed of nests of mature-looking hepatocytes rimmed by clusters of small oval-shaped cells with hyperchromatic nuclei, a high nucleocytoplasmic ratio, and variable expression of CK7/19 and stemness markers (CD56/NCAM, EpCAM, and CD133).

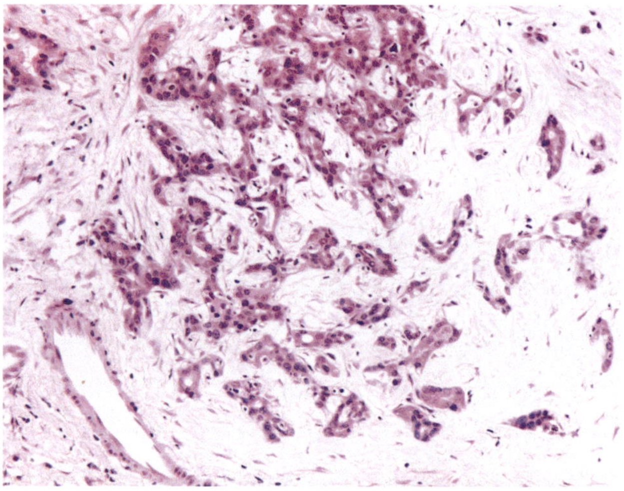

Fig. 14.78 Cholangiolocellular subtype of combined hepatocellular-cholangiocarcinoma with stem cell features. Tumour cells are arranged in a tubular and antler-like pattern in marked fibrous stroma. The cholangiolocellular subtype of combined HCC-CC with stem cell features is composed of a tubular, cord-like, and antler-like growth of small oval-shaped cells in fibrous stroma, resembling canals of Hering/bile ductules (cholangioles). The tumour cells possess hyperchromatic nuclei and a high nucleocytoplasmic ratio. Nuclear pleomorphism typically is mild, but mucin production is absent. Stemness markers (CD56/NCAM, EpCAM, and CD133) are variably expressed. More differentiated areas with classic HCC or classic cholangiocarcinoma morphology frequently are observed at the periphery of these tumours.

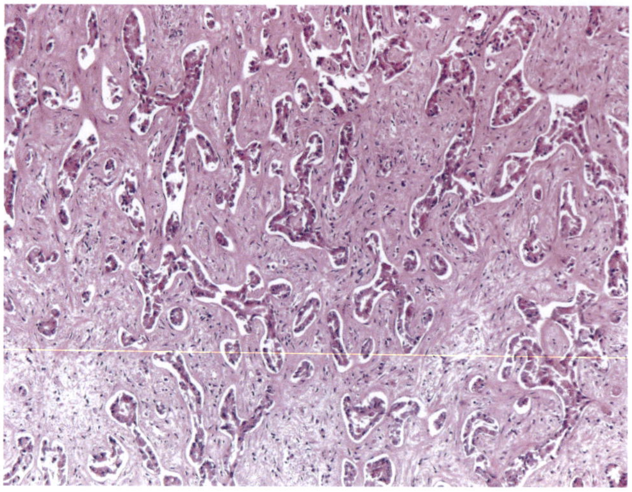

Fig. 14.79 Cholangiolocellular subtype of combined hepatocellular-cholangiocarcinoma with stem cell features. Tumour cells are arranged in a tubular and antler-like pattern in marked fibrous stroma. The cholangiolocellular subtype of combined HCC-CC with stem cell features previously was classified as a variant of cholangiocarcinoma (cholangiolocarcinoma). It may mimic a ductular reaction, but cytologic atypia is (at least focally) present and neutrophils, which normally accompany ductular reaction, are absent.

14.4 Other Epithelial Neoplasms

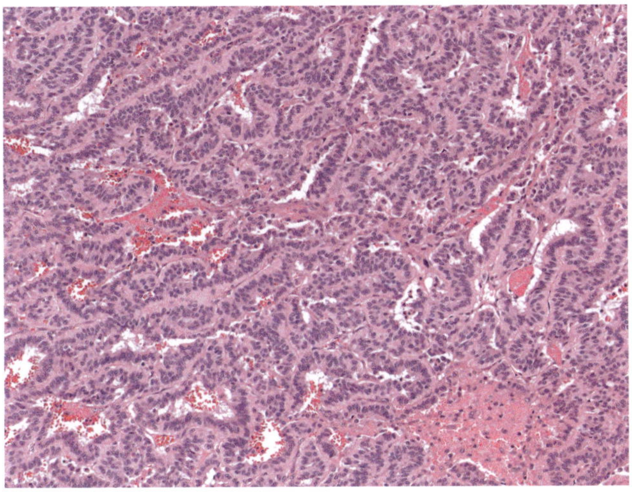

Fig. 14.80 Hepatic carcinoid. There are trabeculae of tumour cells with rich vasculature. The tumour cells exhibit uniform nuclei, "salt-and-pepper" chromatin, and inconspicuous nucleoli. Primary hepatic carcinoid is uncommon, with fewer than 100 cases reported in the literature. It usually affects middle-aged patients, with a slight female predilection (male-to-female ratio of 1:1.4). Patients may present with nonspecific symptoms, including abdominal pain, abdominal mass, fatigue, and weight loss. Carcinoid syndrome (skin flushing, abdominal pain, and diarrhoea) is rare.

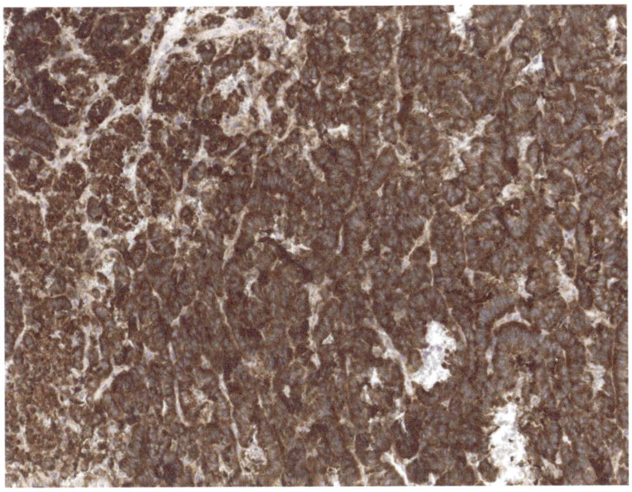

Fig. 14.81 Hepatic carcinoid. These tumour cells are immunoreactive to the neuroendocrine marker synaptophysin. Primary hepatic carcinoid should be distinguished from the more common metastatic carcinoid or well-differentiated neuroendocrine tumour from other sites, noticeably the gastrointestinal tract, pancreas, and lung. There is no histologic difference between primary and metastatic carcinoid. Clinicoradiologic correlation is crucial to establish the definite diagnosis. Their true existence is questioned, as they may represent metastatic spread from small occult extrahepatic tumours.

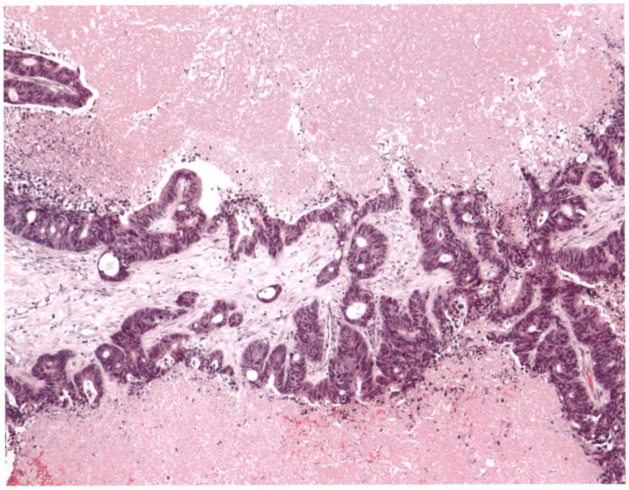

Fig. 14.82 Metastatic colorectal adenocarcinoma. Irregular, complex malignant glands are associated with confluent tumour necrosis. Metastatic carcinoma is the commonest hepatic neoplasm in Western countries. However, metastatic lesions are less frequent than primary hepatic malignancy in Southeast Asia and sub-Saharan Africa because of a high incidence of HCC, shorter life expectancy, and lower incidence of certain malignancies (e.g., colorectal and pulmonary carcinoma). The liver is a common organ of metastasis disseminated through vascular spread (both systemic arterial and portal venous systems), lymphatic spread, and peritoneal deposition.

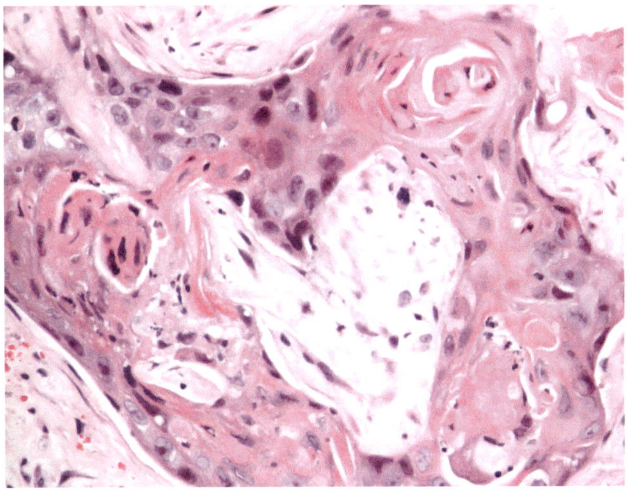

Fig. 14.83 Metastatic squamous cell carcinoma. An irregular nest of keratinising squamous cell carcinoma is present. Metastatic carcinoma is the commonest secondary hepatic neoplasm, followed by malignant melanoma. Haematolymphoid malignancy, sarcoma, and germ cell tumour less frequently metastasise to the liver. The large intestine, stomach, and breasts are the most frequent primary sites of metastatic carcinoma to the liver.

15 Nonepithelial Liver Neoplasms

With the exception of cavernous haemangioma, mesenchymal tumours are rare. They may affect children and adults, and many are very similar histologically to their extrahepatic counterparts. They may be associated with other congenital abnormalities in children or other conditions (e.g., Epstein-Barr virus [EBV], HIV infections) but they usually do not occur in the context of chronic liver disease. They are divided in this chapter into benign mesenchymal tumours, malignant mesenchymal tumours, and haematolymphoid malignancies.

15.1 Benign Mesenchymal Neoplasms

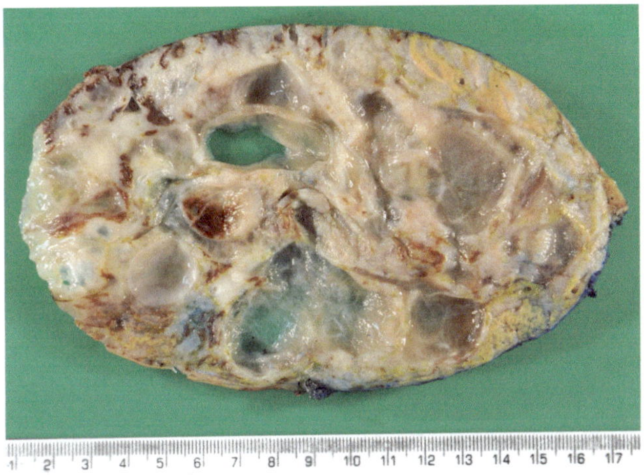

Fig. 15.1 Mesenchymal hamartoma. A solid and cystic tumour contains gelatinous mucoid material within cystic spaces. Mesenchymal hamartoma is the second commonest benign tumour in children after haemangioma. It accounts for 12% and 8% of all liver tumours and tumour-like lesions before the ages of 2 years and 21 years, respectively. More than 95% of patients present before the age of 5 years. A male predominance (70%) is observed in paediatric cases, in contrast to a female predominance in adult cases. Association with other congenital abnormalities is uncommon but has been described in congenital heart disease, intestinal malrotation, oesophageal atresia with or without an annular pancreas, biliary atresia, exomphalos, Beckwith-Wiedemann syndrome, and placental mesenchymal dysplasia.

A.W.H. Chan et al., *Atlas of Liver Pathology*, Atlas of Anatomic Pathology,
DOI 10.1007/978-1-4614-9114-9_15, © Springer Science+Business Media New York 2014

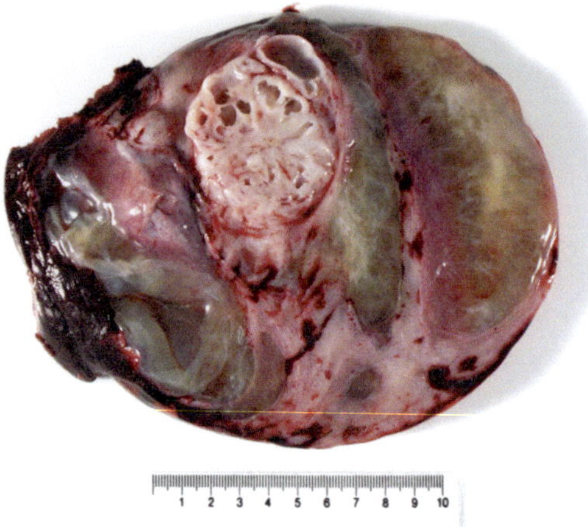

Fig. 15.2 Mesenchymal hamartoma. Mesenchymal hamartoma is located more commonly in the right lobe (75%) and may be pedunculated from the inferior surface of the liver in 20% of cases. Its size is highly variable and may reach 30 cm in its greatest dimension and 3 kg in weight. It typically is a circumscribed, unencapsulated mass with both solid and cystic components. Cystic spaces do not communicate with the biliary tree. Its numbers vary from a few to multiple and range from a few millimetres to a few centimetres. Young infants usually have more solid and less cystic tumours.

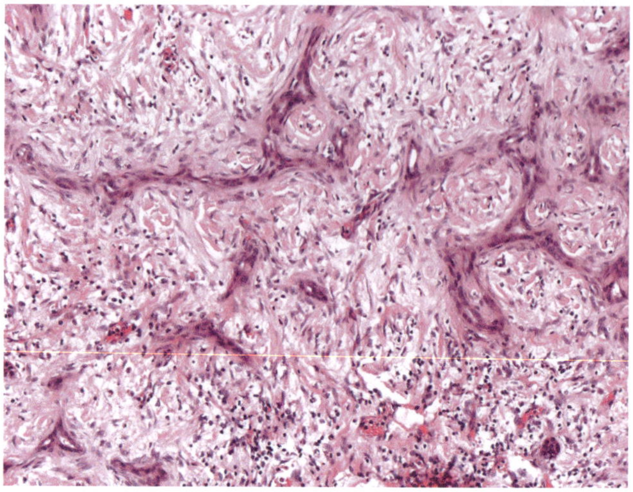

Fig. 15.4 Mesenchymal hamartoma. Bile ductules exhibit ductal-plate malformation configuration in a fibromyxoid stroma. Mesenchymal hamartoma traditionally is considered a hamartomatous lesion, but it may represent a neoplastic process as evidenced by rare malignant transformation into embryonal sarcoma and the presence of aberrant cytogenetic alternations.

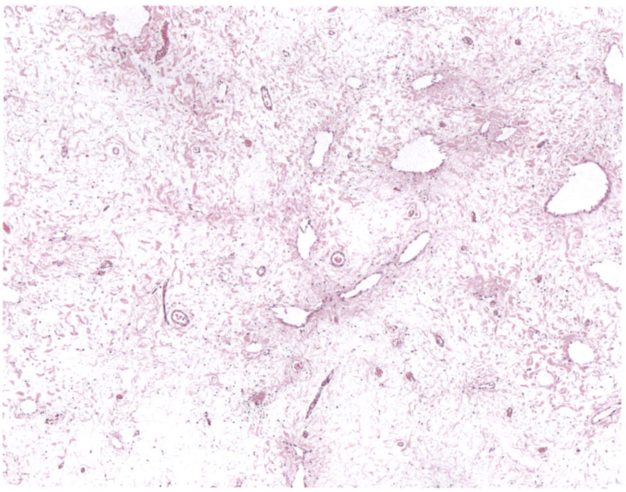

Fig. 15.3 Mesenchymal hamartoma. A loose myxoid stroma contains cystic spaces of varied sizes and blood vessels. Mesenchymal hamartomas are composed of disorganised mesenchymal and epithelial components microscopically. The stroma is (fibro)myxoid and contains a variable number of epithelial-lined cysts and nonepithelialized cystic spaces. Smaller cysts are lined by biliary-type epithelium, whereas larger cysts usually are devoid of an epithelial lining and represent stromal cystic degeneration. Variable amounts of fibroblasts, myofibroblasts, collagen fibres, blood vessels, bile ductules, and islands of hepatocytes are scattered within the tumour. Foci of extramedullary haematopoiesis are common findings in more than 85% of cases. Immunoreactivity towards bcl-2 is common in both epithelial and mesenchymal components.

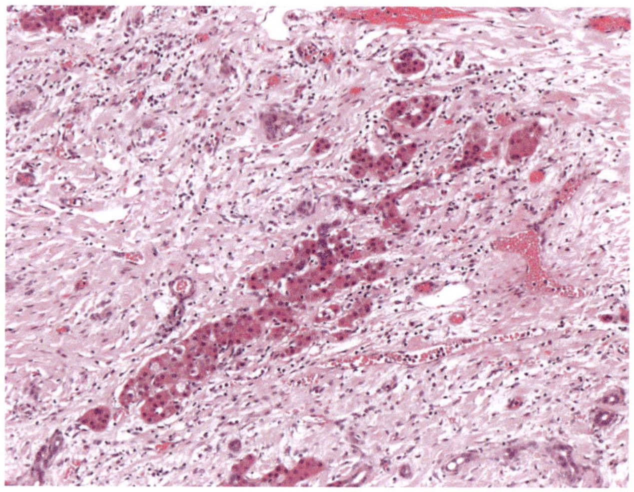

Fig. 15.5 Mesenchymal hamartoma. Islands of normal-looking hepatocytes without normal lobular architecture are present in a fibromyxoid stroma. Exceptional cases may present with a markedly elevated serum α-fetoprotein level, raising the possibility of hepatoblastoma as a differential diagnosis clinically. Moreover, the solid and cystic appearance of mesenchymal hamartomas on imaging also makes embryonal sarcoma a differential diagnosis radiologically. However, the histopathologic differentiation of mesenchymal hamartoma from hepatoblastoma and embryonal sarcoma usually is straightforward. Occasionally, mesenchymal hamartomas may contain very prominent angiomatous components and must be distinguished from infantile haemangioma. Identification of characteristic epithelial and mesenchymal components in mesenchymal hamartoma, in addition to angiomatous components, points to the correct diagnosis.

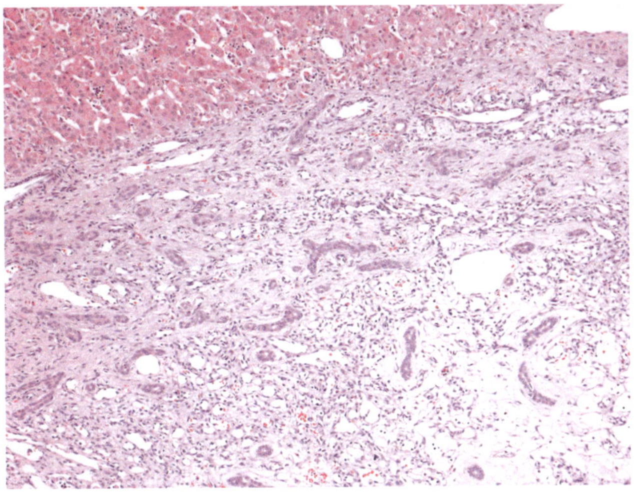

Fig. 15.6 Infantile haemangioma. Capillary-like small vascular channels are associated with entrapped bile ducts and ductules at the edge of the lesion. Infantile haemangioma, formerly known as infantile haemangioendothelioma, accounts for 40% and 20% of all liver tumours and tumour-like lesions before the ages of 2 years and 21 years, respectively. About 90% of cases present before the first 6 months and more frequently affect females (63%). Rare cases of "infantile" haemangioma or capillary-type haemangioma have been found in adults. Coincidental haemangiomas in the skin or other sites are reported in 11% to 87% of patients. Rare associations with diaphragmatic hernia, Beckwith-Wiedemann syndrome, and Cornelia de Lange syndrome have been reported.

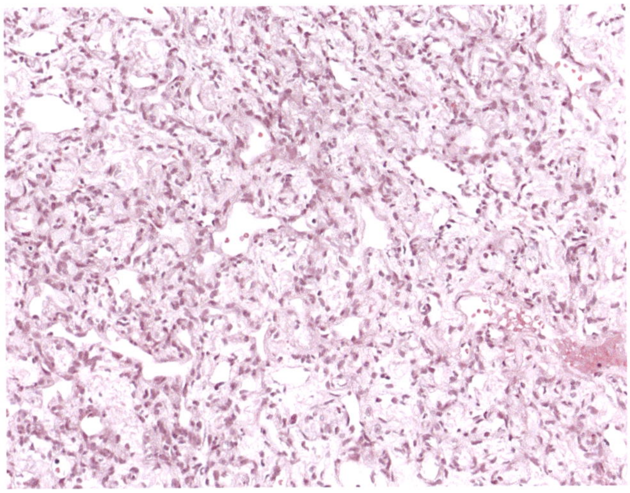

Fig. 15.8 Infantile haemangioma. Capillary-like small vascular channels are lined by a single layer of plump bland endothelial cells. The differential diagnoses include congenital vascular malformation with capillary proliferation, angiosarcoma, and mesenchymal hamartoma with a prominent angiomatous component. Immunoreactivity towards glucose transporter 1 (GLUT1) in infantile haemangioma distinguishes it from GLUT1-negative congenital vascular malformation. Infantile haemangioma historically was classified into two types. Type 1 tumour was referred to as conventional infantile haemangioma. Type 2 tumour was characterised by hyperchromatic and pleomorphic atypical endothelial cells with multilayering, papillary projection, and often kaposiform spindle cell components, and now is more appropriately regarded as an angiosarcoma.

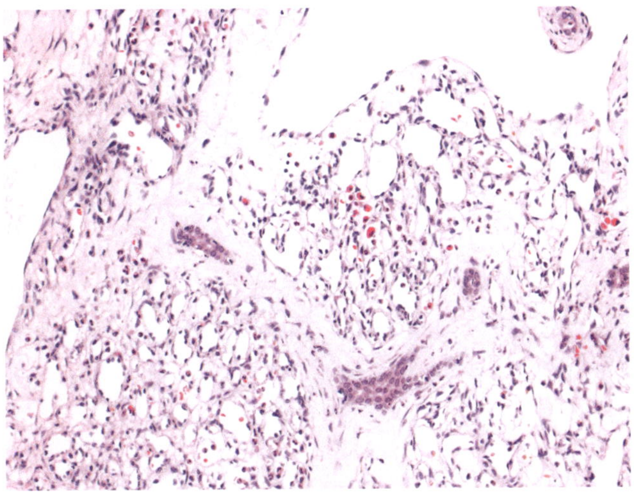

Fig. 15.7 Infantile haemangioma. Capillary-like small vascular channels and a few dilated vascular spaces are present. Infantile haemangioma may be solitary (55%) or multiple (45%) and occur anywhere throughout the liver. Histologically, the periphery of the tumour is composed of numerous capillary-like vascular channels lined by a single layer of plump bland endothelial cells. Intertwining stroma usually is scanty. Entrapped hepatocytes and bile ducts not uncommonly are found in the advancing edge of the tumour. The central portion of the lesion is composed predominantly of larger cavernous vascular spaces lined by attenuated endothelial cells, and more supporting fibrous stroma. Thrombosis, haemorrhage, infarction, fibrosis, and dystrophic calcification are signs of regression. Foci of extramedullary haematopoiesis also may be found.

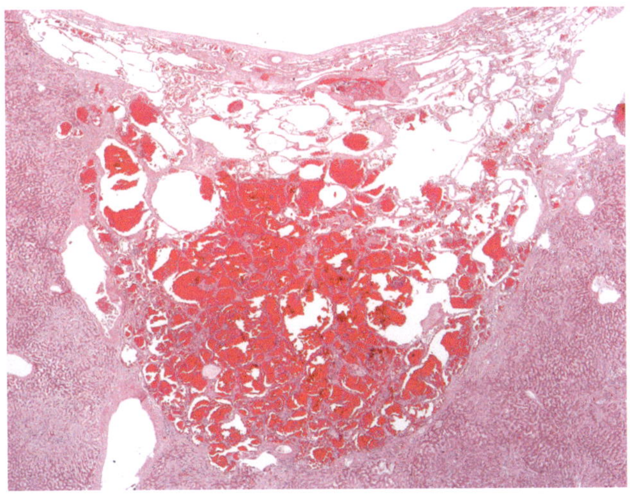

Fig. 15.9 Cavernous haemangioma. A benign vascular tumour is composed of multiple cavernous vascular spaces of varying sizes, separated by fibrous septa. Cavernous haemangioma is the commonest benign liver tumour, affecting up to 20% of the general population. It occurs at all ages but most frequently in young adult women. Nearly 90% of cavernous haemangiomas are solitary. The remaining cases represent multiple haemangiomas and the rare diffuse hepatic haemangiomatosis. Their size ranges from a few millimetres to lesions replacing most of the liver, but most haemangiomas are less than 4 cm. Diffuse hepatic haemangiomatosis occurs predominantly during infancy and is associated with haemangiomatosis of other organs. Rare cases of isolated diffuse hepatic haemangiomatosis without extrahepatic involvement in adults have been reported.

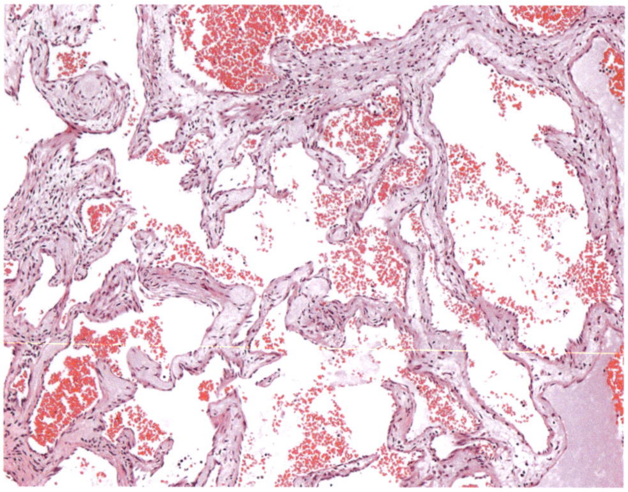

Fig. 15.10 Cavernous haemangioma. Variable-sized vascular spaces are separated by fibrous septa of varied thickness and lined by a single layer of attenuated endothelial cells. These lesions are composed of vascular spaces of varied sizes separated by fibrous septa and lined by a single layer of flat, bland endothelial cells. Most cases are well demarcated, but some may entrap bile ducts and extend into the liver parenchyma as in infantile haemangiomas. Thrombosis, fibrosis, and dystrophic calcification also may be found. Sclerosed haemangiomas are composed of obliterated vessels in sclerotic hyalinized stroma, and those vessels may require elastic stain to be highlighted. Diffuse hepatic haemangiomatosis is characterised by extensive replacement and infiltration of liver parenchyma by numerous cavernous haemangiomas.

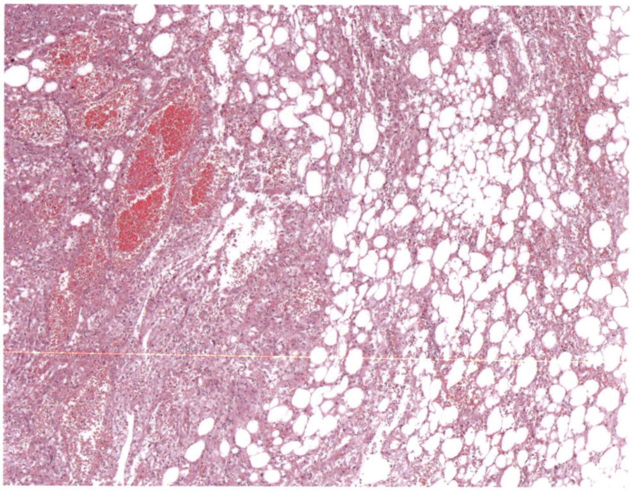

Fig. 15.12 Angiomyolipoma. All three components of angiomyolipoma are present and admixed together: thick-walled vessels, smooth muscle, and adipose tissue. Angiomyolipomas have a wide spectrum of histologic appearance. According to the predominant components, angiomyolipoma is classified into mixed, lipomatous (>70% adipose tissue), myomatous (<10% adipose tissue), and angiomatous types. However, it should be emphasised that smooth muscle cells are the only diagnostic component, and their immunoreactivity towards melanocytic markers (HMB45, Melan-A, and MiTF1) is the hallmark feature. The adipose tissue component is composed mainly of mature adipocytes and, rarely, lipoblast-like cells. The vascular component consists of abnormal vessels showing tortuosity and thick walls. Extramedullary haematopoiesis is another frequent and characteristic finding.

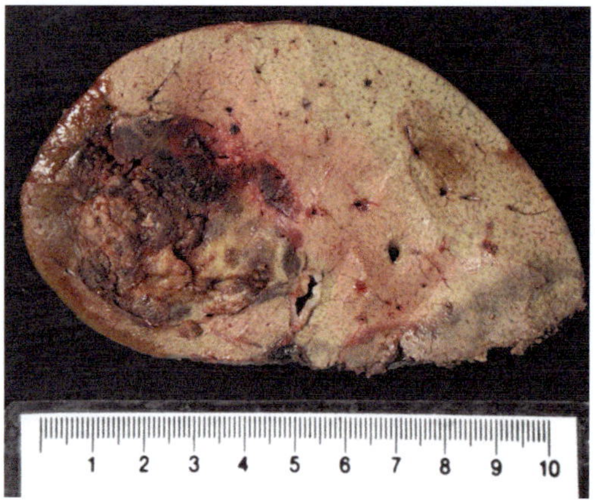

Fig. 15.11 Angiomyolipoma. A circumscribed tumour has variegated cut surfaces containing haemorrhagic regions and yellowish fatty regions. Angiomyolipomas belong to a family of tumours of perivascular epithelioid cells (PEComas). They affect a wide range of age groups, with a mean age of about 50 years. The female-to-male ratio is between 2:1 and 6:1. About 5% to 10% of cases are associated with tuberous sclerosis, in which there often is coexisting renal angiomyolipoma and usually multiple hepatic tumours. Otherwise, angiomyolipoma typically is solitary (>90%) and ranges in size from 0.1 to >36 cm. It is a circumscribed, unencapsulated tumour with a variegated appearance depending on the various proportions of vascular (dark brownish), smooth muscle (firm tan to whitish), and fatty tissue (soft yellowish) components. Haemorrhage and necrosis may be found in larger tumours.

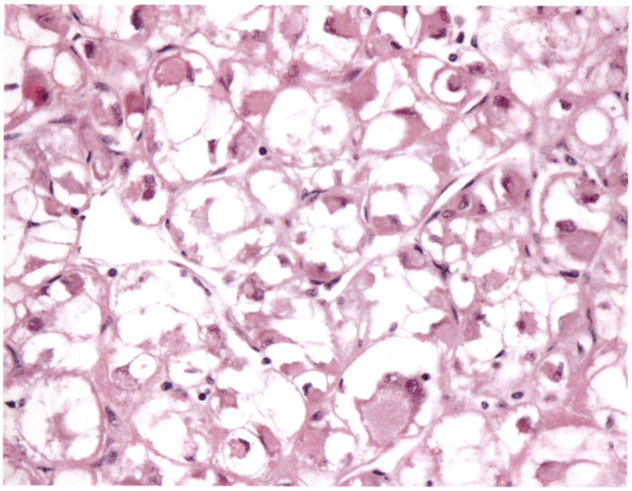

Fig. 15.13 Angiomyolipoma. There are sheets and trabeculae of epithelioid smooth muscle cells separated by a sinusoid-like vasculature. The smooth muscle cells exhibit perinuclear condensation of eosinophilic granular cytosol, leaving a clear cytoplasm at the periphery. Their nuclei are round to oval with a single, distinct nucleolus. The smooth muscle cells are mainly epithelioid cells arranged in sheets and, less commonly, spindle cells arranged in fascicles. The nuclei are round to oval with a single nucleolus. Nuclear pleomorphism is common, but mitosis is exceedingly rare. The epithelioid smooth muscle cells may be clear (sugar cells), oncocytic, or pleomorphic. The pleomorphic variant contains bizarre or multinucleated cells with a preserved nucleocytoplasmic ratio and no mitotic activity.

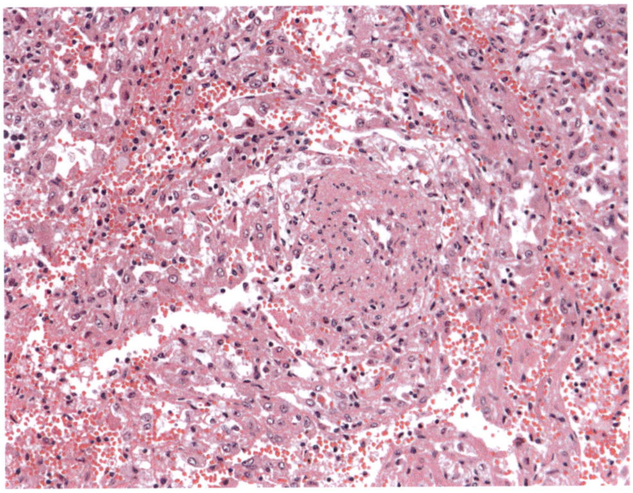

Fig. 15.14 Angiomyolipoma. A thick-walled vessel is surrounded by whorls of plump spindle eosinophilic smooth muscle cells. Diagnosis of the myomatous type of angiomyolipoma may be challenging. Tumours containing predominantly epithelioid cells with scattered pleomorphic cells and a trabecular growth pattern may be misinterpreted as hepatocellular carcinomas. On the other hand, those containing predominantly spindle cells may mimic sarcomas. To differentiate angiomyolipoma from its mimickers, immunohistochemical stains for melanocytic markers are helpful, as is a detailed search for the other two components and extramedullary haematopoiesis in angiomyolipoma.

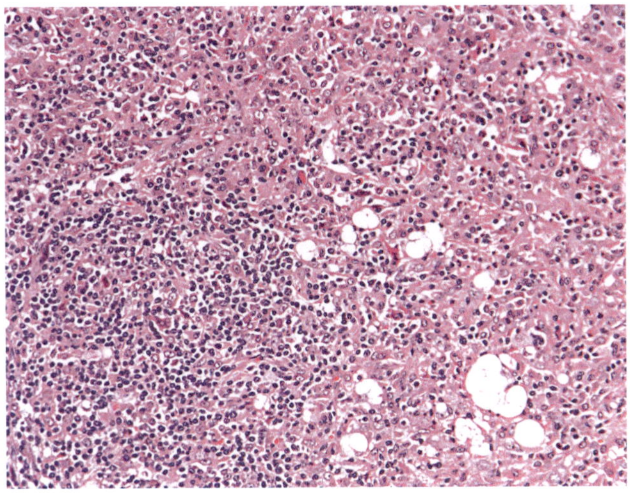

Fig. 15.16 Angiomyolipoma. A diffuse inflammatory infiltrate is seen within sheets of plump spindle-shaped smooth muscle cells, scattered adipocytes, and lipoblast-like cells. The inflammatory variant accounts for only 3% of all angiomyolipomas. It does not differ clinically from conventional angiomyolipoma but may mimic inflammatory pseudotumour (IPT) and IPT-like follicular dendritic cell tumour histopathologically. A rare variant of so-called invasive or malignant angiomyolipoma has been described. There is no consensus regarding the diagnostic criteria for malignancy, but suggested histologic features include monotypic epithelioid morphology, marked nuclear atypia, increased mitosis, and necrosis. Metastasis is the only commonly accepted feature, but these tumours may be associated with multicentricity of the lesions rather than genuine malignant transformation.

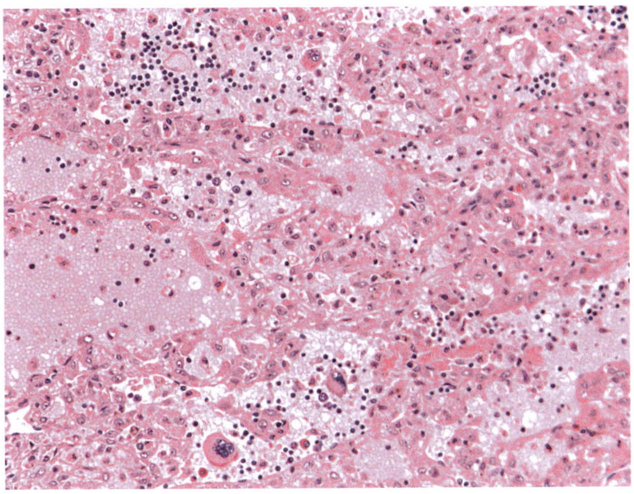

Fig. 15.15 Angiomyolipoma. Sheets and fascicles of plump smooth muscle cells are separated by irregular cystic blood-filled spaces (peliosis). Some extramedullary haematopoietic cells and several pleomorphic multinucleated smooth muscle cells are found within blood-filled spaces. Angiomyolipomas may exhibit unusual growth patterns, namely trabecular, pelioid, and inflammatory. The trabecular pattern shows epithelioid smooth muscle cells in trabeculae with intervening sinusoids lined by endothelial cells and at least partial loss of the reticulin framework. The pelioid pattern has dilated cystic blood-filled spaces without an endothelial lining and often is associated with haemorrhage. The inflammatory pattern has a varied appearance ranging from multiple reactive lymphoid follicles to diffuse inflammatory infiltrate with stromal sclerosis.

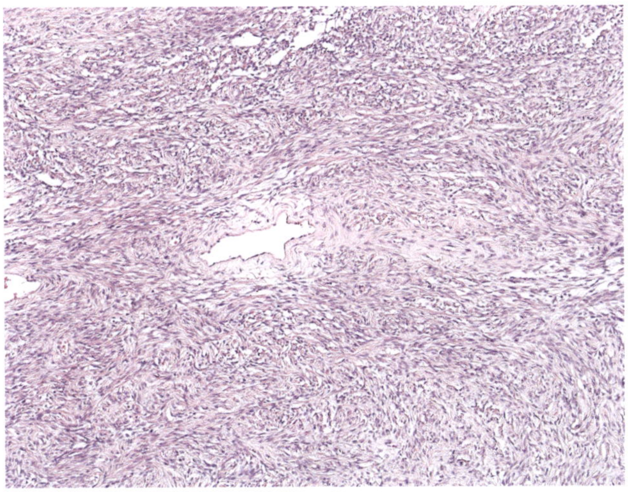

Fig. 15.17 Solitary fibrous tumour. It is a rare primary hepatic neoplasm, with fewer than 40 reported cases. It affects a wide range of age groups (16–84 years), with a mean age of 55 years. Solitary fibrous tumour ranges in size from 2 to 32 cm. It is composed of bland, uniform spindle cells in a fibrous stroma and often is arranged in alternating hypocellular and hypercellular areas. Hyalinized, somewhat keloidal collagen and branching haemangiopericytoma-like vessels commonly are found, giving rise to what is described as a patternless pattern. Immunohistochemically, these lesions consistently express CD34 and variably express CD99 and bcl-2. Histologic features suggesting malignancy include infiltrative margins, high cellularity, prominent cellular pleomorphism, increased mitosis (more than four mitoses per 10 high-power fields [HPF]), and necrosis.

15.2 Malignant Mesenchymal Neoplasms

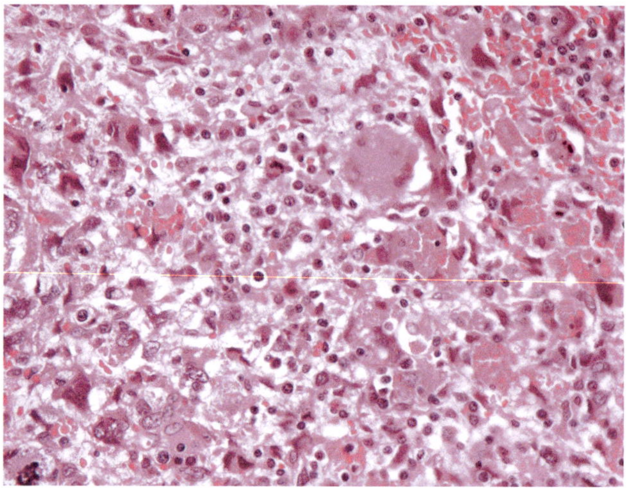

Fig. 15.18 Embryonal sarcoma. Highly pleomorphic and giant tumour cells are present. Embryonal sarcoma, also known as undifferentiated sarcoma and malignant mesenchymoma, is the third commonest primary malignant paediatric liver tumour, accounting for 9% to 15% of cases. Most cases (>75%) occur between the ages of 6 and 15 years, but rare cases have been reported in adults up to the age of 73 years. No sex predilection is observed. Embryonal sarcomas range in size from 10 to 20 cm. They are well-demarcated but unencapsulated solid and cystic tumours with a variegated cut surface containing solid, glistening whitish areas; cystic gelatinous areas; necrosis; and haemorrhage.

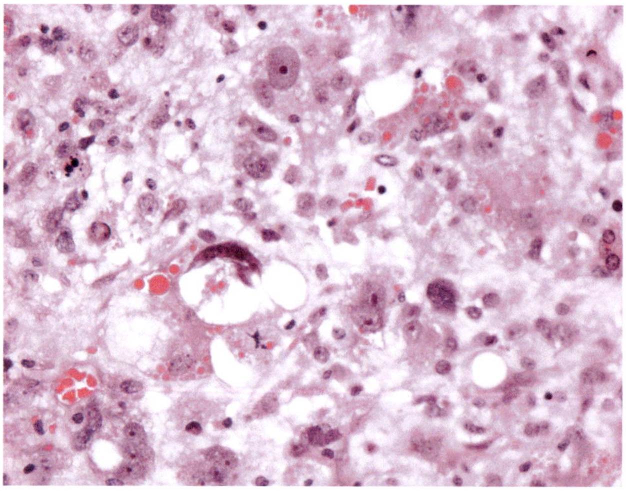

Fig. 15.19 Embryonal sarcoma. Multiple extracellular and intracytoplasmic eosinophilic hyaline globules are present. Embryonal sarcoma consists of medium-sized to large spindle, stellate, and giant tumour cells in a loose fibromyxoid stroma. Marked nuclear pleomorphism and hyperchromasia, as well as frequent mitotic figures, are typical findings. Extracellular and intracytoplasmic eosinophilic hyaline globules of varying sizes are a characteristic feature. These globules are periodic acid-Schiff positive and diastase resistant and are immunoreactive for vimentin, albumin, immunoglobulin, α_1-antitrypsin, and/or α_1-antichymotrypsin. Entrapped hepatocytes and bile ducts occasionally are found in the periphery of the tumour. Focal areas with storiform growth, branching haemangiopericytoma-like vessels, small undifferentiated cells, and osteoid formation may be encountered.

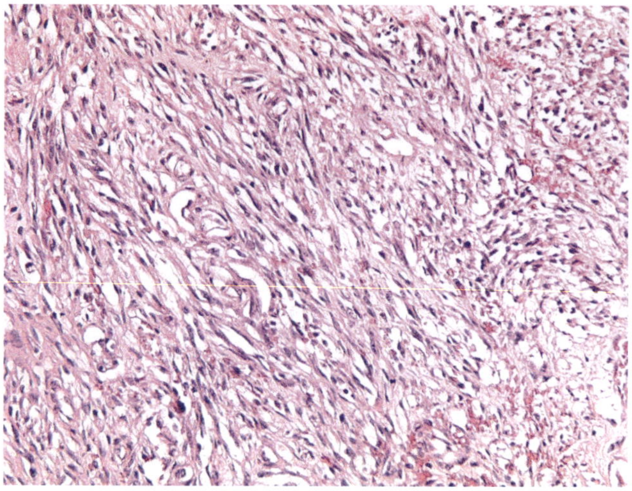

Fig. 15.20 Kaposi sarcoma. Fascicles of spindle cells are associated with many slit-like spaces and focal haemorrhage. Hepatic Kaposi sarcoma is found normally as part of disseminated disease in immunocompromised individuals, particularly patients with AIDS. It typically is manifest as multiple red-brownish nodules in the portal and periportal regions, varying in size from a few millimetres to up to 7 cm. Histologically, Kaposi sarcoma is composed of fascicles of spindle cells associated with slit-like vascular spaces, haemorrhage, and haemosiderin deposition. Intracytoplasmic hyaline globules and focal lymphoplasmacytic infiltrate are typical findings. Peliotic foci often are found at the periphery. The tumour cells are immunoreactive for CD31, CD34, D2-40, and, most importantly, human herpesvirus 8 (HHV-8).

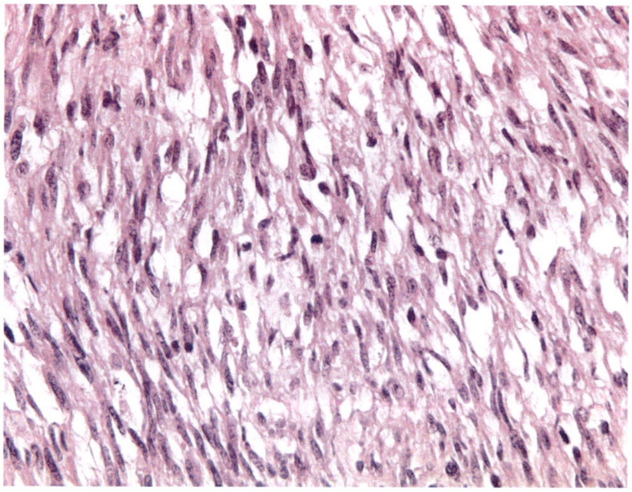

Fig. 15.21 Kaposi sarcoma. Fascicles of spindle cells are associated with slit-like spaces. The differential diagnosis includes other spindle cell hepatic neoplasms. EBV-associated smooth muscle tumour is a particularly important differential diagnosis in immunosuppressed patients; these smooth muscle tumours are variably positive for desmin and smooth muscle actin and by in situ hybridization for EBV-encoded RNA (EBER). Peliotic foci of Kaposi sarcoma may mimic bacillary peliosis hepatis in AIDS patients. Demonstration of clumps of bacteria by Warthin-Starry stain and immunostaining for *Bartonella* is diagnostic for bacillary peliosis hepatis.

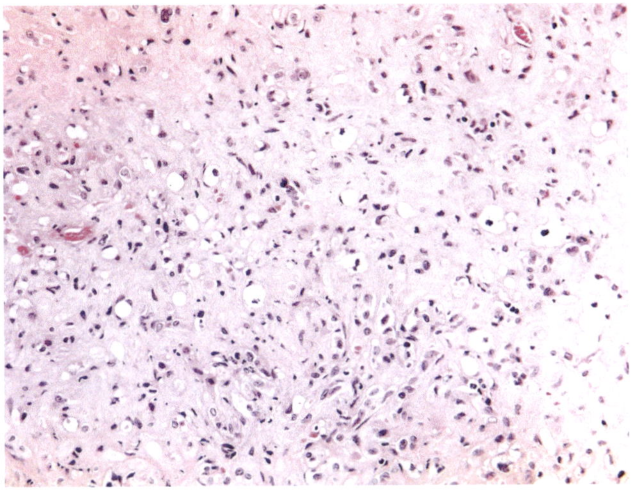

Fig. 15.22 Epithelioid haemangioendothelioma. Small groups of epithelioid cells with vacuolated cytoplasm are seen within in a chondromyxoid stroma. A few intracytoplasmic vacuoles contain blood cells. Epithelioid haemangioendothelioma is a rare hepatic tumour with an incidence of <0.1 per 100,000. It affects a wide range of age groups (3–86 years), with a mean age of 42 years. The female-to-male ratio is 3:2. Epithelioid haemangioendotheliomas often are multifocal (70%), with multiple firm to rubbery, whitish, discrete lesions ranging from 0.2 to 14 cm.

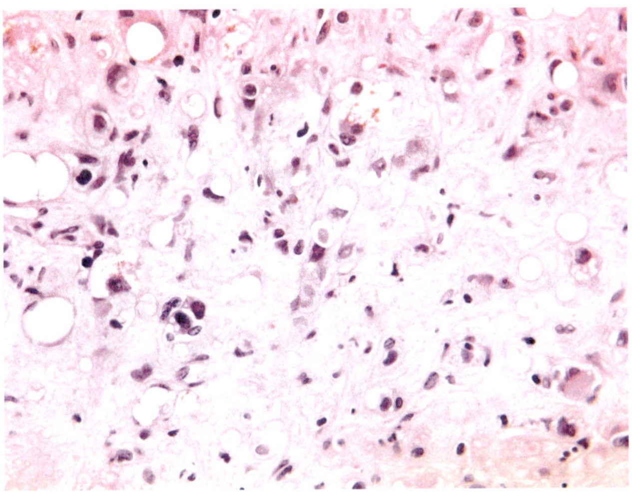

Fig. 15.23 Epithelioid haemangioendothelioma. Individual tumour cells and small groups of epithelioid cells with vacuolated cytoplasm are set within a chondromyxoid stroma. The tumour cells are predominantly epithelioid, with intracytoplasmic vacuoles sometimes containing blood cells. Dendritic cells with interdigitating processes, as well as intermediate cells, also are found. At the periphery, tumour cells often infiltrate into the adjacent hepatic sinusoids and may occlude blood vessels (terminal venules and portal veins). The tumour cells are immunoreactive towards CD31, CD34, D2-40, and, rarely, cytokeratin. Differential diagnoses include metastatic signet ring carcinoma and tumours with a fibrous stroma, including cholangiocarcinoma, scirrhous hepatocellular carcinoma, and sclerosed haemangioma. On biopsy samples, sclerosed areas may be mistaken for centrilobular fibrous obliteration.

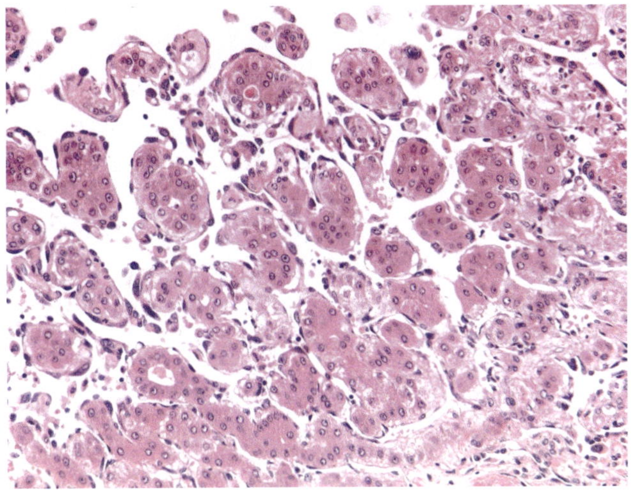

Fig. 15.24 Angiosarcoma. Malignant endothelial cells with hyperchromatic and pleomorphic nuclei grow along hepatic sinusoids. The entrapped hepatocytes show variably regenerating activity with pseudoacinar formation, mimicking hepatocellular carcinoma. Angiosarcoma is the commonest primary hepatic malignant mesenchymal tumour, accounting for 2% of all hepatic neoplasms. It commonly affects patients at 60 to 70 years of age but also is known to occur in younger patients. The male-to-female ratio is 3:1. Angiosarcoma is known to be associated with exposure to vinyl chloride, arsenic, androgenic steroids, and, historically, thorotrast (colloid thorium oxide, used as a radiologic contrast medium between the 1930s and 1950s).

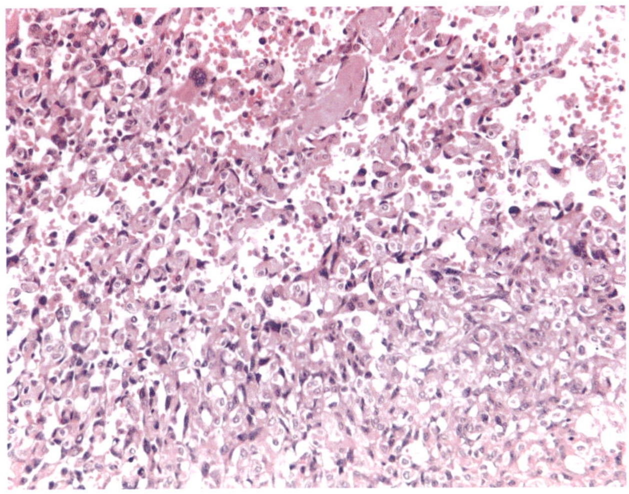

Fig. 15.25 Angiosarcoma. Multiple pseudo-papillae are covered by malignant endothelial cells with hyperchromatic and pleomorphic nuclei. Angiosarcomas often are multicentric tumours composed of greyish white to haemorrhagic nodules, ranging in millimetres to several centimetres. Histologically, a sinusoidal growth pattern is typical and characterised by malignant endothelial cells with marked nuclear atypia and frequent mitoses, growing along dilated sinusoids and separated by residual atrophic or hyperplastic hepatocytes. Other growth patterns include irregular anastomosing, blood-filled vascular channels, cavernous spaces, pseudo-papillary structures, and solid strands and sheets. Thrombosis, infarction, and haemorrhage also are found commonly.

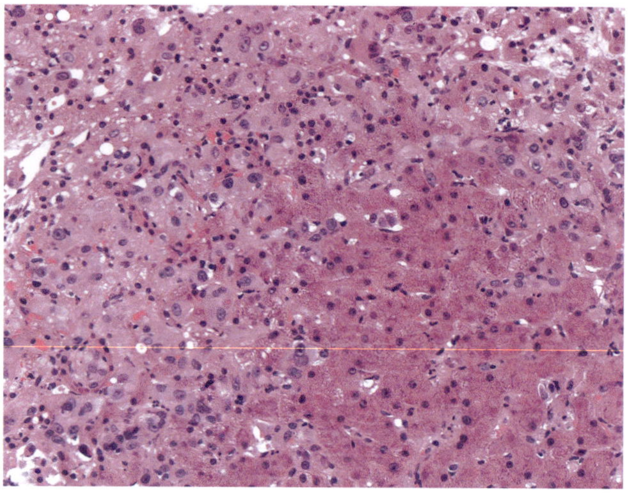

Fig. 15.26 Epithelioid angiosarcoma. Epithelioid malignant tumour cells infiltrate into hepatic sinusoids. The tumour cells exhibit large pleomorphic nuclei, prominent nucleoli, and abundant pale eosinophilic cytoplasm. No fibrous or chondromyxoid stroma is associated. Epithelioid angiosarcoma is a variant of angiosarcoma and mimics carcinoma and epithelioid haemangioendothelioma. Occasionally, immunoreactivity for cytokeratins in such tumours is misleading and makes the distinction from carcinoma more difficult. However, identification of intracytoplasmic vacuoles containing blood cells and immunostains for endothelial markers help differentiate angiosarcoma from carcinoma. A prominent infiltrative or solid growth pattern and the absence of fibrous or chondromyxoid stroma favour the diagnosis of epithelioid angiosarcoma over epithelioid haemangioendothelioma.

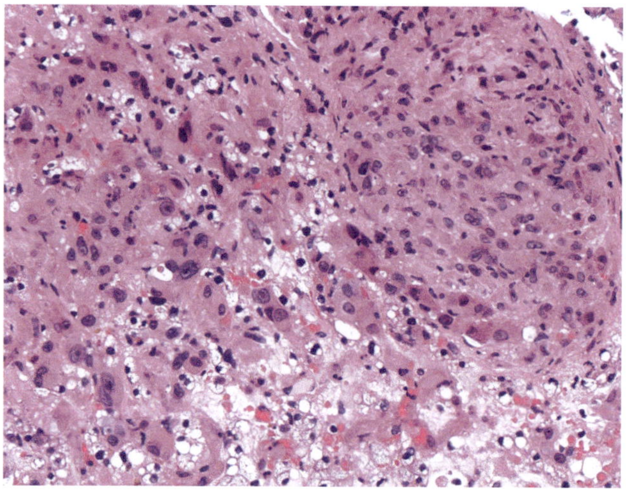

Fig. 15.27 Epithelioid angiosarcoma. Epithelioid and plump spindle-shaped malignant tumour cells form solid nodules and strands without an associated fibrous or chondromyxoid stroma. Rare intracytoplasmic vacuoles containing blood cells and immunostains for CD31 and CD34 confirm their endothelial nature.

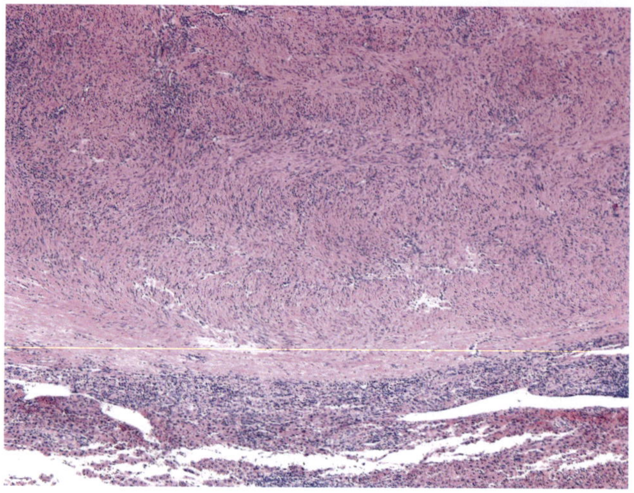

Fig. 15.28 Epstein-Barr virus–associated smooth muscle tumour. Smooth muscle tumour cells are arranged in interlacing fascicles and admixed with lymphoid infiltrate. Almost all conventional leiomyosarcomas are metastatic, whereas EBV-associated smooth muscle tumours may be primary hepatic neoplasms. EBV-associated smooth muscle tumour affects three main groups of immunocompromised patients: those with congenital immunodeficiency, those with HIV infection, and organ transplant/autoimmune disease patients on immunosuppression. EBV-associated smooth muscle tumours tend to be multifocal. This characteristic multifocal property initially was thought to represent metastatic tumour spread but has been shown by clonality analysis to be multiple synchronic independent tumour formation of multifocal EBV-associated smooth muscle tumour.

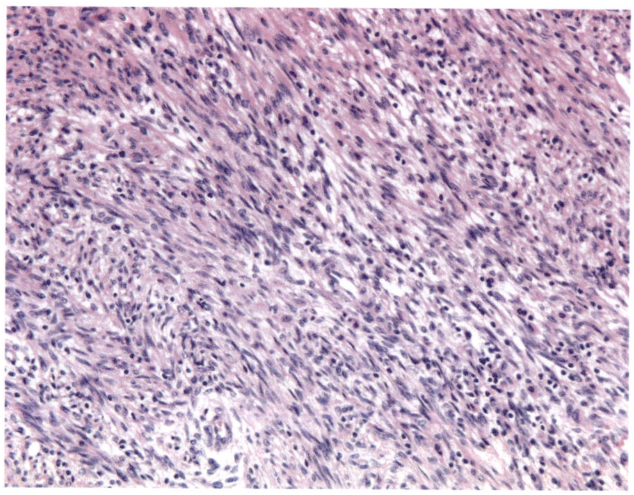

Fig. 15.29 Epstein-Barr virus–associated smooth muscle tumour. Smooth muscle tumour cells are arranged in interlacing fascicles and admixed with a lymphoid infiltrate. These tumours are composed of intersecting fascicles of monomorphic spindle smooth muscle cells with minimal to mild cytologic atypia. Mitotic activity varies, with an average of fewer than three mitoses per 10 HPF. Occasional, more primitive, round myoid cells with irregular nuclear contours are found in half the cases. A variable intratumoral lymphoid infiltrate is found in most cases. Coagulative tumour necrosis and myxoid change are infrequent findings. Differential diagnoses include other primary and metastatic hepatic spindle neoplasms. Kaposi sarcoma is an essential differential diagnosis in immunosuppressed patients, and those spindle cells are positive for CD31, CD34, and HHV-8.

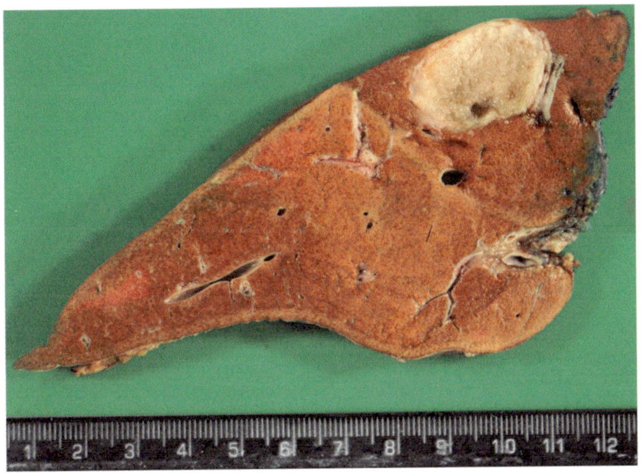

Fig. 15.30 Metastatic gastrointestinal stromal tumour. A well-circumscribed, firm, whitish tumour is present in the subscapular region. Metastatic sarcomas are uncommon, and most originate from either gastrointestinal stromal tumours (positive for c-kit/CD117 and DOG1 in >95% and CD34 in 70%) or uterine leiomyosarcomas (positive for desmin and smooth muscle actin). Sarcomatoid carcinoma, notably from renal primary tumour, and carcinosarcoma, such as malignant mixed müllerian tumour of the female genital tract, also can metastasise to the liver and may exhibit a predominantly sarcomatous growth pattern.

15.3 Haematolymphoid Neoplasms

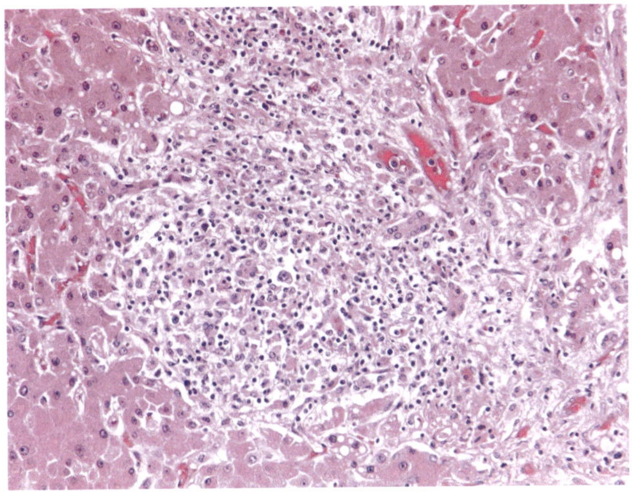

Fig. 15.31 Classic Hodgkin lymphoma. A portal tract is expanded by atypical lymphoid infiltrate and accompanied by bile duct injury and a ductular reaction. The infiltrate is composed of scattered large lymphoid cells with vesicular nuclei and prominent nucleoli, in the background of small lymphocytes and histiocytes. Primary hepatic lymphoma is rare and accounts for 0.016% of all lymphomas. Secondary hepatic involvement in Hodgkin lymphoma is found in up to 55% of cases in postmortem series.

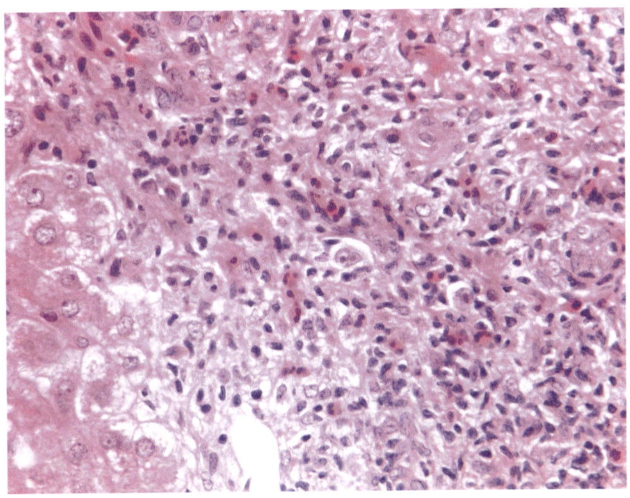

Fig. 15.32 Classic Hodgkin lymphoma. A binucleated Reed-Sternberg cell with prominent nucleoli is present in a background of a polymorphous inflammatory infiltrate containing small lymphocytes, histiocytes, eosinophils, and neutrophils. Hodgkin lymphoma primarily infiltrates the portal tracts, with occasional additional parenchymal tumour nodules (10%) and sinusoidal infiltration (10%). Polymorphous portal inflammatory infiltrates of lymphocytes, plasma cells, and eosinophils are common but nonspecific. Identification of Reed-Sternberg cells or their variants is diagnostic. Epithelioid granulomas are found in 6% to 12% of patients, but these may be related to a host response to the tumour or previous lymphangiogram rather than to direct tumoural involvement. Their prognostic significance is controversial. Peliosis hepatis and sinusoidal dilatation are common and associated with the presence of systemic symptoms.

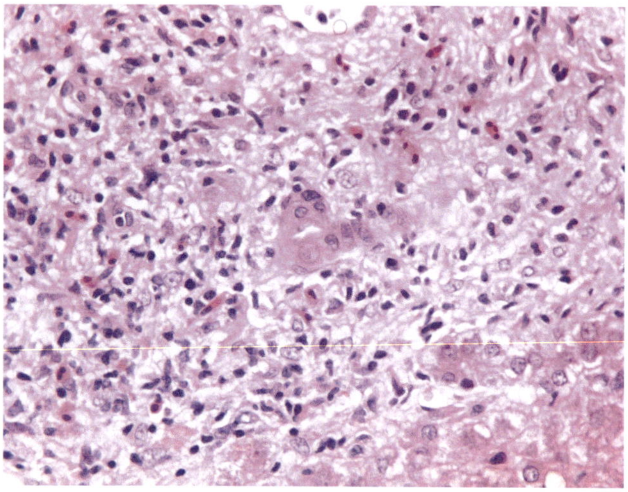

Fig. 15.33 Classic Hodgkin lymphoma. A bile duct shows epithelial disarray and regenerative change. Up to 15% of patients with Hodgkin lymphoma develop jaundice. It may be mild and related to haemolysis or a paraneoplastic syndrome or may be more severe and related to extensive hepatic tumoural involvement or a postchemotherapeutic response. Histologically, bland cholestasis may be observed in the paraneoplastic syndrome (treatment-related hyperbilirubinaemia). Bile duct lymphoepithelial lesions, characterised by ducts being surrounded and infiltrated by tumour cells, resulting in bile duct injury and obliteration, are observed in 20% of cases. Ductopaenia or vanishing bile duct syndrome also may occur but appears to be reversible in at least one third of patients.

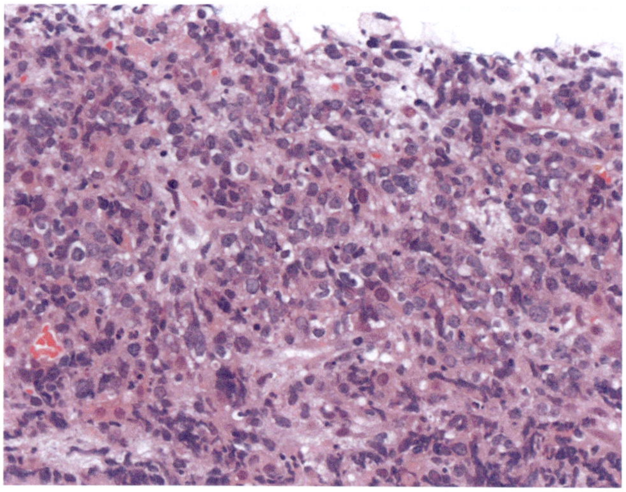

Fig. 15.34 Primary diffuse large B-cell lymphoma. An atypical lymphoid infiltrate forms a tumour mass and is composed of large lymphoid cells with vesicular nuclei and distinct nucleoli. The tumour cells are immunoreactive for CD20. Diffuse large B-cell lymphomas account for 80% to 90% of primary hepatic lymphomas. Primary hepatic lymphoma typically affects middle-aged patients, with a mean age of 50 years. The male-to-female ratio is 2:1. Most primary hepatic lymphomas are idiopathic, but some are associated with hepatitis B virus, hepatitis C virus, or EBV. The tumour typically presents as a solitary mass or multiple nodules, and occasionally there is diffuse hepatomegaly without a discrete lesion.

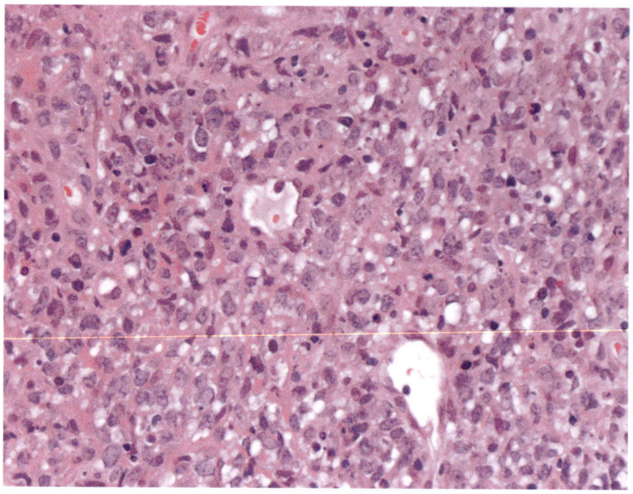

Fig. 15.35 Primary diffuse large B-cell lymphoma. The atypical lymphoid infiltrate forms a tumour mass and is composed of large lymphoid cells with vesicular nuclei and distinct nucleoli. Diffuse large B-cell lymphoma presents predominantly with tumour nodules distributed diffusely throughout the liver parenchyma (77%), with some cases also showing portal infiltration (30%) or sinusoidal spread (13%). Bile duct lymphoepithelial lesions are present in 3% of cases. T-cell/histiocyte-rich large B-cell lymphoma, a variant of diffuse large B-cell lymphoma, presents as either a mixed portal and sinusoidal infiltrate or discrete tumour nodules. These tumours may show atypical granuloma formation; foci of necrosis are seen frequently. Malignant B cells may be few and surrounded by the reactive component, but can be identified by immunohistochemistry for B-cell markers (CD20, CD79a, PAX-5, or Oct-2).

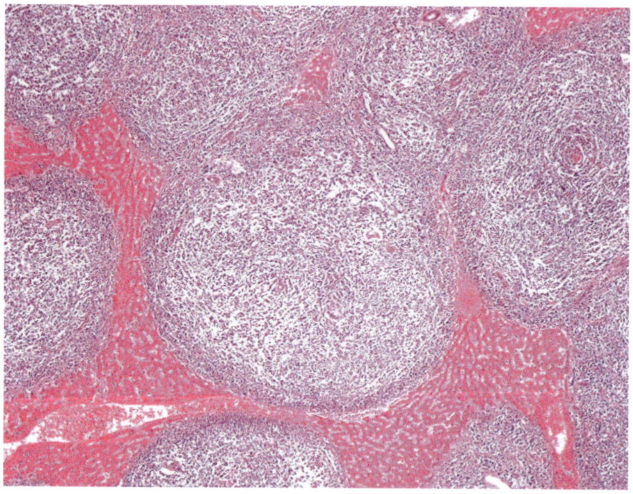

Fig. 15.36 Marginal zone lymphoma of mucosa-associated lymphoid tissue (MALT lymphoma). Portal tracts are markedly expanded by an atypical lymphoid infiltrate. MALT lymphoma is the second most common primary hepatic lymphoma. However, secondary spread from a MALT lymphoma of gastrointestinal tract origin or a splenic marginal zone lymphoma is more frequent. MALT lymphoma is characterised by dense portal atypical lymphoid infiltrates (89%) with frequent sinusoidal spread (44%) and bile duct lymphoepithelial lesions (44%). Although bile duct lymphoepithelial lesions are typical of MALT lymphoma, they are not entirely specific, because Hodgkin lymphoma and diffuse large B-cell lymphoma may contain such a lesion in 20% and 3% of cases, respectively. Primary hepatic MALT lymphoma frequently is associated with a translocation of *IGH* and *MALT1*, t(11;18)(q21;q21).

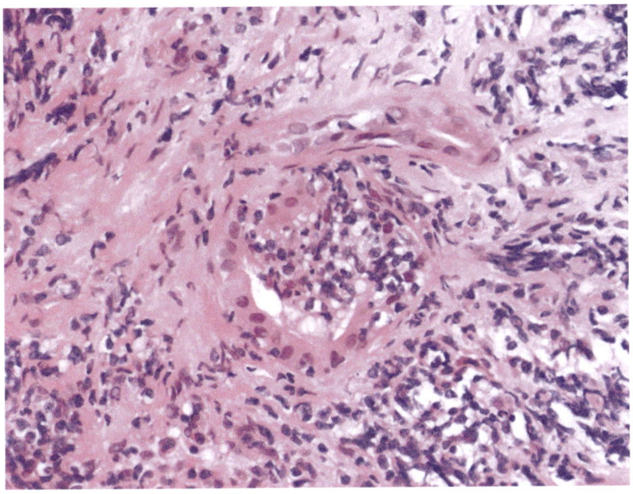

Fig. 15.37 Marginal zone lymphoma of mucosa-associated lymphoid tissue. A bile duct is infiltrated by small, atypical lymphoid cells (lymphoepithelial lesion). Other low-grade B-cell lymphomas with secondary hepatic involvement include chronic lymphocytic leukaemia, follicular lymphoma, and mantle cell lymphoma. Hepatic infiltration signifies stage IV disease. Pathologically, MALT lymphoma primarily shows portal infiltration, with some cases also demonstrating sinusoidal spread and parenchymal tumour nodules.

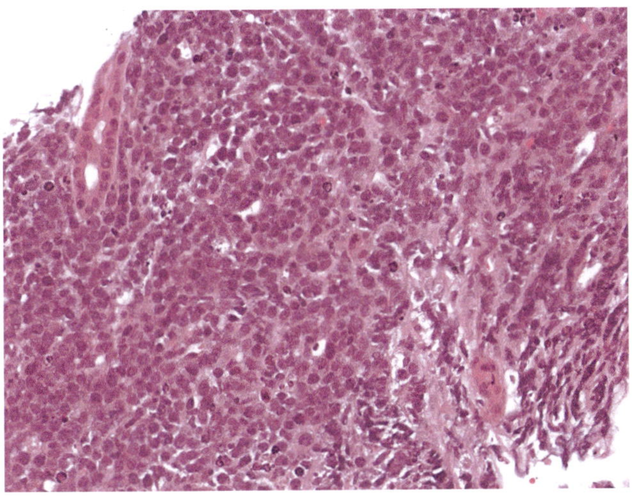

Fig. 15.38 Burkitt lymphoma. Atypical lymphoid cells infiltrate the portal tracts and liver parenchyma to form a mass lesion. The tumour cells are medium-sized cells with coarse chromatin, tiny nucleoli, small amounts of cytoplasm, and frequent apoptosis. They are immunoreactive for CD20 and CD10 but negative for bcl-2 and terminal deoxynucleotidyl transferase (TdT). The proliferation index by Ki67/MIB-1 approaches 100%. A starry sky pattern with tangible macrophages scattered in the background of atypical lymphoid cells is characteristic. Primary hepatic Burkitt lymphoma is very rare, whereas secondary hepatic involvement is observed in up to 71% of cases. Pathologically, Burkitt lymphoma typically presents as parenchymal tumour nodules and occasionally subcapsular infiltration, probably secondary to direct spread from the peritoneum. Their doubling time can be extremely fast.

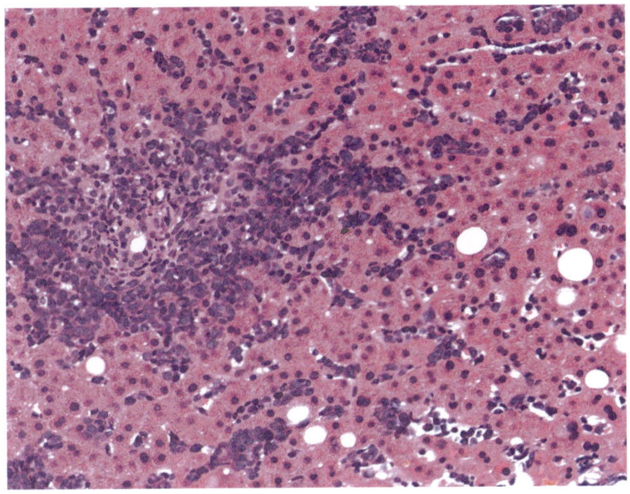

Fig. 15.39 B-cell acute lymphoblastic leukaemia. The atypical haematolymphoid cells infiltrate portal tracts and sinusoids. The tumour cells are medium-sized cells with fine chromatin, inconspicuous nucleoli, and scant cytoplasm and are immunoreactive for Oct-2 and TdT. Leukaemia may involve the liver in the advanced stages of disease. Leukaemic cells typically exhibit diffuse sinusoidal infiltration, except in chronic lymphocytic and acute lymphoblastic leukaemia, which often involve the portal tracts as low-grade lymphoma does. Hairy cell leukaemia is a mature B-cell neoplasm accounting for 2% to 3% of all leukaemic cases. It is characterised by tumour cells infiltrating hepatic sinusoids and may produce multiple peliosis-like lesions with tumour cells adherent to their walls. An abundant clear cytoplasm with "hairy" projections is characteristic but easily overlooked in haematoxylin and eosin–stained sections.

16 Obstetric Liver Disease

Up to 3 % of all gestations are complicated by various liver diseases. Some of these are unique to pregnancy, whereas others are either coincidental with pregnancy or associated with preexisting chronic liver diseases. Severe liver diseases in pregnancy are rare but may lead to significant morbidities and even mortality for both mother and fetus/infant. The major pregnancy-related liver diseases comprise intrahepatic cholestasis of pregnancy, acute fatty liver of pregnancy, toxaemia of pregnancy, HELLP syndrome (haemolysis, elevated liver enzymes, and low platelet count), hepatic infarction and rupture, and hyperemesis gravidarum.

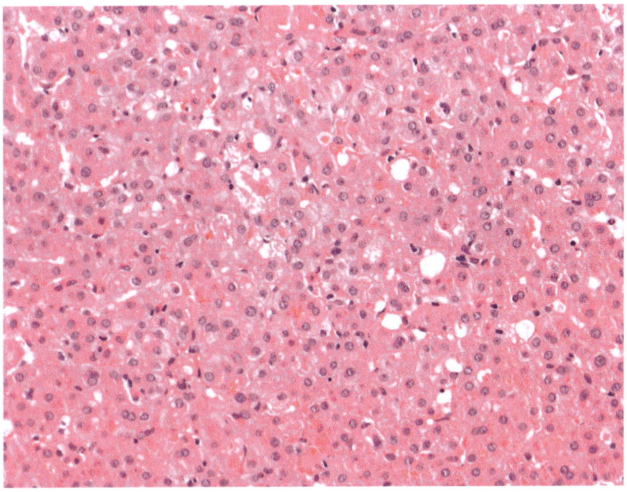

Fig. 16.1 Intrahepatic cholestasis of pregnancy. Bilirubinostasis is present in dilated canaliculi, the cytoplasm of hepatocytes, and Kupffer cells, with minimal necroinflammatory activity (bland cholestasis). Intrahepatic cholestasis of pregnancy affects about 0.3 % to 5.6 %, 0.5 % to 1.5 %, and 6 % of all gestations in the United States, Europe, and China, respectively. Women with this disorder tend to have a recurrence in subsequent pregnancies and to develop cholestasis with oral contraceptives, and have a higher risk of developing chronic liver or biliary diseases. It currently is recognised that this disorder is associated with defects of bile acid transporter proteins, including multidrug resistance 3 (MDR3; encoded by *ABCB4*) and bile salt export pump (BSEP; encoded by *ABCB11*).

A.W.H. Chan et al., *Atlas of Liver Pathology*, Atlas of Anatomic Pathology,
DOI 10.1007/978-1-4614-9114-9_16,

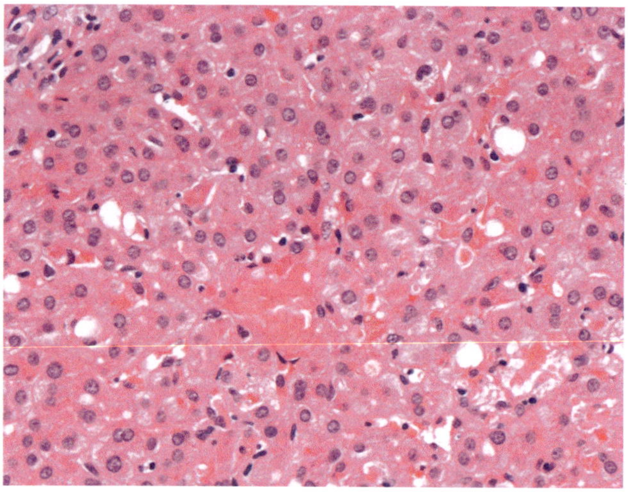

Fig. 16.2 Intrahepatic cholestasis of pregnancy. Bilirubinostasis is present in the dilated canaliculi, cytoplasm of hepatocytes, and Kupffer cells, with negligible necroinflammatory activity (bland cholestasis). Although intrahepatic cholestasis of pregnancy seldom requires a liver biopsy to establish the diagnosis, the typical histologic feature is one of bland cholestasis, with a perivenular-predominant distribution. However, this form of cholestasis also might be associated with drug-induced liver injury, sepsis, shock, paraneoplastic syndrome, early large duct obstruction, and benign recurrent intrahepatic cholestasis.

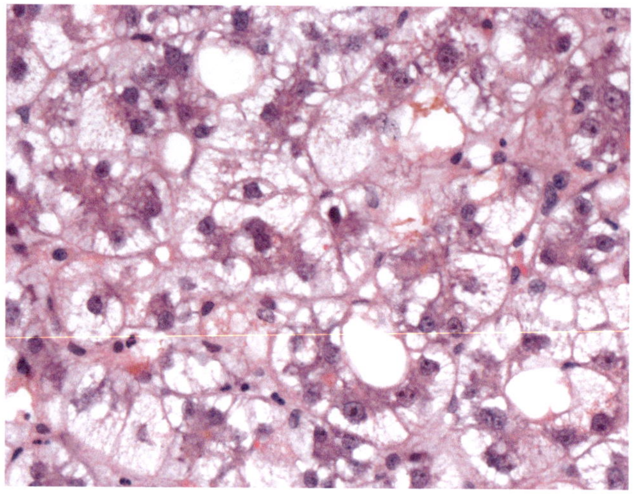

Fig. 16.4 Acute fatty liver of pregnancy. The hepatocytes are distended by multiple minute fat droplets (microvesicular steatosis), imparting a swollen and foamy appearance. Tinges of bilirubin pigments also are present in the cytoplasm of hepatocytes. Microvesicular steatosis, predominantly periportal sparing, is the hallmark of acute fatty liver disease. Other histologic findings include bilirubinostasis, ceroid-laden Kupffer cells, a mild mononuclear inflammatory infiltrate in lobules and portal tracts, and, rarely, sinusoidal fibrin deposition and haemorrhage. Other causes of microvesicular steatosis, such as acute alcoholic foamy degeneration; drug/toxin-induced liver injury; and toxaemia of pregnancy/HELLP syndrome need to be considered.

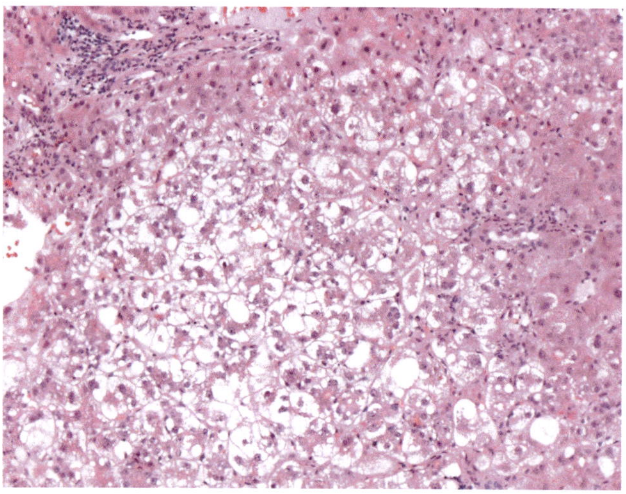

Fig. 16.3 Acute fatty liver of pregnancy. A large group of hepatocytes exhibit cytoplasmic enlargement and clearing resulting from the accumulation of multiple minute fat droplets (microvesicular steatosis). Acute fatty liver of pregnancy is a rare liver complication, affecting 0.005 % to 0.014 % of all pregnancies. Its risk factors include multiple pregnancies, nulliparity, and previous acute fatty liver of pregnancy. It usually occurs in the third trimester but is seen rarely in the second trimester and after delivery. Acute fatty liver of pregnancy is one of the mitochondriopathies. Its exact pathogenesis is uncertain, but it may be associated with concurrent fetal fatty acid oxidation defects and placental mitochondrial dysfunction.

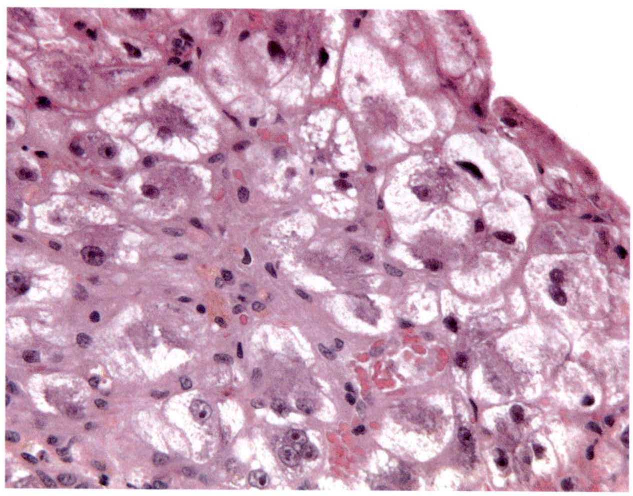

Fig. 16.5 Acute fatty liver of pregnancy. Among pregnancy-related liver diseases, microvesicular steatosis is not pathognomonic for acute fatty liver of pregnancy, because it also is associated with toxaemia of pregnancy and HELLP syndrome. On the other hand, haemorrhage, sinusoidal fibrin deposition, and necrosis, which are common pathologic features of toxaemia of pregnancy and HELLP syndrome, may be present to a mild degree in acute fatty liver of pregnancy. Moreover, up to half of patients with acute fatty liver of pregnancy present with hypertension and proteinuria.

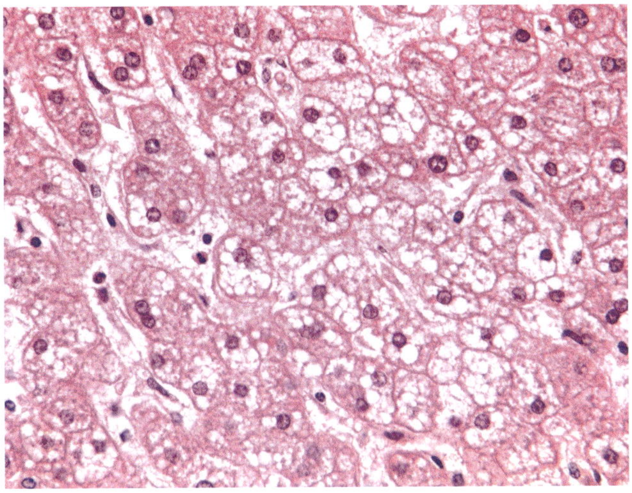

Fig. 16.6 Acute fatty liver of pregnancy. The hepatocytes are distended by multiple small fat droplets, with nondisplaced, centrally located nuclei (microvesicular steatosis). Microvesicular steatosis is distinguished from its mimickers, namely ballooning degeneration, feathery degeneration, and glycogen-rich hepatocytes, by the presence of discrete fat droplets. However, these fat droplets may be so small (Figs. 16.3–16.5) that their identification is difficult. An oil red O stain can highlight these fine fat droplets.

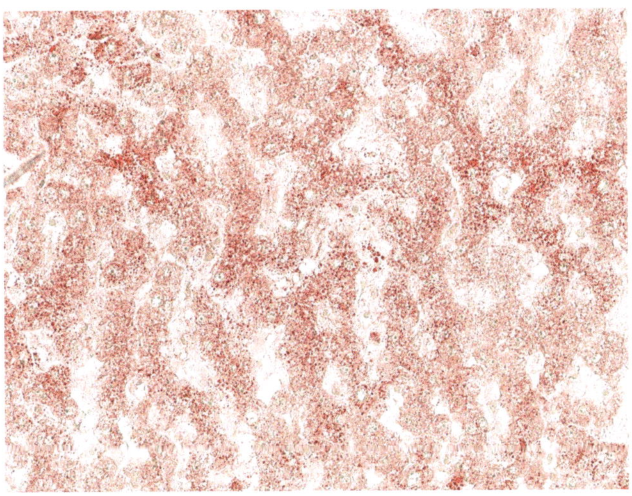

Fig. 16.7 Acute fatty liver of pregnancy (oil red O stain). Multiple minute fat droplets are highlighted in the hepatocytes. Fat droplets in microvesicular steatosis may be so tiny that the affected hepatocytes show a vaguely foamy cytoplasm or even have an apparently normal appearance. The oil red O stain is crucial in such cases to make the diagnosis. However, it requires a frozen section of the specimen (preferably fresh) before paraffin embedding. Thus, it is not performed routinely but may be prepared optimally if the clinician alerts the pathologist before sending the specimen of a suspected case.

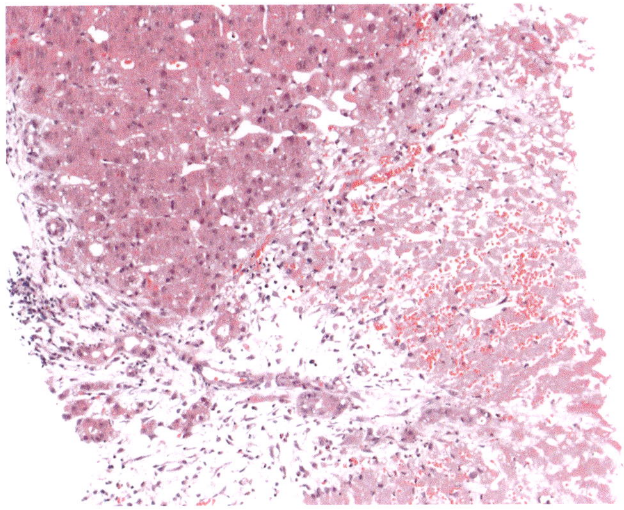

Fig. 16.8 Toxaemia of pregnancy/HELLP syndrome. Haemorrhagic necrosis is noted in the periportal region. Toxaemia of pregnancy/preeclampsia, which complicates over 5 % of all pregnancies, is characterised by hypertension and proteinuria after 20 weeks of gestation and/or within 48 hours after delivery. Eclampsia is a severe form of the disease spectrum with central nervous system involvement often presenting with seizures. Infarction, haematoma, and rupture are rare hepatic complications. Abnormal trophoblastic implantation, endothelial dysfunction, imbalance of vasodilators and vasoconstrictors, and an imbalance of angiogenic and antiangiogenic factors have been implicated in the pathogenesis of toxaemia. The associated liver injury may be related to insufficient hepatic perfusion and aberrant CD95 signalling.

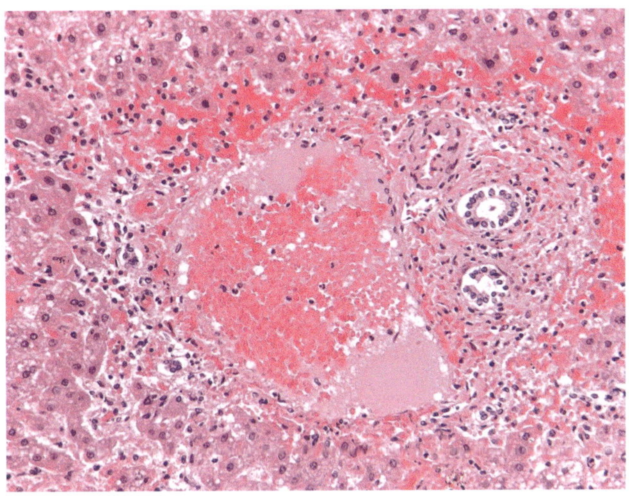

Fig. 16.9 Toxaemia of pregnancy/HELLP syndrome. The presence of portal vein fibrin thrombosis is associated with periportal haemorrhage. HELLP syndrome (haemolysis, elevated liver enzymes, and low platelets) affects 0.2 % to 0.6 % of all pregnancies. It is thought to be in the spectrum of pregnancy-induced hypertensive diseases that includes toxaemia of pregnancy. About 2 % to 12 % and up to 30 % of patients with preeclampsia and eclampsia, respectively, develop HELLP syndrome.

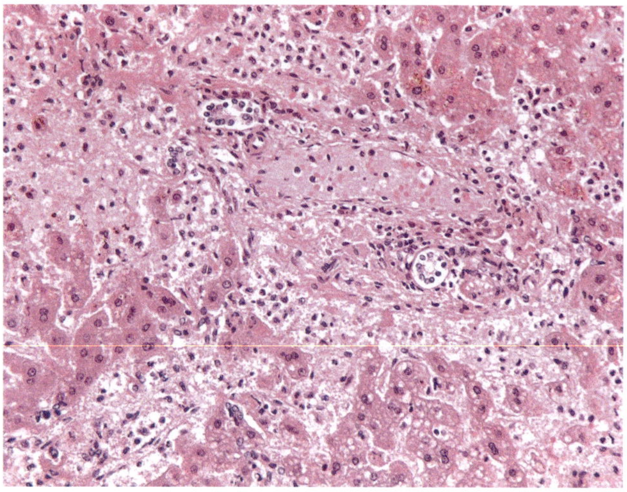

Fig. 16.10 Toxaemia of pregnancy/HELLP syndrome. Haemorrhagic necrosis of periportal hepatocytes and sinusoidal fibrin deposition are present. Periportal necrosis with haemorrhage and sinusoidal fibrin deposition is characteristic of toxaemia of pregnancy. The liver in some cases of HELLP syndrome also may have such histologic features, but many cases demonstrate only nonspecific reactive hepatitis. Other conditions with a predominantly periportal haemorrhagic necrosis include disseminated intravascular coagulation, drug/toxin-induced liver injury (e.g., from iron, phosphorus, or cocaine), acute hepatitis A, and small-for-size syndrome in liver allografts.

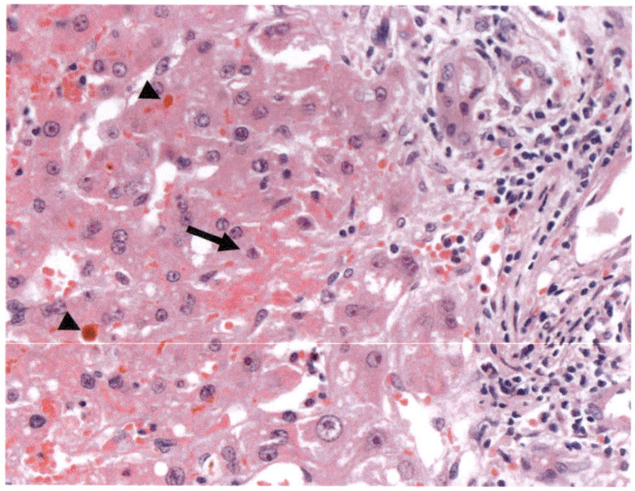

Fig. 16.11 Toxaemia of pregnancy/HELLP syndrome. Sinusoidal fibrin deposition (*arrow*) and canalicular bilirubinostasis (*arrowheads*) are observed in the periportal region. Bilirubinostasis and mild microvesicular steatosis also may be found in toxaemia of pregnancy and HELLP syndrome. In contrast to toxaemia of pregnancy and HELLP syndrome, intrahepatic cholestasis of pregnancy exhibits bland cholestasis without any associated necrosis, haemorrhage, or fibrin deposition. Acute fatty liver of pregnancy may share similar clinical manifestations and histologic features with toxaemia of pregnancy and HELLP syndrome, requiring proper clinical correlation for their differentiation.

17 Transplantation Pathology

The histopathologist is involved in many stages of the liver transplantation process, including evaluation of the: (1) donor liver prior to transplantation, (2) native liver removed at transplantation, (3) baseline graft status, and 4) posttransplantation graft. The type of posttransplant complication depends on various factors, including time post transplantation, primary liver condition, and the patient's age. For example, acute rejection affects the graft early, whereas recurrent disease occurs later. Like other types of liver disorders, the severity of rejection can be graded semiquantitatively, the commonest system used being the Banff scheme. Table 17.1 gives a brief summary of graft complications.

Graft-versus-host disease (GVHD), sinusoidal obstruction syndrome/veno-occlusive disease, and drug- or viral-induced hepatitis are the most common causes of liver injury in haemopoietic transplant patients. These are described at the end of the chapter.

Table 17.1 Graft Complications

Hours/days/weeks	Primary nonfunction
	Hyperacute rejection
	Preservation/reperfusion injury
	Rejection (acute/hyperacute)
	Vascular/biliary complications
Weeks/months	Rejection (acute/late)
	Vascular/biliary complications
	Infections
	Recurrent disease
	Posttransplant lymphoproliferative disorders (PTLD)
Months/years	Rejection (late/chronic)
	Chronic idiopathic hepatitis
	Vascular/biliary complications
	De novo diseases
	Recurrent disease
	Infections
	Posttransplant lymphoproliferative disorders (PTLD)
	Other neoplasms

A.W.H. Chan et al., *Atlas of Liver Pathology*, Atlas of Anatomic Pathology,
DOI 10.1007/978-1-4614-9114-9_17, © Springer Science+Business Media New York 2014

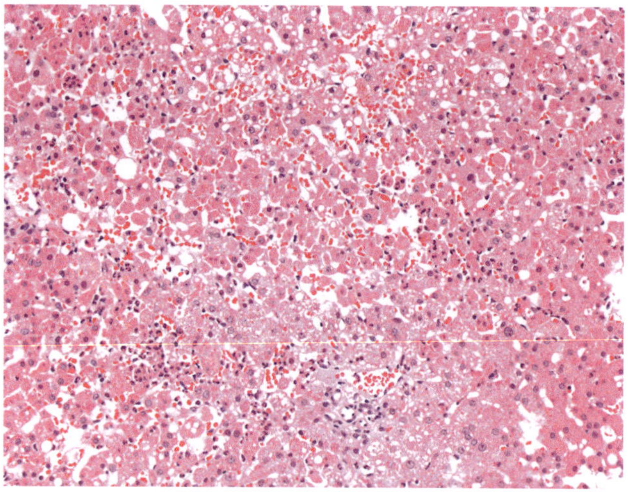

Fig. 17.1 Preservation–reperfusion injury. Clusters of detached, rounded, necrotic hepatocytes are accompanied by a neutrophilic infiltrate, mild sinusoidal congestion, and mild steatosis. Perfusion–reperfusion injury usually presents within the first week after transplantation. Clinical manifestations vary from asymptomatic mild elevations of liver enzymes to severe primary graft dysfunction. Its underlying pathogenesis is associated with damage to hepatocytes, biliary epithelial cells, and endothelial cells from warm and cold ischaemia and activation of Kupffer cells in reperfusion. Mild cases resolve over weeks, whereas severe cases involve a prolonged cholestatic period for weeks to months or may necessitate retransplantation.

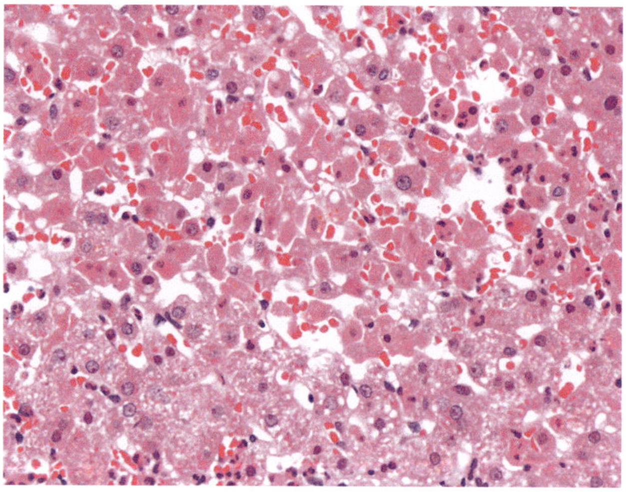

Fig. 17.2 Preservation–reperfusion injury. In preservation–reperfusion injury, varying degrees of hepatocyte damage characterised by ballooning degeneration, detachment and rounding of hepatocytes, necrosis, and apoptosis are noted. The extent ranges from mild (zone 3) to severe (confluent, particularly in subcapsular regions). A sinusoidal neutrophilic infiltrate is intimately associated with damaged hepatocytes. Bilirubinostasis, a mild ductular reaction, and lipopeliosis (accumulation of fat globules in the spaces of Disse due to ruptured fat globules of damaged hepatocytes) are additional findings. In contrast to hyperacute rejection, there is an absence of extensive haemorrhagic necrosis, vascular thrombi, and fibrinoid necrosis of blood vessels.

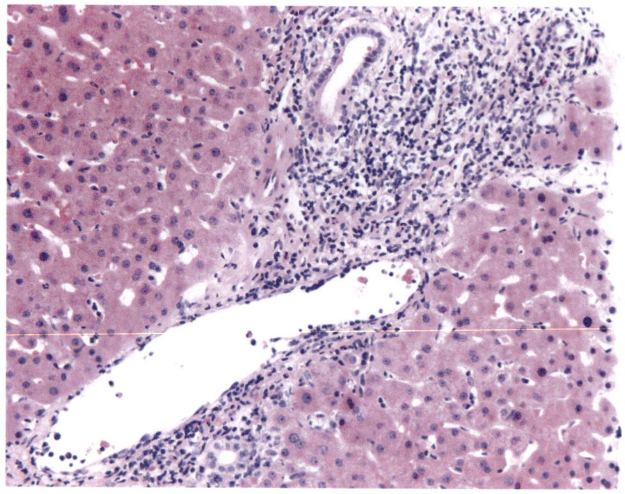

Fig. 17.3 Acute rejection. A portal tract is expanded by a dense, mixed inflammatory infiltrate. Endothelitis of the portal vein also is present. Acute rejection is the commonest cause of early allograft failure and usually presents within the first month after transplantation. About 20% to 40% of recipients experience one or more episodes of acute rejection, which manifests as fever, right upper quadrant pain, and a cholestatic pattern of deranged liver function. The hallmark pathologic features of acute rejection are a mixed portal inflammatory infiltrate, bile duct damage, and endothelitis.

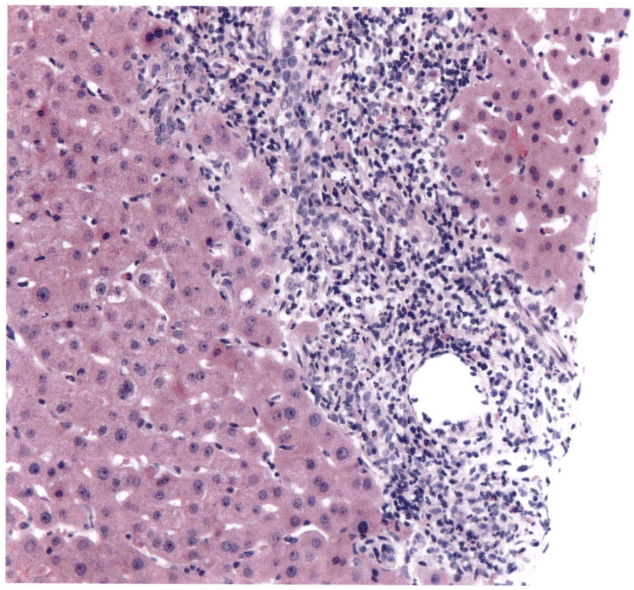

Fig. 17.4 Acute rejection. A portal tract is expanded by a dense, mixed inflammatory infiltrate. Mild endothelitis of the portal vein and bile duct damage also are present. The portal tracts are expanded initially by a lymphocytic and subsequently by a mixed inflammatory infiltrate. The latter is composed of small lymphocytes, activated "blast" lymphoid cells, neutrophils, and eosinophils. The presence of prominent eosinophils or significant interface hepatitis indicates a more severe form of acute rejection. Portal granulomas typically are not present.

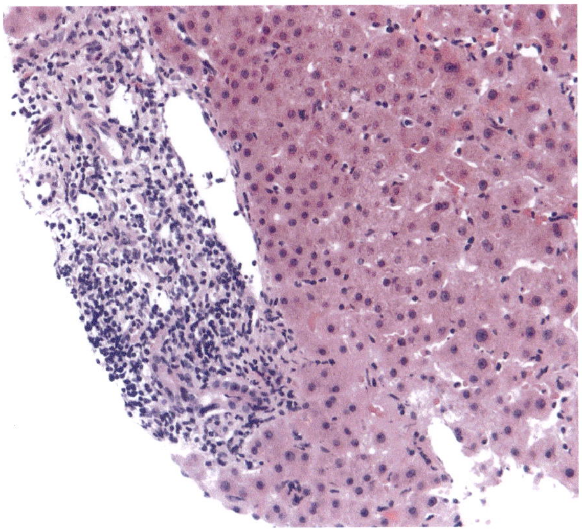

Fig. 17.5 Acute rejection. Acute rejection must be distinguished from other inflammatory processes. Portal lymphoid follicles and mild steatosis are more suggestive of recurrent hepatitis C. A lobular lymphoid infiltrate and atypical lymphoid cells expressing Epstein-Barr virus (EBV)–latent membrane protein 1 (LMP1)/EBV-encoded RNA (EBER) indicate EBV-related disease. A significant lymphoplasmacytic infiltrate, prominent interface hepatitis, and lobular activity suggest recurrent or de novo autoimmune hepatitis. Recurrent or de-novo disease affects the graft usually a few months after transplant. At this stage, rejection (late rejection) manifests as a more hepatitic injury, with a "toned-down" portal infiltrate, often minimal or no endotheliitis, and lobular involvement in the form of central perivenulitis. For this reason, late rejection is more difficult to differentiate from recurrent or de-novo disease. The so-called "chronic idiopathic hepatitis of the graft," which may be associated with progressive graft fibrosis, overlaps in appearance with late rejection, recurrent, and de-novo disease.

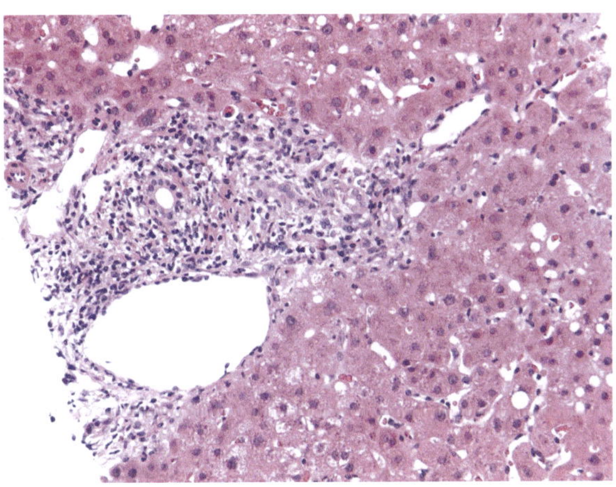

Fig. 17.6 Acute rejection. An injured interlobular bile duct is seen in which there is epithelial disarray and a lymphocytic infiltrate. Bile duct damage is another salient feature of acute rejection and is characterised by cytoplasmic vacuolation, apoptosis, and regenerative changes, with an intraepithelial lymphocytic and/or neutrophilic infiltrate. A ductular reaction and even "acute cholangitis" (intraluminal neutrophilic accumulation) may be present. Acute cellular rejection should be distinguished from other biliary processes, such as ischaemic cholangitis, biliary stricture, and recurrent biliary disease. The presence of endothelitis and mixed portal inflammation with activated "blast" lymphoid cells favours acute rejection, in the early post-transplant phase.

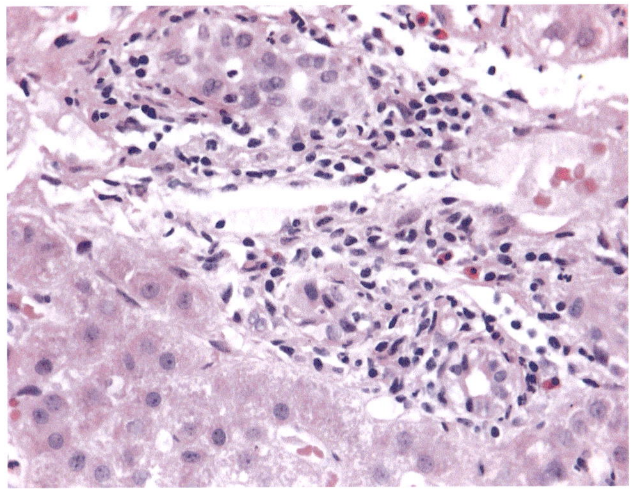

Fig. 17.7 Acute rejection. Note the epithelial vacuolation and lymphocytic infiltrate. Portal oedema, significant acute cholangitis, a prominent ductular reaction, and biloma (rarely observed in biopsy samples) would be more suggestive of biliary stricture or acute large duct obstruction from some other cause.

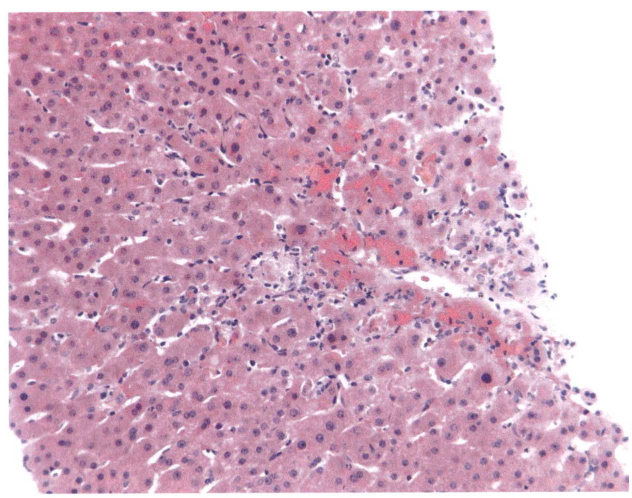

Fig. 17.8 Acute rejection. A terminal hepatic venule shows a subendothelial inflammatory infiltrate, which is associated with perivenular congestion and confluent hepatocellular necrosis. Endothelitis, also referred to as endotheliitis and endothelialitis, is characterised by a subendothelial inflammatory infiltrate with lifting and disruption of the endothelial lining. Portal veins and terminal hepatic venules commonly are affected, whereas hepatic arteries rarely are involved. Although endothelitis usually is considered a characteristic feature of acute rejection, it is not entirely pathognomonic because mild endothelitis is often observed in autoimmune hepatitis, primary biliary cirrhosis, viral hepatitis, and posttransplant lymphoid proliferative disease. A coexisting mixed portal inflammation with activated "blast" lymphoid cells or bile duct damage secures the diagnosis of acute cellular rejection.

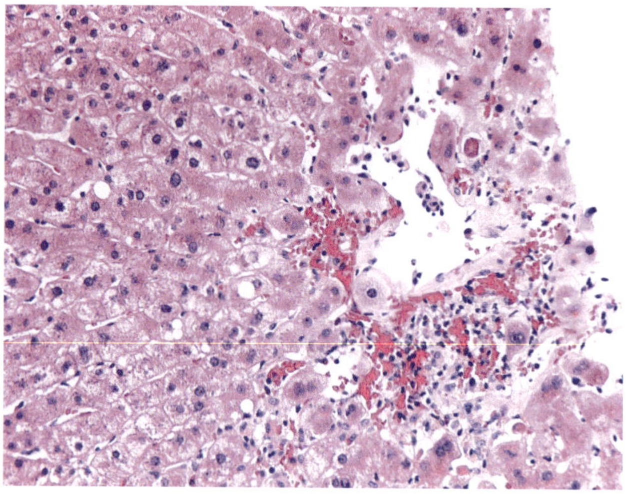

Fig. 17.9 Acute rejection. Central perivenulitis is seen associated with perivenular confluent hepatocellular necrosis. Coexisting central perivenulitis and mixed portal inflammation and/or bile duct damage indicate a more severe form of acute rejection and are associated with a poorer response to conventional immunosuppressants and a higher chance of rapid progression to chronic rejection. Isolated central perivenulitis without significant mixed portal inflammation and bile duct damage is regarded as a manifestation of late rejection (>3 months after transplantation). It affects up to one third of patients receiving transplants. A hepatitic pattern of deranged liver function is the usual biochemical manifestation. Most of these patients respond to augmentation of the immunosuppression.

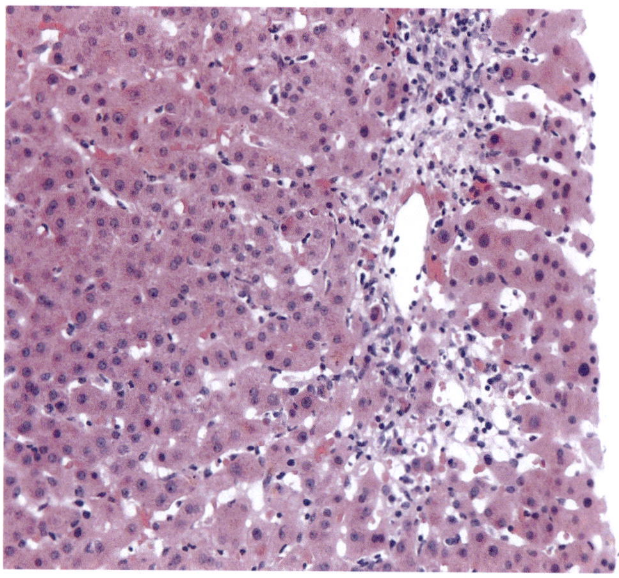

Fig. 17.10 Acute rejection. This image shows central perivenulitis with a lymphoplasmacytic infiltrate and perivenular confluent hepatocellular necrosis. Isolated central perivenulitis as a manifestation of acute or late rejection needs to be differentiated from other causes of perivenular injury, and in particular ischaemia, as it tends to affect the centrilobular region. De novo or recurrent autoimmune hepatitis also are associated with perivenular injury. Recurrent hepatitis C tends to affect the lobule more diffusely, usually in the form of necroinflammatory foci, with apoptotic bodies and steatosis. Portal inflammation with lymphoid aggregate formation later in the course of the disease complete the pattern.

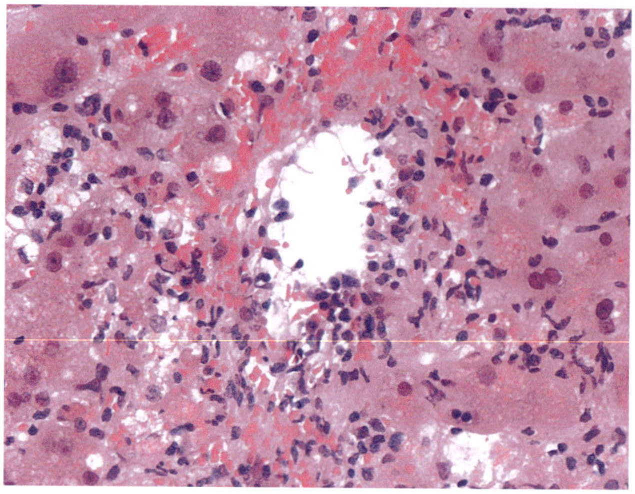

Fig. 17.11 Central perivenulitis with marked disruption of a terminal hepatic venule associated with perivenular necrosis and congestion. Late rejection occurs more than 3 to 6 months after transplantation. Isolated central perivenulitis is regarded as a manifestation of late rejection, and its appearance overlaps with that of de novo autoimmune hepatitis and idiopathic chronic hepatitis.

GLOBAL ASSESSMENT	CRITERIA
Indeterminate	Portal inflammatory infiltrate that fails to meet the criteria for the diagnosis of acute cellular rejection
Mild (Grade I)	Rejection infiltrate in a minority of the portal tracts, that is mild and confined within the portal tracts
Moderate (Grade II)	Rejection infiltrate expands most or all of the portal tracts
Severe (Grade III)	Rejection infiltrate expands most or all of the portal tracts with spillover into periportal parenchyma, and moderate to severe perivenular inflammation with perivenular necrosis

Fig. 17.12 Banff schema for grading liver allograft rejection (global assessment). The Banff schema is a consensus document created by an international panel of hepatopathologists, hepatologists, surgeons, and scientists. After establishing a diagnosis of acute cellular rejection, an overall rejection grade can be assigned to mild, moderate, or severe cases. The indeterminate category is reserved for low-grade or early acute cellular rejection failing to meet the criteria (at least two of three cardinal features: mixed portal inflammatory infiltrate, bile duct damage, and endothelitis).

CATEGORY	CRITERIA	SCORE
Portal inflammation	Mostly lymphocytes infiltrate but not noticeably expand a minority of the portal tracts	1
	Mixed inflammatory cells expand most or all the portal tracts	2
	Mixed inflammatory cells markedly expand most or all the portal tracts with spillover into periportal parenchyma	3
Bile duct damage	A minority of the bile ducts are infiltrated by inflammatory cells and show mild reactive changes	1
	Most or all the bile ducts are infiltrated by inflammatory cells and some show prominent reactive changes	2
	Most or all the bile ducts are infiltrated by inflammatory cells and show prominent reactive changes	3
Endothelitis	Subendothelial inflammation of a minority of the portal vein/ terminal hepatic venules	1
	Subendothelial inflammation of most or all of the portal vein/ terminal hepatic venules	2
	Subendothelial inflammation of most or all of the portal vein/ terminal hepatic venules with central perivenulitis	3

Fig. 17.13 Banff schema for grading liver allograft rejection (rejection activity index). After establishing a diagnosis of acute cellular rejection and assigning an overall rejection grade, a rejection activity index can be calculated by summation of the individual component scores.

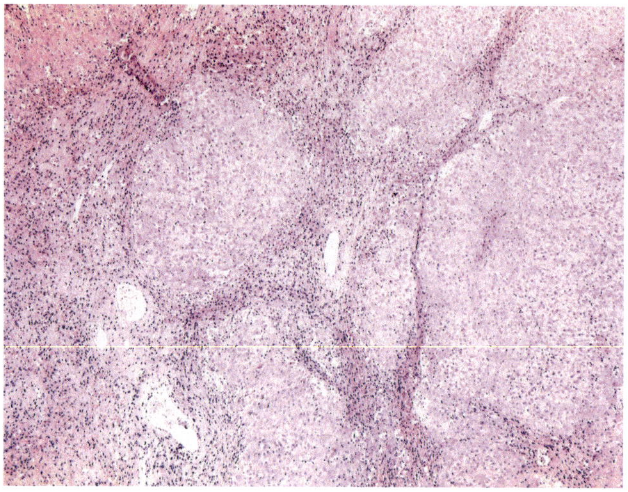

Fig. 17.14 Late rejection progressed to bridging fibrosis and bile duct loss, with signs of chronic rejection. Ductopaenia without any significant ductular reaction is noted. Chronic rejection has declined in allograft patients, from up to 20% previously to 2% to 3% currently, because of improved immunosuppression. It usually presents within 6 months after transplantation and follows multiple episodes of acute rejection, an episode of refractory acute rejection, or less commonly, insidiously without any preceding acute rejection. Progressive jaundice with cholestatic liver function derangement is the typical clinical manifestation.

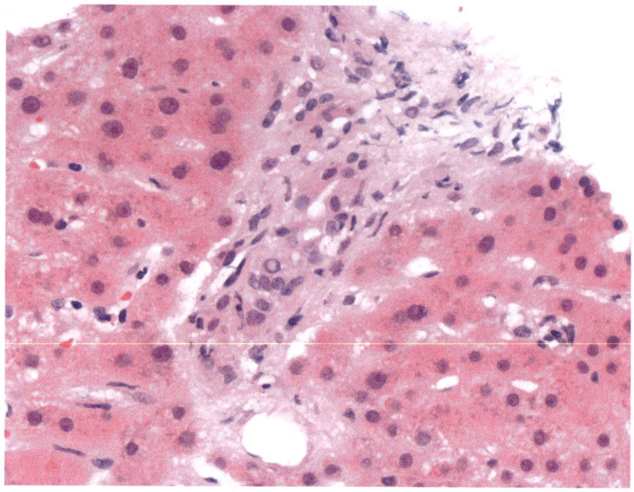

Fig. 17.16 Chronic rejection. Cholangiocytes show degenerate changes, but the accompanying inflammatory infiltrate is mild. Early chronic rejection typically is devoid of a ductular reaction, cholate stasis, or significant portal inflammation.

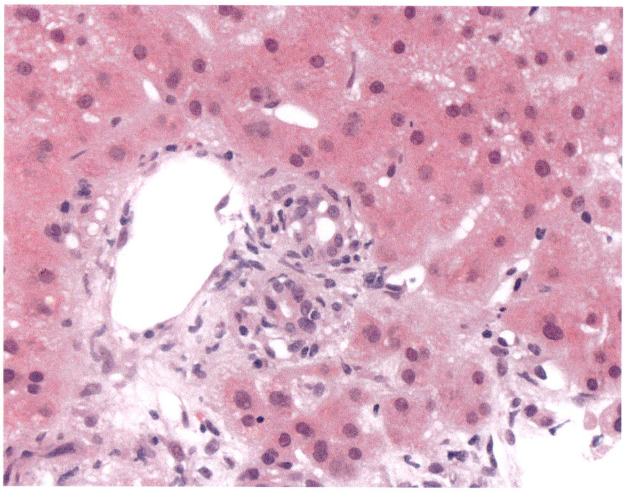

Fig. 17.15 Chronic rejection. Degenerative changes of bile ducts are evidenced by epithelial attenuation, uneven nuclear spacing, and nuclear hyperchromasia and loss. The pathologic processes of chronic rejection mainly affect the bile ducts and hepatic arteries. Affected small interlobular bile ducts exhibit degenerative changes, with epithelial attenuation, uneven nuclear spacing, nuclear hyperchromasia and loss, an increased nucleocytoplasmic ratio, and cytoplasmic eosinophilia. Bile duct loss is present in less than 50% and at least 50% of portal tracts in early and late chronic rejection, respectively. A ductular reaction typically is absent. In early chronic rejection, arteries show focal foam cell accumulation; and in the latter, there may be mural fibrosis in late chronic rejection.

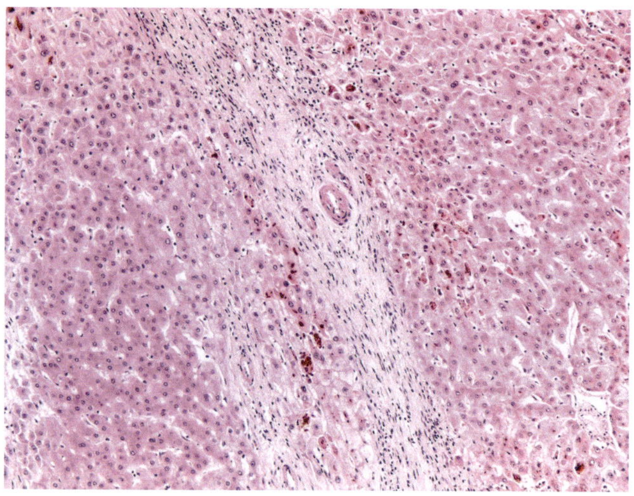

Fig. 17.17 Chronic rejection. A fibrous septum contains an unpaired hepatic arteriole without an accompanying interlobular bile duct (ductopaenia). Bilirubinostasis is present in periseptal hepatocytes and Kupffer cells. A ductular reaction is absent. Progressive damage to small interlobular bile ducts in chronic rejection leads to loss of interlobular bile ducts. Bile duct loss is present in less than 50% and at least 50% of portal tracts in early and late chronic rejection, respectively.

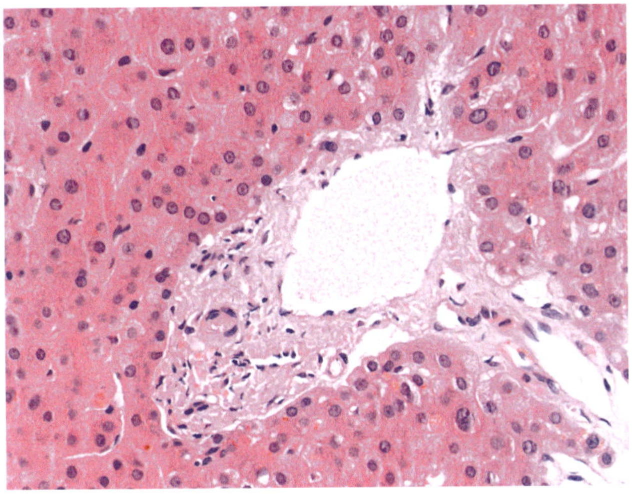

Fig. 17.18 Chronic rejection. A portal tract contains an unpaired hepatic arteriole without an accompanying interlobular bile duct (ductopaenia). Chronic rejection is characteristically devoid of a ductular reaction, cholate stasis, or significant portal inflammation, as opposed to other forms of biliary injury like ischaemic biliary strictures, or recurrent primary sclerosing cholangitis or recurrent primary biliary cirrhosis.

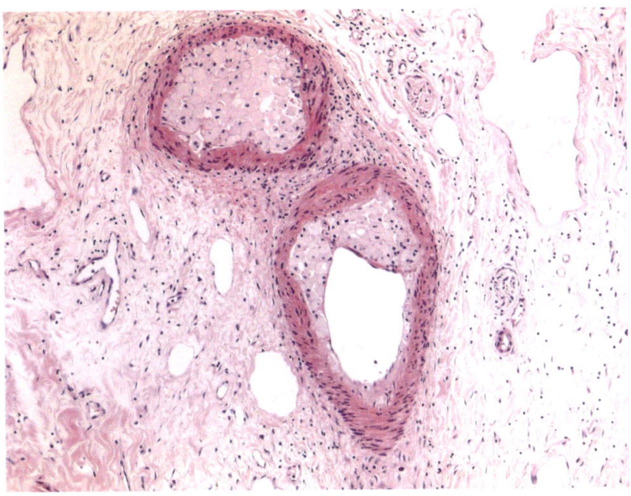

Fig. 17.19 Chronic rejection. Subintimal foamy histiocytes accumulate in a medium-sized hepatic artery, causing occlusion of the lumen. Medium-sized to large hepatic arteries exhibit subintimal foam cell accumulation. Intimal inflammation without luminal compromise is typical in early chronic rejection, whereas luminal narrowing with fibrointimal proliferation is characteristic for late chronic rejection. However, foam cell obliterative arteriopathy is uncommonly represented in biopsy specimens.

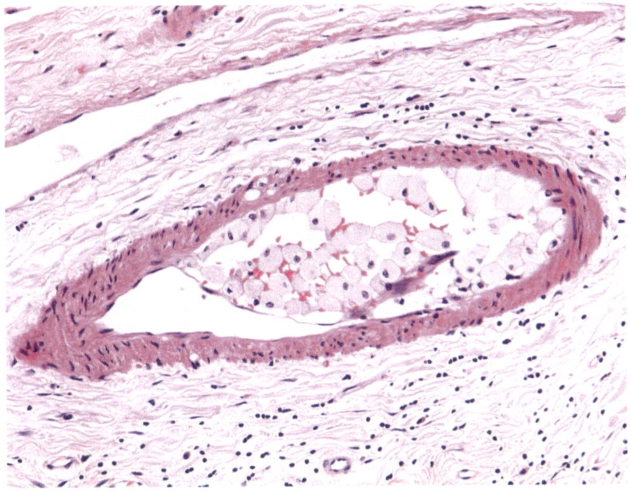

Fig. 17.20 Chronic rejection. Subintimal foamy histiocytes accumulate in a medium-sized hepatic artery. Other pathologic changes in early chronic rejection include mild perivenular necroinflammation, spotty necrosis, and perivenular fibrosis, whereas those in late chronic rejection are marked bilirubinostasis, sinusoidal foam cell accumulation, focal obliteration of terminal hepatic venules, and bridging fibrosis. Perivenular necrosis and fibrosis are regarded as consequences of foam cell obliterative arteriopathy. The presence of significant spotty necrosis in an otherwise typical chronic rejection sometimes may be designated as "transition" hepatitis. It may represent a transitional phase from acute or late rejection to chronic rejection, or a distinctive chronic hepatitis-like pattern of chronic rejection. Jaundice with hepatitic liver function derangement is the usual clinical presentation.

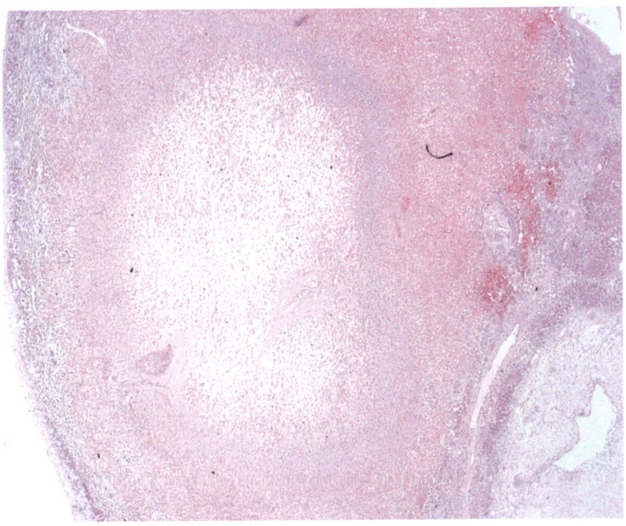

Fig. 17.21 Hepatic artery thrombosis. There is a large area of hepatic necrosis secondary to vascular occlusion by hepatic artery thrombosis. Hepatic artery thrombosis is the commonest vascular complication in liver allografts. It affects 2.5% to 11% of patients receiving transplants, particularly children and patients receiving reduced-size grafts. Anastomotic stenosis of the hepatic artery, kinking of the hepatic artery, and splenic arterial steal syndrome are other vascular complications occurring in liver allografts.

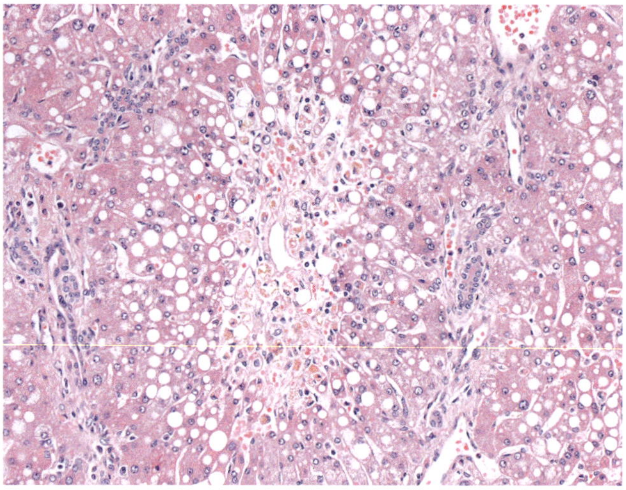

Fig. 17.22 Hepatic artery thrombosis. Mild perivenular necrosis is present in a background of marked steatosis. Hepatic artery thrombosis may manifest as hepatocellular necrosis. The necrotic areas are highly variable in size (small confluent perivenular necrosis to large multiacinar necrosis) and distribution. Because of the patchy distribution, liver biopsy is not a reliable tool for evaluating the severity of ischaemic injury.

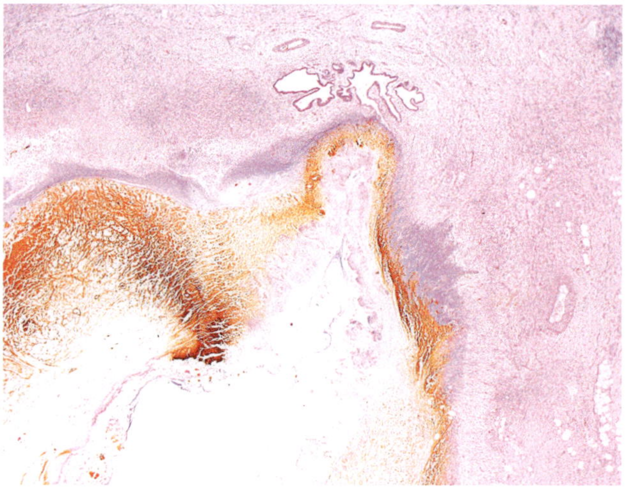

Fig. 17.23 Hepatic artery thrombosis. A large perihilar bile duct shows extensive ischaemic necrosis with leakage of bile into the necrotic wall. Ischaemic cholangitis is a complication of hepatic artery thrombosis, because the biliary tree depends entirely on arterial perfusion, as opposed to the dual portal-arterial supply to the hepatic plates. Acute ischaemic cholangitis is manifest by ulceration, ischaemic necrosis, extravasation of bile into the necrotic wall and surrounding liver parenchyma, and even abscess formation. Chronic ischaemic cholangitis is characterised by fibro-obliterative changes of bile ducts with periductal "onion-skin" concentric fibrosis. Differentiation between ischaemic cholangitis, biliary stricture, and recurrent primary sclerosing cholangitis is difficult on histologic grounds alone.

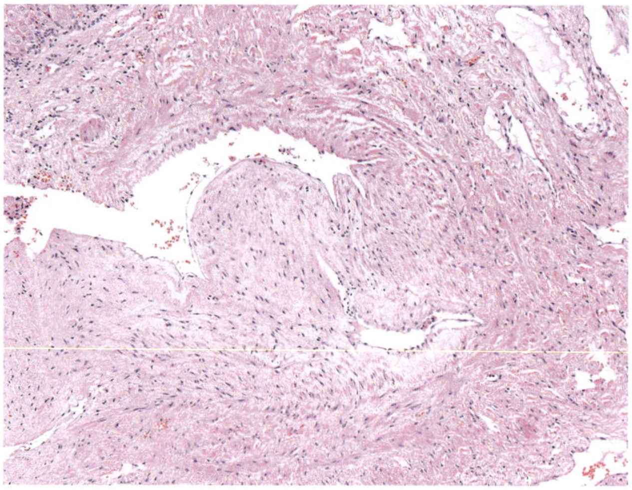

Fig. 17.24 Portal vein thrombosis. A thrombosed large portal vein shows partial recanalization. Portal vein thrombosis and stenosis are uncommon. Early portal vein thrombosis is associated with early graft dysfunction and failure, whereas late thrombosis may manifest as non-cirrhotic portal hypertension.

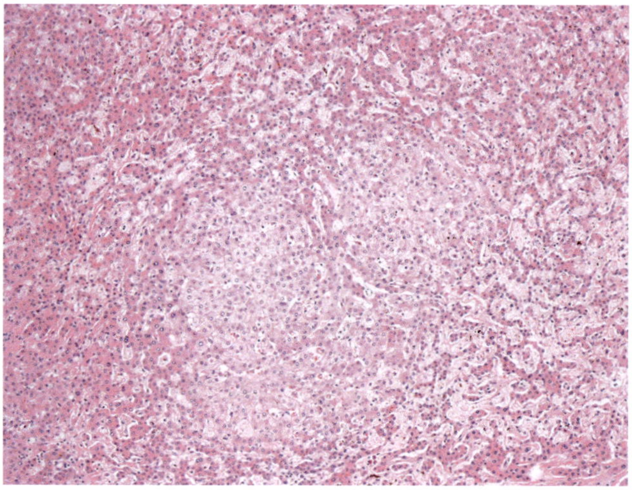

Fig. 17.25 Nodular regenerative hyperplasia associated with portal vein thrombosis in an allograft. Parenchymal nodular change is present without any fibrosis. Nodular regenerative hyperplasia is the commonest structural change in late allograft biopsies; others include irregular thickening of hepatocyte plates, sinusoidal fibrosis, and sinusoidal congestion and dilatation. Structural changes are reported in 1.3% to 82% of late allograft biopsies and may be caused by portal or hepatic venopathy, drug-induced liver injuries, or rejection-associated injury to the sinusoidal or vascular endothelium.

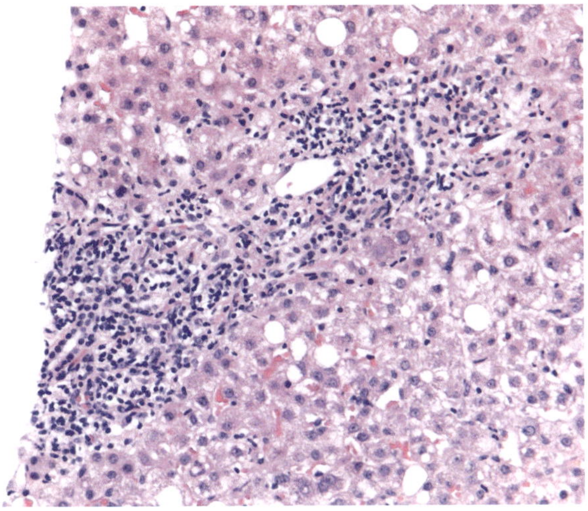

Fig. 17.26 Recurrent hepatitis C. A moderate portal, predominantly lymphocytic infiltrate is present, with mild interface hepatitis and mild steatosis. More than 90% of patients undergoing transplantation for chronic hepatitis C develop recurrent disease. Pathologic manifestations of recurrent hepatitis C include acute hepatitis, chronic hepatitis, and a form of fibrosing cholestatic hepatitis. Acute hepatitis C, which is uncommon in the native liver, is manifest by lobular disarray with ballooning degeneration and apoptosis. Varying degrees of sinusoidal lymphocytosis and portal lymphocyte-predominant inflammation may be present. Bile duct damage, endothelitis, and even central perivenulitis also may be found.

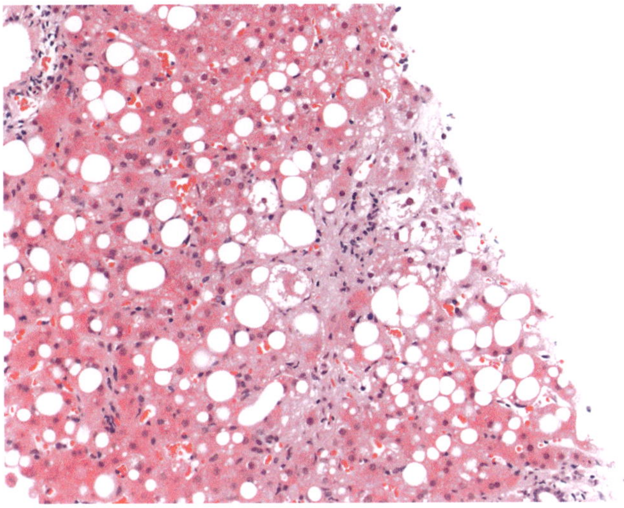

Fig. 17.28 Recurrent steatohepatitis. Many ballooned hepatocytes are present within a background of marked steatosis. Alcoholic liver disease (ALD) and nonalcoholic fatty liver disease (NAFLD) recur in 10% to 30% and 20% to 40% of patients receiving transplants, respectively. Resumption of alcohol is common, but alcoholic hepatitis, advanced fibrosis, and cirrhosis are relatively uncommon and confined to heavy recidivist drinkers. Insulin resistance associated with immunosuppressive agents exacerbates preexisting risk factors for NAFLD. The pathologic features of ALD and NAFLD are similar to those in the native liver.

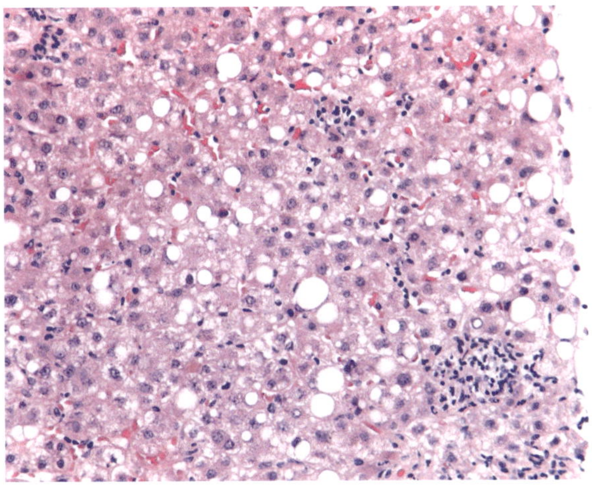

Fig. 17.27 Recurrent viral hepatitis C. Scattered foci of spotty necrosis and apoptosis are accompanied by mild steatosis. Portal lymphoid follicles tend to be less frequent in recurrent hepatitis C compared with that occurring in the native liver, whereas lobular necroinflammatory activity often tends to be more significant. In contrast to chronic rejection, a mild ductular reaction usually is evident, but degenerative changes of bile ducts and ductopaenia typically are absent. Progression to cirrhosis is common and observed in 10% to 30% and 50% of patients within 5 years and 10 years, respectively. The variant of fibrosing cholestatic hepatitis seen with recurrent hepatitis C virus is characterised by variable combinations of portal, periportal, and pericellular fibrosis; a ductular reaction; ballooning degeneration; bilirubinostasis; and steatosis.

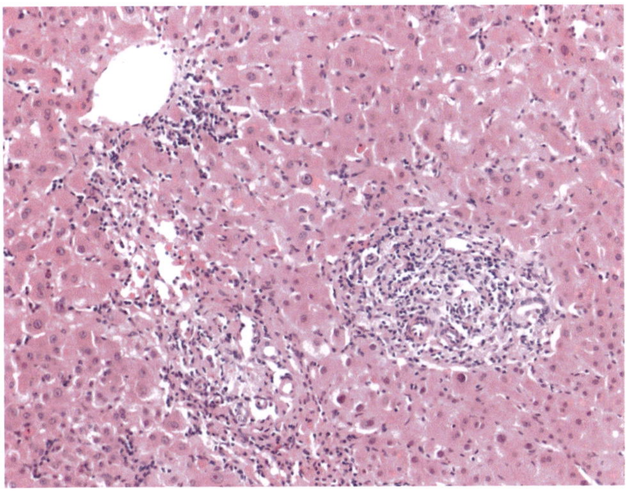

Fig. 17.29 Recurrent autoimmune hepatitis. Bridging necrosis is accompanied by a moderate portal lymphocyte-predominant infiltrate, central perivenulitis, and lobular inflammation. Autoimmune hepatitis relapses in 20% to 30% of patients undergoing transplantation, particularly those with suboptimal immunosuppression. Most cases present after 1 year of transplantation. High titres of autoantibodies (antinuclear antibody [ANA], anti–smooth muscle antigen [SMA]) and hypergammaglobulinaemia are common findings resembling autoimmune hepatitis in patients not receiving transplants. However, serum autoantibodies are unreliable diagnostic markers because they persist after transplantation, even without recurrent disease.

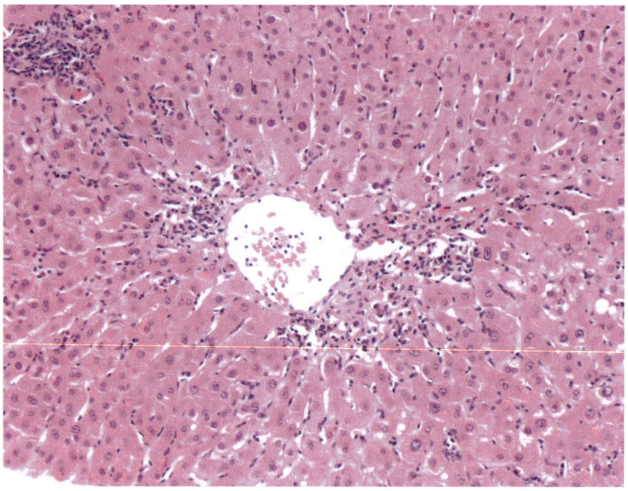

Fig. 17.30 Recurrent autoimmune hepatitis. Central perivenulitis is manifest by perivenular necrosis and inflammation. Moderate lobular necroinflammatory activity also is present. Recurrent autoimmune hepatitis is characterised pathologically by portal plasma cell–rich infiltrate with varying degrees of interface hepatitis, lobular necroinflammatory activity, and central perivenulitis. Isolated central perivenulitis may precede the other, more distinctive pathologic features of recurrent autoimmune hepatitis. About 20% to 40% of recurrent autoimmune hepatitis cases progress to cirrhosis and graft failure, but the incidence has declined because of prompt recognition and optimal immunosuppression.

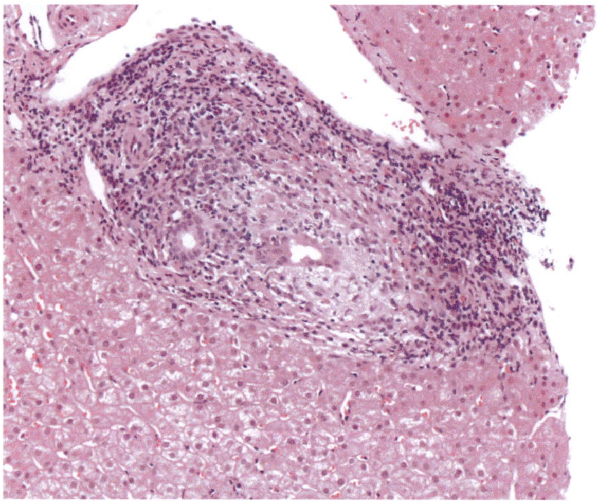

Fig. 17.31 Recurrent primary biliary cirrhosis. A florid duct lesion is characterised by cholangiocyte injury with a surrounding dense lymphohistiocytic infiltrate. Many plasma cells and occasional eosinophils also are present in the portal tract. About 20% to 50% of patients undergoing transplantation for primary biliary cirrhosis develop recurrent disease, usually after 1 year following transplantation. Most cases are asymptomatic, with normal liver enzymes. Serum antimitochondrial antibodies are an unreliable diagnostic marker because they persist after transplantation, even in the absence of recurrent disease. Less than 1% of recurrent primary biliary cirrhosis cases progress to cirrhosis and graft failure.

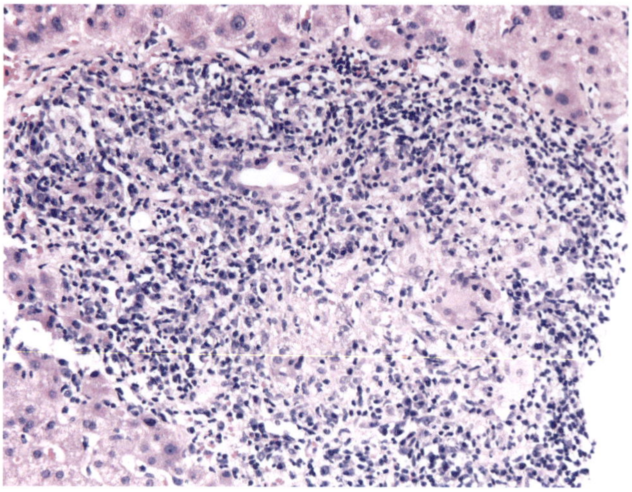

Fig. 17.32 Recurrent primary biliary cirrhosis. A damaged bile duct is surrounded by dense lymphoplasmacytic infiltrate and a noncaseating epithelioid granuloma. Recurrent primary biliary cirrhosis is histologically similar to that in the native liver. Variable degrees of bile duct damage from a florid duct lesion to lymphocytic cholangitis may be seen, accompanied by portal mononuclear infiltrate, portal granuloma, ductular reaction, ductopaenia, and cholate stasis. Although the florid duct lesion is pathognomonic, it is found in only up to 30% of cases. In contrast to acute cellular rejection, portal inflammation and bile duct damage tend to be more localised and endothelitis typically is absent or, at most, mild. Compared with chronic rejection, there tends to be more significant portal inflammation, and a ductular reaction frequently is present.

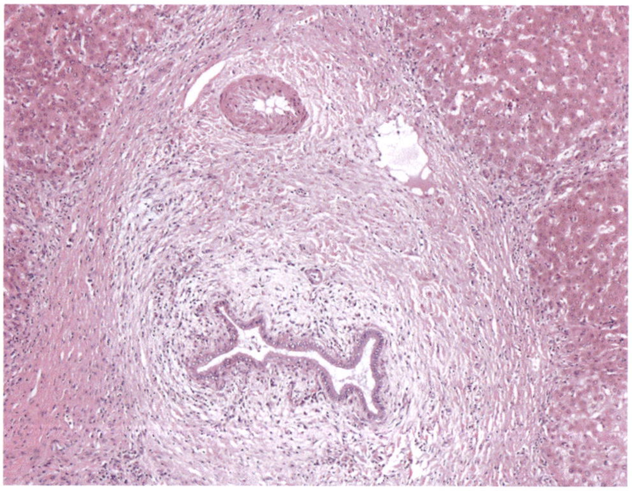

Fig. 17.33 Recurrent primary sclerosing cholangitis. A medium-sized bile duct with an irregular contour is seen, with periductal onion-skin concentric fibrosis and oedema and a mild portal lymphocytic infiltrate. About 20% to 30% of cases undergoing transplantation for primary sclerosing cirrhosis recur, usually after 1 year following transplantation. Patients normally present with clinical features of chronic cholestasis and repeated episodes of acute cholangitis. Up to 10% of recurrent primary sclerosing cholangitis cases progress to cirrhosis and graft failure.

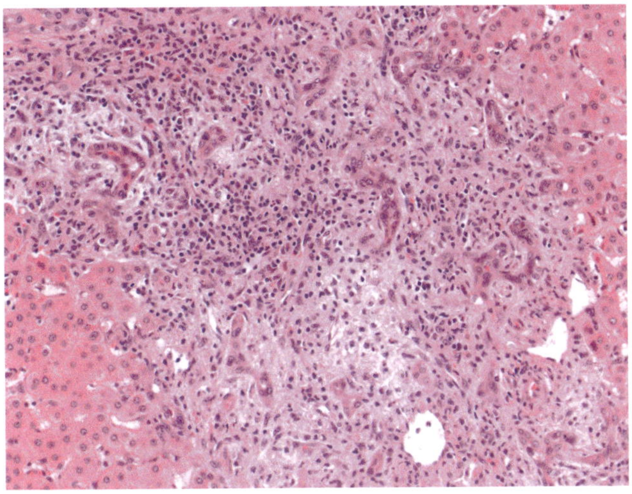

Fig. 17.34 Recurrent primary sclerosing cholangitis. A moderate ductular reaction is present in a portal tract devoid of an interlobular bile duct. Recurrent primary sclerosing cholangitis is pathologically similar to that in the nontransplanted liver. It is characterised by fibro-obliterative change of bile ducts with varying degrees of portal mixed inflammation, xanthogranulomatous inflammation, ductular reaction, ductopaenia, cholate stasis, and portal vein phlebitis. Degenerative epithelial changes of small bile ducts are seen more often in chronic rejection, but recurrent small duct primary sclerosing cholangitis may show similar features. However, distinction between recurrent primary sclerosing cholangitis and secondary sclerosing cholangitis is impossible by histology alone.

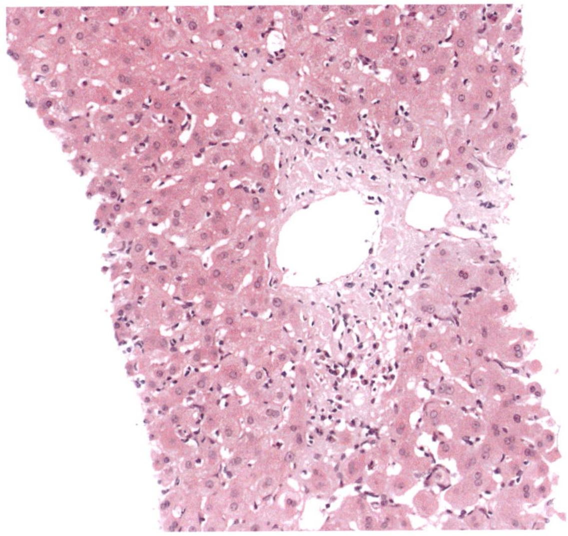

Fig. 17.36 De novo autoimmune hepatitis. Prominent perivenular fibrosis and necrosis are accompanied by a mild lymphoplasmacytic infiltrate. De novo autoimmune hepatitis is characterised pathologically by a portal plasma cell–rich infiltrate with a variable degree of interface hepatitis, lobular necroinflammatory activity, and central perivenulitis. Lobular changes often are more marked and frequent than those of autoimmune hepatitis in patients not receiving transplants. Portal and perivenular fibrosis may be present. Some regard de novo autoimmune hepatitis, along with idiopathic chronic hepatitis of the graft as histologic variants of late rejection.

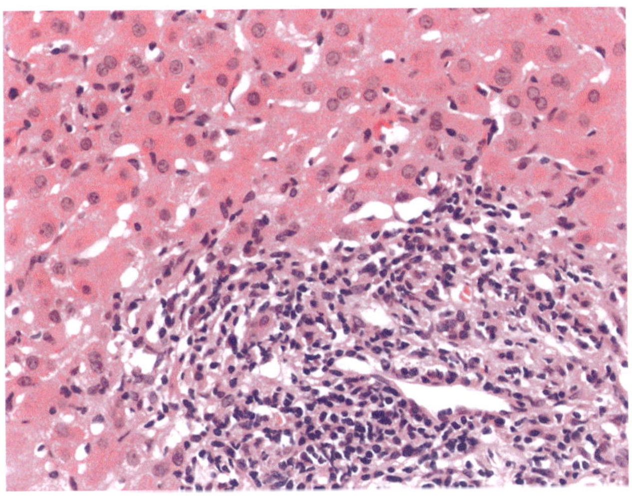

Fig. 17.35 De novo autoimmune hepatitis. A dense portal lymphoplasmacytic infiltrate is accompanied by moderate interface hepatitis. De novo autoimmune hepatitis, also referred to as plasma cell hepatitis, occurs in 1% to 2% and 5% to 10% of adults and children receiving liver allografts, respectively. Most cases present after 1 year of transplantation. High titres of autoantibodies (ANA and SMA) and hypergammaglobulinaemia are common findings resembling autoimmune hepatitis in patients who have not undergone transplantation.

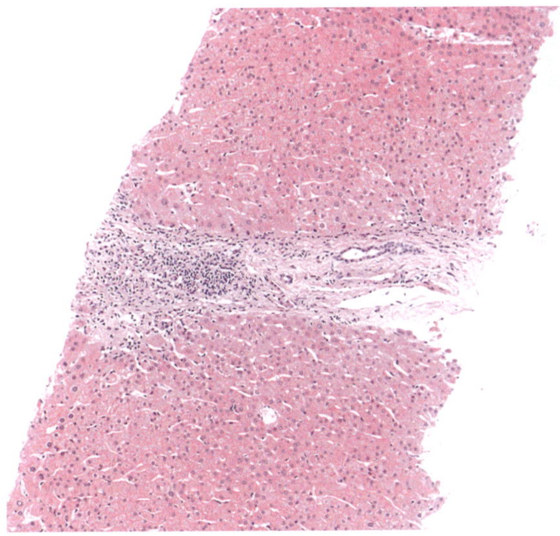

Fig. 17.37 Idiopathic chronic hepatitis. A moderate portal lymphocyte-predominant infiltrate is present with minimal interface hepatitis. Idiopathic chronic hepatitis is a diagnosis of exclusion and comprises unexplained chronic hepatitis in the allograft. Its prevalence increases progressively from 20% to 30% during the first 3 years to more than 60% at 10 years post transplantation. Histologically, it is characterised by a portal mononuclear infiltrate with varying degrees of interface hepatitis, lobular necroinflammatory activity, and, in some cases, central perivenulitis. Progression to bridging fibrosis and cirrhosis is a common long-term sequel.

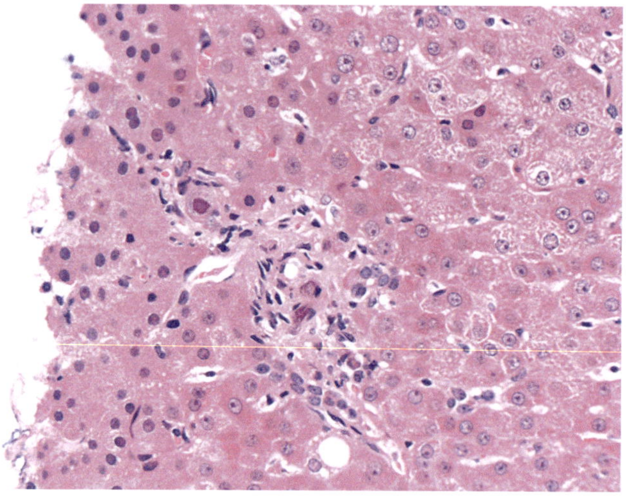

Fig. 17.38 Cytomegalovirus (CMV) hepatitis. A periportal hepatocyte contains a large eosinophilic intranuclear inclusion. CMV hepatitis has been reported in 4% to 34.6% of liver allografts, but its incidence has been reduced markedly by the use of antiviral prophylaxis. It usually occurs 4 to 12 weeks after transplantation but may present 1 year or more after discontinuation of prophylactic treatment currently. The characteristic viral inclusion is pathognomonic for CMV and may be found in endothelial cells, bile duct epithelial cells, and hepatocytes. The affected cell shows cytomegaly with a large eosinophilic intranuclear inclusion surrounded by a clear halo. Basophilic cytoplasmic inclusions also may be found. Immunostaining for CMV is confirmatory.

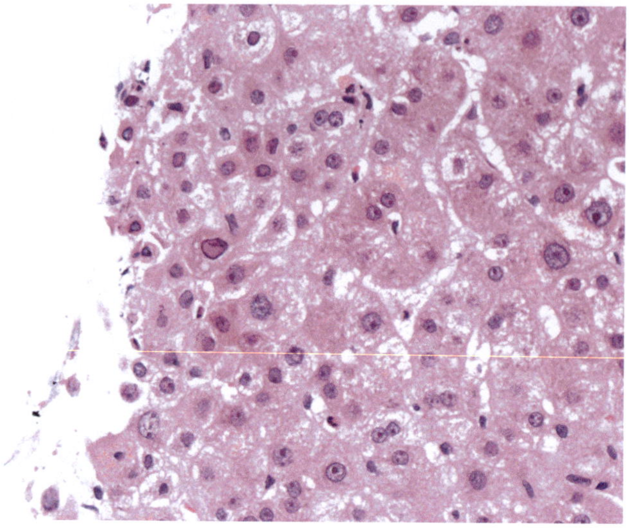

Fig. 17.40 Herpes simplex virus hepatitis. Several hepatocytes contain ground-glass intranuclear viral inclusions (Cowdry B) with chromatin margination. Herpes zoster virus (HZV), a member of Herpesviridae, rarely affects liver allografts. It produces a pathologic picture and viral inclusions similar to those of HSV. Immunostaining for HZV confirms the diagnosis. On the other hand, human herpesvirus 6 (HHV-6), another member of Herpesviridae, affects up to 80% of liver allografts. It is associated with concurrent rejection, CMV hepatitis, or opportunistic fungal infections. Histologically, HHV-6 hepatitis is characterised by a moderate portal lymphocyte-predominant infiltrate, spotty necrosis, and lobular microabscess. The definitive diagnosis is established by immunoreactivity of HHV-6 in portal lymphocytes.

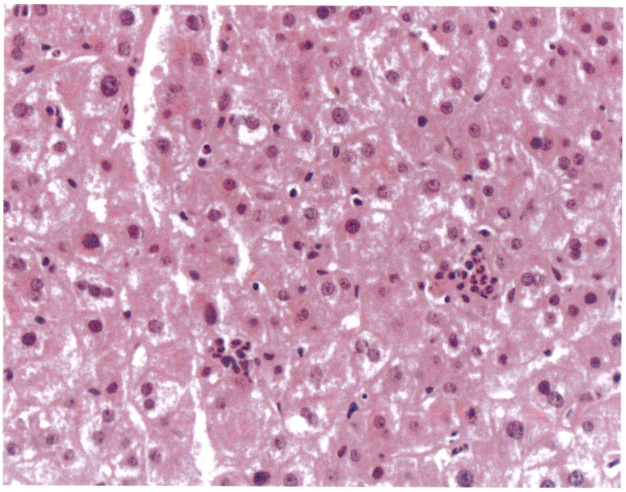

Fig. 17.39 Cytomegalovirus hepatitis. Two small clusters of neutrophils (microabscesses) are present. Lobular microabscess formation is a typical feature of CMV hepatitis. Clusters of neutrophils usually surround a necrotic hepatocyte or hepatocyte with viral inclusion. Lobular microabscesses, however, are not entirely specific and may be found in other infections, graft ischaemia, biliary obstruction, cholangitis, sepsis, and "surgical" hepatitis. However, it has been suggested that a significant number of microabscesses (more than nine) may indicate CMV hepatitis. Lymphocyte-predominant portal inflammation, spotty necrosis, apoptotic hepatocytes, ballooning degeneration, and Kupffer cell hyperplasia are other histologic features of CMV hepatitis, resembling other acute hepatitides.

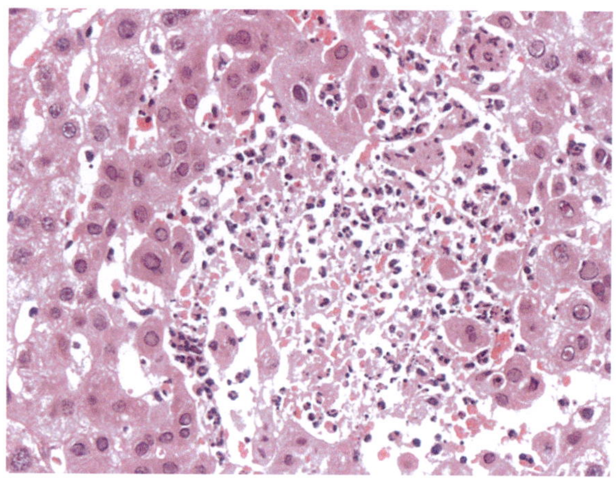

Fig. 17.41 Herpes simplex virus (HSV) hepatitis. Confluent necrosis of hepatocytes is accompanied by a neutrophilic infiltrate. Most residual hepatocytes show a large eosinophilic intranuclear inclusion surrounded by a clear halo (Cowdry A) or a ground-glass intranuclear viral inclusion (Cowdry B) with chromatin margination. HSV hepatitis is a rare opportunistic viral infection in liver allograft patients and is characterised by punched-out areas of confluent necrosis surrounded by viable hepatocytes with characteristic viral inclusions. Syncytial multinucleated hepatocytes also may be found. Immunostaining for HSV confirms the diagnosis. Adenovirus hepatitis is an uncommon opportunistic viral infection in liver allograft patients, particularly paediatric patients. It may resemble HSV hepatitis morphologically, but it is distinguished by the smudgy intranuclear viral inclusions and positive immunostaining for adenovirus.

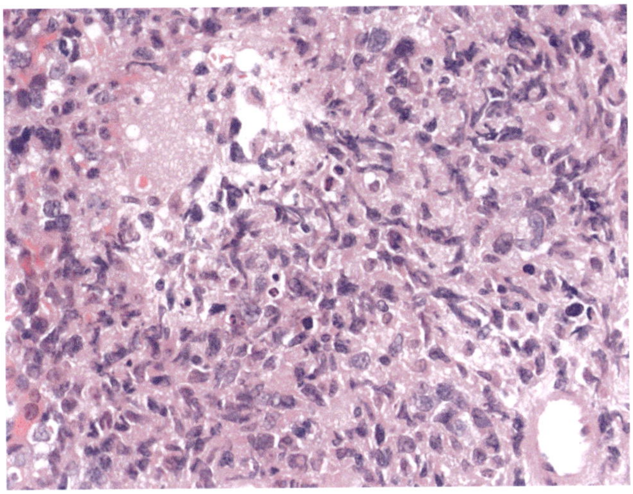

Fig. 17.42 Epstein-Barr virus–associated posttransplant lymphoproliferative disease (PTLD). A portal tract is markedly expanded by markedly atypical lymphoid cells with irregularly enlarged nuclei. Mature small lymphocytes and plasma cells are absent. In the liver allograft, EBV may manifest as EBV hepatitis or PTLD. EBV hepatitis usually occurs within 6 months after transplantation and is asymptomatic in most cases. Pathologically, it is characterised by a diffuse sinusoidal lymphocytic infiltrate with occasional atypical activated lymphoid cells. Apoptotic hepatocytes, steatosis, noncaseating epithelioid granulomas and portal atypical lymphoid infiltrate also are present. Demonstration of EBV in infiltrated lymphoid cells by immunostaining for EBV-LMP or in situ hybridization for EBER is diagnostic.

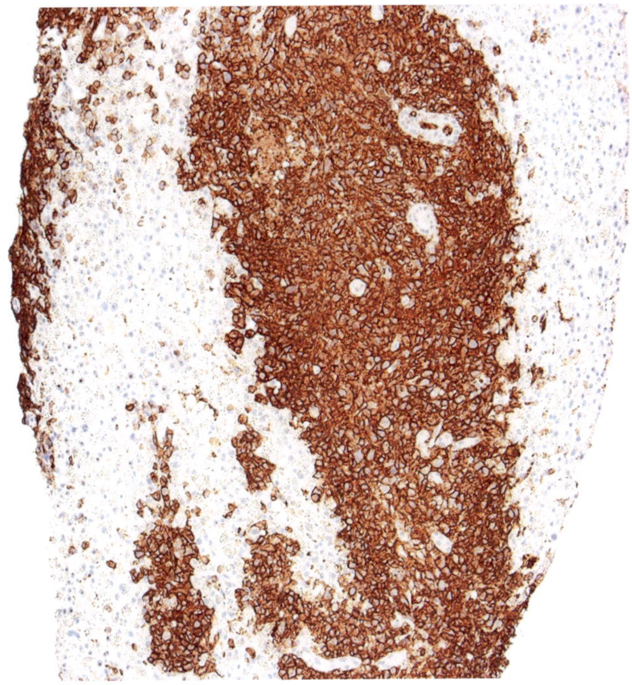

Fig. 17.43 Epstein-Barr virus–associated posttransplant lymphoproliferative disease (CD20 stain). The infiltrating lymphoid cells are composed solely of atypical B cells. PTLD complicates 2% to 3% and up to 10% of adults and children with liver transplants, respectively. It comprises a full spectrum of proliferation of primarily B cells (rarely, T cells or natural killer cells), including (1) early lesions (plasmacytic hyperplasia, infectious mononucleosis–like PTLD), (2) polymorphic PTLD, (3) monomorphic PTLD, and (4) classic Hodgkin lymphoma–type PTLD. Such lymphoid proliferation is driven mainly by EBV but rarely may be associated with CMV or hepatitis virus C.

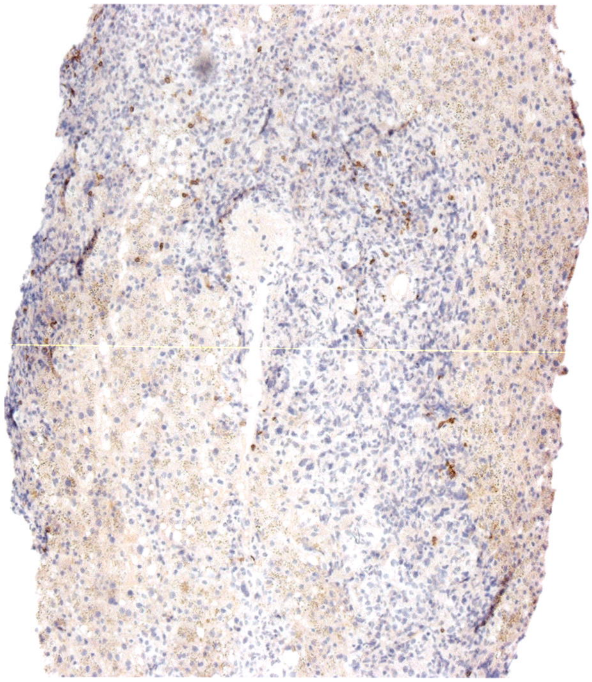

Fig. 17.44 Epstein-Barr virus–associated posttransplant lymphoproliferative disease (CD3 stain). Only scanty small reactive T cells are present. Early lesions of hepatic PTLD are characterised by a diffuse portal infiltrate of small lymphocytes and plasma cells. Polymorphic PTLD is characterised by diffuse portal infiltration showing a full spectrum of B-cell maturation with portal tract effacement. Monomorphic PTLD essentially is a non-Hodgkin lymphoma or plasma cell neoplasm and is subclassified according to the lymphoma it resembles. Diffuse large B-cell lymphoma and Burkitt lymphoma are the most common monomorphic PTLDs, whereas plasmacytoma, myeloma, peripheral T-cell lymphoma–not otherwise specified and hepatosplenic T-cell lymphoma are other, rarer forms of monomorphic PTLD. Classic Hodgkin lymphoma–type PTLD is the rarest form of PTLD.

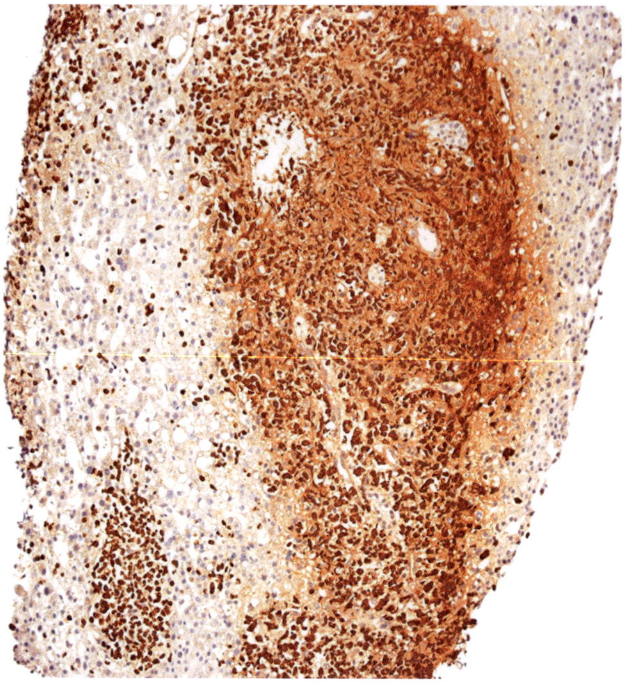

Fig. 17.45 Epstein-Barr virus–associated posttransplant lymphoproliferative disease (in situ hybridization for EBER). The atypical lymphoid cells are EBV positive. Demonstration of EBV in infiltrated lymphoid cells by immunostaining for EBV-LMP or in situ hybridization for EBER is essential to establish EBV-associated PTLD. Most of the lesional cells in early lesions, polymorphic PTLD, and classic Hodgkin lymphoma–type PTLD express EBV. However, EBV positivity is highly variable in monomorphic PTLD. Hence, the absence of EBV in non-Hodgkin lymphoma or plasma cell neoplasm arising in a liver allograft does not preclude monomorphic PTLD. Demonstration of scanty EBV-positive cells in the absence of an appropriate lymphoid proliferation is not diagnostic of PTLD.

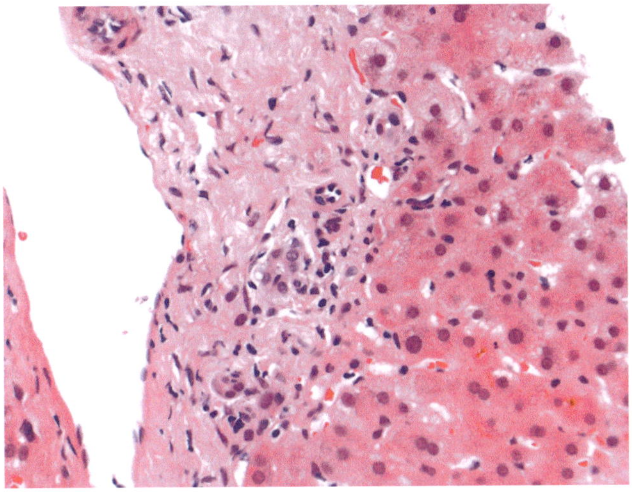

Fig. 17.46 Graft-versus-host disease. An interlobular bile duct shows degenerative changes with nuclear enlargement, hyperchromasia, and irregularity of the cholangiocytes. Mild canalicular bilirubinostasis is noted in periportal hepatocytes. GVHD is a complication commonly seen in haemopoietic cell transplantation and rarely found in solid organ transplantation. Traditionally, it was divided into acute and chronic forms, depending on an arbitrary cutoff onset time of 100 days. Currently, it is believed that the acute and chronic forms are better categorised according to clinical and pathologic manifestations. Hepatic GVHD mostly is a component of multiorgan GVHD, with accompanying skin and gastrointestinal involvement, and only rarely is a standalone, single-organ disease. Jaundice with a cholestatic liver function derangement is the typical clinical presentation.

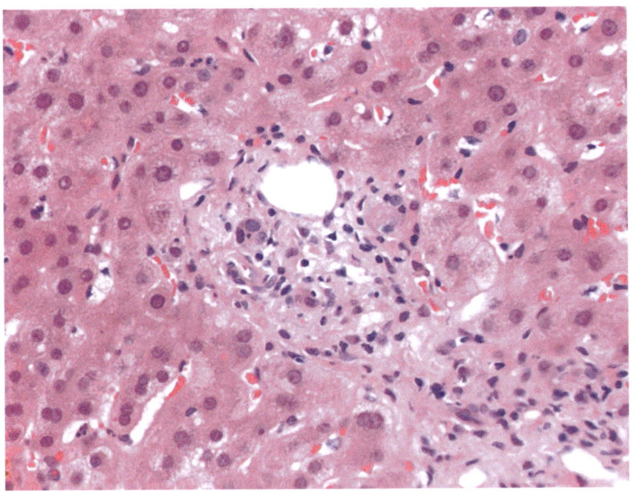

Fig. 17.47 Graft-versus-host disease. An interlobular bile duct shows epithelial degenerative changes with nuclear enlargement, hyperchromasia, and irregularity. A mild lymphocytic infiltration into the bile duct is present. Bile duct damage is the hallmark of hepatic GVHD. It usually is present extensively throughout the entire liver, but its severity may vary from portal tract to portal tract. It is characterised by epithelial degenerative injury. A mild portal chronic inflammatory infiltrate is an additional nonspecific finding. Mild endothelitis of the portal vein also is an uncommon but more specific histologic feature of severe hepatic GVHD.

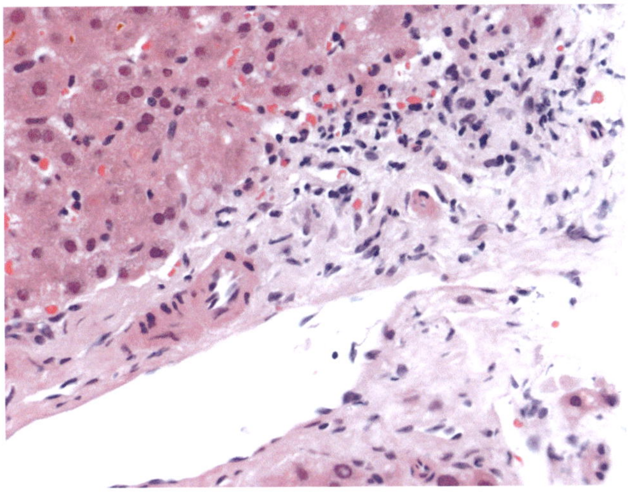

Fig. 17.48 Graft-versus-host disease. A mild lymphoplasmacytic infiltrate is present in a portal tract devoid of an interlobular bile duct (ductopaenia). Canalicular bilirubinostasis is noted in periportal hepatocytes. As hepatic GVHD progresses, bile duct damage may result in ductopaenia. In contrast to other chronic biliary diseases, ductular reaction or biliary fibrosis is not a prominent feature of hepatic GVHD. However, a mild ductular reaction may be present in up to 80% of cases. Biliary fibrosis and even cirrhosis may develop in a minority of cases.

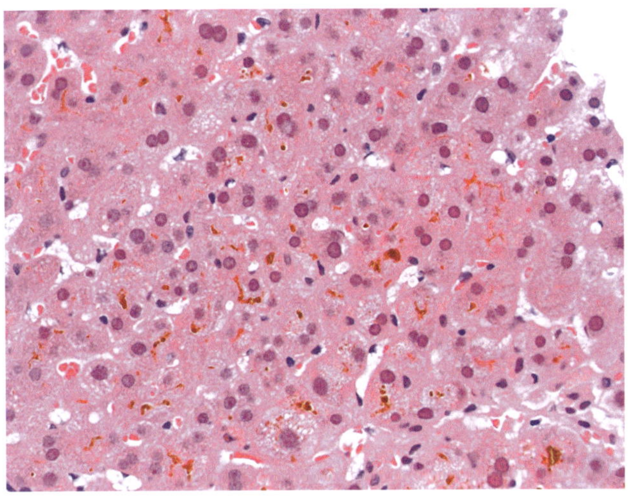

Fig. 17.49 Graft-versus-host disease. Extensive canalicular and intracytoplasmic bilirubinostasis is present. A varying degree of bilirubinostasis is observed in hepatic GVHD associated with the bile duct damage. Spotty necrosis and apoptotic hepatocytes are nonspecific lobular changes and typically are mild. An uncommon hepatitic variant of GVHD is characterised by prominent lobular necroinflammatory activity histologically and hepatitic liver function derangement biochemically. Mild endothelitis of terminal hepatic venules is seen in some cases of severe hepatic GVHD.

Index

A

Acute fatty liver
  fat droplets and oil red O stain, 223
  hepatocytes, 222
  microvesicular steatosis, 223
  mitochondriopathies, 222
  toxaemia, 222
Adrenal–hepatic fusion, 47
AIH. *See* Autoimmune hepatitis (AIH)
AIH-PBC overlap syndrome. *See* Autoimmune hepatitis-primary biliary cirrhosis (AIH-PBC) overlap syndrome
AIH-PSC. *See* Autoimmune hepatitis-primary sclerosing cholangitis (AIH-PSC)
Alagille syndrome, 46
Alcoholic hepatitis, 7, 21, 71, 73, 74, 86, 233
Alcoholic liver disease
  cirrhosis, 71, 76
  ductular reaction, 74
  foamy degeneration, 72
  giant mitochondria, 75
  hepatitis, 73
  pericellular fibrosis, 75
  perivenular fibrosis, 75
  sclerosing hyaline necrosis, 74
  siderosis, 75
  steatosis, 72
Amino acid metabolism disorders
  hereditary tyrosinaemia, 60
  urea cycle defects and related diseases, 61
Anatomic and vascular anomalies
  adrenal–hepatic fusion, 47
  ataxia telangiectasia, 48
  congenital intrahepatic portosystemic venous shunt, 48
  HHT, 48
  pancreatic heterotopia, 47
Ancillary tests
  immunohistochemistry, 15
  immunostain
    CD34, 17
    CD56/NCAM, 16
    CD56/neural cell adhesion molecule, 16
    cytokeratin 8/18 (CK8/18), 15
    cytokeratin 19 (CK19), 15, 16
    glypican-3 (GPC3), 17
    hepatitis B surface antigen, 15
    hepatocyte paraffin-1 (HepPar-1), 16
    pCEA, 16
    serum amyloid A (SAA), 17
    in situ hybridization, EBER, 17
Angiomyolipoma
  components, 212
  diagnosis, myomatous type, 213
  diffuse inflammatory infitrate, 213
  epithelioid smooth muscle cells, 212
  haemorrhage and necrosis, 212
  hepatic sinusoids, 215
  malignant endothelial cells, 215
  multiple pseudo-papillae, 215
  peliosis, 213
  perivascular epithelioid cells, 212
Angiosarcoma, 215
α1-Antitrypsin (A1AT) deficiency, 58, 59
Apoptosis, 24, 51, 73, 78, 88, 140, 150, 233
Ataxia telangiectasia, 48
Autoimmune cholangitis, 126, 128, 153
Autoimmune hepatitis (AIH)
  bridging necrosis, 142
  diagnostic criteria, 139, 144, 147
  emperipolesis, 141
  epithelial disarray and lymphocytic infiltration, 141
  epithelioid granuloma, 147
  extensive ballooning degeneration, 143
  histologic features, 142
  histologic remission, 143
  lobular disarray, 141, 142
  lymphoplasmacytic infiltrate, 140
  overlap syndromes, 139, 147
  perivenular confluent necrosis, 142
  plasma cell–rich interface, 140
  portal lymphoplasmacytic infiltrate, 140
  portal–periportal activity, Scheuer grading, 144
  regenerative nodule, cirrhotic liver, 140
  Scheuer grading, lobular activity, 145
  Scheuer staging, 146
  syncytial multinucleated hepatocytes, 143
Autoimmune hepatitis-primary biliary cirrhosis (AIH-PBC) overlap syndrome, 147
Autoimmune hepatitis-primary sclerosing cholangitis (AIH-PSC), 147

B

Bacillus Calmette-Guérin (BCG), 108
Bacterial infection
  pyogenic abscess, 106
  sepsis
    bland cholestasis, 106
    ductular cholestasis, 105
Banff schema, 229

A.W.H. Chan et al., *Atlas of Liver Pathology*, Atlas of Anatomic Pathology,
DOI 10.1007/978-1-4614-9114-9,

B-cell acute lymphoblastic leukaemia, 219
BCG. *See* Bacillus Calmette-Guérin (BCG)
Benign mesenchymal tumours
  Mesenchymal hamartoma
  angiomyolipoma (*see* Angiomyolipoma)
  bile ductules, 210
  cavernous haemangioma
    hepatic, 211
    size, 211
    variable-sized vascular spaces, 212
    vascular tumour, 211
  components, 210
  infantile haemangioma, 211
  location and size, 210
  loose myxoid stroma, 210
  solid and cystic tumour, 209
  solitary fibrous tumour, 213
Bile acid and bilirubin metabolism disorders
  Crigler-Najjar disease, 38, 67
  Gilbert syndrome, 67
  intrahepatic cholestasis, 66
  PFIC, 66, 67
Biliary atresia, 46–47
Biliary cirrhosis, 37, 68, 69, 128. *See also* Primary biliary cirrhosis (PBC)
Biliary disease
  acute large duct obstruction, 157
  cholangiocarcinoma, 159
  chronic large duct obstruction, 157
  description, 149
  IgG4, 159, 160
  langerhans cell histiocytosis (*see* Langerhans cell histiocytosis)
  PBC (*see* Primary biliary cirrhosis (PBC))
  PSC (*see* Primary sclerosing cholangitis (PSC))
  sarcoidosis, 161, 162
Biliary epithelial neoplasms
  AJCC TNM system, perihilar cholangiocarcinoma, 203
  bile duct adenoma and differential diagnoses, 198
  intrahepatic cholangiocarcinoma (*see* Intrahepatic cholangiocarcinoma)
  MCN (*see* Mucinous cystic neoplasm (MCN))
  serous microcystic adenoma
    glycogen, 199
    renal cell carcinoma, 200
Biliary intraepithelial neoplasia (BilIN)
  characteristics, 175
  intrahepatic bile ducts, 175
  three-tiered grading system, 175
BilIN. *See* Biliary intraepithelial neoplasia (BilIN)
Budd-Chiari syndrome
  dilated sinusoids and extravasation, 165
  hepatic veins, 166
  hepatoportal sclerosis, 165
  liver biopsy, 166
  prominent sinusoidal dilatation, 166
  thrombosis, 165
Burkitt lymphoma, 219

C
Carbohydrate metabolism disorders
  galactosaemia, 57
  GSD, 55, 56
  hepatocellular adenoma, 56
  hereditary fructose intolerance, 57
  Mauriac syndrome, 58
Caroli disease, 44–45
Cellular damage
  apoptosis, 24
  apoptotic body, 25
  ballooning degeneration, 23, 24
  bile duct damage, 27
  bridging necrosis, 26
  confluent necrosis, 25
  ductopaenia, 28
  feathery degeneration, 24
  hepatocytes and cholangiocytes, 23
  panacinar/panlobular necrosis, 26, 27
  parenchymal extinction, 27
  spotty necrosis, 25
CESD. *See* Cholesterol ester storage disease (CESD)
Choledochal cyst, 45, 157, 200
Cholestatic injury
  acute
    drugs and toxins, 127
    focal necrosis and scattered eosinophils, 126
    perivenular necrosis, 126
  bland
    drugs and toxins, 126
    herbal medication, 125
    jaundice and pruritus, 125
    marked hepatocellular and canalicular bilirubinostasis, 125
  chronic
    drugs and toxin, 128
    ductopaenia, 128
    trifluoperazine, 128
Cholesterol ester storage disease (CESD), 64
Chronic hepatitis B
  features, 87
  ground-glass hepatocytes, 87
  HBsAg stain, 87
  interface, 88
  orcein stain, 87
  portal inflammation, 87
  spotty necrosis and apoptotic bodies, 88
Chronic hepatitis C
  autoantibodies and mimic autoimmune hepatitis, 90
  autoimmune mechanisms, 90
  focal epithelial disarray, interlobular bile duct, 89
  macrophages, refractile foreign bodies, 90
  macrovesicular and mediovesicular steatosis, 89
  portal lymphoid follicles, 89
  sinusoidal lymphocytes, 89
Chronic viral hepatitis
  Ishak score
    confluent necrosis, 97, 98
    interface hepatitis, 96
    portal inflammation, 99
    spotty necrosis, 98
  METAVIR score
    lobular necrosis, 94
    piecemeal and lobular necrosis, 95
    piecemeal necrosis, 94
  necroinflammatory activity and fibrosis, 91
  Scheuer's grading
    lobular activity, 93
    portal–periportal activity, 92
  picrosirius red stain, 99
  staging
    fibrosis, 100
    picrosirius red stain, 99
Ciliated foregut cyst, 44, 115, 179, 182, 183
Cirrhosis
  alcoholic, 71, 76
  biliary (*see* Biliary cirrhosis)

biliary-type pattern, 51
cholangiocarcinoma, 185
macronodular, 71
micronodular, 71
multiple regenerative nodules, 56, 65
parenchymal extinction, 26
regenerative nodules, 50
venocentric, 165
Classic Hodgkin lymphoma
binucleated Reed-Sternberg cell, 217
epithelial disarray and regenerative change, bile duct, 219
infiltration, 217
paraneoplastic syndrome, 219
Coagulative necrosis, 167
Combined hepatocellular–cholangiocarcinoma (HCC-CC)
components, 204
definition, 204
differentiation, 204
ductular reaction, 206
HepPar-1 and CK19, 205
mature-hepatocytes rim, 206
nuclear pleomorphism, 206
prognosis, 204
small oval-shaped cells, 205
stem cell features, 204, 205
stemness markers, 205
types, 205
Congenital hepatic fibrosis, 42–43
Congenital intrahepatic portosystemic venous shunt, 48
Copper metabolism disorders, 53–54
Crigler-Najjar disease, 67–68
Cystic fibrosis, 68–69
Cytomegalovirus (CMV) hepatitis, 101, 236

D
Developmental abnormality
fibrocystic liver disease and choledochal cyst, 41–45
intrahepatic bile ducts and biliary atresia, 46–47
miscellaneous anatomic and vascular anomalies, 47–48
normal
bile duct development, 39, 40
extramedullary haematopoiesis, 40
infant, 40, 41
Drug-induced liver injury
cholestatic (*see* Cholestatic injury)
diagnosis, 119
differential diagnosis, 119
enzyme induction, 136
lipofuscin deposition, 137
morbidity and mortality, 119
necroinflammatory (*see* Necroinflammatory injury)
neoplasm and tumour-like lesions, 135–136
portal macrophages pigments, liver biopsy, 137
pseudo-ground-glass inclusion, thioguanine, 136
steatosis and steatohepatitis (*see* Steatosis and steatohepatitis)
vascular lesions, 132–134

E
Embryonal sarcoma, 214
Endoplasmic reticulum storage disorders, 58–59
Epithelial liver neoplasm
biliary (*see* Biliary epithelial neoplasms)
chronic biliary inflammation, 185
combined HCC-CC (*see* Combined hepatocellular–cholangiocarcinoma (HCC-CC))
definition, 185
definition, cholangiocarcinomas, 185
HCA (*see* Hepatocellular adenoma (HCA))
HCC (*see* Hepatocellular carcinoma (HCC))
hepatic carcinoid, 207
metastatic colorectal adenocarcinoma, 207
metastatic squamous cell carcinoma, 207
types, 185
Epithelioid angiosarcoma, 216
Epithelioid granuloma, 22
Epithelioid haemangioendothelioma, 215
EPP. *See* Erythropoietic protoporphyria (EPP)
Epstein-Barr virus (EBV)
EBER, 17, 227
hepatitis, 102
infection, 21, 109, 113
PTLD, 236–238
smooth muscle tumour, 216
Erythropoietic protoporphyria (EPP), 69–70
Extramedullary haematopoiesis, 40

F
Fatty liver disease
alcoholic, 71–76
focal fatty change, 84
nonalcoholic, 76–83
steatosis, 71
Fibrinoid necrosis, 167, 168
Fibrin ring granuloma, 22
Fibrocystic liver disease
Caroli disease, 44, 45
congenital hepatic fibrosis, 42, 43
description, 41
polycystic liver disease, 43–44
solitary bile duct cyst, 44
von Meyenburg complex, 41, 42
Fibrosing cholestatic hepatitis B, 88
Fibrosis
bridging, 37
cirrhosis, 37
pericellular, 36
periductal, 36
perivenular and pericellular, 36
portal and periportal, 36
FNH. *See* Focal nodular hyperplasia (FNH)
Foamy macrophage aggregates, 23
Focal fatty change, 84
Focal nodular hyperplasia (FNH)
glutamine synthetase, 180
haemangioma, 179
hepatic lobules, 179
radiating fibrous septa, 180
Fungal infection
aspergillosis, 110
candidiasis, 110
cryptococcal, 111
cryptosporidiosis, 113–114
elements, 110
histoplasmosis, 111
identification, 110
immunostains, 110
malaria, 112–113
Pneumocystis jiroveci, 112
size and morphology, 110
tropical splenomegaly syndrome, 113
visceral leishmaniasis, 114
zygomycosis, 112

G
Galactosaemia, 57, 60, 186
Gaucher disease, 62, 63
Genetic disorders, intrahepatic cholestasis, 66
Giant mitochondria, 11, 23, 28–30, 75, 77, 79
Gilbert syndrome, 67
Glycogen storage disease (GSD)
  defective enzymes and gene loci, 55
  hepatocellular adenoma, 56
  type I, 55
  type IV, 56
Grade 2 parenchymal siderosis, 75
Graft-*versus*-host disease (GVHD), 225, 238, 239
GSD. *See* Glycogen storage disease (GSD)
GVHD. *See* Graft-*versus*-host disease (GVHD)

H
Haematolymphoid malignancies
  B-cell acute lymphoblastic leukaemia, 219
  Burkitt lymphoma, 219
  MALT lymphoma (*see* Marginal zone lymphoma of mucosa-associated lymphoid tissue (MALT lymphoma))
  primary diffuse large B-cell lymphoma, 218
Haemorrhagic cyst, 179, 183
Handling and histochemical staining, liver tissue
  Gordon-Sweets reticulin stain, 12
  liver biopsy (*see* Liver biopsy)
  "liver panel", 10
  Masson trichrome stain, 11
  oil red O stain, 14
  Orcein stain, 13
  PAS stain, 13, 14
  Perls stain, 12, 13
  picrosirius red stain, 11
HCA. *See* Hepatocellular adenoma (HCA)
HCC. *See* Hepatocellular carcinoma (HCC)
HCC-CC. *See* Combined hepatocellular–cholangiocarcinoma (HCC-CC)
Helminth infection
  cestodes, 115
  classification, 115
  clonorchiasis and opisthorchiasis, 116–117
  echinococcosis, 115
  schistosomiasis, 116
  visceral larva migrans, 117
Hepatic artery thrombosis, 231–232
Hepatic carcinoid, 207
Hepatoblastoma
  AFP expression, 190
  extramedullary haematopoietic cells, 190
  fibroblastic mesenchymal component, 190
  macrotrabeculae, 190
  mitosis, 189
  mixed fetal and embryonal epithelial components, 189
  post chemotherapy, 191
  primary malignant hepatic neoplasm, 189
  trabeculae fetal hepatocytes, 189
  translocation, β-catenin, 191
Hepatocellular adenoma (HCA)
  bland hepatocytes, trabeculae, 186
  glycogen storage disease and β-catenin-activated, 187
  haemorrhagic tumour, noncirrhotic liver, 186
  hepatic angiomyolipoma, 188
  hepatoblastoma (*see* Hepatoblastoma)
  hepatocellular carcinoma (*see* Hepatocellular carcinoma (HCC))
  lesional hepatocytes, 188
  L-FABP, HNF1α-inactivated, 187
  neoplasm and tumour-like lesions, 135
  phenotype and genotype, 186
  serum amyloid A and C-reactive protein, 188
  solitary, 186
  telangiectatic focal nodular hyperplasia, 188
  transarterial chemoembolisation, 196
Hepatocellular carcinoma (HCC)
  bile production, 194
  CD34 stain, 197
  cirrhotic livers, 172
  compact, 193
  extensive investigations, 171
  fibrolamellar, 195
  fibrous pseudo-capsule, necrotic tumour, 191
  glypican-3 stain, 197
  immunoreactivity, 196
  lymphocytes, 195
  Mallory-Denk bodies, 194
  massive, 192
  multiple nodules, 192
  neoplasm and tumour-like lesions, 135
  nodular, 191, 192
  pale bodies, 194–195
  pleomorphic, 194
  pseudoacinar pattern, 193
  sarcomatoid, 196
  scirrhous, 195
  steatotic/steatohepatitic, 193
  TNM system, 197
  trabecular pattern, 192
  tumour cells with clear cytoplasm, 193
  vascular invasion, 196
Hepatoportal sclerosis, 164, 165
Hepatotropic viral hepatitis
  acute
    ballooned hepatocytes and mild sinusoidal lymphocytic infiltrate, 85
    cellular swelling, 86
    liver failure, 86
    lobular inflammation, 86
    residual ballooned hepatocytes, 86
  chronic hepatitis B (*see* Chronic hepatitis B)
  chronic hepatitis C (*see* Chronic hepatitis C)
  chronic hepatitis D, 90–91
  fibrosing cholestatic hepatitis B, 88
Hereditary haemochromatosis, 50–51
Hereditary haemorrhagic telangiectasia (HHT), 48
Hereditary tyrosinaemia, 60
Herpes simplex virus (HSV) hepatitis, 103, 238
HHT. *See* Hereditary haemorrhagic telangiectasia (HHT)
High-grade dysplastic nodule
  cytologic changes, 173
  dysplastic nodule, 173, 174
  hepatocytes, 174
  unpaired/nontriad arterioles, 174

I
Infantile haemangioma, 211
Inflammation
  epithelioid granuloma, 22
  fibrin ring granuloma, 22
  foamy macrophage aggregates, 23

lipogranuloma, 23
lobular epithelioid granulomas, 22
lobular inflammation, hepatocellular damage, 21, 22
morphologic changes categories, liver injury, 19
portal inflammation
atypical lymphoid infiltrate, 21
eosinophil rich, 20
interface hepatitis, 21
lymphocyte predominant, 19–20
neutrophil rich, 20
plasma cell rich, 20
Inflammatory pseudotumour
fibroblasts and myofibroblasts, 181
hepatic tumour, 182
Interface hepatitis, 21
Intracellular/extracellular accumulations
amyloidosis, 34
α1-antitrypsin globules, 30
bilirubinostasis, 32
ceroid/ lipofuscin, 32
copper-associated protein, 33
ductular cholestasis, 32
giant mitochondria, 30
glycogenated nuclei, 31
glycogen-rich hepatocytes, 29
ground-glass hepatocytes, 31
intracellular hyaline bodies, 30
intrahepatic depositions, 28
iron (Perls stain), 33
lipofuscin, 32
macrovesicular and "mediovesicular" steatosis, 29
macrovesicular steatosis, 28
Mallory-Denk bodies, 30
microvesicular steatosis, 29
pale bodies, 31
Intraductal papillary neoplasm
cholangiocarcinoma, 176
cystic ductal dilatation, 177
immunophenotypes, 176
phenotypes, 176
Intrahepatic bile ducts, 46
Intrahepatic cholangiocarcinoma
AJCC TNM system, 203
irregular and angulated glands, fibrous stroma, 201
lymphoepithelioma-like, 202
mass-forming and periductal-infiltration, 200
mucoepidermoid, 202
multiple tan-coloured tumour masses, noncirrhotic liver, 200
periductal-infiltration, 200
sarcomatoid type, 202
signet ring cells, 201
von Meyenburg complexes and bile duct adenomas, 201
white tumour, cirrhotic liver, 200
Intrahepatic cholestasis, 221, 222
Iron metabolism disorders
hereditary haemochromatosis, 50, 51
hereditary iron overload, 50
neonatal haemochromatosis, 52
secondary iron overload, 52
Ischaemic necrosis, 167

K
Kaposi sarcoma, 214, 216

L
Langerhans cell histiocytosis
bile ducts, 160, 161
Birbeck granules, 160, 161
hepatic involvement, 160
Lipogranuloma, 22, 23, 73, 78
Liver biopsy
adequacy, 11
fixation, 9
request form, 9
samples, 8
wrapping, 10
Lobular epithelioid granulomas, 22
Lysosomal storage disorders
CESD, 64
Gaucher disease, 63
hepatic involvement, 62
Niemann-Pick disease, 63

M
Macrovesicular steatosis, 71–73, 75–77, 84
MAI. *See Mycobacterium avium-intracellulare* (MAI)
Malignant mesenchymal tumours
angiosarcoma, 215
EBV-associated smooth muscle tumour, 216
embryonal sarcoma, 214
epithelioid angiosarcoma, 216
epithelioid haemangioendothelioma, 215
Kaposi sarcoma, 214
metastatic gastrointestinal stromal tumour, 217
Mallory-Denk bodies, 77
MALT lymphoma. *See* Marginal zone lymphoma of mucosa-associated lymphoid tissue (MALT lymphoma)
Marginal zone lymphoma of mucosa-associated lymphoid tissue (MALT lymphoma)
gastrointestinal tract origin, 218
portal infltration, 219
primary hepatic, 218
Mauriac syndrome, 58
MCN. *See* Mucinous cystic neoplasm (MCN)
Metabolic liver disease
amino acid metabolism disorders, 60–61
bile acid and bilirubin metabolism, 66–68
carbohydrate metabolism disorders, 55–58
copper metabolism disorders, 53–54
cystic fibrosis, 68–69
endoplasmic reticulum storage disorders, 58–59
EPP, 69–70
iron metabolism disorders, 50–52
lysosomal storage disorders, 62–64
primary mitochondrial hepatopathy, 64–65
Metastatic colorectal adenocarcinoma, 207
Metastatic gastrointestinal stromal tumour, 217
Metastatic squamous cell carcinoma, 207
Microvesicular steatosis, 71, 72
Mucinous cystic neoplasm (MCN)
high-grade intraepithelial neoplasia, 199
invasive carcinoma, 199
low-grade intraepithelial neoplasia
architectural and cytologic atypia, 199
categories, 198
cyst-formation, 198
ovarian-type mesenchymal stroma, 198
progestrogen receptor [PR] stain, 199
single layer, multilobular cyst, 198

Mycobacterial infection
  BCG, 108
  MAI, 108
  mycobacterium tuberculosis
    hepatic, 107
    necrotizing epithelioid granulomas, 107
    Ziehl-Neelsen stain, 107
Mycobacterium avium-intracellulare (MAI), 108

N
Necroinflammatory injury
  acute hepatic necrosis
    diclofenac, 122
    drugs and toxins, 121, 122
    ferrous sulphate, 120
    halothane, 120
    mild zone 3 hepatocytic hydropic swelling, 122
    paracetamol, 119
    rifampicin, 120
    spotty necrosis, 122
  hepatic granulomas
    drugs and toxins, 123
    epithelioid, 123
    genuine, 123
    liver injury, 123
Neonatal haemochromatosis (NH), 52
Neoplasm and tumour-like lesions
  angiosarcoma, 136
  cholangiocarcinoma, 135
  focal nodular hyperplasia, 135
  hepatocellular carcinoma (HCC), 135
Neoplasm-like liver lesions
  ciliated foregut cyst, 182, 183
  cystic neoplasm, 179
  FNH, 179, 180
  haemorrhagic cyst, 183
  inflammatory pseudotumour, 181, 182
  large regenerative nodule, 181
  nodular regenerative hyperplasia, 179, 180
  solitary bile duct cyst, 182
NH. *See* Neonatal haemochromatosis (NH)
Niemann-Pick disease, 63
Nodular regenerative hyperplasia, 164, 179, 180, 232
Nonalcoholic fatty liver disease
  cirrhosis, 81
  giant mitochondria, 79
  lipogranuloma, 78
  macrovesicular steatosis, 76
  mild lymphocytic infiltrate, 79
  mild parenchymal siderosis, 80
  nuclear clear vacuolation, 79
  portal and periportal fibrosis, 80
  sinusoidal lymphohistiocytic infiltrate, 78
  spotty necrosis, 78
  staging, 82, 83
  steatohepatitis, 77, 78, 81, 82
  zone 3 pericellular fibrosis, 80
Nonepithelial liver neoplasm
  children, 209
  haematolymphoid malignancies (*see* Haematolymphoid malignancies)
  malignant mesenchymal tumours (*see* Malignant mesenchymal tumours)
  mesenchymal hamartoma (*see* Mesenchymal hamartoma)
  types, 209
Nonhepatotropic viral hepatitis
  adenovirus, 101
  cytomegalovirus, 101–102
  Epstein-Barr virus, 102
  herpes simplex virus, 103
  parvovirus B19 infection, 103
Nonviral infectious liver disease
  bacterial (*see* Bacterial infection)
  component, 105
  fungal (*see* Fungal infection)
  heminths (*see* Heminth infection)
  mycobacterial (*see* Mycobacterial infection)
  rickettsial, 109
Normal liver landmarks
  classic lobular architecture, 1, 4
  hepatic vein, 1, 3
  parenchyma, 1
  perivenular region, 1, 3
  portal tract, 1, 2
  Rappaport acinar architecture, 1, 4
  terminal hepatic venule, 1, 3
Normal variants and artefacts
  adolescent's liver, 5
  drying artefact, 5, 7
  elderly individual liver, 5, 6
  immersion, saline, 5, 7
  infant liver, 5, 6
  subcapsular liver, 5
  surgical hepatitis, 7

O
Obliterative portal venopathy, 164
Obstetric liver disease
  acute fatty liver (*see* Acute fatty liver)
  description, 221
  intrahepatic cholestasis, 221, 222
  toxaemia, pregnancy/HELLP syndrome (*see* Toxaemia, pregnancy/HELLP syndrome)

P
Pancreatic heterotopia, 47
Parvovirus B19 infection, 103
Paucity, intrahepatic bile ducts, 46–47
PBC. *See* Primary biliary cirrhosis (PBC)
pCEA. *See* Polyclonal carcinoembryonic antigen (pCEA)
Pericellular fibrosis, 36, 75
Periductal fibrosis, 36
Perivenular fibrosis, 36, 75
PFIC. *See* Progressive familial intrahepatic cholestasis (PFIC)
Polyclonal carcinoembryonic antigen (pCEA), 16, 196, 201, 204
Polycystic liver disease, 43–44
Portal and periportal fibrosis, 36
Portal vein thrombosis, 163, 164
Premalignant lesion
  BilIN. (*see* Biliary intraepithelial neoplasia (BilIN))
  dysplastic nodule, 173
  HCC, 171
  hepatocellular carcinoma, 174
  high-grade dysplastic nodule, 173, 174
  hyperplastic biliary epithelial cells, 175

intraductal papillary neoplasm, 176, 177
iron-free foci, 172
large cell change, 172
low-grade dysplastic nodule, 173
oncocytic focus, 172
small cell change, 172
Primary biliary cirrhosis (PBC)
autoimmune cholangitis, 153
chronic cholate stasis, 152
cirrhotic liver, 150
damaged bile ducts, 150
ductopaenia, 152
epithelioid granuloma, 151
florid duct lesion, 150
interface hepatitis, 152
moderate ductular reaction, 151
noncaseating epithelioid granulomas, 151
prominent ductular reaction, 151
staging systems, 153
Primary hepatolithiasis/recurrent pyogenic cholangitis
atrophic liver segment, 157
bile duct, 159
calculi, 158
segmental and septal bile ducts, 158
stone-containing bile ducts and bile duct contains, 158
Primary mitochondrial hepatopathy, 64–65
Primary sclerosing cholangitis (PSC)
ductopaenia, 156
ductular reaction, 155
epithelial lining, 154
interlobular bile ducts, 155
"onion-skin", 154
periseptal hepatocytes, 156
regenerative nodules, 156
septal bile duct, 154
xanthogranulomatous inflammation, duct ulceration and bile extravasation, 155
Progressive familial intrahepatic cholestasis (PFIC), 66–67
PSC. *See* Primary sclerosing cholangitis (PSC)

R

Regeneration
ductular reaction, 35
hepatocyte rosette, 34
mitotic activity, 35
ploidy, 35
twin-cell plate, 34
Rickettsial diseases, 109

S

Sarcoidosis
hepatic sarcoidosis, 161
interlobular duct, 162
systemic granulomatous disease, 161
Sclerosed haemangiomas, 212
Sclerosing hyaline necrosis, 74
Seronegative autoimmune hepatitis, 147, 148
Sinusoidal dilatation, 168
Solitary bile duct cyst, 44, 182
Solitary fibrous tumour, 213
Steatohepatitis. *See also* Steatosis and steatohepatitis
ballooning degeneration, hepatocytes, 73
nonalcoholic, 73, 74, 77, 78, 81–83
Steatosis and steatohepatitis
amiodarone, 130
drugs and toxins, 131
macrovesicular, 129
methotrexate, 130
microvesicular, 129
stellate cell lipidosis and hypertrophy, vitamin A, 130

T

TNM system. *See* Tumour-node-metastasis (TNM) system
Toxaemia, pregnancy/HELLP syndrome
haemorrhagic necrosis, 223
periportal necrosis, 224
portal vein fibrin thrombosis, 223
sinusoidal fibrin deposition, 224
Transplantation pathology
acute rejection, 226–228
Banff schema, grading liver allograft rejection, 229
central perivenulitis, 228
chronic rejection, 230–231
CMV hepatitis, 236
de novo autoimmune hepatitis, 235
EBV-associated PTLD, 236–238
graft complications, 225
GVHD, 238–239
hepatic artery thrombosis, 231–232
HSV hepatitis, 238
idiopathic chronic hepatitis, 235
late rejection, 230
nodular regenerative hyperplasia, 232
portal vein thrombosis, 232
preservation-reperfusion injury, 226
recurrent autoimmune hepatitis, 233–234
recurrent hepatitis C, 233
recurrent primary sclerosing cholangitis, 234, 235
recurrent steatohepatitis, 233
recurrent viral hepatitis, 233
Tumour-node-metastasis (TNM) system
biliary epithelial neoplasms, 203
HCC, epithelial neoplasms, 197
intrahepatic cholangiocarcinoma, 203

U

Urea cycle defects, 61

V

Vascular disorders
acute hepatic artery thrombosis, 167
acute sinusoidal obstruction syndrome, 169
Budd-Chiari syndrome. (*see* Budd Chiari syndrome)
chronic sinusoidal obstruction syndrome, 170
coagulative necrosis, 167
fibrinoid necrosis, 167, 168
hepatoportal sclerosis, 164, 165
ischaemic necrosis, 167
liver parenchyma, 163
nodular regenerative hyperplasia, 164
obliterative portal venopathy, 164
peliosis hepatis, 169
portal and hepatic vein thrombosis, 163
portal vein thrombosis, 163, 164
sinusoidal dilatation, 168
sinusoidal obstruction syndrome, 163

Vascular lesions
  nodular regenerative hyperplasia, 132–133
  sinusoidal dilatation and peliosis
    azathioprine, 133
    drugs and toxins, 134
    oral, 133
  sinusoidal obstruction syndrome
    acute Budd-Chiari syndrome, 132
    chemotherapeutic agent, 132
    chemotherapy, 132
    drugs and toxins, 132
  vasculitis, phenytoin, 134
Viral liver disease
  biopsy, 85
  chronic (*see* Chronic viral hepatitis)
  hepatotropic (*see* Hepatotropic viral hepatitis)
  nonhepatotropic (*see* Nonhepatotropic viral hepatitis)
von Meyenburg complex, 41, 42

W

Wilson disease, 53–54

X

Xanthogranulomatous inflammation, 155, 181, 235

MIX
Papier aus verantwortungsvollen Quellen
Paper from responsible sources
FSC® C105338

If you have any concerns about our products,
you can contact us on
ProductSafety@springernature.com

In case Publisher is established outside the EU,
the EU authorized representative is:
Springer Nature Customer Service Center GmbH
Europaplatz 3, 69115 Heidelberg, Germany

Printed by Libri Plureos GmbH
in Hamburg, Germany